Strategic Health Technology

Strategic Health Technology

Editor: Tandy Rocco

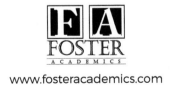

www.fosteracademics.com

www.fosteracademics.com

Cataloging-in-Publication Data

Strategic health technology / edited by Tandy Rocco.
    p. cm.
Includes bibliographical references and index.
ISBN 978-1-64646-626-9
1. Medical technology. 2. Public health--Technological innovations.
3. Medical innovations. 4. Biomedical engineering. I. Rocco, Tandy.
R855.3 .S77 2023
610.285--dc23

Foster Academics,
118-35 Queens Blvd., Suite 400,
Forest Hills, NY 11375, USA

ISBN 978-1-64646-626-9 (Hardback)

Contents

Preface

This book has been an outcome of determined endeavour from a group of educationists in the field. The primary objective was to involve a broad spectrum of professionals from diverse cultural background involved in the field for developing new researches. The book not only targets students but also scholars pursuing higher research for further enhancement of the theoretical and practical applications of the subject.

The technologies or medical devices that have been designed or developed using IT systems, algorithms, artificial intelligence (AI), cloud or blockchain, which are meant for supporting the healthcare organizations fall under the umbrella of healthcare technology. The advancement of technology has led to the adoption of medical equipment and technologies such as electronic health records (EHRs) and diagnostic imaging machines. EHRs have substituted the paper medical records thus making it easier to access and organize the medical records, reports and other healthcare data. Technology solutions help in increasing the productivity as they maintain collaboration across systems and manage costs. Healthcare interoperability across diverse and fragmented healthcare systems significantly reduces the total cost of care by minimizing the number of unnecessary or repeated tests which ultimately help the clinicians make faster diagnoses. It further automates the process of measuring and capturing data of patient care to spot the specific issues that need improvement. This book outlines the processes and applications of strategic heath technology. It traces the progress in this field and highlights some of its key concepts and applications. This book includes contributions of experts and scientists which will provide innovative insights into this field.

It was an honour to edit such a profound book and also a challenging task to compile and examine all the relevant data for accuracy and originality. I wish to acknowledge the efforts of the contributors for submitting such brilliant and diverse chapters in the field and for endlessly working for the completion of the book. Last, but not the least; I thank my family for being a constant source of support in all my research endeavours.

Editor

FluMob: Enabling Surveillance of Acute Respiratory Infections in Health-Care Workers *via* Mobile Phones

May Oo Lwin[1]*, Chee Fu Yung [2], Peiling Yap[3], Karthikayen Jayasundar[1], Anita Sheldenkar[1], Kosala Subasinghe[1], Schubert Foo[1], Udeepa Gayantha Jayasinghe[4], Huarong Xu[3], Siaw Ching Chai[3], Ashwin Kurlye[4], Jie Chen[2] and Brenda Sze Peng Ang[3]

[1] Wee Kim Wee School of Communication and Information, Nanyang Technological University (NTU), Singapore, Singapore, [2] KK Women's and Children's Hospital (KKH), Singapore, Singapore, [3] Tan Tock Seng Hospital (TTSH), Singapore, Singapore, [4] Institute of Media Innovation (IMI), Singapore, Singapore

*Correspondence:
May Oo Lwin
tmaylwin@ntu.edu.sg

Singapore is a hotspot for emerging infectious diseases and faces a constant risk of pandemic outbreaks as a major travel and health hub for Southeast Asia. With an increasing penetration of smart phone usage in this region, Singapore's pandemic preparedness framework can be strengthened by applying a mobile-based approach to health surveillance and control, and improving upon existing ideas by addressing gaps, such as a lack of health communication. FluMob is a digitally integrated syndromic surveillance system designed to assist health authorities in obtaining real-time epidemiological and surveillance data from health-care workers (HCWs) within Singapore, by allowing them to report influenza incidence using smartphones. The system, integrating a fully responsive web-based interface and a mobile interface, is made available to HCW using various types of mobile devices and web browsers. Real-time data generated from FluMob will be complementary to current health-care- and laboratory-based systems. This paper describes the development of FluMob, as well as challenges faced in the creation of the system.

Keywords: mobile-health, influenza, mobile phones, application, health-care workers, surveillance

INTRODUCTION

Seasonal influenza affects nearly 20–25% of the Singapore population (1). The all-cause mortality attributable to influenza stands at 14.8 per 100,000 person-years, making the burden comparable to other temperate countries (2). Globally, it is estimated that there were approximately 284,500 respiratory and cardiovascular deaths associated with the 2009 influenza pandemic (3). Due to Singapore's geographical location, pandemic threats from respiratory infectious diseases continue to persist, e.g., avian influenza A subtype viruses (H5N1 and H7N9) in Shanghai, China, and the Middle East respiratory syndrome coronavirus in the Middle East, in addition to seasonal influenza. The true impact of influenza often stretches beyond the viral illness itself and contributes to other disease burden by causing complications in patients with preexisting conditions (i.e., cardiovascular diseases or cardiopulmonary disease).

Economic modeling has recently demonstrated that the treatment-only strategy for influenza resulted in a mean number of 690 simulated deaths, 13,950 hospital days, an equivalent of 2.5 million workdays lost, and a mean economic cost of USD$469.8 million per year (4). Southeast Asia is acknowledged as a hotspot for emerging infectious diseases (5), and Singapore—as a travel and health hub of the region—faces a constant risk of pandemic outbreaks. The 2003 severe acute respiratory syndrome outbreak proved to be a huge burden on Singapore's economy, costing US$570 million and resulting in unprecedented rates of unemployment at 5.5% (6, 7). Existing and potential threats highlight the importance of having robust surveillance and health communication systems present, which can forewarn people, detect unusual signals and provide health education in an efficient and cost-effective manner.

Given the absence of an efficient surveillance system that addresses challenges within hospitals in Singapore, this paper reports the design and development of a prototype integrated mobile-health participatory influenza surveillance system entitled FluMob. Following a review of literature on information and communication technology (ICT) approaches to addressing influenza tracking and surveillance, we describe FluMob's architecture, followed briefly by the methodologies used to recruit and retain users. Finally, we present the challenges the research team faced in the various phases of the implementation of the intervention, and lessons learnt, which will be useful to public health researchers and practitioners involved in similar initiatives or interventions in the future.

RELATED LITERATURE

Participatory epidemiology (PE) is a concept that has increasingly been used in health surveillance in recent years. It uses community involvement to improve the understanding and control of diseases and was most prominently brought to attention by work conducted in Africa investigating animal health from information gathered by local farmers (8).

With the proliferation of Internet and mobile phone usage, ICT has played a significant role in the development of PE for disease surveillance, health monitoring, and information sharing; enabling both individuals at the point of care and stakeholders such as health authorities and health providers to be directly linked to the communities they served. Platforms such as "Outbreaks Near Me" and "Ushahidi" have been effective in optimizing the collaboration between ICT and health surveillance (9). Communication through ICT such as mobile phone messaging has also been used to influence health behaviors by encouraging healthy eating and exercise (10), adhering to medication recommendations (11), and promoting the cessation of smoking (12). With the increase of mobile phone usage, health-care workers (HCWs) in developing countries are now able to effectively collect health data in a quick and economical way (13).

Collecting real-time surveillance data provide the foundation for any pandemic preparedness program, but current approaches continue to rely on traditional methods with minimal use of new technology or social engagement. For example,

existing infrastructure for influenza surveillance and epidemiology are focused on health-care institutions providing clinical reports of acute respiratory infections as well as laboratory-based confirmed influenza cases (14). These methods usually rely on the symptomatic person visiting a health-care facility, and such systems can be made less efficient by poor health-seeking behavior and delays in disease notifications. Despite their strengths, the setup and maintenance of these systems can be costly, particularly in developing countries (13). During the 2009 H1N1 pandemic, public health bodies worldwide faced difficulties and delays in ramping up such traditional surveillance systems (15).

To address the limitations of routine surveillance systems during pandemic H1N1 in 2009, a number of countries such as the UK urgently developed Internet-based systems to be used by the public (16). These have shown good results and continue to be used for routine seasonal influenza. Other approaches have included the development and use of population web searches on influenza-related terms to help predict an outbreak of infectious disease (17). However, despite early acclaim during pandemic outbreaks, systems such as Google Flu trends have been shown to be too sensitive to media reports, resulting in difficult to control biases, particularly during normal influenza seasons (18, 19).

More recently, Lwin et al. (20) reported the application of the PE approach to the conceptual and technological development of a mobile-based crowd-surveillance application called Mo-Buzz for use by public health inspectors and the general public to address dengue outbreaks in Sri Lanka. Other similar initiatives have adopted this approach to bolster the public health management of asthma, and natural disasters such as earthquakes (9). While most of these efforts send health alerts or enable people to report disease experiences, they offer little by way of telling the user how exactly to prevent or protect oneself from the outbreak. Singapore's pandemic preparedness framework—confronted by a significant influenza burden and looming threat of emerging infectious diseases—can be strengthened by utilizing the mobile-based PE approach and improve upon existing ideas by addressing clear gaps (such as a lack of health communication).

The rapid development and innovation of new and affordable tablet devices, digital applications, and geographic information systems have become easily accessible to the Singaporean population, with nearly 90% smartphone penetration. Therefore, Singapore is best positioned to spearhead the development of this public health innovation in the region and to scientifically evaluate its impact on population groups at risk from influenza. These technologies can be integrated to design an innovative dynamic system where health authorities obtain real-time epidemiological and surveillance data from HCWs within Singapore who report disease incidence using smartphones.

The data generated from such a system with its significant time advantage could detect clusters of diseases and could be used as early warning signals for emerging influenza outbreaks within the hospital context, allowing public health authorities to initiate further investigations. The above literature emphasizes how real-time surveillance has become increasingly important in investigating infectious diseases such as influenza, which remains a social and economic burden. Given that smartphones are becoming more widespread in developing countries due to decreasing costs and increasing availability, pandemic preventative programs need to focus on integrating social media to streamline influenza surveillance, treatment, and health communication.

DEVELOPMENT OF FluMob

Technical Specifications

The FluMob system blends ubiquitous access to the Internet, and the simple portability of mobile phones to create a digitally integrated syndromic surveillance system. The system, integrating a fully responsive web-based interface and a mobile interface, is made available to HCWs using various types of mobile devices and web browsers. The ease and convenience in using application software on their mobile phones will allow users to provide reports of non-specific syndromes such as influenza-like illness (ILI) on a weekly basis. The near real-time data generated from the system will be complementary to current health-care- and laboratory-based systems in assisting with streamlining hospital outbreak response among HCWs and informing vaccine policy. **Figure 1** shows the overall system architecture of FluMob. The application supports two mediums of data input (web browsers and mobile phones) that are fed into a central server and are subsequently generated as reports to be analyzed.

The FluMob application consists of mobile operating systems (Android and iOS) and a responsive web portal. These applications are integrated into a central database using common web services. Central servers hold the business logics related to the FluMob application and the report analysis module. Once users are registered in the system, they have to log in with user identifications and passwords. There are no identified constraints in the application, and it is a simple, user-friendly process. All required data will be stored in an encrypted manner for security and confidentiality purposes.

Operating Environment

The operating environment of FluMob can be divided into two components: *software environment (SE)* and *hardware environment (HE)*.

The SE is the collection of software required to operate the application, and those used in the FluMob application are Windows server 2008 R2, Apache/2.4.17, PHP Version 5.5.30, MySQL 5.6, Android studio, and xCode for iOS development.

The HE refers to the set of hardware required to deploy the application. The FluMob central server is configured with Core2 Intel Xeon Processor with four cores, 8 GB of random-access memory, and 500 GB of storage space. The main server supports any number of web clients. Based on the initial system prototype, more than 100 clients are expected, and the system was tested with 500 dummy clients. The system supported 100 concurrent users without any technical malfunctions. The maximum number of sever connections was restricted to 100

connections, which proved to be sufficient, as database servers will be configured to allow connection pooling. There are no specific security mechanisms added to the client application, but predefined private keys to communicate with central servers have been implemented.

PARTICIPANT ENGAGEMENT

Figure 2 shows the use case diagram for FluMob. New users are first required to register with the system to define their profiles. The login system provides functionality for users to view the FAQs associated with the system and allows them to make changes to their profile information and reset their passwords. At a predetermined schedule, users are notified to log into the system and carry out the routine survey. At any time, users can view all their past survey returns and changes over time. The accumulated survey results are analyzed and made available to the administrator of the system for further actions.

The FluMob system is being tested and used by consenting participants from Tan Tock Seng Hospital (TTSH) and KK Women's and Children's Hospital (KKH). TTSH has a Communicable Disease Centre and is the designated hospital to handle and manage outbreaks of novel diseases. KKH is a women's and children's hospital, with a large inpatient and outpatient pediatric patient workload. The research is being conducted using standard research practice and ethics guidelines. An optimal sample size of 278 was calculated for the study's statistical validation representing the health-care workforce using G*Power analysis (21). However, factoring in attrition rates, the researchers aim to recruit 700 HCWs. Participants, who include clinical and non-clinical HCW across these two hospitals, are required to be no less than 21 years old, and own smartphones installed with either iOS or Android software. Hospital staff at all departments were invited to download the app *via* mass emails. Upon responding, users are given a link to the relevant software app store to download the free app. Once the app is loaded on the mobile phone, each user is first asked to register by filling a form capturing demographic, lifestyle details, and medical history. **Figure 3** shows the screenshots of the mobile application on a typical screen.

Clinical and social scientists from collaborating institutions developed and collated a range of questions to capture data relating to HCW demographics, lifestyle, influenza virus symptoms, and prevention. FluMob registration requires participants to fill in a form capturing demographic details (e.g., date of birth, sex, and ethnicity), workplace information (e.g., hospital name, job category, and department), information about family (e.g., how many people in different age groups), lifestyle behaviors (e.g., mode of transport to work and frequency of eating at food centers), medical history (e.g., vaccination records and disease profiles), as well as technology use and acceptance (e.g., usage of mobile phone, Internet, and mobile applications). The questions serve as a baseline for researchers to understand the lifestyle patterns and technology consumption among local HCWs. Descriptive analyses could potentially assist in the development of policies for disease monitoring and preventive measures. The data collected at registration can also be used for analytics at a

4

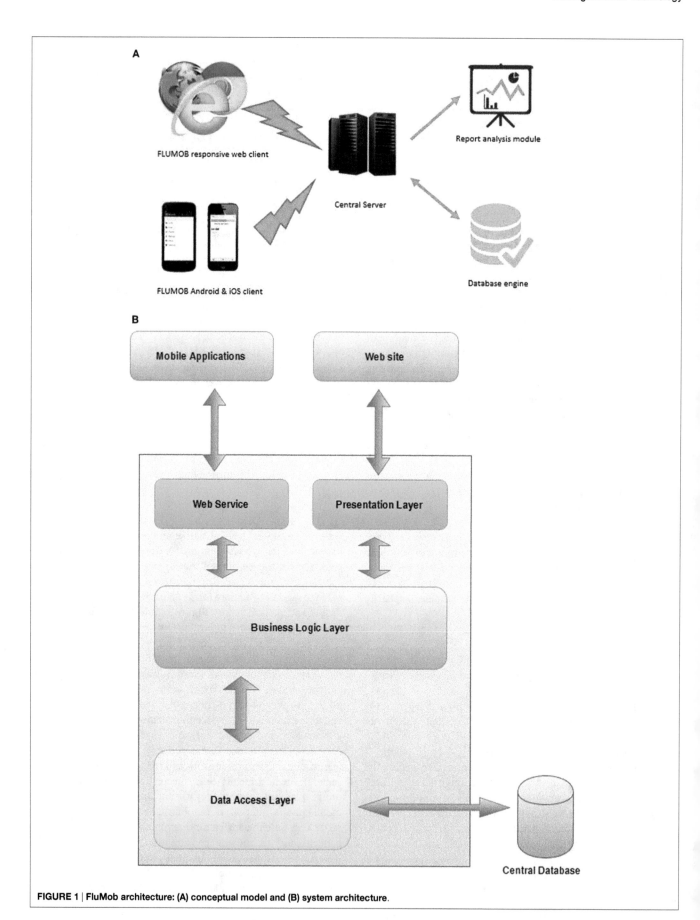

FIGURE 1 | FluMob architecture: (A) conceptual model and (B) system architecture.

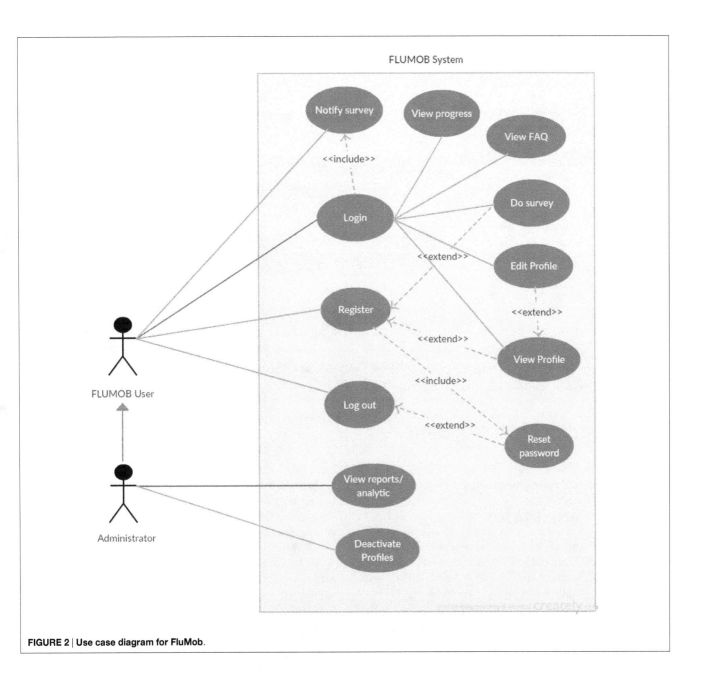

FIGURE 2 | Use case diagram for FluMob.

later stage to identify any potential relationship between demographics, lifestyle behaviors, medical history, and vulnerability to influenza.

Health-care workers are prompted to submit weekly health reports on whether they have ILI symptoms, a dichotomous "yes-or-no" question is first presented to the users to capture the presence of ILI symptoms after they have chosen their ward/ location of duty. If users answer "no," they will then receive a "thank you" note for submission and can immediately resume their daily work tasks or activities. Conversely, when users have declared having ILI symptoms, they will be asked to specify their symptoms from a list, which includes fever, cough, muscle/joint pain, vomiting, diarrhea, and others. After which, users will then need to provide further information regarding the illness, such

as the date of onset and end of symptoms, body temperature, whether they have fever, medical services visited, medication taken as well as some medical leave-related questions. Finally, they will be asked to rate their health status on the day itself on a scale of 0–100.

This component was designed to enhance surveillance efforts with real-time information about ILI episodes among the clinical and non-clinical staff in both hospitals. The reports are submitted on mobile phones or web browsers to assist the research team in detecting potential influenza outbreaks within the hospital. Users are provided with incentives after submitting a certain amount of reports. As soon as a user has submitted the report, the information is stored in a data repository, which allows clinicians and researchers to gather real-time crowd-sourced information for

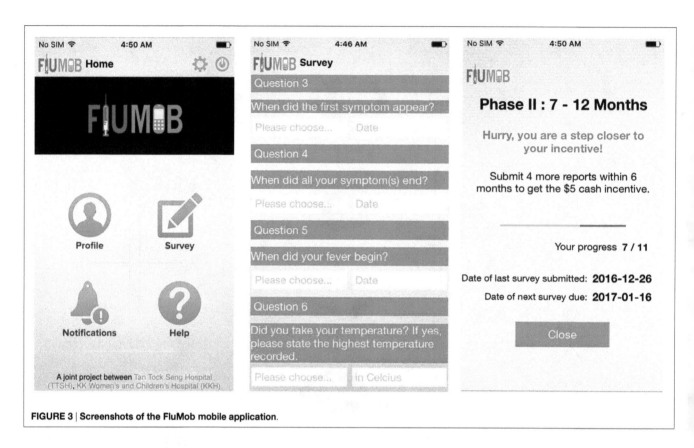

FIGURE 3 | Screenshots of the FluMob mobile application.

clinical analytics so as to inform strategies for disease surveillance, prevention, and management.

PROGRESS AND STATUS

The Android version of the application was introduced to the health workers at TTSH and KKH in May 2016, and saw over 50 HCWs from TTSH signing up for the study within the first week. The iOS version was launched later in June 2016, and there are currently more than 200 iOS users who have installed the FluMob application. At this stage, the team has steadily recruited almost 700 participants. Of these, approximately 50% are regularly submitting weekly reports.

CHALLENGES AND LEARNING EXPERIENCES

A number of challenges were faced in the development and implementation of the system. This section will look at the challenges faced, and how they were addressed and resolved by the team. The first trial was encountered during the development phase of the application. The most recent data available (22) show that the Android (i.e., Samsung S-series) software for mobile phones dominates the Singaporean market, holding 65.58% of the market share, whereas iOS (i.e., Apple iPhones) holds 27.24%.

Therefore, the technical expertise of the research team focused only on the development of Android-based applications and outsourced the development of the iOS version to an external development specialist. Due to the demands of the project and

other unforeseen circumstances, the study was first launched only with the Android application, and interested IOS individuals had to be put on waiting list for more than a month. When the IOS version was finally released and individuals on the wait list were re-contacted, a lot of the initial interests had waned leading to only 75% of them being successfully recruited into the study.

To prevent the coding and programming issues described earlier, a platform where both Android and iOS mobile phone applications can be developed simultaneously can be considered in the future. A software called Appcelerator Titanium (23) can be used to create a full-featured iOS application using JavaScript and can automatically convert the JavaScript code into Objective-C code, which is a requirement of coding for iOS mobile applications. Creating the Android version of the same application is also simplified as the Titanium software will convert the JavaScript code into Java and create an application suitable for the Android Marketplace.

The second challenge pertained to the type and number of survey questions that were to be included in both the registration and the weekly reports sections of the FluMob application. The researchers were faced with the arduous task of filtering through numerous survey questions that effectively measured demographic variables (i.e., socioeconomic status, sex, and age) and overall health of the participant (i.e., smoking status). Sifting through previously published peer-reviewed literature took time, and numerous meetings were required to settle on the questions which were to be included.

This issue was resolved by meeting frequently, and by using scales that have been previously tested and established in their

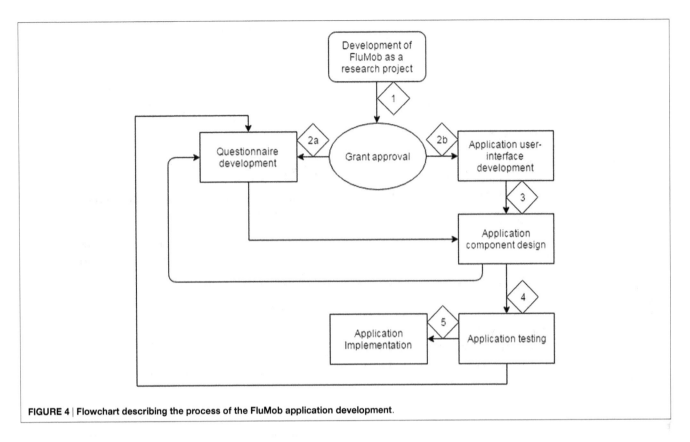

FIGURE 4 | Flowchart describing the process of the FluMob application development.

efficacy at measuring ILI symptoms. The team also resolved differences in opinion in an objective, evidence-based manner, which allowed for more empirical formulation of survey questions. The question list was pilot tested on a small sample ($N = 10$) of participants from TTSH. This allowed for feedback to be collected and amendments made prior to the large-scale implementation of the application.

The final challenge arose in the form of inter-organizational and transdisciplinary research. The research team comprises of clinician scientists, social scientists, and research engineers, hailing from several different institutions; Nanyang Technological University, KKH, TTSH, National University of Singapore, and National Public Health Laboratory. **Figure 4** shows the flowchart visualizing the work flow involved in developing the FluMob application.

In **Figure 4**, the diamond-shaped boxes with numerical values describe the order of the process. As shown in the chart, the idea for the development of the application is the first step, after which grant writing and submission ensue. After approval, the team splits into two groups; the clinical/social science groups (2a) and the research engineering group (2b). After the development of the user interface of the application, the research engineer team should bring the application into its testing phase (3). However, frequent revisions to the application pertaining to both the design and the survey questions were made by the clinical/social science team. This resulted in multiple phases of component design and testing (4), which inherently delayed the implementation of the application (5).

The research team resolved the issue of constant iterations of the survey by completing full scale testing within 1 week and freezing any changes that could be made to the application a week prior to launch. The final version of the survey was fully agreed upon by both clinical and social scientists and allowed for a measurement of the full spectrum of variables that permitted all the research hypotheses to be tested effectively. The nature of having experts of varied specializations gave project a larger research scope, limited to not just social science or clinical science. This is an example of how transdisciplinary research can be both an advantage and a disadvantage to the implementation of such a research project.

DISCUSSION AND FUTURE DEVELOPMENT

The completion of the study period will see detailed data analysis, which includes an analysis of the weekly reports and cases identified for follow-up. The registration questions will serve as a baseline for researchers to understand the lifestyle patterns and technology consumption among local HCWs. Descriptive analyses will also yield valuable data and could potentially assist in the development of policies for disease monitoring and preventive measures. The data collected at registration can also be used for analytics at a later stage to identify any potential relationship between demographics, lifestyle behaviors, medical history, and vulnerability to influenza.

At the next stage, our plan is to incorporate health education messaging and communication. The present system allows for users to select the option to enable or disable notifications and avoids broadcasting of messages, instead electing to personalize reminder messages for each user. The research team wants to build on this and is considering including, in a subsequent version of FluMob, a health education messaging service that will send out health educational messages to users when they report having flu-like symptoms. For example, if a user were to report fever as a symptom, a notification would be sent to the user to encourage them to wear a mask, avoid contact with others, or to see a doctor. Two areas of academic inquiry are being considered by the research team; the first tests the efficacy of more tailored messages, and the second studies the effects of various modalities of communicating health messages.

The FluMob study is currently under deployment with participants in both hospitals where data are being collated, the results of which will be analyzed in the near term future. At of the time of writing, recruitment numbers are still increasing, and weekly influenza reports from HCWs are being steadily submitted. The research team is presently building upon the knowledge gained to create a novel integrated syndromic surveillance system for general public use, which they hope will further address the gaps in disease prevention on a wider national and regional scale, and streamline influenza surveillance to reduce the burden of emerging infectious diseases.

AUTHOR CONTRIBUTIONS

ML, BA, CFY, PY, and SF were involved in the conceptualization of the paper and the overall editing. KJ, AS, and KS wrote the main sections of the paper. HX and CJ were involved in data collection in their respective hospitals. UJ, AK, and KS were involved in the technical development of the application. SC was the overall coordinator for the project.

ACKNOWLEDGMENTS

The authors would like to acknowledge the contribution of larger team members: Vincent Chow from the National University of Singapore, Raymond Lin and Cui Lin who are involved in the laboratory work at the NPHL (National Public Health Laboratory) as well as Gentatsu Lim in research assistance during the early parts of the project.

FUNDING

This research was supported by the Singapore Ministry of Health's National Medical Research Council under its Communicable Diseases—Public Health Research Grant (CDPHRG13NOV020).

REFERENCES

1. Ng TP, Pwee KH, Niti M, Goh LG. Influenza in Singapore: assessing the burden of illness in the community. *Ann Acad Med Singapore* (2002) 31(2):182–8.
2. Chow A, Ma S, Ling AE, Chew SK. Influenza-associated deaths in tropical Singapore. *Emerg Infect Dis* (2006) 12(1):114. doi:10.3201/eid1201.050826
3. Dawood FS, Iuliano AD, Reed C, Meltzer MI, Shay DK, Cheng PY, et al. Estimated global mortality associated with the first 12 months of 2009 pandemic influenza A H1N1 virus circulation: a modelling study. *Lancet Infect Dis* (2012) 12(9):687–95. doi:10.1016/S1473-3099(12)70121-4
4. Lee VJ, Tok MY, Chow VT, Phua KH, Ooi EE, Tambyah PA, et al. Economic analysis of pandemic influenza vaccination strategies in Singapore. *PLoS One* (2009) 4(9):e7108. doi:10.1371/journal.pone.0007108
5. Coker RJ, Hunter BM, Rudge JW, Liverani M, Hanvoravongchai P. Emerging infectious diseases in Southeast Asia: regional challenges to control. *Lancet* (2011) 377(9765):599–609. doi:10.1016/S0140-6736(10)62004-1
6. Henderson JC, Ng A. Responding to crisis: severe acute respiratory syndrome (SARS) and hotels in Singapore. *Int J Tourism Res* (2004) 6(6):411–9. doi:10.1002/jtr.505
7. Lee JW, McKibbin WJ. Estimating the global economic costs of SARS. *Learning from SARS: Preparing for the Next Disease Outbreak: Workshop Summary*. (2004).
8. Catley A. Use of participatory epidemiology to compare the clinical veterinary knowledge of pastoralists and veterinarians in East Africa. *Trop Anim Health Prod* (2006) 38(3):171–84. doi:10.1007/s11250-006-4365-9
9. Kass-Hout TA, Alhinnawi H. Social media in public health. *Br Med Bull* (2013) 108(1):5–24. doi:10.1093/bmb/ldt028
10. Haapala I, Barengo NC, Biggs S, Surakka L, Manninen P. Weight loss by mobile phone: a 1-year effectiveness study. *Public Health Nutr* (2009) 12(12):2382–91. doi:10.1017/S1368980009005230
11. Cocosila M, Archer N, Haynes RB, Yuan Y. Can wireless text messaging improve adherence to preventive activities? Results of a randomised controlled trial. *Int J Med Inform* (2009) 78(4):230–8. doi:10.1016/j.ijmedinf.2008.07.011
12. Free C, Knight R, Robertson S, Whittaker R, Edwards P, Zhou W, et al. Smoking cessation support delivered via mobile phone text messaging (txt2stop): a single-blind, randomised trial. *Lancet* (2011) 378(9785):49–55. doi:10.1016/S0140-6736(11)60701-0
13. Blaya JA, Fraser HS, Holt B. E-health technologies show promise in developing countries. *Health Aff* (2010) 29(2):244–51. doi:10.1377/hlthaff.2009.0894
14. Briand S, Mounts A, Chamberland M. Challenges of global surveillance during an influenza pandemic. *Public Health* (2011) 125(5):247–56. doi:10.1016/j.puhe.2010.12.007
15. Lipsitch M, Finelli L, Heffernan RT, Leung GM, Redd SC; 2009 H1N1 Surveillance Group. Improving the evidence base for decision making during a pandemic: the example of 2009 influenza A/H1N1. *Biosecur Bioterror* (2011) 9(2):89–115. doi:10.1089/bsp.2011.0007
16. Tilston NL, Eames KT, Paolotti D, Ealden T, Edmunds WJ. Internet-based surveillance of influenza-like-illness in the UK during the 2009 H1N1 influenza pandemic. *BMC Public Health* (2010) 10(1):650. doi:10.1186/1471-2458-10-650
17. Eysenbach G. Infodemiology: tracking flu-related searches on the web for syndromic surveillance. *AMIA Annual Symposium Proceedings*. (Vol. 2006), Washington, DC: American Medical Informatics Association (2006). 244 p.
18. de Lange MM, Meijer A, Friesema IH, Donker GA, Koppeschaar CE, Hooiveld M, et al. Comparison of five influenza surveillance systems during the 2009 pandemic and their association with media attention. *BMC Public Health* (2013) 13(1):881. doi:10.1186/1471-2458-13-881
19. Ginsberg J, Mohebbi MH, Patel RS, Brammer L, Smolinski MS, Brilliant L. Detecting influenza epidemics using search engine query data. *Nature* (2009) 457(7232):1012–4. doi:10.1038/nature07634
20. Lwin MO, Vijaykumar S, Fernando ON, Cheong SA, Rathnayake VS, Lim G, et al. A 21st century approach to tackling dengue: crowdsourced surveillance, predictive mapping and tailored communication. *Acta Trop* (2014) 130:100–7. doi:10.1016/j.actatropica.2013.09.021
21. Faul F, Erdfelder E, Buchner A, Lang AG. Statistical power analyses using G* power 3.1: tests for correlation and regression analyses. *Behav Res Methods* (2009) 41(4):1149–60. doi:10.3758/BRM.41.4.1149
22. NETMARKETSHARE. *Market Share Statistics for Internet Technologies*. (2016). Available from: https://www.netmarketshare.com/
23. Brousseau C. *Creating Mobile Apps with Appcelerator Titanium*. Packt Publishing Ltd (2013).

2

Bleeding Risk in Patients Using Oral Anticoagulants Undergoing Surgical Procedures in Dentistry

Natália Karol de Andrade[1], Rogério Heládio Lopes Motta[1]*, Cristiane de Cássia Bergamaschi[2], Luciana Butini Oliveira[3], Caio Chaves Guimarães[1], Jimmy de Oliveira Araújo[1] and Luciane Cruz Lopes[2]

[1] Division of Pharmacology, Anesthesiology and Therapeutics, Faculdade São Leopoldo Mandic, Instituto de Pesquisas São Leopoldo Mandic, Campinas, Brazil, [2] Pharmaceutical Science Graduate Course, University of Sorocaba, Sorocaba, Brazil, [3] Division of Paediatric Dentistry, Faculdade São Leopoldo Mandic, Instituto de Pesquisas São Leopoldo Mandic, Campinas, Brazil

*Correspondence:
Rogério Héladio Lopes Motta
rogerio.motta@slmandic.edu.br

The management of patients who undergo dental surgical procedures and receive oral anticoagulant therapy requires particular attention due to the risk of bleeding that may occur during the procedure. Bleeding rates in these trans- or post-operative patients tend to be unpredictable. The aim of this study was to conduct a systematic review in order to assess the risk of bleeding during and after performing oral surgery in patients administered oral anticoagulants compared with a group that discontinued anticoagulant therapy. For the purposes of this review, we searched the databases of the Cochrane Central Register of Controlled Trials (CENTRAL), MEDLINE (*via* Ovid), EMBASE (*via* Ovid), and the Virtual Health Library (VHL) from inception of the database to December 2018. The primary outcome was defined as the occurrence of local bleeding during and after oral surgical procedures. Four reviewers, independently and in pairs, screened titles and abstracts for full-text eligibility. Data regarding participant characteristics, interventions, and design and outcomes of the included studies were extracted. The data were pooled using random-effects meta-analyses and described as risk ratios (RRs) with a 95% confidence interval (95% CI). The confidence for the pooled estimates was ascertained through the Grading of Recommendations Assessment, Development, and Evaluation (GRADE) approach, and the protocol of this review was recorded in PROSPERO (CRD42017056986). A total of 58 eligible studies were identified, of which three randomized controlled trials were included in the meta-analysis, covering a total of 323 adult participants, among whom 167 were taking anticoagulants at the time they underwent dental surgery. Of these patients, 14.2% had reported bleeding. The risk of bleeding was found to be one to almost three times greater in patients taking warfarin compared with patients who discontinued the use of anticoagulant during the trans-operative period (RR = 1.67, 95% CI = 0.97 to 2.89) and in the post-operative period (RR = 1.44, 95% CI = 0.71 to 2.92), although the quality of evidence was very low. The results indicate that there is no evidence that the use of anticoagulants eliminates the risk of bleeding during surgical dental procedures.

Keywords: oral surgery, oral anticoagulant, bleeding, safety, systematic review, meta-analysis

INTRODUCTION

The routine use of oral anticoagulants is related to hemostatic imbalance between clotting and blood anticoagulation, and significant variations in this relationship may increase the risk of hemorrhage or thromboembolism (Dahlback, 2000; Leiria et al., 2007; Barco et al., 2013; Harter et al., 2015; Yeh et al., 2015; Gerzson et al., 2016).

Anticoagulants can be classified according to their route of administration. Oral anticoagulants include vitamin K antagonists, such as warfarin, that inhibit factors II, VII, IX, and X of the coagulation cascade; new oral anticoagulants that directly inhibit thrombin (coagulation cascade factor II), such as dabigatran; and those that inhibit factor Xa, such as rivaroxaban. A commonly used parenteral anticoagulant is low molecular weight heparin (Barco et al., 2013; Lijfering and Tichellar, 2018).

The increasing use of these medications raises the probability of anticoagulant therapy in patients undergoing dental treatment. Thus, it is necessary to promote safe and preventive treatment in order to avoid complications and comorbidities in these patients (Thacil and Gagg, 2015).

According to the Guidelines of the American College of Chest Physicians (2012), the desirable value of the International Normative Ratio (INR) for patients taking oral anticoagulants is between 2 and 3. When this index indicates anomalies, treatment should be adjusted by the health professional in charge, in order to maintain the patient in a favorable health condition while promoting good short- and long-term prognoses.

Some studies have demonstrated that exodontias performed in patients with a recommendable INR range can be safely conducted without oral anticoagulant interruption or antiplatelet drugs (Campbell et al., 2000; Barrero et al., 2002; Aframian et al., 2007; Morimoto et al., 2008; Goodchild and Donaldson, 2009; Nematullah et al., 2009; Bajkin et al., 2015).

Although previous systematic reviews have assessed the risk of bleeding during oral surgical procedures in patients using oral anticoagulants (Dunn and Turpie, 2003; Madrid and Sanz, 2009; Nematullah et al., 2009; Diermen et al., 2013; Kämmerer et al., 2015; Yang et al., 2016; Shi et al., 2017), the safety of performing dental surgical procedures remains uncertain, on account of the various methodological discrepancies or inconsistencies in these studies. For example, the findings reported by Nematullah et al. (2009) and Madrid et al. (2009) were not restricted to dental surgeries, whereas Diermen et al. (2013) did not perform a meta-analysis of the results, and Kämmerer et al. (2015), Yang et al. (2016), and Shi et al. (2017) used observational studies instead of clinical trials and did not restrict INR values. Furthermore, none of these systematic reviews used GRADE (Grading of Recommendations Assessment, Development and Evaluation), a tool that is routinely used to evaluate the quality of a body of evidence and the strength of recommendations of the findings.

The present review aims to answer the following PICO question: "What is the risk of bleeding in patients who take oral anticoagulants and will undergo oral surgical procedures with or without antithrombotic therapy interruption?" Accordingly, by conducting this systematic review, we aim to determine the risk of bleeding during and after dental surgery in patients undergoing anticoagulant therapy, as well as providing guidance that will assist dental professionals in making informed clinical decisions.

METHODS

Protocol and Registration

This systematic review was conducted in accordance with the recommendations described in the Cochrane Handbook for Systematic Reviews of Interventions (Moher et al., 2009). The study was performed in accordance with the checklist of PRISMA (Preferred Reporting Items for Systematic Reviews and Meta-Analyses) (Moher et al., 2009; Higgins and Green, 2011). The protocol of this review has been recorded in PROSPERO (International Prospective Register of Systematic Reviews) (protocol CRD42017056986) (http://www.crd.york.ac.uk/PROSPERO) (Motta et al., 2017).

Eligibility Criteria
Study Selection Criteria

Studies considered eligible for inclusion were randomized controlled trials (RCT) involving adult volunteers of both genders, users of oral anticoagulants (vitamin K antagonists, factor Xa inhibitors, or direct thrombin inhibitors), and requiring dental surgeries such as exodontias and dental implants. Included studies were also required to have an experimental group containing participants who were submitted to dental surgeries without interruption of anticoagulant therapy and a control group containing participants who were submitted to dental surgeries with interruption of anticoagulant therapy.

Exclusion Criteria

Exclusion criteria included studies in which patients under combined anticoagulant therapy (oral anticoagulant associated with a platelet antiaggregant) represented more than 20% of the sample; studies in which the population was not clearly representative (e.g., patients presenting different bleeding risks due to recent episodes of stroke and recent ablation surgeries); and/or an INR value higher or lower than the desirable range between 2 and 3 in more than 20% of the sample.

Outcomes Assessed

Included studies should have reported one of the following outcomes: trans-operative or post-operative local bleeding measured at least 48 h after oral surgical intervention. The definition of bleeding was accepted as described in each study. Oral complications (infections, implant failures, and healing problems at the surgical site) were considered as secondary outcomes.

Search for Primary Studies
Electronic Databases

For the purposes of the review, we performed searches for eligible studies in CENTRAL (Cochrane Central Register of Controlled Trials) part of The Cochrane Library and MEDLINE (via Ovid), and EMBASE (via Ovid) and VHL (Virtual Health Library) databases from the inception of the database until

December 2018, without restrictions relating to language or year of publication. The management of the references (listing and removal of duplicates) was carried out using Endnote X8 software.

Other Search Resources

Two reviewers (NA and CB) performed a manual search by reading the reference lists of each selected study or citations found in secondary studies in order to verify potentially eligible studies.

Search Strategies

For search purposes, the terms describing the risk of bleeding and oral surgical procedure were combined. The search was conducted using MeSH (Medical Subject Headings) terms for each minor oral surgical procedure (oral surgery, exodontias, and dental implant installation), risk of hemorrhagic events and their synonyms, and several oral anticoagulants (vitamin K antagonists and new oral anticoagulants). The search strategy was adapted for each database and is described in **Supplementary Material A**.

Study Selection

Four reviewers (NA and CB; LO and JA), working independently and in pairs (as indicated), selected potentially relevant titles and abstracts, to which the eligibility criteria were applied. The full texts of potentially eligible studies were obtained, and two reviewers (NA and RM) independently assessed the eligibility of each study. All disagreements were resolved through consensus.

Data Extraction

Initially, four reviewers (RM and CG; LO and NA), working independently and in pairs, extracted the data from two articles, and a consensus was reached. Discordances were resolved by consensus, and contentious issues were discussed with a third reviewer (LL).

The same reviewers, independently and in pairs, extracted data and recorded information regarding patients, methods, interventions, outcomes, and absence of significant results. A data extraction sheet was used in accordance with the instruction manual prepared by the lead author of this review (NA).

Assessment of the Risk of Bias

The Cochrane Collaboration tool was used to evaluate the risk of bias (Altman et al., 1990; Higgins and Green, 2011). All reviewers, independently and in pairs, assessed the risk of bias for each clinical trial according to randomization; allocation concealment; blinding of the patient, the healthcare professional, and the outcome assessors; reporting of incomplete outcomes; and selective reporting of outcomes and imbalance in baseline measurements of the sample.

For each domain, the reviewers assigned response options of "definitely yes," "probably yes," "probably not," or "definitely not," with "definitely yes" and "probably yes" ultimately indicating a low risk of bias and "definitely not" and "probably not" indicating a high risk of bias (Akl et al., 2013). In cases of disagreement, a consensus was reached through discussion or consultation with a third author (LL).

Data Synthesis

Analysis was performed for each anticoagulant and outcome of interest. Confidence in the findings was determined by estimates for each body of evidence. For studies that reported dichotomous outcomes, the relative risk (RR) was calculated combined with a 95% confidence interval (95% CI).

Continuous outcomes were not considered. However, if available they would be described according to the information available in the published protocol of this review (Motta et al., 2017). Details regarding the methods adopted for data synthesis can be found in the same protocol. The random effects associated with meta-analysis were determined using STATA Software (version 10.1).

Quality of Evidence

The quality of the evidence was independently assessed (confidence in estimates of the effect) for each outcome reported using the GRADE system (Guyatt et al., 2011a; Guyatt et al., 2011b). In this approach, randomized trials that were initially considered to have a high quality of evidence may have their quality status diminished according to assessment of one or more of the following five categories of limitation: risk of bias (assessed for each study as described previously), inconsistency, indirect evidence, imprecision, and publication bias (Guyatt et al., 2013a, Guyatt et al., 2013b).

The heterogeneity was also evaluated in association with the estimates of the effects using a χ^2 test and the I^2 statistic (Higgins and Thompson, 2002) and was classified as follows: 0% to 25% (low heterogeneity), 50% (moderate heterogeneity), and 75% (high heterogeneity) (Higgins and Thompson, 2002).

RESULTS

Literature Search Results

From our searches within the aforementioned four databases, we extracted 2,266 publications for consideration, of which 70 articles were duplicates. Accordingly, a total of 2,196 publications were deemed to be potentially eligible. A further 26 publications were identified through manual searches. Of these studies, 58 were considered to fulfil the eligibility criteria established for this review, three of which were included in the qualitative synthesis (Campbell et al., 2000; Evans et al., 2002; Al-Mubarak et al., 2007), and two (Evans et al., 2002; Al-Mubarak et al., 2007) were included in the meta-analysis (**Figure 1**).

Synthesis Results

The characteristics of the three studies subjected to qualitative synthesis are shown in **Table 1**. These studies evaluated 348 users of oral anticoagulants, most of whom were using vitamin K antagonists. The studies, however, did not present information relating to the underlying diseases that justified the prescription of anticoagulants. All studies compared the risk of bleeding in patients undergoing oral surgical procedures with or without interruption (a few days prior to the dental procedure) of anticoagulant therapy but did not report other outcomes. The

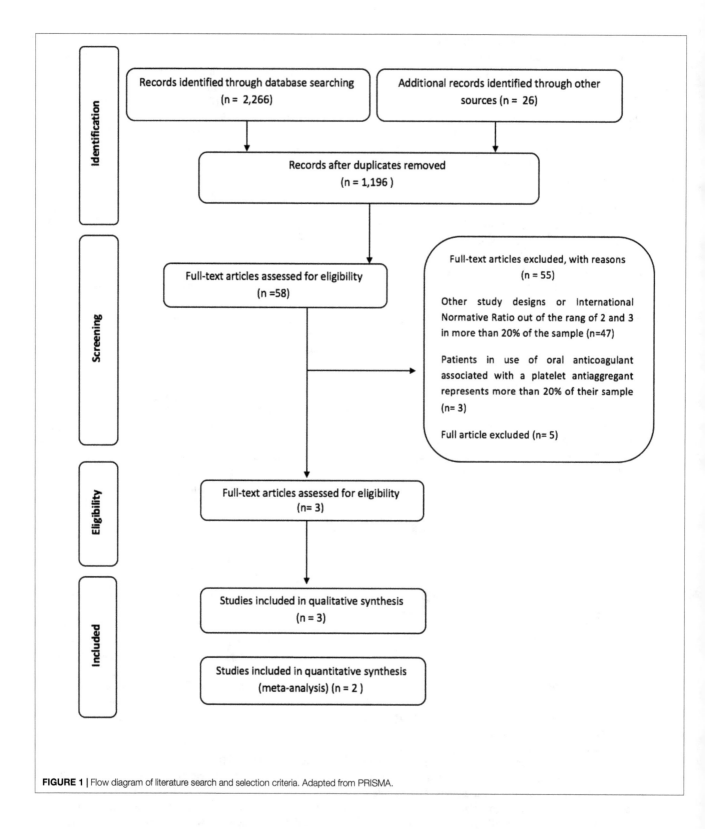

FIGURE 1 | Flow diagram of literature search and selection criteria. Adapted from PRISMA.

list of excluded studies and the reasons for their exclusion are presented in **Supplementary Material B**. Local hemostatic measures, such as compression with gauze and sutures (Campbell et al., 2000; Evans et al., 2002; Al-Mubarak et al., 2007) and

sutured oxidized cellulose sponges, were used in the surgical beds in order to control bleeding (Evans et al., 2002).

Two of the three studies provided details of patient follow-up during the first week of the post-operative periods. In the third

TABLE 1 | Characteristics of included studies.

Study characteristics	Campbell et al. (2000)	Evans et al. (2002)	Al-Mubarak et al. (2007)
Sample (n = 348)	25	109	214
Women (%)	NR	33%	67%
Country	USA	United Kingdom	Saudi Arabia
Anticoagulant type	Not specified	Warfarin	Warfarin
Outcome assessed	Bleeding before and after surgery	Bleeding before and after surgery	Bleeding before and after surgery
Follow-up (days)	2	7	7
Surgical procedures (n = 345)	22 exodontias (simple or several), 2 alveoloplasties and 1 labial frenectomy	109 exodontias (simple or several)	214 exodontias (simple or several)
Use of hemostatic measures	gauze compression and suture	gauze compression, oxidized cellulose, sponges and suture	Gauze compression and suture
Multicentric study	No	Yes	No
Concomitant drugs	No	Yes (antibiotics)	No
Industry funding	No	No	No

VKA, vitamin K antagonist; INR, International Normative Ratio.

study by Campbell et al. (2000), the results indicated a 2-day follow-up time, although this was not stated explicitly in the text.

The study conducted by Evans et al. (2002) reported the concomitant use of other drugs during the research period, in which some patients received antibiotic prophylaxis. None of the studies received industrial funding. Although all three studies reported the primary outcome "local bleeding," none reported secondary outcomes.

Campbell et al. (2000) performed a qualitative evaluation of the bleeding associated with minor oral surgeries in patients with VKA (the study does not specify the anticoagulant). Bleeding was assessed in terms of "surgical sponge weight" in the pre- and post-operative periods. In this regard, it was considered that each gram of blood is equivalent to a volume of 1 ml, and accordingly the volume of blood lost in the pre- and post-operative periods was determined from the difference in sponge weight. Twenty-five patients were allocated to one of two groups (mean INR of 2.0 ± 0.5): the "experimental group" (n = 12) in which patients' use of anticoagulants before and after surgical procedures was maintained, and the "control group" (n = 13) in which anticoagulant use was interrupted 72 to 96 h before the surgical intervention. None of the patients presented trans- or post-operative bleeding requiring any therapeutic intervention, and there was no significant difference in blood loss between the groups. Although the authors have suggested the need for additional investigations, they also consider that it would be possible to perform minor oral surgical procedures in patients taking oral anticoagulants without additional pharmacological interventions.

Evans et al. (2002) evaluated the risk of bleeding in 109 individuals taking warfarin, who underwent simple and multiple exodontia. Bleeding was assessed by the use of gauze, which the patient was instructed to bite on for a period of 10 min. If the hemostatic measures were not sufficient to contain the bleeding, the event was considered as "immediate bleeding." Patients were randomly assigned to one of the two study groups by allocation concealment (57 to the experimental group and 52 to the control group). Individuals in the experimental group continued using warfarin, whereas those in the control group interrupted the use of warfarin 2 days prior to the surgical procedure. All surgical beds were covered with oxidized cellulose sponges, and the

patients were sutured. The patients were instructed to bite a gauze pad for 10 min. If such local hemostatic measures were not sufficient to contain bleeding, it was considered "immediate bleeding." Twenty-two patients presented complications related to bleeding (post-surgery only), 15 (26%) of whom were in the experimental group and seven (13.5%) (n = 7) were in the control group. The study thus indicates the possible heightened risk of complications associated with bleeding when warfarin is maintained. In most cases, however, these events can be controlled by administering local treatment.

Al-Mubarak et al. (2007) evaluated the incidence of post-operative hemorrhage in patients taking warfarin (dose of 2 to 10 mg daily) undergoing exodontia. The bleeding was assessed by the use of gauze on which the patient was instructed to bite for a period of 6 to 10 min. If these hemostatic measures were not sufficient to contain the bleeding, the event was considered as bleeding. Additionally, the volunteers were followed for up to 7 days in order to verify the presence of hemorrhagic sites (evaluated in terms clot formation and the local repair process). A total of 214 patients were randomly divided into four groups. Patients in groups 1 and 3 interrupted warfarin intake (2 days before the surgical procedure): group 1 (n = 48, mean INR 1.8 and no suture) and group 3 (n = 56, mean INR 1.9 and with suture). Patients in groups 2 and 4 maintained warfarin use: group 2 (n = 58, mean INR 2.4 and without suture) and group 4 (n = 52, mean INR 2.7 and with suture). All patients received gauze compression for 6 to 10 min and were followed for up to 7 days. It was observed that among the patients in groups 1 and 2, 12% (n = 6) and 21% (n = 12) presented trans-operative hemorrhagic events, respectively. During the post-operative period, 4% (n = 2) of the patients in group 1 and 3% (n = 2) in group 2 presented bleeding.

Risk of Bias Assessment

As shown in **Figures 2** and **3**, the three included studies had a high risk bias. However, the three studies did not provide sufficient data regarding the randomization process to enable an evaluation of potential selection bias (Campbell et al., 2000; Al-Mubarak et al., 2007). Evans et al. (2002), however, describe the generation of random sequences of patients in the groups.

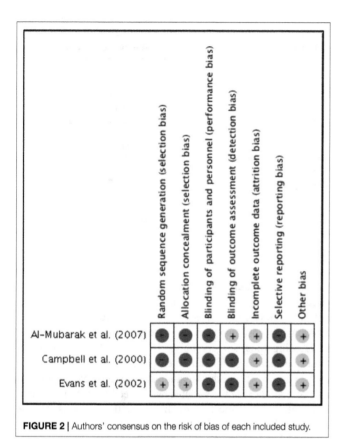

FIGURE 2 | Authors' consensus on the risk of bias of each included study.

although they did not clearly describe how the procedure was performed.

Furthermore, none of the studies clarified whether there was follow-up loss, although all included studies described the evaluated outcomes. However, apparently, all patients enrolled in the studies initiated and completed the proposed treatments.

The incidence of thromboembolic events among patients who interrupted anticoagulant therapy was not assessed in clinical trials. Other secondary outcomes, such as bruising, ecchymoses, or post-operative infections, may have been considered by the studies; however, these were not reported. None of the studies presented the protocol record, which would have enabled us to infer the risk of uncertain bias.

None of the included studies obtained industrial funding, and based on a reading of the studies, no other problems were identified in addition to those already mentioned; thus, we assume that the studies were free of other potential sources of bias.

Results of Evaluated Outcome and Quality of Evidence

Random-effects meta-analysis revealed no statistically significant difference between the groups that continued or interrupted the use of anticoagulants. Nevertheless, the results have demonstrated a one to almost three times greater bleeding risk in patients taking warfarin compared with patients who discontinued the use of anticoagulant in the trans-operative (RR = 1.67, 95% CI = 0.97 to 2.89) and post-operative (RR = 1.44, 95% CI = 0.71 to 2.92) periods (**Figure 4**). Sub-group analyses were not possible due to the low number of studies included.

The quality of evidence according to GRADE (**Table 2**) concerning "bleeding risk" (the main outcome) in both trans- and post-operative periods was considered very low, which indicates a very small confidence in the estimated effect. Furthermore, we also noted that the studies were associated with a high risk of bias, and thus the relative estimate of results may not be reliable. We did, however, observe an overlap in the confidence intervals of the studies, and therefore, the inconsistency was considered

In the studies reported by Campbell et al. (2000) and Al-Mubarak et al. (2007), concealment of the allocation was not guaranteed, and none of the studies provided sufficient information in order for us to determine whether there was blinding of the patients or of those involved in the research, which may have caused detection bias, as the outcomes evaluated are likely to be influenced by the absence of blinding. Only Al-Mubarak et al. (2007) provided an indication that there was blinding of the professionals who evaluated the outcomes,

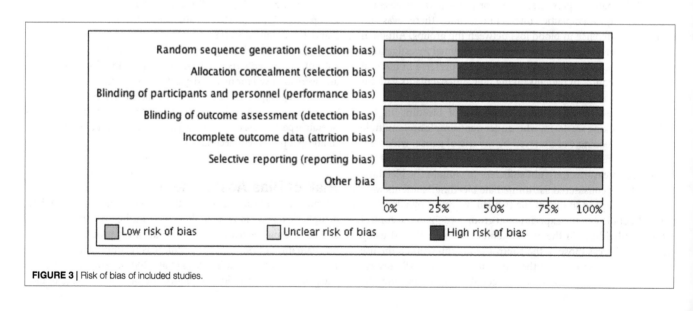

FIGURE 3 | Risk of bias of included studies.

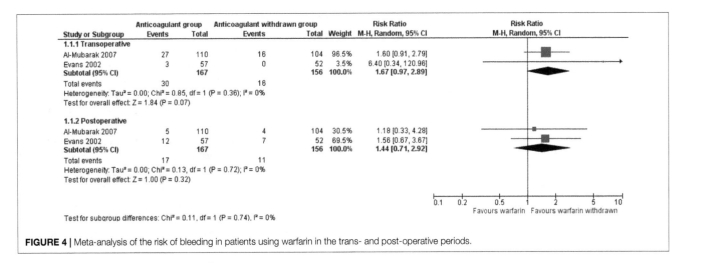

FIGURE 4 | Meta-analysis of the risk of bleeding in patients using warfarin in the trans- and post-operative periods.

unimportant. Moreover, low heterogeneity was observed between the results.

The included studies presented details of interventions and outcomes of interest, and therefore the evidence was considered direct. Considerable imprecision was noted with regard to the number of total events and the small number of samples, in addition to the wide confidence intervals with no true effect.

Although each of the included studies reported few bleeding events, the lack of any details on other meaningful outcomes, including the incidence of thromboembolism or local complications, limits the scope of the clinical decision making, such as the interruption or maintenance of antithrombotic therapy prior to dental surgical procedures. The absence of such details may suggest a publication bias.

DISCUSSION

Excessive trans-or post-operative bleeding is a negative outcome in dentistry that limits several surgical interventions, and in this regard, an evaluation of the risk of bleeding in users of oral anticoagulants may contribute to minimizing the complications experienced by dental patients.

In this study, we evaluated the risk of bleeding in patients using oral anticoagulants who underwent dental surgical procedures. For the purposes of the descriptive analysis, we performed a detailed assessment of three relevant studies (Campbell et al., 2000; Evans et al., 2002; Al-Mubarak et al., 2007), two of which were included in the meta-analysis (Evans et al., 2002; Al-Mubarak et al., 2007).

The assessments undertaken in the present review are restricted to warfarin, for which no recent RCTs have been published. Although our meta-analysis indicates an increased risk of bleeding when patients maintain the use of this anticoagulant, the findings of the assessed studies present very poor-quality evidence, which represents a constraint in terms of making any definite recommendations.

It is noteworthy, however, that apart from bleeding, no other important relevant outcomes, such as ecchymoses and thromboembolism, were reported in the trials included in this review and therefore could not be evaluated. Further, we were unable to perform sub-group analyses, on account of the small number of studies included. Given that the frequency of thromboembolic events is an important outcome for assessing safe antithrombotic therapy interruption, the absence of any report on this outcome in clinical trials may suggest bias due to the selective reporting of outcomes.

According to the guidelines of the American College of Chest Physicians Holbrook et al. (2012), a safe INR for dental interventions ranges from 2 to 3. This INR range has not always been considered as an eligibility criterion in previous studies, as comparisons are difficult and a larger amplitude of INR becomes an inconclusive factor, particularly for those patients who are users of vitamin K antagonists. In the present study we used patient INR values ranging from 2 to 3 as an inclusion criterion for clinical trials, which necessarily limited the number of studies we were able to select for the review. In addition to the INR interval adopted by the studies, other disparities were observed in the systematic reviews previously published on this subject (Dunn and Turpie, 2003; Madrid and Sanz, 2009; Diermen et al., 2013; Kämmerer et al., 2015; Yang et al., 2016; Shi et al., 2017), which accordingly highlight the relevance of the present study.

In a systematic review conducted by Dunn and Turpie (2003), the authors identified a low incidence of thromboembolic events in patients who had discontinued anticoagulant therapy (1.6% of patients). However, this finding was based on a consideration of both medical and oral procedures. Moreover, the authors of this review did not assess the risk of bias or the quality of the evidence of the findings.

Some systematic reviews have indicated that there is no difference in the risk of bleeding among patients who interrupt and those who maintain anticoagulant therapy prior to undergoing surgical procedures (Madri and Sanz, 2009; Yang et al., 2016), which corroborates the findings of the present study. However, the findings of Kämmerer et al. (2015) and Shi et al. (2017) have indicated an increased risk of bleeding in patients who maintain anticoagulant therapy during the period in which they undergo dental procedures. Nevertheless, they concluded that such complications can be

TABLE 2 | Quality of study evidence according to Grading of Recommendations Assessment, Development, and Evaluation (GRADE).

# of studies	Study type	Measured parameters					Number of patients		Effect		Quality	Outcome importance/relevance
		Risk of bias	Inconsistency	Indirectness evidence	Imprecision	Other considerations	Used oral anticoagulants	Did not use oral anticoagulants	Relative risk (95% CI)	Absolute risk (95% CI)		
Bleeding risk (transoperative)												
2	Randomized clinical trials	Very severe[a]	Not severe	Not severe	Severe[b]	None	30/167 (18.0%)	16/156 (10.3%)	1.67 (0.97 to 2.89)	69/1,000 (3 to 194)	⊕○○○ very low	CRITICAL
Bleeding risk (postoperative)												
2	Randomized clinical trials	Very severe[a]	Not severe	Not severe	Severe[b]	None	17/167 (10.2%)	11/156 (7.1%)	1.44 (0.71 to 2.92)	31/1,000 (20 to 135)	⊕○○○ very low	CRITICAL

RR, relative risk; 95% CI, 95% confidence interval. [a]Al-Mubarack's study presented a risk of bias for randomization, concealment of allocation and blinding and the Evans' study presented problems in blinding. [b]Number of total events is small and the confidence interval is wide with no effect.

readily treated using local hemostatic measures. However, none of these studies included only RCTs, and none took INR values into account.

Kämmerer et al. (2015) emphasized that the risk of potentially fatal thromboembolism due to interruption of anticoagulant therapy outweighs the risk of post-operative bleeding episodes. The authors suggest that minor procedures, such as exodontias and dental implants, can be safely performed if the INR is within the therapeutic range and local hemostatic measures are used.

Diermen et al. (2013) evaluated the level of evidence and grade of recommendation (regardless of study design and including clinical practice guidelines) of studies that examined the risk of discontinuing treatment with antiplatelet agents and anticoagulants prior to oral surgical procedures. The results indicated that antithrombotic therapy should not be interrupted for simple dental procedures.

Although the review performed by Yang et al. (2016) also included the studies of Evans et al. (2002) and Al-Mubarak et al. (2007), it was essentially a qualitative analysis and considered other study designs in addition to RCTs. The authors suggested that patients who maintain oral anticoagulant therapy are not at any greater risk of bleeding after dental extractions than are patients who have discontinued oral anticoagulant therapy.

Strengths and Limitations of This Study

The present study was carried out with methodological accuracy, including an evaluation of the risk of bias and an assessment of the quality of evidence, which have not featured in the previously published systematic reviews of this topic (Dunn and Turpie, 2003; Madrid and Sanz, 2009; Nematullah et al., 2009; Diermen et al., 2013; Kämmerer et al., 2015; Yang et al., 2016; Shi et al., 2017). Thus, we have explicitly highlighted the eligibility criteria, the comprehensive database search, and the independent and paired evaluation of each study. Moreover, the use of GRADE made it possible to evaluate the strength and the quality of the body of evidence in relation to the effect of bleeding risk.

The specific criteria used for the selection of included studies do, however, represent a limiting factor for the findings of this review, owing to our requirement regarding the methodological quality of the RCT. This, nevertheless, highlights the necessity for a greater number of primary studies on this subject, with greater methodological accuracy in order to increase the reliability of the findings.

Implications for Clinical Practice and Future Research

Our findings have revealed that there is no statistical difference in the risk of bleeding in warfarin users undergoing dental surgery without anticoagulant therapy interruption compared with those who discontinue the therapy. However, due to the poor quality evidence, the most appropriate practice with respect to whether oral anticoagulant therapy should be interrupted remains uncertain. Meticulous methodological quality should be encouraged with regard to answering the question posed at the outset, in addition to emphasizing the use of INR as a standardized criterion for future research.

On the basis of our findings, we recommend dental surgical planning based on a diagnosis of the general health condition of the patient. This diagnosis implies the accomplishment of a comprehensive anamnesis, including the diseases involved and use of the drugs related to blood hemostasis. This evaluation should additionally include the request for a complete blood exam and determine whether the patient is decompensated or presents comorbidities that contribute to a greater risk associated with the surgical procedures. Moreover, it is important that they be referred to the doctor in charge for a more specific opinion and classification of risk.

To date there have been no RCTs that have evaluated the outcomes of interest of this research in relation to new oral anticoagulants. Given this scenario, new studies with variable control and the use of standardized methods for determining outcomes should be developed.

CONCLUSION

The findings of this analysis indicate that there is no evidence of a greater risk of bleeding in patients using oral anticoagulants who undergo surgical dental procedures. However, the findings should be interpreted with caution and new studies on the subject should be initiated.

AUTHOR CONTRIBUTIONS

NA is the main investigator and led the development and the writing of the manuscript. LL, RM, and CB are the project managers and co-investigators, who contributed to the development, writing, and revision of the manuscript. LO, CG, and JA are co-investigators and contributed to the development and revision of the manuscript. All authors have read and approved the final manuscript.

ACKNOWLEDGMENTS

We thank the researchers Professors Marcus Tolentino Silva and Lauren Giustti Mazzei for their support in the data analysis.

REFERENCES

Aframian, D. J., Lalla, R. V., and Peterson, D. E. (2007). Management of dental patients taking common hemostasis-altering medications. Oral Surg. Oral Med. Oral Pathol. Oral Radiol. Endod. 103 (Suppl 1), S45e1–S4511. doi: 10.1016/j.tripleo.2006.11.011

Akl, E. A., Johnston, B. C., Alonso-Coello, P., Neumann, I., Ebrahim, S., Briel, M. et al., (2013). Addressing dichotomous data for participants excluded from trial analysis: a guide for systematic reviewers. PLOS One 8(2), e57132 doi: 10.1371/journal.pone.0057132

Al-Mubarak, S., Al-Ali, N., Abou-Rass, M., Al-Sohail, A., Robert, A., Al-Zoman, K., et al. (2007). Evaluation of dental extractions, suturing and INR on postoperative bleeding of patients maintained on oral anticoagulant therapy. Br. Dent. J. 203 (7), E15. doi: 10.1038/bdj.2007.725

Altman, R., Alarcón, G., Appelrouth, D., Bloch, D., Borenstein, D., Brandt, K., et al. (1990). The American College of Rheumatology criteria for the classification and reporting of osteoarthritis of the hand. Arthritis Rheum. 33 (11), 1601–1610. doi: 10.1002/art.1780331101

Bajkin, B. V., Vujkov, S. B., Milekic, B. R., and Vuckovic, B. A. (2015). Risk factors for bleeding after oral surgery in patients who continued using oral anticoagulant therapy. J. Am. Dent. Assoc. 46 (6), 375–381. doi: 10.1016/j.adaj.2015.01.017

Barco, S., Cheung, Y. W., Eikelboom, J. W., and Coppens, M. (2013). New oral anticoagulants in elderly patients. Best Pract. Res. Clin. Haematol. 26 (2), 215–224. doi: 10.1016/j.beha.2013.07.011

Barrero, V. M., Knezevic, M., Tapia, M. M., Viejo, L. A., Orengo, V. J. C., García, J. F., et al. (2002). Oral surgery in patients undergoing oral anticoagulant therapy. Med. Oral. 7 (1), 63–66, 67–70.

Campbell, J. H., Alvarado, F., and Murray, R. A. (2000). Anticoagulation and minor oral surgery: should the anticoagulation regiment be altered? J. Oral. Maxillofac. Surg. 58, 131–135. doi: 10.1016/S0278-2391(00)90324-0

Dahlback, B. (2000). Blood coagulation. Lancet 355 (9215), 1627–1632. doi: 10.1016/S0140-6736(00)02225-X

Diermen, D., Waal, I., and Hoogstraten, J. (2013). Management recommendations for invasive dental treatment in patients using oral antithrombotic medication, including novel oral anticoagulants. Oral Surg. Oral Med Oral Pathol. Oral Radiol. 116 (6), 709–716. doi: 10.1016/j.oooo.2013.07.026.

Dunn, A. S., and Turpie, A. G. (2003). Perioperative management of patients receiving oral anticoagulants: a systematic review. Arch. Intern. Med. 163 (8), 901–908. doi: 10.1001/archinte.163.8.901

Evans, I. L., Sayers, M. S., Gibbons, A. J., Price, G., Snooks, H., and Sugar, A. W. (2002). Can warfarin be continued during dental extraction? Results of a randomized controlled trial. Br. J. Oral Maxillofac. Surg. 40 (3), 248–252. doi: 10.1054/bjom.2001.0773

Gerzson, A. S., Grassi, L., Lopes, L. A. Z., and Gallicchio, L. H. H. (2016). Cirurgias odontológicas em pacientes sob terapia com antiagregante plaquetário e anticoagulante oral: revisão de literatura. J. Clin. Dent. Res. 13 (2), 98–105. doi: 10.14436/2447-911x.13.2.098-105.oar

Goodchild, J. H., and Donaldson, M. (2009). An evidence-based dentistry challenge: treating patients on WF (Coumadin). Dent. Implantol. Update. 20, 1–8.

Guyatt, G. H., Oxman, A. D., Kunz, R., Woodcock, J., Brozek, J., Helfand, M., et al. (2011a). GRADE Working Group. GRADE guidelines: 7. Rating the quality of evidence—inconsistency. J. Clin. Epidemiol. 64 (12), 1294–1302. doi: 10.1016/j.jclinepi.2011.03.017

Guyatt, G. H., Oxman, A. D., Montori, V., Vist, G., Kunz, R., Brozek, J., et al. (2011b). GRADE guidelines: 5. Rating the quality of evidence—publication bias. J. Clin. Epidemiol. 64 (12), 1277–1282. doi: 10.1016/j.jclinepi.2011.01.011

Guyatt, G. H., Thorlund, K., Oxman, A. D., Walter, S. D., Patrick, D., Furukawa, T. A., et al. (2013a). GRADE guidelines: 13. Preparing summary of findings tables and evidence profiles—continuous outcomes. J. Clin. Epidemiol. 66 (2), 173–183. doi: 10.1016/j.jclinepi.2012.08.001

Guyatt, G., Eikelboom, J. W., Akl, E. A., Crowther, M., Gutterman, D., Kahn, S. R., et al. (2013b). A guide to GRADE guidelines for the readers of JTH. J. Thromb. Haemost. 1 (8), 1603–1608. doi: 10.1111/jth.12320

Harter, K., Levine, M., and Henderson, S. O. (2015). Anticoagulation drug therapy: a review. West J. Emerg. Med. 16 (1), 11–17. doi: 10.5811/westjem.2014.12.22933

Higgins, J. P. T., and Green, S. (2011). Cochrane handbook for systematic reviews of interventions version 5.1.0. The Cochrane Collaboration.

Higgins, J. P., and Thompson, S. G. (2002). Quantifying heterogeneity in a meta-analysis. Stat. Med. 21, 1539–1558. doi: 10.1002/sim.1186

Holbrook, A., Schulman, S., Witt, D.M., Vandvik, P.O., Fish, J., Kovacs, M.J., (2012). Evidence-based management of anticoagulant therapy: Antithrombotic Therapy and Prevention of Thrombosis, 9th ed: American College of Chest Physicians Evidence-Based Clinical Practice Guidelines. Chest. 141 (2 Suppl), e152S–e184S. doi: 10.1378/chest.11-2295

Kämmerer, P. W., Frerich, B., Liese, J., Scheignitz, E., and Al-Nawas, B. (2015). Oral surgery during therapy with anticoagulants: a systematic review. Clin. Oral Investig. 19 (2), 171–180. doi: 10.1007/s00784-014-1366-3

Leiria, T. L., Pellanda, L. C., Magalhães, E., and Lima, G. G. (2007). Comparative study of a portable system for prothrombin monitoring using capillary blood against venous blood measurements in patients using oral anticoagulants: correlation and concordance. *Arq. Bras. Cardiol.* 89 (1), 1–5. doi: 10.1590/S0066-782X2007001300001

Lijfering, W. M., and Tichelaar, Y. I. G. V. (2018). Direct oral anticoagulant use and risk ofperioperative bleeding: Evidence of absence or absence of evidence? *Res. Pract. Thromb. Haemost.* 2 (2), 182–185. doi: 10.1002/rth2.12084.

Madrid, C., and Sanz, M. (2009). What influence do anticoagulants have on oral implant therapy? A systematic review. *Clin. Oral Impl. Res.* 20 (4), 96–106. doi: 10.1111/j.1600-0501.2009.01770.x

Moher, D., Liberati, A., Tetzlaff, J., Altman, D. G., and Group, PRISMA (2009). Preferred reporting items for systematic reviews and meta-analyses: the PRISMA statement. *PLoS Med.* 6 (7), e1000097. doi: 10.1371/journal.pmed.1000097

Morimoto, Y., Niwa, H., and Minematsu, K. (2008). Hemostatic management of tooth extractions in patients on oral antithrombotic therapy. *J. Oral Maxillofac. Surg.* 66, 51–57. doi: 10.1016/j.joms.2007.06.655

Motta, R. H. L., Bergamaschi, C. C., de Andrade, N. K., Guimaraes, C. C., Ramacciato, J. C., and Araújo, J. O. (2017). Bleeding risk in patients using oral anticoagulants submitted to surgical procedures in dentistry: a systematic review protocol. *BMJ Open.* 7 (12), e019161. doi: 10.1136/bmjopen-2017-019161

Nematullah, A., Alabousi, A., Blanas, N., Douketis, J. D., and Sutherland, S. E. (2009). Dental surgery for patients on anticoagulant therapy with warfarin: a systematic review and meta-analysis. *J. Can. Dent. Assoc.* 75 (1), 41.

Shi, Q., Xu, J., Zhang, T., Zhang, B., and Liu, H. (2017). Post-operative bleeding risk in dental surgery for patients on oral anticoagulant therapy: a meta-analysis of observational studies. *Front. Pharmacol.* 8, 58. doi: 10.3389/fphar.2017.00058

Thachil, J., and Gagg, J. (2015). Problem-Based Review: Non Vitamin K Antagonist Oral Anticoagulants for the Acute Physician. *Acute Med.* 14 (2), 83–89.

Yang, S., Shi, Q., Liu, J., Li, J., and Xu, J. (2016). Should oral anticoagulant therapy be continued during dental extraction? A meta-analysis. *BMC Oral Health* 16 (1), 81. doi: 10.1186/s12903-016-0278-9

Yeh, C. H., Hogg, K., and Weitz, J. I. (2015). Overview of the new oral anticoagulants: opportunities and challenges. *Arterioscler. Thromb. Vasc. Biol.* 35 (5), 1056–1065. doi: 10.1161/ATVBAHA.115.303397

3

Use Profile of Magnesium Sulfate in Anesthesia in Brazil

Ismar Lima Cavalcanti[1,2]*, Fernando Lopes Tavares de Lima[2], Mario Jorge Sobreira da Silva[2], Rubens Antunes da Cruz Filho[3], Estêvão Luiz Carvalho Braga[1] and Nubia Verçosa[4]

[1] Department of General and Specialized Surgery, Anesthesiology, Fluminense Federal University, Niterói, Brazil, [2] Coordination for Education, Brazilian National Cancer Institute (INCA), Rio de Janeiro, Brazil, [3] Department of Clinical Medicine, Fluminense Federal University, Niterói, Brazil, [4] Department of Surgery, Anesthesiology, Federal University of Rio de Janeiro, Rio de Janeiro, Brazil

Correspondence:
Ismar Lima Cavalcanti
ismarcavalcanti@gmail.com

Objectives: The use of magnesium sulfate in the perioperative period has several benefits, including analgesia, inhibition of the release of catecholamines and prevention of vasospasm. The aim of this survey was to provide an overview of the use of magnesium sulfate in anesthesia.

Method: This was a prospective descriptive cross-sectional study. An online questionnaire was sent to 9,869 Brazilian anesthesiologists and trainees. The questionnaire comprised closed questions mainly regarding the frequency, clinical effects, adverse events, and doses of magnesium sulfate used in anesthesia.

Results: Of the 954 doctors who responded to the survey, 337 (35.32%) reported using magnesium sulfate in anesthesia. The most commonly cited clinical effects for the use of magnesium sulfate in anesthesia were (*n*/%): postoperative analgesia (245/72.70%), reduction of anesthetic consumption (240/71.21%) and prevention and treatment of preeclampsia and seizures in eclampsia (220/65.28%). The most frequently reported adverse events were hypotension (187/55.48%), residual neuromuscular blockade (133/39.46%), hypermagnesemia (30/8.90%), and intravenous injection pain (26/7.71%). The intravenous doses of magnesium sulfate used in most general anesthesia inductions were between 30 and 40 mg.kg^{-1}.

Conclusions: Magnesium sulfate is an important adjuvant drug in the practice of anesthesia, with several clinical effects and a low incidence of adverse events when used at recommended doses.

Keywords: anesthetics (MeSH), analgesics, magnesium sulfate, survey, adverse events

INTRODUCTION

Magnesium is the fourth most common ion in the body, and it participates in several cellular processes, including protein synthesis, neuromuscular function and stability of nucleic acid, as well as regulating other electrolytes such as calcium and sodium. Magnesium acts as a cofactor in protein synthesis, neuromuscular function and stability and the function of nucleic acids. It is a component of adenosine 5-triphosphatases and an endogenous regulator of other electrolytes. It is a calcium antagonist because it is a non-competitive inhibitor of calcium channels with inositol triphosphate. Magnesium modulates sodium and potassium currents and, as a consequence, interferes with the transmembrane potential. It is a central nervous system depressant, antagonizing N-methyl-D-aspartate (NMDA) and inhibiting the release of catecholamines (Herroeder et al., 2011).

Some studies have shown that the use of magnesium sulfate as an adjunct in anesthesia reduces intraoperative consumption of anesthetics (Koinig et al., 1998; Seyhan et al., 2006; Ryu et al., 2008; Forget and Cata, 2017). It also provides better analgesia and reduces the amount of morphine used in the postoperative period (Mentes et al., 2008; Dabbagh et al., 2009; Hwang et al., 2010). Studies in clinical practice have demonstrated the inhibitory effects of magnesium on the release of catecholamines (Herroeder et al., 2011) through better hemodynamic control during laryngoscopy (Puri et al., 1998; Shin et al., 2011) and pneumoperitoneum insufflation for videolaparoscopy (Mentes et al., 2008). Magnesium sulfate also reduces levels of noradrenaline and vasopressin during anesthesia (Jee et al., 2009).

Other benefits of using intraoperative magnesium have been reported, including hemodynamic control in surgeries for resection of pheochromocytoma (James and Cronjé, 2004), reduced incidence of atrial fibrillation in myocardial revascularization surgeries (Toraman et al., 2001), and prevention of vasospasm (Wong et al., 2006) and neurological protection after subarachnoid hemorrhage (Schmid-Elsaesser et al., 2006). The attenuation of the release of catecholamines by the adrenal glands and antagonism to calcium in smooth muscle cells of arterioles are possible mechanisms of action (Herroeder et al., 2011).

The clinical duration of nondepolarizing neuromuscular blockers is prolonged with the use of magnesium sulfate in anesthesia (Fuchs-Buder et al., 1995; Kussman et al., 1997; Czarnetzki et al., 2010; Rotava et al., 2013). Magnesium interferes with neuromuscular function by reducing the conductance of calcium in presynaptic membranes, decreasing the amount of acetylcholine released by motor neurons (Herroeder et al., 2011). It may also reduce post-synaptic sensitivity to acetylcholine or have a direct effect on the membrane potential of muscle cells (Del Castillo and Engbaek, 1954).

This survey was conducted to contribute evidence on the use of magnesium sulfate as adjunct of anesthesia due to its potential clinical benefits.

The primary objective of this study was to know the use profile of Magnesium Sulfate in Anesthesia in Brazil.

MATERIALS AND METHODS

The descriptive study was approved by the Research Ethics Committee of the Fluminense Federal University, Niterói, RJ, Brazil (CAAE 35038614.0.0000.5243, opinion 884.839, dated 11/13/2014). The informed consent form was signed electronically.

All the anesthesiologists and trainees members of Brazilian Society of Anesthesiology in 2015 were invited to participate. A self-administered electronic questionnaire was sent via e-mail to 9,869 potential participants of the research using the Survey Monkey software. The invitation was sent by 3 times with the 10-day interval between them.

We did not find in the literature a data collection instrument on the subject of this research. The lead researcher created the

electronic questionnaire used in this research, composed of 10 closed questions that addressed the following aspects: duration of practice of anesthesiology, use of magnesium sulfate and other anesthesia adjuvants, indications, complications and doses of magnesium sulfate in anesthesia (**Figure 1**).

The instrument was pre-tested in two stages. In the first stage, the relevance of the instrument was evaluated and was carried out by the researchers themselves. In the second stage, the questionnaire was evaluated by 8 anesthesiologists and the results were used to create the final version of the questionnaire used in the research.

Data were analyzed using descriptive statistics. The original data can be accessed in the **Supplementary Table 1**.

RESULTS

Survey responses were received from 945 (9.57%) participants. The length of time of anesthesia practice among the respondents is shown in **Table 1**.

Of the 945 anesthesiologists who responded to this survey, 331 (35.02%) reported using magnesium sulfate in anesthesia. The frequency of use of adjuvant drugs in anesthesia is described in **Table 2**.

The number and percentage of clinical effects (n/%) for the use of magnesium sulfate in anesthesia were (in descending order, more than one response per participant allowed): postoperative analgesia (242/73,11%), reduction of anesthetic consumption (237/71.60%), prevention and treatment of preeclampsia and seizures in eclampsia (218/65.86%), prevention and treatment of arrhythmias (175/52.87%), reduction of the dose of neuromuscular blockers (168/50.75%), prevention of postoperative chronic pain (167/50.45%), bronchodilation (165/49.84%), prevention of hyperalgesia post remifentanil use (160/48.34%), hypomagnesemia prevention in large surgeries (128/38.67%), induced systemic arterial hypotension (112/33.83%), brain protection (95/28.70%), sedation (86/25.98%), reduction of surgical bleeding or reduction of perioperative blood replacement (74/22.35%), management of pheochromocytoma (72/21.75%), prevention and treatment of agitation in emergence from general anesthesia (64/19.33%), inhibition of preterm birth (59/17.82%), prevention of myocardial ischemia (54/16.31%), prevention and treatment of shivering (50/15.10%), facilitation of tracheal intubation without the use of neuromuscular blocker agent (44/13.29%), reduction of nausea and vomiting (39/11.78%), prevention and treatment of laryngospasm (38/11.48%), control of fasciculation and myalgia after succinylcholine (31/9.36%), prevention of myoclonus after intravenous injection of etomidate (24/7.25%), treatment of tetanus (20/6.04%), adjuvant in spinal anesthesia (19/5.74%), decrease in platelet aggregation (14/4.23%), attenuation of the sympathetic response to tracheal intubation (1/0.30%) and extension of duration of motor block on subdural anesthesia (1/0,30%).

All anesthesiologists reported using the intravenous route (331/100.00%) to administer magnesium sulfate. Other routes were used less frequently: muscular (16/4.83%), nerve plexus

Questionnaire - Use of Magnesium Sulphate in Anesthesia in Brazil

1. Duration as anesthesiologist:

( ) 1 to 5 years   ( ) 6 to 10 years   ( ) 11 to 15 years   ( ) 6 to 20 years   ( ) more than 20 years

2. Do you use magnesium sulfate in anesthesia?
( ) yes   ( ) not

3. Except for magnesium sulfate, which of the adjuvants do you use in anesthesia? (More than one answer is possible)
( ) clonidine   ( ) dexmedetomidine   ( ) ketamine   ( ) lidocaine   ( ) other   ( ) I do not use anesthesia adjuvants

If you use magnesium sulfate, please answer the following questions:

4. What is the clinical effect (s) for the use of magnesium sulphate during anesthesia? (More than one answer is possible)
( ) prevention of myocardial ischemia
( ) brain protection
( ) reduction of the dose of neuromuscular blocker
( ) attenuation of sympathetic response to tracheal intubation
( ) postoperative analgesia
( ) decreased anesthetic consumption
( ) inhibition of preterm birth
( ) prevention and treatment of preeclampsia and seizures in eclampsia;
( ) bronchodilation
( ) adjuvant in spinal anesthesia
( ) prevention / treatment of cardiac arrhythmias
( ) handling of pheochromocytoma
( ) prevention of hypomagnesemia in large surgeries
( ) decreased platelet aggregation
( ) prevention / treatment of laryngospasm
( ) prevention of myoclonus after venous injection of etomidate
( ) prevention of chronic postoperative pain
( ) facilitation of tracheal intubation without the use of neuromuscular blocker
( ) control of fasciculation and myalgia after succinylcholine
( ) prevention of hyperalgesia after use of remifentanil
( ) prevention / treatment of shivering
( ) reduction of surgical bleeding
( ) reduction of perioperative blood replacement
( ) tetanus treatment
( ) reduction of nausea and vomiting
( ) induced hypotension
( ) sedation
( ) prevention / agitation treatment on awakening from anesthesia
( ) prevention / treatment of chronic pain
( ) other

5. Which route (s) do you use to administer magnesium sulfate? (More than one answer is possible)
( ) intravenous   ( ) intramuscle   ( ) spinal   ( ) nerve plexus   ( ) intravenous regional   ( ) surgical wound infiltration

6. Which of the adverse events of using magnesium sulfate in anesthesia have you witnessed? (More than one answer is possible)
( ) residual neuromuscular blockade   ( ) intravenous injection pain   ( ) respiratory depression   ( ) systemic arterial hypotension
( ) hypermagnesemia   ( ) other

7. In the case of observed adverse events, how do you classify them in terms of severity? (More than one answer is possible)
( ) mild   ( ) moderate   ( ) severe   ( ) death

8. What is the intravenous dose you often use in inducing general anesthesia? (only one answer)
( ) <30 mg.kg^{-1} ( ) 30 to 40 mg.kg^{-1} ( ) 40 to 50 mg.kg^{-1} ( ) 50 to 60 mg.kg^{-1} ( ) > 60mg.kg^{-1} ( ) I do not use inducing doses

9. What venous dose do you often use to maintain general anesthesia? (only one answer)
( ) <30 mg.kg^{-1} ( ) 30 to 40 mg.kg^{-1} ( ) 40 to 50 mg.kg^{-1} ( ) 50 to 60 mg.kg^{-1} ( ) > 60mg.kg^{-1} ( ) I do not use maintenance doses

10. Doses used for sedation?
( ) <30 mg.kg^{-1} ( ) 30 to 40 mg.kg^{-1} ( ) 40 to 50 mg.kg^{-1} ( ) 50 to 60 mg.kg^{-1} ( ) > 60mg.kg^{-1}
( ) I do not use magnesium sulfate for sedation

FIGURE 1 | Electronic questionnaire used in research "Use of Magnesium Sulfate in Anesthesia in Brazil." Brazil, 2015.

TABLE 1 | Distribution of anesthesiologists that answered the questionnaire (n = 945) by the duration of anesthesia practice (n, %).

Time of practice of anesthesia	n	%
Trainee	135	14.29
1–5 years	240	25.40
6–10 years	116	12.27
11–15 years	83	8.78
16–20 years	82	8.67
21 years or more	289	30.59

Brazil, 2015.

TABLE 2 | Frequency of use of adjuvant drugs in anesthesia (n, %).

Adjuvant drug	n	%
Clonidine	805	85.19
Ketamine	689	72.91
Lidocaine	614	64.97
Dexmedetomidine	417	44.12
Magnesium sulfate	331	35.02
No use of adjuvant	39	4.13

More than one response per participant was possible (n = 945). Brazil, 2015.

TABLE 3 | Frequency of adverse events during use of magnesium sulfate witnessed at least once by the anesthesiologist.

Adverse events	n	%
Systemic arterial hypotension	184	55.59
Residual neuromuscular blockade	131	39.57
Hypermagnesemia	28	8.45
Intravenous injection pain	22	6.64
Respiratory depression	22	6.64
Heat sensation	4	1.20
Bradycardia	4	1.20
Facial/cervical flushing	2	0.60
Tachycardia	2	0.60
Intense sedation	2	0.60
Cardiac arrhythmia	1	0.30
Prolonged emergence from anesthesia	1	0.30
Myocardial depression	1	0.3
None	40	12.08

More than one response per participant was possible (n = 331). Brazil, 2015.

TABLE 4 | Rate of intensity level of adverse events witnessed by anesthesiologists using magnesium sulfate anesthesia (n = 305).

	N	%
Mild	225	73.78
Moderate	71	23.27
Severe	9	2.95

Brazil, 2015.

TABLE 5 | Magnesium sulfate intravenous doses most commonly used in the induction of general anesthesia and sedation (n = 331).

	Doses	n	%
Induction of general anesthesia	$<30\,mg.kg^{-1}$	55	16.61
	$30–40\,mg.kg^{-1}$	114	34.45
	$40–50\,mg.kg^{-1}$	47	14.20
	$50–60\,mg.kg^{-1}$	9	2.71
	No use for induction of general anesthesia	106	32.03
Sedation	$<30\,mg.kg^{-1}$	58	17.52
	$30–40\,mg.kg^{-1}$	28	8.46
	$40–50\,mg.kg^{-1}$	10	3.02
	$50–60\,mg.kg^{-1}$	1	0.30
	No use for sedation	234	70.70

Brazil, 2015.

some adverse events were reported as severe, i.e., respiratory depression (4), hypotension (4), residual curarisation (4), hypermagnesemia (2) and bradycardia (1).

Table 5 shows the dosages of intravenous magnesium sulfate commonly used for induction of general anesthesia and sedation.

DISCUSSION

Little or no scientific literature exists that reports on surveys on the use of magnesium sulfate in anesthesia.

Approximately 10% of those who received the invitation to participate completed the survey, specifically, 945 anesthesiologists. Several medical polls have reported similar response rates (Naguib et al., 2010; Locks et al., 2015). Low adherence of participants can be explained by the electronic method used for data collection.

Duration of Anesthesia Practice of the Survey Participants

In the present survey, anesthesiologists with more than 20 years of anesthesia practice (30.59%) reported using magnesium sulfate in anesthesia and sedation most frequently; this group was followed by those with between 1 and 5 years of clinical practice (25.40%). The frequent use of magnesium sulfate among the more experienced anesthesiologists may stem from common use in certain specialties, particularly obstetrics. The high frequency of use of magnesium sulfate among the younger group of anesthesiologists may be result of the recent attention being paid

(6/1.81%), spinal (3/0.90%), regional intravenous anesthesia (3/0.90%), wound infiltration (2/0.60%), inhalation (2/0.60%), and oral (1/0.30%).

Table 3 shows the frequency of adverse events during use of magnesium sulfate witnessed at least once by the anesthesiologist. The most commonly reported were hypotension, residual neuromuscular blockade, hypermagnesemia, intravenous injection pain, and respiratory depression.

Of the adverse events reported, 73.78% of the cases were considered of mild gravity (see **Table 4**). It should be noted that to this drug, as well as the introduction of multimodal analgesic and anesthesia techniques (Czarnetzki et al., 2010; Herroeder et al., 2011; Shin et al., 2011; Rotava et al., 2013).

Adjuvant Drugs in Anesthesia

Anesthesia adjuvants are agents that are administered in association with anesthetics to increase effectiveness, improve delivery, or decrease required dosage. The survey showed that the drug most commonly used in Brazil as an anesthesia adjuvant is clonidine (85.18%); magnesium sulfate (35.02%) ranks fifth among the medicines included as possible survey responses.

Giovannitti et al. (2015) postulated that agonists of the α-2 adrenergic receptors, including clonidine and dexmedetomidine, are important tools in the arsenal of modern anesthesia because of their ability to induce calm without causing respiratory depression. They also promote cardiovascular stability and reduce anesthetic requirements.

The drug reported as the second most frequently used adjuvant was ketamine. Bakan et al. (2014) conducted a randomized clinical trial and showed that ketamine, when associated with remifentanil in total intravenous anesthesia in children, is well suited to rigid bronchoscopic procedures.

Although this survey found that lidocaine ranked third on the list of most used drugs, Kranke et al. (2015), in a systematic review, reported that there is only little or moderate evidence that a continuous infusion of lidocaine has an impact on pain intensity, especially in the early postoperative period, or on postoperative nausea. There is limited evidence that it has consequences in other clinical outcomes, such as gastrointestinal recovery, length of hospital stay and opioid use (Kranke et al., 2015).

Gupta et al. (2006) demonstrated that magnesium sulfate has anesthetic, analgesic and muscle relaxing effects and significantly reduces the need for anesthetic drugs and neuromuscular blockers.

Clinical Effects of Magnesium Sulfate in Anesthesia

As noted in this survey, there is a wide range of clinical effects for the use of magnesium sulfate in anesthesia. The great variety of clinical effects could be explained by the substantial involvement of magnesium in the physiology of various organs and systems.

Magnesium participates in over 325 cellular enzyme systems and is the second most abundant intracellular cation after potassium. Magnesium participates in numerous physiological and homeostatic functions, such as binding of hormone receptors, the transmembrane flow of ions, regulation of adenylate cyclase, calcium release, muscle contraction, cardiac excitability, neuronal activity, control of vasomotor tone and release of neurotransmitters, blood pressure and peripheral blood flow. Mg^{2+} modulates and controls the input of cell Ca^{2+} and Ca^{2+} release from the sarcoplasmic reticulum (Altura, 1994).

Magnesium is essential in the transfer, storage and utilization of energy in cells. The intracellular level of free Mg^{2+} ($[Mg^{2+}]i$) regulates intermediate metabolism, synthesis and structure of DNA and RNA, cell growth, reproduction and membrane structure (Altura and Altura, 1996).

Dubé and Granry (2003) cited the therapeutic use of magnesium in the following anesthesia, intensive care and emergency situations: prevention and treatment of hypomagnesemia, induction of anesthesia, control of pheochromocytoma, cardiac arrhythmias, preeclampsia and eclampsia, perioperative analgesia, asthma, myocardial infarction, hypertensive crisis, and insulin resistance.

Roscoe and Ahmed conducted a postal survey of cardiac anesthetists in the United Kingdom, to determine the extent of magnesium sulfate ($MgSO_4$) use and the main indications for its administration. The most common indications for administration were arrhythmia prophylaxis and treatment, myocardial protection and treatment of hypomagnesemia (Roscoe and Ahmed, 2003).

All the clinical effects for the use of magnesium sulfate in anesthesia presented by the anesthesiologists participating in this survey have been reported in other publications, including various systematic reviews and meta-analyses, although some of them are still subjects of controversy Beşogul et al., 2009; Gozdemir et al., 2010; Rhee et al., 2012; Abdulatif et al., 2013; Rotava et al., 2013; Agrawal et al., 2014; Ahsan et al., 2014; Crowther et al., 2014; Kahraman and Eroglu, 2014; Kew et al., 2014; Marzban et al., 2014; Rodrigo et al., 2014; Srebro et al., 2014; Uludag et al., 2014; Berhan and Berhan, 2015; Kim et al., 2015; Safavi et al., 2015; Vigil-De Gracia and Ludmir, 2015; Demiroglu et al., 2016; Green, 2016; Griffiths and Kew, 2016; Jangra et al., 2016; Juibari et al., 2016; Maged et al., 2016; Naghipour et al., 2016; Rodríguez-Rubio et al., 2016, 2017; Soltani et al., 2016; Thomas and Behr, 2016; Ulm et al., 2016; Vendrell et al., 2016; Xie et al., 2016, 2017; Brookfield et al., 2017; Haryalchi et al., 2017; Kutlesic et al., 2017; Lecuyer et al., 2017; McKeown et al., 2017; Mendonca et al., 2017; Salaminia et al., 2018; Zhang et al., 2018.

Adverse Events of Magnesium Sulfate Use and Classification of Intensity

Herroeder et al. (2011) reported that the vasodilator effect of magnesium is the likely cause of burning or heat sensations in the body. Prolonged PR and QT intervals as well as atrioventricular blockage may occur. Toxicity occurs with the administration of venous doses greater than 30 g or with plasma concentrations above 14.4 mg/dl (Herroeder et al., 2011). Hypermagnesemia is manifested by abolition of tendon reflex; treatment consists of calcium gluconate, furosemide furosemide and hemodialysis (Herroeder et al., 2011).

In this survey, 2.95% of respondents reported severe complications from the use of magnesium sulfate. It is worth mentioning that the occurrence of severe adverse events is of fundamental importance, demonstrating that the administration of magnesium sulfate is not risk free. As in the present research, Herroeder et al. (2011) related as severe adverse events from the use of magnesium sulfate: arterial hypotension, bradycardia, muscle weakness, and respiratory depression. The results of our survey demonstrated similar results. Despite the occurrence of reports of serious AEs, the use of magnesium sulfate can be safe in recommended doses with close monitoring of patients (Kutlesic et al., 2017).

Marret and Ancel (2016) used magnesium sulfate in obstetric patients at an initial venous dose of 4 g followed by 1 g/h, without exceeding the cumulative total dose of 50 g. In their analysis of short and medium-term outcomes, they found no serious maternal adverse effects nor adverse effects on the newborns.

Griffiths and Kew (2016) observed few adverse effects when intravenous magnesium sulfate was used for treatment of asthma in children in the emergency department.

Wilson et al. (2014) realized a retrospective cohort study to evaluated the tolerability and safety of high doses of intravenous magnesium sulfate for tocolysis in preterm labor. The frequency of severe adverse events was 5.3% while in our survey it was 2.95%. This difference can be explained because all patients in the study received high doses of magnesium sulfate. They concluded that side effects occurred in 9 out of 10 patients and were considered severe for 1 out of every 20 pregnant women.

Intravenous Dose of Magnesium Sulfate Most Frequently Used in Induction of General Anesthesia and Sedation

Germano Filho et al. (2015), in a randomized controlled study, demonstrated a significant increase in magnesium plasma concentrations after infusions of 40 mg.kg^{-1} solution containing magnesium sulfate among ASA 1 or 2 patients. This confirmed that this dose is capable of increasing magnesium serum levels.

The magnesium sulfate doses reported in this survey are in accordance with those found in other publications. There are reports of magnesium sulfate induction doses in general anesthesia from 15 mg.kg^{-1} to 75 mg.kg^{-1} (Beşogul et al., 2009; Gozdemir et al., 2010; Rotava et al., 2013; Kahraman and Eroglu, 2014; Rodrigo et al., 2014; Honarmand et al., 2015; Rower et al., 2017) and doses up to 50 mg.kg^{-1} in sedation (Lecuyer et al., 2017).

We observed that the Brazilian anesthesiologist uses magnesium sulfate rationally. Clinical effects, doses and routes of administration are found in the literature.

This survey describes the wide range of purposes magnesium sulfate is used for in anesthesia in Brazil. Although anesthesiologists have free access to the use of magnesium sulfate, research data have shown that the drug has been used primarily in those indications approved by the Health Authorities and/or supported by critical evaluation of systematic reviews and meta-analyzes. The frequency of its use is related to the amount and strength of evidence of its effects reported in the literature.

This survey has some limitations. Only Brazilian anesthesiologists participated in the study. Further, the participation of the anesthesiologists was voluntary; those who agreed to participate are likely those most interested in the use of magnesium sulfate in anesthesia. This may have created bias that could interfere with the generalization of the responses to the full population of anesthesia specialists. Only 10% effectively responded to the survey, that the results may thus be biased. The questionnaire was not validated.

We conclude that magnesium sulfate is among the five most commonly used adjuvants in anesthesia, along with clonidine, ketamine, lidocaine and dexmedetomidine. Several clinical effects for magnesium sulfate were reported, especially postoperative analgesia, reduction of anesthetic consumption and the prevention and treatment of preeclampsia and eclampsia seizures. Hypotension, residual neuromuscular blockade, hypermagnesemia and pain on intravenous injection were the most frequent adverse events and, in general, were considered mild. Magnesium sulfate intravenous doses used in most general anesthesia induction were between 30 and 40 mg.kg^{-1}.

AUTHOR CONTRIBUTIONS

IC, FL, and MS designed the study and performed the experiments, IC, RCF, EB, and NV analyzed the data and wrote the manuscript.

FUNDING

The study was supported by the Fluminense Federal University, Niterói, Brazil and Brazilian Society of Anesthesiology, Rio de Janeiro, Brazil. There was no funding source for this study.

REFERENCES

Abdulatif, M., Ahmed, A., Mukhtar, A., and Badawy, S. (2013). The effect of magnesium sulphate infusion on the incidence and severity of emergence agitation in children undergoing adenotonsillectomy using sevoflurane anaesthesia. Anaesthesia 68, 1045–1052. doi: 10.1111/anae.12380

Agrawal, A., Agrawal, S., and Payal, Y. S. (2014). Effect of continuous magnesium sulfate infusion on spinal block characteristics: a prospective study. Saudi J. Anaesth. 8, 78–82. doi: 10.4103/1658-354X.125945

Ahsan, B., Rahimi, E., Moradi, A., and Rashadmanesh, N. (2014). The effects of magnesium sulphate on succinylcholine-induced fasciculation during induction of general anaesthesia. J. Pak. Med. Assoc. 64, 1151–1153.

Altura, B. M. (1994). Introduction: importance of Mg in physiology and medicine and the need for ion selective electrodes. Scand. J. Clin. Lab. Invest. Suppl. 217, 5–9. doi: 10.1080/00365519409095206

Altura, B. M., and Altura, B. T. (1996). Role of magnesium in patho-physiological processes and the clinical utility of magnesium ion selective electrodes. Scand. J. Clin. Lab. Invest. Suppl. 224, 211–234. doi: 10.3109/00365519609088642

Bakan, M., Topuz, U., Umutoglu, T., Gundogdu, G., Ilce, Z., Elicevik, M., et al. (2014). Remifentanil-based total intravenous anesthesia for pediatric rigid bronchoscopy: comparison of adjuvant propofol and ketamine. Clinics 69, 372–377. doi: 10.6061/clinics/2014(06)01

Berhan, Y., and Berhan, A. (2015). Should magnesium sulfate be administered to women with mild pre-eclampsia? A systematic review of published reports on eclampsia. J. Obstet. Gynecol. Res. 41, 831–842. doi: 10.1111/jog.12697

Beşogul, Y., Gemalmaz, H., and Aslan, R. (2009). Effects of preoperative magnesium therapy on arrhythmias and myocardial ischemia during off-pump coronary surgery. Ann. Thorac. Med. 4, 137–139. doi: 10.4103/1817-1737.53355

Brookfield, K. F., Elkomy, M., Su, F., Drover, D. R., and Carvalho, B. (2017). Optimization of maternal magnesium sulfate administration for fetal neuroprotection: application of a prospectively constructed pharmacokinetic model to the BEAM cohort. *J. Clin. Pharmacol.* 57, 1419–1424. doi: 10.1002/jcph.941

Crowther, C. A., Brown, J., McKinlay, C. J., and Middleton, P. (2014). Magnesium sulphate for preventing preterm birth in threatened preterm labour. *Cochr. Datab. Syst. Rev.* 15:CD001060. doi: 10.1002/14651858.CD001060.pub2

Czarnetzki, C., Lysakowski, C., Elia, N., and Tramèr, M. R. (2010). Time course of rocuronium-induced neuromuscular block after pre-treatment with magnesium sulphate: a randomised study. *Acta Anaesthesiol. Scand.* 54, 299–306. doi: 10.1111/j.1399-6576.2009.02160.x

Dabbagh, A., Elyasi, H., Razavi, S. S., Fathi, M., and Rajaei, S. (2009). Intravenous magnesium sulfate for post-operative pain in patients undergoing lower limb orthopedic surgery. *Acta Anaesthesiol. Scand.* 53, 1088–1091. doi: 10.1111/j.1399-6576.2009.02025.x

Del Castillo, J., and Engbaek, L. (1954). The nature of the neuromuscular block produced by magnesium. *J. Physiol.* 124, 370–384. doi: 10.1113/jphysiol.1954.sp005114

Demiroglu, M., Ün, C., Ornek, D. H., Kici, O., Yildirim, A. E., Horasanli, E., et al. (2016). The effect of systemic and regional use of magnesium sulfate on postoperative tramadol consumption in lumbar disc surgery. *Biomed Res. Int.* 2016:3216246. doi: 10.1155/2016/3216246

Dubé, L., and Granry, J. C. (2003). The therapeutic use of magnesium in anesthesiology, intensive care and emergency medicine: a review. *Can. J. Anaesth.* 50, 732–746. doi: 10.1007/BF03018719

Forget, P., and Cata, J. (2017). Stable anesthesia with alternative to opioids: Are ketamine and magnesium helpful in stabilizing hemodynamics during surgery? A systematic review and meta-analyses of randomized controlled trials. *Res Clin Anaesthesiol.* 31, 523–531. doi: 10.1016/j.bpa.2017.07.001

Fuchs-Buder, T., Wilder-Smith, O. H., Borgeat, A., and Tassonyi, E. (1995). Interaction of magnesium sulphate with vecuronium-induced neuromuscular block. *Br. J. Anaesth.* 74, 405–409. doi: 10.1093/bja/74.4.405

Germano Filho, P. A., Cavalcanti, I. L., Barrucand, L., and Verçosa, N. (2015). Effect of magnesium sulphate on sugammadex reversal time for neuromuscular blockade: a randomised controlled study. *Anaesthesia* 70, 956–961. doi: 10.1111/anae.12987

Giovannitti, J. A., Thoms, S. M., and Crawford, J. J. (2015). Alpha-2 adrenergic receptor agonists: a review of current clinical applications. *Anesth. Prog.* 62, 31–38. doi: 10.2344/0003-3006-62.1.31

Gozdemir, M., Usta, B., Demircioglu, R. I., Muslu, B., Sert, H., and Karatas, O. F. (2010). Magnesium sulfate infusion prevents shivering during transurethral prostatectomy with spinal anesthesia: a randomized, double-blinded, controlled study. *J. Clin. Anesth.* 22, 184–189. doi: 10.1016/j.jclinane.2009.06.006

Green, R. H. (2016). Asthma in adults (acute): magnesium sulfate treatment. *Clin. Evid.* 01:1513

Griffiths, B., and Kew, K. M. (2016). Intravenous magnesium sulfate for treating children with acute asthma in the emergency department. *Cochr. Datab. Syst. Rev.* 4:Cd011050. doi: 10.1002/14651858.CD011050.pub2

Gupta, K., Vohra, V., and Sood, J. (2006). The role of magnesium as an adjuvant during general anaesthesia. *Anaesthesia* 61, 1058–1063. doi: 10.1111/j.1365-2044.2006.04801.x

Haryalchi, K., Abedinzade, M., Khanaki, K., Mansour Ghanaie, M., and Mohammad Zadeh, F. (2017). Whether preventive low dose magnesium sulphate infusion has an influence on postoperative pain perception and the level of serum beta-endorphin throughout the total abdominal hysterectomy. *Rev. Esp. Anestesiol. Reanim.* 64, 384–390. doi: 10.1016/j.redar.2016.11.009

Herroeder, S., Schönherr, M. E., De Hert, S. G., and Hollmann, M. W. (2011). Magnesium—essentials for anesthesiologists. *Anesthesiology* 114, 971–993. doi: 10.1097/ALN.0b013e318210483d

Honarmand, A., Safavi, M., Badiei, S., and Daftari-Fard, N. (2015). Different doses of intravenous magnesium sulfate on cardiovascular changes following the laryngoscopy and tracheal intubation: a double-blind randomized controlled trial. *J. Res. Pharm. Pract.* 4, 79–84. doi: 10.4103/2279-042X.154365

Hwang, J. Y., Na, H. S., Jeon, Y. T., Ro, Y. J., Kim, C. S., and Do, S. H. (2010). I.V. infusion of magnesium sulphate during spinal anaesthesia improves postoperative analgesia. *Br. J. Anaesth.* 104, 89–93. doi: 10.1093/bja/aep334

James, M. F., and Cronjé, L. (2004). Pheochromocytoma crisis: the use of magnesium sulfate. *Anesth. Analg.* 99, 680–686. doi: 10.1213/01.ANE.0000133136.01381.52

Jangra, K., Malhotra, S. K., Gupta, A., and Arora, S. (2016). Comparison of quality of the surgical field after controlled hypotension using esmolol and magnesium sulfate during endoscopic sinus surgery. *J. Anaesthesiol. Clin. Pharmacol.* 32, 325–328. doi: 10.4103/0970-9185.173400

Jee, D., Lee, D., Yun, S., and Lee, C. (2009). Magnesium sulphate attenuates arterial pressure increase during laparoscopic cholecystectomy. *Br. J. Anaesth.* 103, 484–489. doi: 10.1093/bja/aep196

Juibari, H. M., Eftekharian, H. R., and Arabion, H. R. (2016). Intravenous magnesium sulfate to deliberate hypotension and bleeding after bimaxillary orthognathic surgery; a randomized double-blind controlled trial. *J. Dent.* 17, 276–282.

Kahraman, F., and Eroglu, A. (2014). The effect of intravenous magnesium sulfate infusion on sensory spinal block and postoperative pain score in abdominal hysterectomy. *Biomed Res. Int.* 2014:236024. doi: 10.1155/2014/236024

Kew, K. M., Kirtchuk, L., and Michell, C. I. (2014). Intravenous magnesium sulfate for treating adults with acute asthma in the emergency department. *Cochr. Datab. Syst. Rev.* 28:CD010909. doi: 10.1002/14651858.CD010909

Kim, J. E., Shin, C. S., Lee, Y. C., Lee, H. S., Ban, M., and Kim, S. Y. (2015). Beneficial effect of intravenous magnesium during endoscopic submucosal dissection for gastric neoplasm. *Surg. Endosc.* 29, 3795–3802. doi: 10.1007/s00464-015-4514-1

Koinig, H., Wallner, T., Marhofer, P., Andel, H., Hörauf, K., and Mayer, N. (1998). Magnesium sulfate reduces intra- and postoperative analgesic requirements. *Anesth. Analg.* 87, 206–210.

Kranke, P., Jokinen, J., Pace, N. L., Schnabel, A., Hollmann, M. W., Hahnenkamp, K., et al. (2015). Continuous intravenous perioperative lidocaine infusion for postoperative pain and recovery. *Cochr. Datab. Syst. Rev.* 16:CD009642. doi: 10.1002/14651858.CD009642.pub2

Kussman, B., Shorten, G., Uppington, J., and Comunale, M. E. (1997). Administration of magnesium sulphate before rocuronium: effects on speed of onset and duration of neuromuscular block. *Br. J. Anaesth.* 79, 122–124. doi: 10.1093/bja/79.1.122

Kutlesic, M. S., Kutlesic, R. M., and Mostic-Ilic, T. (2017). Magnesium in obstetric anesthesia and intensive care. *J. Anesth.* 31, 127–139. doi: 10.1007/s00540-016-2257-3

Lecuyer, M., Rubio, M., Chollat, C., Lecointre, M., Jégou, S., Leroux, P., et al. (2017). Experimental and clinical evidence of differential effects of magnesium sulfate on neuroprotection and angiogenesis in the fetal brain. *Pharmacol. Res. Perspect.* 5, e00315. doi: 10.1002/prp2.315

Locks, G. D. F., Cavalcanti, I. L., Duarte, N. M., Da Cunha, R. M., and De Almeida, M. C. (2015). Use of neuromuscular blockers in Brazil. *Braz. J. Anesthesiol.* 65, 319–325. doi: 10.1016/j.bjan.2015.03.001

Maged, A. M., Hashem, A. M., Gad Allah, S. H., Mahy, M. E., Mostafa, W. A., and Kotb, A. (2016). The effect of loading dose of magnesium sulfate on uterine, umbilical, and fetal middle cerebral arteries Doppler in women with severe preeclampsia: a case control study. *Hypertens. Pregnancy* 35, 91–99. doi: 10.3109/10641955.2015.1116552

Marret, S., and Ancel, P. (2016). Neuroprotection for preterm infants with antenatal magnesium sulphate. *J. Gynecol. Obstet. Biol. Reprod.* 45, 1418–1433. doi: 10.1016/j.jgyn.2016.09.028

Marzban, S., Haddadi, S., Naghipour, M. R., Sayah Varg, Z., and Naderi Nabi, B. (2014). The effect of intravenous magnesium sulfate on laryngospasm after elective adenotonsillectomy surgery in children. *Anesth. Pain Med.* 4:e15960. doi: 10.5812/aapm.15960

McKeown, A., Seppi, V., and Hodgson, R. (2017). Intravenous magnesium sulphate for analgesia after caesarean section: a systematic review. *Anesthesiol. Res. Pract.* 2017:9186374. doi: 10.1155/2017/9186374.

Mendonca, F. T., de Queiroz, L. M., Guimaraes, C. C., and Xavier, A. C. (2017). Effects of lidocaine and magnesium sulfate in attenuating hemodynamic response to tracheal intubation: single-center, prospective, double-blind, randomized study. *Rev. Bras. Anestesiol.* 67, 50–56. doi: 10.1016/j.bjane.2015.08.004

Mentes, O., Harlak, A., Yigit, T., Balkan, A., Balkan, M., Cosar, A., et al. (2008). Effect of intraoperative magnesium sulphate infusion on pain relief after laparoscopic cholecystectomy. *Acta Anaesthesiol. Scand.* 52, 1353–1359. doi: 10.1111/j.1399-6576.2008.01816.x

Naghipour, B., Faridaalaee, G., Shadvar, K., Bilehjani, E., Khabaz, A. H., and Fakhari, S. (2016). Effect of prophylaxis of magnesium sulfate for reduction of postcardiac surgery arrhythmia: randomized clinical trial. *Ann. Card. Anaesth.* 19, 662–667. doi: 10.4103/0971-9784.191577

Naguib, M., Kopman, A. F., Lien, C. A., Hunter, J. M., Lopez, A., and Brull, S. J. (2010). A survey of current management of neuromuscular block in the United States and Europe. *Anesth. Analg.* 111, 110–119. doi: 10.1213/ANE.0b013e3181c07428

Puri, G. D., Marudhachalam, K. S., Chari, P., and Suri, R. K. (1998). The effect of magnesium sulphate on hemodynamics and its efficacy in attenuating the response to endotracheal intubation in patients with coronary artery disease. *Anesth. Analg.* 87, 808–811.

Rhee, E., Beiswenger, T., Oguejiofor, C. E., and James, A. H. (2012). The effects of magnesium sulfate on maternal and fetal platelet aggregation. *J. Matern. Fetal Neonatal Med.* 25, 478–483. doi: 10.3109/14767058.2011.584087

Rodrigo, C., Fernando, D., and Rajapakse, S. (2014). Pharmacological management of tetanus: an evidence-based review. *Crit Care* 18:217. doi: 10.1186/cc13797

Rodríguez-Rubio, L., Del Pozo, J. S. G., Nava, E., and Jordan, J. (2016). Interaction between magnesium sulfate and neuromuscular blockers during the perioperative period. A systematic review and meta-analysis. *J. Clin. Anesth.* 34, 524–534. doi: 10.1016/j.jclinane.2016.06.011

Rodríguez-Rubio, L., Nava, E., Del Pozo, J. S. G., and Jordán, J. (2017). Influence of the perioperative administration of magnesium sulfate on the total dose of anesthetics during general anesthesia. A systematic review and meta-analysis. *J. Clin. Anesth.* 39, 129–138. doi: 10.1016/j.jclinane.2017.03.038

Roscoe, A., and Ahmed, A. B. (2003). A survey of peri-operative use of magnesium sulphate in adult cardiac surgery in the UK. *Anaesthesia* 58, 363–365. doi: 10.1046/j.1365-2044.2003.03082_1.x

Rotava, P., Cavalcanti, I. L., Barrucand, L., Vane, L. A., and Verçosa, N. (2013). Effects of magnesium sulphate on the pharmacodynamics of rocuronium in patients aged 60 years and older: a randomised trial. *Eur. J. Anaesthesiol.* 30, 599–604. doi: 10.1097/EJA.0b013e328361d342

Rower, J. E., Liu, X., Yu, T., Mundorff, M., Sherwin, C. M., and Johnson, M. D. (2017). Clinical pharmacokinetics of magnesium sulfate in the treatment of children with severe acute asthma. *Eur. J. Clin. Pharmacol.* 73, 325–331. doi: 10.1007/s00228-016-2165-3

Ryu, J. H., Kang, M. H., Park, K. S., and Do, S. H. (2008). Effects of magnesium sulphate on intraoperative anaesthetic requirements and postoperative analgesia in gynaecology patients receiving total intravenous anaesthesia. *Br. J. Anaesth.* 100, 397–403. doi: 10.1093/bja/aem407

Safavi, M., Honarmand, A., Sahaf, A. S., Sahaf, S. M., Attari, M., Payandeh, M., et al. (2015). Magnesium sulfate versus lidocaine pretreatment for prevention of pain on etomidate injection: a randomized, double-blinded placebo controlled trial. *J. Res. Pharm. Pract.* 4, 4–8. doi: 10.4103/2279-042X.150044

Salaminia, S., Sayehmiri, F., Angha, P., Sayehmiri, K., and Motedayen, M. (2018). Evaluating the effect of magnesium supplementation and cardiac arrhythmias after acute coronary syndrome: a systematic review and meta-analysis. *BMC Cardiovasc. Disord.* 18:129. doi: 10.1186/s12872-018-0857-6

Schmid-Elsaesser, R., Kunz, M., Zausinger, S., Prueckner, S., Briegel, J., and Steiger, H. J. (2006). Intravenous magnesium versus nimodipine in the treatment of patients with aneurysmal subarachnoid hemorrhage: a randomized study. *Neurosurgery* 58, 1054–1065. doi: 10.1227/01.NEU.0000215868.40441.D9

Seyhan, T. O., Tugrul, M., Sungur, M. O., Kayacan, S., Telci, L., Pembeci, K., et al. (2006). Effects of three different dose regimens of magnesium on

propofol requirements, haemodynamic variables and postoperative pain relief in gynaecological surgery. *Br. J. Anaesth.* 96, 247–252. doi: 10.1093/bja/aei291

Shin, Y. H., Choi, S. J., Jeong, H. Y., and Kim, M. H. (2011). Evaluation of dose effects of magnesium sulfate on rocuronium injection pain and hemodynamic changes by laryngoscopy and endotracheal intubation. *Korean J. Anesthesiol.* 60, 329–333. doi: 10.4097/kjae.2011.60.5.329

Soltani, H. A., Hashemi, S. J., Montazeri, K., Dehghani, A., and Nematbakhsh, M. (2016). The role of magnesium sulfate in tracheal intubation without muscle relaxation in patients undergoing ophthalmic surgery. *J. Res. Med. Sci.* 21:96. doi: 10.4103/1735-1995.193168

Srebro, D. P., Vuckovic, S., Vujovic, K. S., and Prostran, M. (2014). Anti-hyperalgesic effect of systemic magnesium sulfate in carrageenan-induced inflammatory pain in rats: influence of the nitric oxide pathway. *Magnes. Res.* 27, 77–85. doi: 10.1684/mrh.2014.0364

Thomas, S. H., and Behr, E. R. (2016). Pharmacological treatment of acquired QT prolongation and torsades de pointes. *Br. J. Clin. Pharmacol.* 81, 420–427. doi: 10.1111/bcp.12726

Toraman, F., Karabulut, E. H., Alhan, H. C., Dagdelen, S., and Tarcan, S. (2001). Magnesium infusion dramatically decreases the incidence of atrial fibrillation after coronary artery bypass grafting. *Ann. Thorac. Surg.* 72, 1256–1261. doi: 10.1016/S0003-4975(01)02898-3

Ulm, M. A., Watson, C. H., Vaddadi, P., Wan, J. Y., and Santoso, J. T. (2016). Hypomagnesemia is prevalent in patients undergoing gynecologic surgery by a gynecologic oncologist. *Int. J. Gynecol. Cancer* 26, 1320–1326. doi: 10.1097/IGC.0000000000000766

Uludag, E. Ü., Gözükara, I. Ö., Kucur, S. K., Ulug, P., Özdegirmenci, Ö., and Erkaya, S. (2014). Maternal magnesium level effect on preterm labor treatment. *J. Matern. Fetal Neonatal Med.* 27, 1449–1453. doi: 10.3109/14767058.2013.858688

Vendrell, M., Martín, N., Tejedor, A., Ortiz, J. T., Muxí, À., and Taurà, P. (2016). Magnesium sulphate and (123)I-MIBG in pheochromocytoma: two useful techniques for a complicated disease. *Rev. Esp. Anestesiol. Reanim.* 63, 48–53. doi: 10.1016/j.redar.2015.04.001

Vigil-De Gracia, P., and Ludmir, J. (2015). The use of magnesium sulfate for women with severe preeclampsia or eclampsia diagnosed during the postpartum period. *Matern Fetal Neonatal Med.* 28, 2207–2209. doi: 10.3109/14767058.2014.982529

Wilson, M. S., Ingersoll, M., Meschter, E., Bodea-Braescu, A. V., and Edwards, R. K. (2014). Evaluating the side effects of treatment for preterm labor in a center that uses "high-dose" magnesium sulfate. *Am. J. Perinatol.* 31, 711–716. doi: 10.1055/s-0033-1358770

Wong, G. K., Chan, M. T., Boet, R., Poon, W. S., and Gin, T. (2006). Intravenous magnesium sulfate after aneurysmal subarachnoid hemorrhage: a prospective randomized pilot study. *J. Neurosurg. Anesthesiol.* 18, 142–148. doi: 10.1097/00008506-200604000-00009

Xie, M., Li, X. K., and Chen, J. (2016). Effect of magnesium sulphate infusion on emergence agitation in patients undergoing esophageal carcinoma with general anesthesia: a randomized, double-blind, controlled trial. *Nan Fang Yi Ke Da Xue Xue Bao* 36, 1650–1654.

Xie, M., Li, X. K., and Peng, Y. (2017). Magnesium sulfate for postoperative complications in children undergoing tonsillectomies: a systematic review and meta-analysis. *J. Evid. Based Med.* 10, 16–25. doi: 10.1111/jebm.12230

Zhang, J., Wang, Y., Xu, H., and Yang, J. (2018). Influence of magnesium sulfate on hemodynamic responses during laparoscopic cholecystectomy. A meta-analysis of randomized controlled studies. *Medicine* 97:e12747. doi: 10.1097/MD.0000000000012747

4

Outcomes of an International Workshop on Preconception Expanded Carrier Screening: Some Considerations for Governments

Caron M. Molster[1]*[†], Karla Lister[1][†], Selina Metternick-Jones[2], Gareth Baynam[1,3,4,5,6,7,8], Angus John Clarke[9], Volker Straub[10], Hugh J. S. Dawkins[1,11,12,13] and Nigel Laing[14,15]

[1]Office of Population Health Genomics, Public Health Division, Department of Health Western Australia, Perth, WA, Australia, [2]Sir Charles Gairdner Hospital, Perth, WA, Australia, [3]Genetic Services WA, Perth, WA, Australia, [4]School of Paediatrics and Child Health, University of Western Australia, Perth, WA, Australia, [5]Institute for Immunology and Infectious Diseases, Murdoch University, Perth, WA, Australia, [6]Telethon Kids Institute, University of Western Australia, Perth, WA, Australia, [7]Western Australian Register of Developmental Anomalies, Perth, WA, Australia, [8]Spatial Sciences, Department of Science and Engineering, Curtin University, Perth, WA, Australia, [9]Division of Cancer and Genetics, School of Medicine, Cardiff University, Cardiff, UK, [10]Institute of Human Genetics, University of Newcastle upon Tyne, Newcastle upon Tyne, UK, [11]Centre for Comparative Genomics, Murdoch University, Perth, WA, Australia, [12]Centre for Population Health Research, Curtin University, Perth, WA, Australia, [13]School of Pathology and Laboratory Medicine, University of Western Australia, Perth, WA, Australia, [14]Centre for Medical Research, Harry Perkins Institute of Medical Research, University of Western Australia, Perth, WA, Australia, [15]Neurogenetics Unit, Department of Diagnostic Genomics, PathWest Laboratory Medicine, Department of Health Western Australia, Perth, WA, Australia

*Correspondence:
Caron M. Molster
caron.molster@health.wa.gov.au

[†]These authors have contributed equally to this work.

Background: Consideration of expanded carrier screening has become an emerging issue for governments. However, traditional criteria for decision-making regarding screening programs do not incorporate all the issues relevant to expanded carrier screening. Further, there is a lack of consistent guidance in the literature regarding the development of appropriate criteria for government assessment of expanded carrier screening. Given this, a workshop was held to identify key public policy issues related to preconception expanded carrier screening, which governments should consider when deciding whether to publicly fund such programs.

Methods: In June 2015, a satellite workshop was held at the European Society of Human Genetics Conference. It was structured around two design features: (1) the provision of information from a range of perspectives and (2) small group deliberations on the key issues that governments need to consider and the benefits, risks, and challenges of implementing publicly funded whole-population preconception carrier screening.

Results: Forty-one international experts attended the workshop. The deliberations centered primarily on the conditions to be tested and the elements of the screening program itself. Participants expected only severe conditions to be screened but were concerned about the lack of a consensus definition of "severe." Issues raised regarding the screening program included the purpose, benefits, harms, target population, program acceptability, components of a program, and economic evaluation. Participants also made arguments for consideration of the accuracy of screening tests.

Conclusion: A wide range of issues require careful consideration by governments that want to assess expanded carrier screening. Traditional criteria for government decision-making regarding screening programs are not a "best fit" for expanded carrier screening and new models of decision-making with appropriate criteria are required. There is a need to define what a "severe" condition is, to build evidence regarding the reliability and accuracy of screening tests, to consider the equitable availability and downstream effects on and costs of follow-up interventions for those identified as carriers, and to explore the ways in which the components of a screening program would be impacted by unique features of expanded carrier screening.

Keywords: carrier screening, expanded carrier screening, genetic carrier screening, government, public policy

INTRODUCTION

Population-based screening programs are a public health approach implemented by many governments, which usually focus on a specific subpopulation defined by age, sex, and sometimes by ethnicity. Examples include newborn screening, prenatal screening, and screening for breast, bowel, and cervical cancer. In most countries, programs for screening the population to identify carriers of genetic diseases have not yet been adopted by governments. However, the possibility of offering such programs has become more salient in recent years in the wake of technology drivers such as the availability of relatively low cost massively parallel sequencing. Given this, a workshop was held with experts from a number of countries to identify key public policy issues related to preconception expanded carrier screening, which governments should consider before deciding whether to publicly fund such programs.

Carrier screening is a form of genetic testing that is used to determine a couple's risk of having a child with a recessive genetic disorder, when there is no *a priori* risk based on personal or family history (1). The process involves analyzing a sample of blood, or other biological material, for evidence of genetic mutations associated with autosomal-recessive and X-linked conditions. Carriers of autosomal-recessive conditions are people who have one copy of a gene mutation that can cause a condition in their offspring. If two carriers of a mutation in the same gene have children, their offspring have a one in four chance of having the condition. For women who carry a gene mutation associated with an X-linked condition, their children have a 50% chance of inheriting that gene mutation. Male children of these women are usually affected by the condition since they inherit their only copy of the X chromosome from their mother, while female children are usually protected from the condition by the inheritance of a second X chromosome from the father.

The members of a couple may undertake carrier screening simultaneously or sequentially, and screening can be performed in the preconception period or during pregnancy. If offered in the preconception period, carrier screening provides an opportunity to identify individuals who are at risk of having a child affected with a condition, before they become pregnant. Partners can then make informed reproductive choices including: not having a child at all; adoption; preimplantation genetic diagnosis (PGD)

or *in vitro* fertilization (IVF) to avoid having an affected child; or to have a child naturally, with prior knowledge of their risk of having a child with a specific condition. Screening during the preconception period can be considered more favorable than during pregnancy, as it avoids expectant parents being faced with a prenatal diagnosis and possibly a decision on whether to selectively terminate an affected pregnancy as the only way of avoiding the birth of an affected child.

Until recently, carrier screening was generally available for one or a very small number of conditions within ethnic subgroups of the population that have a relatively high prevalence of those conditions. Examples include carrier screening offered to the Ashkenazi Jewish population for Tay–Sachs disease and to Mediterranean populations for beta-thalassemia (2–4). In more recent years, the possibility of expanded carrier screening has emerged. This involves simultaneously screening for carrier status for multiple diseases, which can be offered to all members of a pan-ethnic population, regardless of family history or ancestry (5–7). This has been made feasible through advances in genotyping and genetic sequencing technologies, which enable the concurrent evaluation of genetic mutations for large numbers of recessive diseases, for relatively low additional cost (5). Commercial companies have already developed expanded carrier screening tests that can screen for more than 100 recessive diseases at one time and these are being offered direct-to-consumers at a cost (8, 9). However, only consumers who are willing and can afford to pay for these screening tests are able to undertake them.

For carrier screening to be truly universal, it requires a publicly funded approach to ensure equity of access. To warrant public funding, there needs to be an evidence-based assessment of the appropriateness of expanded carrier screening against a range of predetermined criteria (10). This is because, like all population-based screening programs, carrier screening has the potential to result in harm as well as benefits (11). Therefore, there must be a rigorous assessment before implementing a publicly funded program, to ensure that the benefits outweigh the harms. The "gold standard" criteria for evaluating population-based screening were developed for the World Health Organization over 40 years ago by Wilson and Jungner (12, 13). These screening pioneers suggested assessing evidence against 10 principles that explore four themes: (1) the condition being screened, (2) the test, (3) the treatment, and (4) the screening program.

While the Wilson and Jungner principles are the benchmark for government decision-making in screening, the ways in which they have been applied in practice vary across the globe. This is highlighted through a recent review of the criteria for deciding whether to introduce screening programs in Australia, Canada, Denmark, Finland, France, Germany, Italy, the Netherlands, New Zealand, Sweden, the UK, and the USA (14). Across these countries, Seedat et al. (14) identified 46 unique criteria that were associated with screening in general, most of which related to the screening program (27) as opposed to the condition (7), test (6), and treatment (6). Generally, the reason for expansion beyond the original Wilson and Jungner principles and variation in government decision-making criteria is to ensure processes sufficiently explore the issues most pertinent to each local setting (15, 16).

Despite their continued application to the assessment of screening programs worldwide, the Wilson and Jungner principles do not incorporate the full range of considerations for expanded carrier screening. A key limitation is that the criteria were developed without specific examination of the unique benefits, risks and harms that accompany genetic screening (10). These unique features include that most conditions screened for will be rare and that a genetic test is required that in most cases will produce personal information for both the individual having the test, as well as their genetic relatives. Further, in relation to carrier screening, it does not screen for the presence of a condition, but rather for the presence of gene mutations that might cause a condition in offspring, and the "treatment" following on from carrier screening is thus not an intervention in line with the classic definition. This latter point means that, should an individual be identified as a carrier, there is no treatment required since carriers are generally not affected by the condition for which they are a carrier. Instead, carriers are provided with information that will inform their reproductive choices.

While it is recognized that the Wilson and Jungner principles need further consideration in the context of expanded carrier screening, the Netherlands is so far the only country to have developed criteria specifically for assessing genetic screening including carrier screening (17). For other governments looking to develop relevant criteria, there is a lack of clear, consistent guidance in the literature. At the time our workshop was held, there were two statements of recommendations from professional bodies in the USA regarding expanded carrier screening along with a report by the UK Human Genetics Commission, and recommendations have subsequently been published by the European Society of Human Genetics (ESHG) (1, 7, 18, 19). However, the content of these documents varies considerably, highlighting the current lack of consensus. There is literature that has identified lessons learned and factors for the successful implementation of existing, usually ethnicity-based, carrier screening programs (20–23). Yet, to our knowledge, there has been no systematic evaluation of the extent to which these factors can inform decision-making criteria for assessing expanded carrier screening.

Given the lack of clear, consistent policy and academic guidance on the relevant criteria to assess expanded carrier screening, we believe there is a need for more research to inform governments of the issues they need to consider before implementing expanded carrier screening. In the first instance, best practice public policy development suggests that there is a need to understand the values, expectations, preferences, and concerns of key stakeholders (10). In line with this, we held an international workshop to gain an understanding of which issues experts considered were the most salient for governments to consider. We chose to focus on screening in the preconception period since this is considered to be the best timing for carrier screening to optimize reproductive choice (1, 24).

METHOD

In June 2015, we held a satellite workshop at the ESHG Conference. To reach experts who might want to attend the workshop, a call for expressions of interest was posted on the ESHG Conference website. Invitations were also issued to known experts in fields related to expanded carrier screening, with a request to forward the invitation to other experts who might also be interested in the workshop. These communications included information on the objectives of the workshop. One of the objectives listed was "to contribute to the academic literature on expanded carrier screening," which would be by publishing the outcomes of the workshop in a peer-reviewed journal. The intention to contribute to the academic literature was reiterated in material sent to those who expressed an interest in attending the workshop, as well as at the beginning of the workshop while "setting the scene" and at the end of the workshop in relation to "next steps." By choosing to participate in the workshop, which was a public event, we assumed that participants were giving implied consent to the workshop outcomes being collated, analyzed, and published in academic literature. We considered this a sufficient level of consent, since there would be no identifying information published about the participants and the information obtained from the workshop was neither personal nor private, and could not be linked to an individual but rather were the outcomes of group discussions in a public setting.

The aim of the workshop was to identify expert opinions on the issues that governments should consider when deciding whether or not to implement preconception expanded carrier screening. To achieve this, the workshop was structured around two design features, these being information provision and small group deliberations. The morning session of the workshop involved a series of presentations from nine experts in different fields relevant to expanded carrier screening. These presentations were designed to expose workshop participants to information from outside their field of expertise and to a range of different perspectives on the key issues that government policymakers might face in relation to preconception expanded carrier screening (see **Table 1**). Providing a range of perspectives was considered important as it was recognized that these presentations would likely frame the subsequent deliberations of the small groups.

Following the presentations, participants worked in small groups of between six and eight people to discuss and develop answers to three questions, namely:

1. What are the key factors/issues that governments need to consider when deciding whether or not to implement publicly

TABLE 1 | Range of perspectives covered in workshop presentations.

Role	Focus of presentation
Clinical geneticist	Justifications for offering carrier screening, criteria for assessing public health screening, tensions in the goals of carrier screening, different social and cultural contexts in which screening can be offered, and queries regarding the conditions to screen
Screening policymaker	Criteria that guide government decision-making for population-based screening programs, including the Wilson and Jungner principles, and how these could be applied to preconception expanded carrier screening. Issues such as benefits and harms, public support, understanding the condition, testing, feasibility, and cost
Carrier screening program manager	Population and genetic conditions in Israel, national carrier screening programs, carrier rates in the population
Health economist	How health economics is used in decision-making processes, health technology assessment including cost–benefit analysis and cost-effectiveness, types of healthcare costs, and the kinds of health economic questions that arise in the context of developing screening programs
Health consumer advocate	What conditions to screen, benefits, challenges related to infrastructure, awareness, education, and engaging people
Ethicist	Commercial offers of expanded carrier screening and the range of conditions tested for, criteria to determine "severe" conditions, reproductive decision-making, individual, and social impact
Laboratory scientist	Carrier screening recommendations by professional bodies, test characteristics such as clinical utility and validity and analytic validity, technology that enables expanded carrier screening, condition/mutation selection, pathogenic variants detected and variants of uncertain significance, carrier frequency, education, and counseling
Disability rights advocate	Disability rights objections to expanded carrier screening, reproductive decisions after carrier screening, eugenics, *in vitro* fertilization, discrimination, condition selection
Clinical geneticist	The evolution of reproductive carrier screening, counseling, and education in the past and for expanded carrier screening

funded, whole-population preconception carrier screening programs?

2. What are the benefits of implementing publicly funded whole-population preconception carrier screening programs?
3. What are the risks and challenges of implementing publicly funded whole-population preconception carrier screening programs?

The outcomes for each small group were written down by a scribe on feedback sheets and then orally reported back to the large group. The information recorded by the scribes was subsequently analyzed to identify common themes across all groups, and a summary of these findings is included in this paper.

RESULTS

Forty-one people attended the workshop, representing a range of disciplines including human genetics, clinical genetics, medical

genetics, genetic counseling, primary care, pediatrics, laboratory science, bioethics, population health policy, medical sociology, humanities, health economics, and public health genomics. Participants were largely employed in academia, public health systems, and commercial companies. The outcomes of the small group discussions are presented below, gathered together in line with the Wilson and Jungner themes of the condition, test, treatment, and screening program.

Condition

There was general agreement that only "severe" or "serious" conditions should be included in preconception expanded carrier screening. However, there was concern about the lack of a consensus definition of "severe" and "serious," where the line between "mild" and "severe" should be and why. Some participants suggested "severe" disorders should be defined as early onset conditions where the child dies in the newborn or early childhood periods. There was a belief that screening individuals in line with this definition is (1) less ethically contentious than screening for conditions that do not result in early mortality; (2) avoids perceptions of eugenics; (3) has fewer implications for people living with diseases; and (4) is less vulnerable to the disability rights critique that carrier screening removes normal human diversity.

The lack of a definition of severity was perceived to create confusion regarding which conditions should be screened and the potential for competition between laboratories to offer more and more tests. There was a belief that commercial pressures and technology-led development of expanded carrier screening have the potential to result in a "slippery slope" of offering tests just because they are possible. Thus, participants perceived that a definition of severity, which could be used to determined which conditions to screen, may safeguard against the inappropriate extension of preconception expanded carrier screening programs to include more and more conditions, including "mild" conditions. Another question raised at the workshop was whether participants of a preconception expanded carrier screening program should be able to choose which conditions to be tested for, or whether they could be offered a panel with no option for selecting specific conditions to be tested for.

Test

Participants argued that there is a need for robust up-to-date evidence about tests used in preconception expanded carrier screening. Specifically, evidence is needed on the following: the reliability of the tests (especially the negative predictive value) and their appropriateness for the population; the confidence with which the pathogenicity of the gene mutations has been established; clinical and analytical validity; and residual risk and explanations for variants of unknown significance. It was thought that the tests should have clinical value/utility and public acceptability, and economic factors including the cost of tests need to be considered in deciding which conditions to test for.

Treatment

There were no issues raised in relation to "the treatment" of participants identified as carriers. This undoubtedly relates to the fact that carriers of autosomal-recessive diseases are unaffected by those diseases, and as such they do not need treatment. Carriers of X-linked diseases may sometimes be or become affected, depending upon multiple factors including the pattern of X chromosome inactivation.

Screening Program

For participants, there were many uncertainties around preconception expanded carrier screening and the view that offering a program would be "uncharted waters" in the rapidly changing, dynamic field of genomics. A number of issues were raised regarding aspects of a screening program including the purpose, benefits and harms, target population, program acceptability, components of a program, and economic evaluation.

Clarity of Purpose and Expected Benefits

Participants asserted that it would be important for governments to consider why preconception expanded carrier screening might be implemented as a publicly funded program, and what would be the objectives, motives, rationale, and goals of such a program. In their view, the purpose should be "well framed" with appropriate evidence of benefits and harms and ethical principles (e.g., autonomy and individual rights to informed healthcare choices and to make decisions with as much relevant information as possible). Discussions around the purpose and possible benefits of preconception expanded carrier screening focused on outcomes that might eventuate as a result of program participation. There were two clear perspectives on the overarching purpose or benefits, namely:

- Increased autonomy through increased reproductive choices: the information obtained through preconception expanded carrier screening leads to knowledge of carrier status and this increases the range of reproductive choices, to include not having a child with the conditions screened, or
- Reduced burden of disease: preconception expanded carrier screening could reduce infant mortality and morbidity. This is when identified carriers use the information on their carrier status to make reproductive choices that lead to the prevention or avoidance of children being born with conditions that are "life-threatening," "severe," "serious," "nasty," and "devastating" and with onset during childhood. There was the belief that this would result in fewer sick children being born.

There were tensions between some participants, who held differing views on whether a reduction in disease burden should be a primary goal or a secondary benefit of preconception expanded carrier screening.

Other potential benefits identified by participants included:

- Reduced family burden: the avoidance of births of affected children was linked to the belief that this would result in less distress, anxiety, strain, trauma, suffering, and long-term effects on families, which was then perceived to improve family quality of life. Participants related reduced burden of disease and family burden to the ethical principles of beneficence and prevention of harm.
- Equity of access: this refers to the notion that everyone in the target population should have access to all aspects of

a screening program, including the screening test as well as information provided prior to screening. It was suggested that a government funded program for the whole population would mean less likelihood of a user-pays system. This would enable lower socioeconomic and vulnerable populations to access the program, thereby minimizing health disparities and inequities in access. However, there was some doubt expressed as to whether a preconception expanded carrier screening program would really have the capacity to deliver equitable access.

- Economic value: preconception expanded carrier screening could reduce healthcare expenditure through reducing morbidity and the subsequent need for lifetime care of people who are severely affected by the conditions screened.
- Consumer desire for health information: in making information on carrier status available for those who want it, preconception expanded carrier screening could be beneficial for those people who want as much information as possible related to their health.
- Increased genetics awareness among the public and health professionals: offering a preconception expanded carrier screening program to the whole population could empower people by increasing their knowledge about genetics (genetics literacy) and the fact that everybody is a carrier of something.

Potential Harms

There was a view that preconception expanded carrier screening may increase stigma and discrimination for those identified as carriers, those who opt not to undergo screening and those born with the conditions screened. It was also thought that people living with the conditions screened may be disadvantaged if a reduced incidence of these conditions reduces the incentives to develop treatments and therapies. According to participants, the rights of those who choose not to undergo preconception expanded carrier screening need to be respected. Further, participants felt that there would need to be adequate support for people regardless of the reproductive choice they make following preconception expanded carrier screening.

Participants argued that being identified as a carrier might have financial implications, for example, on insurance premiums, and psychological impacts, such as increased anxiety or false expectations or reassurance that they have been "promised" a healthy baby. Additionally, it was suggested that a government-sponsored preconception expanded carrier screening program might foster the perception of genetic testing being "routine" and that screening is mandated by the government, and thus not voluntary. People may feel social pressure, coercion, or obligation to participate. It might raise questions of government-sponsored eugenics and "where will it end?" A challenge was seen to be providing information and counseling that is "neutral," particularly if there is a "strong incentive" to increase uptake to justify providing the program.

Target Population

The key issues explored by participants included defining the target population, deciding at what age to offer screening, and determining whether screening would be offered to both members of a couple at the same time or to one member of a couple first and only to the other if the first one is a carrier. There was also a perceived need for governments to understand what would motivate or drive decision-making around participation in a pre-conception expanded carrier screening program. Some attendees reflected that the uptake rate for the program has implications for cost-effectiveness, and the extent to which the program could result in benefits such as reduced burden of disease and increased reproductive choice.

Acceptability

Whether preconception expanded carrier screening was "accept-able" was raised by a number of participants. This included whether the general public and target population actually want government funded access to preconception expanded carrier screening, and whether clinicians and politicians would support such a program.

Components of a Program

Participants thought that, if a preconception expanded carrier screening program was to be offered by governments, there should be sufficient resources to invest in an "end to end service." That is, the participants thought a program is not just about the screening test itself. Other components of a program that partici-pants thought important for governments to consider included:

- The provision of information and education to the public, target population, and health professionals. Participants rec-ommended that, as part of a program, information should be provided that would make the aim(s) of the program clear and encapsulate the benefits, risks, harms, consequences, uncer-tainties around genetics and preconception expanded carrier screening, and impact on individuals and society. Further, there was a view that program information should also outline the different conditions screened, testing procedure, interpre-tation of results, and implications. Some workshop participants were concerned that the public might not have the genetic literacy required to understand the information provided including the implications of results, and therefore would be faced with "information burden" or making reproductive decisions based on information that is poorly understood by themselves and/or health professionals. This raised a question around whether preconception expanded carrier screening would actually result in greater autonomy for couples wishing to make reproductive decisions.
- Informed consent. Information provision was linked to being able to provide informed consent to participate in a program. Questions were raised around what is the best way to realize informed consent and whether informed consent was possible if multiple conditions were offered for testing in the program. Linked to the need for informed consent was the need to pro-vide pretest genetic counseling. Workshop participants also thought that posttest genetic counseling was essential to help program participants understand the carrier information they received and make informed decisions about what to do with the information they received.
- Clear care pathways and support for people identified as carriers. This included follow-up care in terms of enabling the

reproductive choices that carriers might want to pursue (e.g., access to IVF or PGD). It was proposed that consideration would need to be given to how the preconception expanded carrier screening program would connect with these other services and what the implications of the program would be for other parts of the health system. According to participants, a preconception expanded carrier screening program needs to be integrated with other programs so that there are no mixed messages and quality is not compromised.
- Collection of data on program participants and program operations. There were concerns around participant privacy and data ownership, protection, confidentiality, sharing, and access.

Questions were also raised by participants around workforce capacity and the impact that a program may have on healthcare providers, how best to start the program, and whether a pilot study would be appropriate.

Economic Evaluation

The resources required to establish a high-quality "end to end" preconception expanded carrier screening program would likely be significant. Participants acknowledged that healthcare systems are experiencing both growing demand and funding ceilings. Consequently they argued there is a need for governments to prioritize spending and consider the opportunity costs of offering a preconception expanded carrier screening program, as opposed to any other program. It was thought that the establishment of a preconception expanded carrier screening program should not take resources away from providing adequate treatment of people who are living with the conditions screened.

There was a perceived need for governments to consider sustainability, cost–benefits, and cost-effectiveness, including direct, indirect, and intangible costs such as anxiety and other psychological harms. However, in making these suggestions, questions arose around how to best do this and what costs and savings should be considered and how can these be measured. In particular, participants questioned the best way to consider savings from reduced births of affected children and reduced long-term support for people living with severe disabilities. Government inertia and the difficulty of estimating costs were seen as inhibitors to investment in a preconception expanded carrier screening program.

DISCUSSION

Workshop findings highlight that there is a wide range of issues that require careful examination by governments that are assess-ing preconception carrier screening, to ensure that the benefits outweigh the harms. Overlaying feedback from the workshop against the original Wilson and Jungner principles demonstrates that these are not a "best fit" for governments to assess precon-ception expanded carrier screening. Given that only Israel has implemented a national program of genetic carrier screening (25) and only the Netherlands has developed tailored decision-making criteria for genetic screening, governments across the globe have further work ahead of them to develop criteria that could inform whether to introduce preconception expanded carrier screening. The workshop findings provide a starting point for governments to begin addressing this policy gap. Specifically, a range of issues have been identified in relation to the conditions to be screened, the tests to be used, and the components that should be incorporated into a preconception carrier screening program.

When considering "the condition," workshop participants agreed that screening should only ever be offered for conditions that are "severe" or "serious." This aligns with the Wilson and Jungner concept of an "important health problem" (12). However, participants recognized that there is no clear, consensus definition of what constitutes "severe," with different suggestions existing in the literature (26, 27). Without a clear definition, it is difficult to determine the scope of conditions that should be considered for inclusion in an expanded screening program. Indeed there is marked disparity in the composition of currently available laboratory panels of conditions for expanded carrier screening (28). From a program perspective, a definition is essential because the number and type of conditions screened has follow-on implications for how the program is implemented. Specifically, it will impact upon components of the program such as information and consent requirements, as well as counseling requirements and treatment or follow-up options. Further, as outlined by workshop participants, the definition of "severe" and thus the conditions screened are likely to impact upon public and clinical perceptions of the program. If a clear definition is not developed, and parameters and safeguards not set, there is the potential for trust in a preconception expanded carrier screening program to be undermined. Therefore, a body of work is needed to consider the definition of "severe." The definition offered by workshop participants is a valid starting point: "early onset conditions where the child dies in the newborn or early childhood period." In excluding conditions that do not result in early mortality, this definition was perceived to be less ethically contentious and to have less of an impact on disability rights.

The workshop discussions around the Wilson and Jungner criteria for "the test" were aligned with the literature reviewed, in terms of the need for the test to be accurate (see **Table 2**). This was in relation to both sensitivity (low false-positives) and specificity (low false-negatives) and also the ability to determine meaningful residual risk for individuals who test negative. The issue of the cost-effectiveness of the tests was also raised by workshop participants, and this would likely be a key consideration for governments within the context of the overall cost-effectiveness of a program.

Workshop participants did not raise any considerations for government in relation to Wilson and Jungner's theme of "the treatment." This demonstrates a lack of salience of this issue for the participants. This could be because care and follow-up for carrier screening does not meet the traditional definition of treatment, since such screening does not result in the identification of people who have conditions. When coupled with the fact that much of the workshop discussion focused on elements of the screening program, the absence of discussion on treatment could also reflect heightened interest in the issue of "how to screen" as opposed to "whether to screen." Nonetheless, the relevance of the Wilson and Jungner criteria associated with "the treatment"

may be queried in relation to preconception expanded carrier screening. The question then becomes whether there are more relevant dimensions that should replace the treatment criterion. For example, instead of the need for treatment being available, should the criterion be to recommend that "interventions are available"? Should the issue of interventions be framed within the context of the reasons for participation in preconception expanded carrier screening, such as "a decision should need to be taken by the person screened" (20) or that "screening should potentially influence the reproductive choices made by at-risk participants" (19)?

In our view, it is essential that governments consider the availability of interventions for preconception expanded carrier screening, and the downstream effects on and costs of providing such interventions. In order for a screening program to be effective and cost-effective, there must be an intervention that can lead to better health outcomes for an individual. Further, the intervention must be effective, available, easily accessible, and acceptable to individuals within the target population (44). Importantly, government consideration should be given to the fact that interventions for individuals identified as carriers are not currently always equitably accessible. For example, IVF and PGD are provided in the private sector within Australia, meaning there can be significant costs to individuals, which may limit access for citizens in lower socioeconomic groups (45, 46). This means that Australia, and other countries where these healthcare services are not equitably accessible, would need to carefully consider its capacity to provide the follow-up interventions required for a population-based approach to preconception expanded carrier screening. Further in relation to equity, consideration would also need to be given to the quality of PGD and IVF services, particularly given concerns regarding false-positive screening results (47, 48), and the fact that the genetics workforce is not keeping pace with the demand for these services (49).

As with the review by Seedat et al. (14) of population-based screening criteria adopted across a number of countries, the findings of the workshop were more likely to focus on considerations relating to "the screening program" as opposed to the condition, test, and treatment. The issues identified in relation to the screening program were largely those that would be relevant to all screening programs, not only preconception expanded carrier screening. These issues included the need for a program that is not just about the test, but rather includes components such as the provision of information and education, informed consent processes, genetic counseling, clear care pathways, data collection, and economic evaluation. There is a need for further exploration of these issues to determine in what ways, if any, these program components would be impacted by the unique features of expanded carrier screening. For example, there was recognition by workshop participants that consent should be informed, but what would be the impact on the ability to obtain informed consent, when expanded carrier screening would test for multiple conditions simultaneously? How would informed consent be defined in this context? Related to this issue, further investigation should examine the impact of preconception expanded carrier screening on the complexity, volume, and financial implications of pretest and posttest counseling (28).

TABLE 2 | Coverage of issues referred to in literature.

Topic area	Issue raised by workshop participants	Issue *not* raised by workshop participants
Condition	– Should be clinically severe (1, 5, 22, 23, 29, 30)	– The impact of the condition on individuals, families, and society needs to be understood (22) – It should be an important health problem (20) – The nature of the condition should influence the reproductive choices made by at-risk participants (19) – Conditions should have a predictable course (23) – The gene mutations that cause the condition should be understood, should have a valid clinical association with the phenotype/severity of the condition, and involve highly penetrant recessive inheritance (5, 7, 19, 29) – There should be a high frequency of carriers in the population (30–32)
Test	– Need to assess test performance and accuracy across all gene mutations assayed (5, 29, 32) – Sensitivity (1, 5, 23, 29, 30, 32) – Specificity (30, 32) – Ability to determine meaningful residual risk for individuals who test negative (7, 19, 33) – Cost-effective (29, 32)	– Non-invasive (32) – Accessible (31) – Straightforward interpretation of results (23) – Highly scalable to avoid limits to universal uptake (5, 32) – Limited to gene mutations that have the highest likelihood of being/are clearly pathogenic (1, 7) – Comply with laboratory guidelines that include quality control (19) – Inexpensive (5, 29, 32)
Treatment		– An effective treatment or intervention should be available for those identified as carriers (5, 20, 23)
Screening program	– A clearly defined purpose and benefits of carrier screening (1, 6, 21, 23, 32, 34) – Understanding of the potential harms of carrier screening, including physical, psychological, psychosocial, social, and ethical, which should all be low compared to benefits (20, 22, 35) – Equity and accessibility (29, 33) – Defining the target population and understanding their needs (23, 29, 36) – Reaching, inviting, recruiting, and informing the target population, and informing and educating the general public, acknowledging that both groups probably having low awareness or knowledge of carrier screening and the diseases screened for (21, 33, 37, 38) – Age to offer and timing of screening (i.e., individuals or couples) (1, 7, 21) – Participation that is voluntary and based on informed consent (1, 7, 20) – Consent processes and the provision of information, education, counseling, and support pre-screen for all participants and post-screen for those with positive test results, particularly about benefits and harms of screening, the test process, possible outcomes, interpretations of results, implications, and management options (1, 7, 20, 29, 30, 33, 34, 38–41) – Education of healthcare providers (1, 7, 21) – Resources and infrastructure, including access to follow-up services such as preimplantation genetic diagnosis and prenatal diagnosis (29, 30, 36, 42) – Public, political, and cultural attitudes toward and acceptability of carrier screening (1, 7, 33, 36) – Economic evaluations, particularly of cost–benefit and cost-effectiveness (1, 7, 21, 22, 32, 34) – Whether the program has been offered in the research setting and/or pilot studies and the outcomes of these studies (22, 31, 42)	– Accredited institutions and appropriately trained professionals (1) – Structure of the healthcare system (public/private) and implications for screening (43) – Monitoring, evaluation/review (21, 43, 44)

In addition to the work that is needed by governments to develop robust decision-making models for assessing preconception expanded carrier screening, researchers should begin to explore a number of issues raised by the workshop participants to inform and complement work in the public policy space. Within local contexts, "societal readiness" for preconception expanded carrier screening could be investigated. While several potential benefits of expanded carrier screening were identified at the workshop, a number of potential harms were also discussed, including concerns around discrimination, eugenics, and people refusing to participate in a program, which could undermine the cost-effectiveness of program delivery. While the UK Human Genetics Commission (18) concluded "there are no specific ethical, legal or social principles that would make preconception genetic testing within the framework of a population screening program unacceptable" (p. 1), this needs to be explored by experts in other local contexts, including the contention expressed by workshop participants around the primary purpose of this screening being reproductive choice and/or reduced burden of disease (50). Further to this, consultation and engagement methodologies could be developed and implemented to assess stakeholder acceptability of preconception expanded carrier screening, including the public, target population, disease associations, clinicians, and laboratory staff. For the target population, this should also include investigation of likely uptake and postscreening decisions around reproductive choices. A recent study in the Netherlands has made initial contributions in the area of citizens/user perceptions of expanded carrier screening (51), while a qualitative study in Sweden has examined healthcare professionals' views on preconception carrier screening (52). This line of work must be extended to further local contexts.

This paper has several limitations. Workshop participants were self-selected and may not be a representative sample of experts relevant to preconception expanded carrier screening. This may impact on the generalizability of the workshop findings. It is also important to note that, in relation to the literature on existing carrier screening programs and recommendations by professional bodies regarding expanded carrier screening, not all of the issues raised in the literature as key success factors or recommendations for implementation were addressed by the participants (see **Table 2**). During the workshop, participants were exposed to a range of perspectives related to preconception expanded carrier screening, which framed the subsequent discussions, and not all perspectives were covered by the workshop presentations. Participant exposure to other perspectives may have resulted in different workshop outcomes. Finally, as noted above, the workshop findings were reasonably high-level and did not drill down to deeper levels of analysis regarding the key issues. Therefore, while the findings provide useful guidance, a more precise exploration of each issue may be required to develop a comprehensive view of the factors governments need to consider when deciding whether to implement preconception expanded carrier screening.

The international workshop was an important opportunity for expert stakeholders in the field of preconception expanded carrier screening to come together to share their values, experiences and knowledge. The workshop outcomes identified benefits, harms, and other key issues that governments should consider when assessing whether to publicly fund preconception expanded carrier screening programs. This is particularly useful since most countries globally do not have decision-making frameworks related to emerging genetic screening options and are at the formative stage of making assessments about preconception expanded carrier screening.

AUTHOR CONTRIBUTIONS

All the authors contributed substantially to the conception and design of the workshop, the acquisition and interpretation of data, have given final approval for the manuscript to be published, and agreed to be accountable for all aspects of the work. CM and KL undertook the data analysis and drafted the manuscript. GB, SM-J, AC, VS, HD, and NL critically revised the manuscript for important intellectual content.

ACKNOWLEDGMENTS

The authors would like to acknowledge the workshop participants for their contributions to the workshop reported in this paper.

FUNDING

This work was financially supported by the Office of Population Health Genomics, Public Health Division, Department of Health Western Australia; Harry Perkins Institute; Life Letters; the European Union Seventh Framework Programme (FP7/2007-2013) under grant agreement No. 305444 (RD-Connect) and 305121 (Neuromics); Australian National Health and Medical Research Council (NHMRC) APP1055319 under the NHMRC–European Union Collaborative Research Grant; and NHMRC Principal Research Fellowship APP1117510.

REFERENCES

1. Henneman L, Borry P, Chokoshvili D, Cornel MC, van El CG, Forzano F, et al. Responsible implementation of expanded carrier screening. *Eur J Hum Genet* (2016) 24:e1–12. doi:10.1038/ejhg.2015.271

2. McCabe LL, McCabe ER. Newborn screening as a model for population screening. *Mol Genet Metab* (2002) 75:299–307. doi:10.1016/S1096-7192(02)00005-7

3. Barlow-Stewart K, Burnett L, Proos A, Howell V, Huq F, Lazarus R, et al. A genetic screening program for Tay-Sachs disease and cystic fibrosis for Australian Jewish high school students. *J Med Genet* (2003) 40:e45. doi:10.1136/jmg.40.4.e45

4. Zlotogora J. Population programs for the detection of couples at risk for severe monogenic genetic diseases. *Hum Genet* (2009) 126:247–53. doi:10.1007/s00439-009-0669-y

5. Bell CJ, Dinwiddie DL, Miller NA, Hateley SL, Ganusova EE, Mudge J, et al. Carrier testing for severe childhood recessive diseases by next-generation sequencing. *Sci Transl Med* (2011) 3:65ra4. doi:10.1126/scitranslmed.3001756

6. Tanner AK, Valencia CA, Rhodenizer D, Espirages M, Da Silva C, Borsuk L, et al. Development and performance of a comprehensive targeted sequencing assay for pan-ethnic screening of carrier status. *J Mol Diagn* (2014) 16:350–60. doi:10.1016/j.jmoldx.2013.12.003

7. Edwards J, Feldman G, Goldberg J, Gregg A, Norton M, Rose N, et al. Expanded carrier screening in reproductive medicine – points to consider. *Obstet Gynecol* (2015) 125:653–62. doi:10.1097/AOG.0000000000000666

8. Borry P, Henneman L, Lakeman P, Ten Kate LP, Cornel MC, Howard HC. Preconceptional genetic carrier testing and the commercial offer directly-to-consumers. *Hum Reprod* (2011) 26:972–7. doi:10.1093/humrep/der042

9. Lazarin G, Haque I. Expanded carrier screening: a review of early implementation and literature. *Semin Perinatol* (2016) 40:29–34. doi:10.1053/j.semperi.2015.11.005

10. Andermann A, Blancquaert I, Dery V. Genetic screening: a conceptual framework for programs and policy-making. *J Health Serv Res Policy* (2010) 15:90–7. doi:10.1258/jhsrp.2009.009084

11. Harris R, Sawaya GF, Moyer VA, Calonge N. Reconsidering the criteria for evaluating proposed screening programs: reflections from 4 current and former members of the U.S. Preventive Services Task Force. *Epidemiol Rev* (2011) 33:20–35. doi:10.1093/epirev/mxr005

12. Wilson JMG, Jungner G. *Principles and Practice of Screening for Disease*. Geneva: World Health Organization (1968). Available from: http://apps.who.int/iris/bitstream/10665/37650/17/WHO_PHP_34.pdf

13. Andermann A, Blancquaert I, Beauchamp S, Déry V. Revisiting Wilson and Jungner in the genomic age: a review of screening criteria over the past 40 years. *Bull World Health Organ* (2008) 86:317–9. doi:10.2471/BLT.07.050112

14. Seedat F, Cooper J, Cameron L, Stranges S, Kandala N, Burton H, et al. *International Comparisons of Screening Policy-Making: A Systematic Review.* Warwick Medical School, The University of Warwick, and PHG Foundation (2014).

15. Metternick-Jones SC, Lister KJ, Dawkins HJS, White CA, Weeramanthri TS. Review of current international decision-making processes for newborn screening: lessons for Australia. *Front Public Health* (2015) 3:214. doi:10.3389/fpubh.2015.00214

16. Jansen M, Metternick-Jones SC, Lister KJ. International differences in the evaluation of conditions for newborn bloodspot screening: a review of scientific literature and policy documents. *Eur J Hum Genet* (2016) 25:10–6. doi:10.1038/ejhg.2016.126

17. Health Council of the Netherlands: Committee Genetic Screening. *Genetic Screening.* The Hague: Health Council (1994). 1994 p.

18. UK Human Genetics Commission. *Increasing Options, Informing Choice: A Report on Preconception Genetic Testing and Screening.* London: Department of Health (2011).

19. Grody WW, Thompson BH, Gregg AR, Bean LH, Monaghan KG, Schneider A, et al. ACMG position statement on prenatal/preconception expanded carrier screening. *Genet Med* (2013) 15:482–3. doi:10.1038/gim.2013.47

20. Henneman L, Poppelaars F, Ten Kate L. Evaluation of cystic fibrosis carrier screening programs according to genetic screening criteria. *Genet Med* (2002) 4:241–9. doi:10.1097/00125817-200207000-00002

21. Castellani C, Macek M Jr, Cassiman J-J, Duff A, Massie J, Ten Kate LP, et al. Benchmarks for cystic fibrosis carrier screening: a European consensus document. *J Cyst Fibros* (2010) 9:165–78. doi:10.1016/j.jcf.2010.02.005

22. Hill MK, Archibald AD, Cohen J, Metcalfe SA. A systematic review of population screening for fragile X syndrome. *Genet Med* (2010) 12:396–410. doi:10.1097/GIM.0b013e3181e38fb6

23. Laberge AM, Watts C, Porter K, Burke W. Assessing the potential success of cystic fibrosis carrier screening: lessons learned from Tay-Sachs disease and β-thalassemia. *Public Health Genomics* (2010) 13:310–9. doi:10.1159/000253122

24. Modra L, Massie R, Delatycki M. Ethical considerations in choosing a model for population-based cystic fibrosis carrier screening. *Med J Aust* (2010) 193:157–60.

25. Zlotogora J, Grotto I, Kaliner E, Gamzu R. The Israeli national population program of genetic carrier screening for reproductive purposes. *Genet Med* (2016) 18:203–6. doi:10.1038/gim.2015.55

26. Lazarin G, Hawthorn F, Collins N, Platt E, Evans E, Haque I. Systematic classification of disease severity for evaluation of expanded carrier screening panels. *PLoS One* (2014) 9:e114391. doi:10.1371/journal.pone.0114391

27. Korngiebel D, McMullen C, Amendola L, Berg J, Davis J, Gilmore M, et al. Generating a taxonomy for genetic conditions relevant to reproductive planning. *Am J Med Genet A* (2016) 170:565–73. doi:10.1002/ajmg.a.37513

28. Yao R, Goetzinger K. Genetic carrier screening in the twenty-first century. *Clin Lab Med* (2016) 36:277–88. doi:10.1016/j.cll.2016.01.003

29. Vallance H, Ford J. Carrier testing for autosomal-recessive disorders. *Crit Rev Clin Lab Sci* (2003) 40:473–97. doi:10.1080/10408360390247832

30. Prior T. Carrier screening for spinal muscular atrophy. *Genet Med* (2008) 10:840–2. doi:10.1097/GIM.0b013e318188d069

31. Muralidharan K, Wilson R, Ogino S, Nagan N, Curtis C, Schrijver I. Population carrier screening for spinal muscular atrophy: a position statement of the Association for Molecular Pathology. *J Mol Diagn* (2011) 13:3–6. doi:10.1016/j.jmoldx.2010.11.012

32. Srinivasan BS, Evans EA, Flannick J, Patterson AS, Change CC, Pham T, et al. A universal carrier test for the long tail of Mendelian disease. *Reprod Biomed Online* (2010) 21:537–51. doi:10.1016/j.rbmo.2010.05.012

33. Ioannou L, McClaren BJ, Massie J, Lewis S, Metcalfe SA, Forrest L, et al. Population-based carrier screening for cystic fibrosis: a systematic review of 23 years of research. *Genet Med* (2014) 16:207–16. doi:10.1038/gim.2013.125

34. Cho D, McGowan ML, Metcalfe J, Sharp RR. Expanded carrier screening in reproductive healthcare: perspectives from genetics professionals. *Hum Reprod* (2013) 28:1725–30. doi:10.1093/humrep/det091

35. Archibald AD, Hickerton CL, Jaques AM, Wake S, Cohen J, Metcalfe SA. "It's about having the choice": stakeholder perceptions of population-based genetic carrier screening for fragile X syndrome. *Am J Med Genet A* (2013) 161:48–58. doi:10.1002/ajmg.a.35674

36. Achterbergh R, Lakeman P, Stemerding D, Moors E, Cornel M. Implementation of preconceptional carrier screening for cystic fibrosis and haemoglobinopathies: a sociotechnical analysis. *Health Policy* (2007) 83:277–86. doi:10.1016/j.healthpol.2007.02.007

37. Poppelaars FAM, Van Der Wal G, Braspenning JCC, Cornel MC, Henneman L, Langendam MW, et al. Possibilities and barriers in the implementation of a preconceptional screening program for cystic fibrosis carriers: a focus group study. *Public Health* (2003) 117:396–403. doi:10.1016/S0033-3506(03)00136-7

38. Archibald AD, Jaques AM, Wake S, Collins VR, Cohen J, Metcalfe SA. "It's something I need to consider": decisions about carrier screening for fragile X syndrome in a population of non-pregnant women. *Am J Med Genet A* (2009) 149A:2731–8. doi:10.1002/ajmg.a.33122

39. Delatycki MB. Population screening for reproductive risk for single gene disorders in Australia: now and the future. *Twin Res Hum Genet* (2008) 11:422–30. doi:10.1375/twin.11.4.422

40. Gross S, Pletcher B, Monaghan K; Professional Practice and Guidelines Committee. Carrier screening in individuals of Ashkenazi Jewish descent. *Genet Med* (2008) 10:54–6. doi:10.1097/GIM.0b013e31815f247c

41. Kim MJ, Kim DJ, Kim SY, Yang JH, Kim MH, Lee SW, et al. Fragile X carrier screening in Korean women of reproductive age. *J Med Screen* (2013) 20:15–20. doi:10.1177/0969141313488364

42. Atkin K, Ahmad WIU. Genetic screening and haemoglobinopathies: ethics, politics and practice. *Soc Sci Med* (1998) 46:445–58.

43. Rosner G, Rosner S, Orr-Urtreger A. Genetic testing in Israel: an overview. *Annu Rev Genomics Hum Genet* (2009) 10:175–92. doi:10.1146/annurev.genom.030308.111406

44. Screening Subcommittee. *Population Based Screening Framework.* Barton: Australian Health Ministers Advisory Council, Commonwealth of Australia (2008). Available from: http://www.cancerscreening.gov.au/internet/screening/publishing.nsf/Content/16AE0B0524753EE9CA257CEE00000B5D7/$File/Final%20Population%20Based%20Screening%20Framework%202016.pdf

45. Reproductive Technology Council. *Preimplantation Genetic Diagnosis (PGD) in Western Australia.* Department of Health, Western Australia (2010). Available from: http://www.rtc.org.au/events/docs/PGD_WA.pdf

46. IVF Australia. *IVF Treatment Costs.* (2016). Available from: http://ivf.com.au/ivf-fees/ivf-costs

47. Dandouh E, Balayla J, Audibert F. Technical update: preimplantation genetic diagnosis and screening. *J Obstet Gynaecol Can* (2009) 37:451–63. doi:10.1016/S1701-2163(15)30261-9

48. SenGupta S, Delhanty J. Preimplantation genetic diagnosis: recent triumphs and remaining challenges. *Expert Rev Mol Diagn* (2012) 12:585–92. doi:10.1586/erm.12.61

49. Kaye C. Genetic service delivery: infrastructure, assessment and information. *Public Health Genomics* (2012) 15:164–71. doi:10.1159/000335552

50. Kihlbom U. Ethical issues in preconception genetic carrier screening. *Ups J Med Sci* (2016) 8:1–4. doi:10.1080/03009734.2016.1189470

51. Holtkamp K, Mathijssen I, Lakeman P, Van Marle M, Dondorp W, Henneman L, et al. Factors for successful implementation of population-based expanded carrier screening: learning from existing initiatives. *Eur J Public Health* (2016):1–6. doi:10.1093/eurpub/ckw110

52. Matar A, Kihlbom U, Höglund A. Swedish healthcare providers' perceptions of preconception expanded carrier screening (ECS) – a qualitative study. *J Community Genet* (2016) 7:2013–4. doi:10.1007/s12687-016-0268-2

5

The Use of Assessment of Chronic Illness Care Technology to Evaluate the Institutional Capacity for HIV/AIDS Management

Andressa Wanneska Martins da Silva[1]*, Micheline Marie Milward de Azevedo Meiners[2], Elza Ferreira Noronha[1] and Maria Inês de Toledo[1]

[1] Tropical Medicine, Faculty of Medicine, University of Brasília, Brasília, Brazil,

[2] College of Pharmacy, Faculty of Ceilândia, University of Brasília, Brasília, Brazil

*Correspondence:
Andressa Wanneska Martins da Silva
wanneska.andressa@gmail.com

The effectiveness of antiretroviral therapy has rendered HIV infection a manageable chronic condition. Currently, the health systems face the challenge of adopting organizational healthcare models capable of ensuring the delivery of comprehensive care. The Chronic Care Model has been reported for its effectiveness, particularly in terms of delivery system design. In this study, the Assessment of Chronic Illness Care (ACIC) questionnaire, a soft technology widely used for other chronic conditions, was employed on a teaching hospital to evaluate healthcare provided to people living with HIV/AIDS. The ACIC technology is a self-explanatory instrument which diagnoses, among the six components of the Chronic Care Model Framework, areas for quality improvements, indicating at the same time, intervention strategies and achievements. These components are *healthcare network organization, delivery system design, self-management support, decision support, clinical information systems,* and *community.* From May to October 2014, the tool was applied to the multidisciplinary teamwork at the points of care identified, as well as to the hospital management board. Respondents broadly rated care as basic. A pronounced contrast was observed from evaluation by management board and health professional staff in some components like *organization of healthcare* and *clinical information system.* The *self-management support* and *delivery system design* were the components best evaluated by the multidisciplinary team. Combined with the array of services offered, the entry points available at the hospital can ensure healthcare comprehensiveness. However, some gaps were detected, precluding the delivery of an effective care. The ACIC was considered an adequate technology to provide knowledge of the gaps, to promote productive discussions and reflections within teams and to indicate actions to achieve improvements on healthcare for people living with HIV/AIDS.

Keywords: Chronic Care Model, ACIC, delivery system design, HIV/AIDS, assessment technology, health evaluation

Abbreviations: ACIC, Assessment of Chronic Illness Care; CCM, Chronic Care Model; HUB, Hospital Universitário de Brasília; IPD, infectious and parasitic disease; PLWHA, people living with HIV/AIDS; SUS, Unified Health System.

INTRODUCTION

In 2017, there were an estimated 37 million PLWHA worldwide and 21.7 million people receiving antiretroviral treatment. In Brazil, there were 880 000 registered cases of AIDS, of which more than 100 000 were pregnant women. Preventive measures have been adopted, including post-exposure prophylaxis, testing campaigns, condom distribution to populations at risk, and implementation of national treatment protocols with free provision of drug therapy. At the end of 2017, 87% of PLWHA had been diagnosed and 75% of all diagnosed were already on antiretroviral therapy (Ministério da Saúde [MS], 2017; United Nations Programme on HIV/AIDS [UNAIDS], 2018; World Health Organization [WHO], 2018).

In 1999, Brazil issued the National Policy for Sexually Transmitted Diseases and AIDS (STD/AIDS), containing guidelines and actions for the National Program of STD/AIDS. Objectives, guidelines and priorities were defined from the perspective of the Unified Healthcare System ("*Sistema Único de Saúde*," SUS) principles – equity, universality, integrality, decentralization and social participation – where the State and society interact in search of health promotion of users. It should be noted that the last three principles sustain SUS, therefore, they must be present in health actions and services (BRASIL, 1999). The National STD/AIDS Program incorporates three coordinated components: (1) Promotion, Protection and Prevention; (2) Diagnosis and Assistance; (3) Institutional Development and Management. Each component is detailed with guidelines, strategies, norms and procedures regarding PLWHA care (BRASIL, 1999).

In 2000, in order to assess the National Policy, the Ministry of Health supported the Qualiaids Research Team to develop and validate a questionnaire, a tool for external assessment based on the Qualiaids Program, as well as its recommendations book, as a monitoring and evaluation mechanism to improve HIV/AIDS, Universidade de São Paulo [USP] (2018). The questionnaire has 84 structure and process indicators and a set of best practice recommendations. The principles and clinical, epidemiological and ethical guidelines of the Program were translated into norms, criteria, indicators and quality standards for the questionnaire elaboration and validation.

Although these efforts have improved prognosis for PLWHA, the challenge to SUS is to adapt the current healthcare model: most PLWHA are retained in the specialized care not being referred to primary care setting. Then, it becomes necessary to change the healthcare model to ensure an effective, comprehensive, multidisciplinary model focused on chronic conditions, aptly integrated with primary healthcare. The traditional model focused in the specialist is unsustainable to the healthcare system (Ministério da Saúde, 2015b).

A global call has been made urging countries to foster research on innovative, optimized management of chronic conditions by healthcare systems, allowing clinical knowledge to be translated to the current healthcare context (World Health Organization [WHO], 2013). The CCM, developed in the United States in the 1990s, identifies six key elements that must function in a coordinated form in order to yield improved healthcare for

chronic conditions. These elements are split into two groups: health systems and community (Improving Chronic Illness Care [ICIC], 2018). In **Figure 1**, we present the CCM model, adapted by us to consider national features from SUS settings, including two additional key elements: *District health plan* and *non-governmental organizations* (Mendes, 2011; Moysés et al., 2012).

In the CCM, changes to the health system should address healthcare network organization, delivery system design, self-management support, decision support, and clinical information systems. The model advocates the establishment of partnerships and the use of resources available in the community to implement the intended changes and align these resources with public policies (Wagner et al., 2005; Mendes, 2011). The CCM implementation can be monitored and evaluated with its own innovative health technology, the ACIC questionnaire (**Supplementary Table 1**), which diagnoses the situation revealing the nature and degree of the improvements required, indicating intervention strategies and measuring the progress achieved after the interventions (Bonomi et al., 2002; Schwab et al., 2014).

The impact of the CCM on a variety of chronic diseases has been reported, including asthma, diabetes, and depression (Improving Chronic Illness Care [ICIC], 2018). Only seven studies, however, have been retrieved on the application of the CCM to HIV/AIDS (Goetz et al., 2008; Drabo et al., 2010; Tu et al., 2013; Clarke et al., 2015; Mahomed and Asmall, 2015; Massoud et al., 2015; Berenguer et al., 2018). These studies reported improved access and adherence to antiretroviral therapy, implementation of pertinent interventions, and increased involvement of PLWHA with their own care, resulting in clinical, immunological, and virological gains. Of note, a systematic review already published compiled data from 16 papers using CCM Framework for people living with HIV (Pasricha et al., 2013). This systematic review aimed to assess the effectiveness of decision support and clinical information system interventions, examining the outcomes: immunological/virological, medical, psychosocial, economic measures. However, the instruments applied for this assessment were others than ACIC. Therefore, the ACIC remains an innovative approach for HIV/AIDS management. Since our last review in 2018, only one study had, in fact, employed this questionnaire to evaluate HIV care (Drabo et al., 2010).

The purpose of the present investigation was to apply a validated Brazilian Portuguese version of the ACIC questionnaire to diagnose the capacity of care to PLWHA at a Brazilian teaching hospital, bringing the high importance of the CCM Framework as a technology which helps the improvement of the quality of care.

MATERIALS AND METHODS

Study Design, Site and Phases

From May to October 2014, this descriptive study was conducted with the staff of points of care for PLWHA and the management board of a Brazilian teaching hospital – HUB.

The entry points, the points of care, and the delivery system design available for PLWHA were identified by interviewing

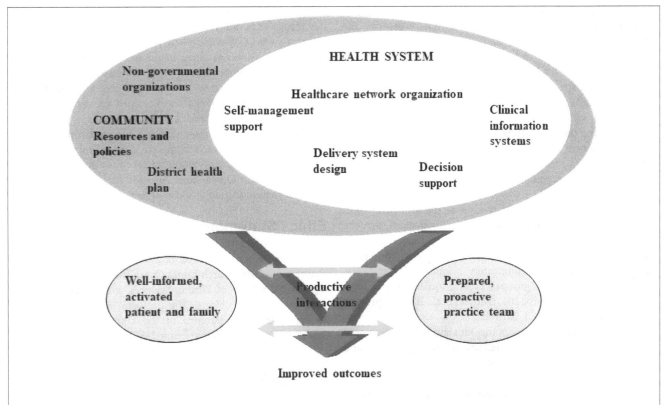

FIGURE 1 | The Chronic Care Model (Wagner, 1998): developed by The MacColl Institute, © ACP-ASIM Journals and Books, reprinted with permission from ACP-ASIM Journals and Books and adapted by authors for SUS.

nutritionists, psychologists, pharmacists, medical interns, and other healthcare professionals. The interviews followed a script comprising three questions concerning PLWHA treated at the HUB: "What are the patient's entry points?", "To which points of care is the patient assigned?", and "To which services is the patient subsequently referred?" In this study, a point of care was defined as any hospital location where PLWHA have their condition directly treated by health professionals (Mendes, 2011).

The term *delivery system design*, defined by Wagner et al. (2005) as *structured reorientation of available healthcare services and interaction between general practitioners and specialists for achieving comprehensive care*, was expressed in our questionnaire as *line of care*, term used in Brazil to represent the reorientation of care flow combined with the relationships that emerge from this flow and are constructed in the light of comprehensiveness (Malta and Merhy, 2010).

In the subsequent phase, the ACIC questionnaire was applied to healthcare professionals at all points of care and to the hospital's managing board in order to allow comparison of the views held by healthcare professionals and institutional leadership.

Evaluation Tools and Data Collection

For this investigation was applied an ACIC questionnaire (version 3.5) from MacColl Institute for Health Care Innovation (2010) previously adapted, translated and validated to Brazilian portuguese by Moysés et al. (2012). This validated questionnaire

was also adapted by the authors for PLWHA according to the hospital context and terminologies. Since Moysés' paper applied ACIC to a primary care context and our work take place in the specialized care scenario, necessary adjustments were made. Also, the term "...chronic conditions" was replaced by "... people living with HIV or PLWHA" along the ACIC tool (Moysés et al., 2012). The questionnaire was applied on different dates for 90 min, on average, to a group of at least three healthcare professionals at different points of care. The answers expressed the group consensus. Within the managing board, only the general manager completed the questionnaire. The researchers acted as facilitators and refrained from interfering with discussions or responses.

How Does the ACIC Questionnaire Work?

The ACIC questionnaire is a self-explanatory instrument which diagnoses, among the six components of CCM Framework, areas for quality improvements, indicating at the same time, intervention strategies and achievements. It covers 35 qualitative indicators divided into seven blocks: one block for each component of the model and an integrative block termed *Integration of CCM components*. These indicators measure processes including technical and interpersonal ones, which can influence the way care is delivered and consequently its success. The interpersonal processes indicators are often ignored because it is not easily available, consisting of limitation in most assessments of quality of care (Donabedian, 1988). In *health system organization*, the questionnaire assesses the management changes that are required to establish a proactive leadership, a healthcare and information flow and incentives to providers and PLWHA. These changes tend to integrate and refine work spaces within the organization (Mendes, 2011; Moysés et al., 2012).

In *delivery system design*, it evaluates how well-defined the tasks are among the health team to ensure a comprehensive and individualized care – adjusted to the social and cultural context of the user. It also measures the system for referral and return-referral which are accountable for linking the points of care (Mendes, 2011).

In *self-management support*, it assesses the knowledge and capability of the user, aiming the patient empowerment – to make decisions, to understand the plan of care and treatment goals; additionally, the service provides emotional support and brings the user to the available community resources, for instance, support groups or peer groups (Epping-Jordan et al., 2004; Wagner et al., 2005; Mendes, 2011; Moysés et al., 2012; Improving Chronic Illness Care [ICIC], 2018).

In *clinical decision support*, the indicators basically focus the use of evidence-based guidelines, training, practical and opportune decisions by the health team, gathering user preferences and health conditions. In addition, the flow of communication between specialists and primary care or interdisciplinary team should improve care (Epping-Jordan et al., 2004; Wagner et al., 2005; Mendes, 2011; Moysés et al., 2012).

In *clinical information system*, it assesses the system of information, including registries, data of individual patients and populations of patients with specific conditions, as well as provides reminders and feedbacks. It should promote, especially, the exchange of information between the various levels of care, leading to a better coordination of information (Epping-Jordan et al., 2004; Wagner et al., 2005; Mendes, 2011; Moysés et al., 2012; Improving Chronic Illness Care [ICIC], 2018).

In *community resources*, it evaluates the implementation of intersectoriality for health, the articulations and partnerships with resources that exist in other sectors of public administration (such as education, sports, social assistance), as well as community organizations (clubs, churches, community centers and support groups such as Alcoholics Anonymous, Narcotics Anonymous, among others) (Wagner et al., 2005). Also, it verifies the District Plan of Health about the resources available to the HIV care (Mendes, 2011; Moysés et al., 2012).

Finally, the ACIC assesses the interrelationship among the six elements of the CCM, linking key elements that contribute to desired clinical and functional outcomes with a positive impact on PLWHA quality of life and health organization effectiveness (Improving Chronic Illness Care [ICIC], 2018).

Criteria for Analysis

The 35 indicators of ACIC are evaluated individually inside of each block. Each indicator measures, on a scale of 0–11, an institution's capacity of care provision for chronic conditions. Scores are grouped into four levels: D (limited, 0–2), C (basic, 3–5), B (reasonably good, 6–8), and A (fully developed, 9–11)

(Bonomi et al., 2002). ACIC guidelines were followed to analyze the results—i.e., for each completed questionnaire, the mean value of each CCM component was calculated and the average of these means was assigned to the questionnaire. To evaluate PLWHA care, a global score was calculated as the average value of the means obtained at the points of care and management board. Also, a global mean was obtained for each component based solely on the points of care.

The value of each component was analyzed considering the means obtained for each component and applying stratified analysis to identify items exhibiting deficits or limitations.

The Microsoft Office Excel 2013 software was employed for the construction of graphs and analyses.

Ethics Statement

This study was carried out in accordance with the recommendations of the Resolution 466/12 of the Brazilian Health Council, Research Ethics Committee of the Universidade de Brasília School of Health Sciences with written informed consent from all subjects. The protocol was approved by the Research Ethics Committee of the Universidade de Brasília School of Health Sciences (permit 278.787).

RESULTS

Delivery System Design and Points of Care

"What are the entry points of PLWHA?", "To which points of care are these patients assigned?", and "To which services are these patients subsequently referred?"

The entry points reported by health professionals were three: the hospital's emergency service, outpatient pharmacy, and psychosocial support center (termed "*Com-Vivência*"). The identified points of PLWHA care were four: the *Com-Vivência*, the outpatient clinic for IPDs, the outpatient pharmacy, and the inpatient unit for IPDs.

Despite ongoing attempts to certify the HUB as an HIV/AIDS referral center for the Federal District, and particularly for the East Region Healthcare Network, none of the respondents reported return-referrals to other health services. This led us to conclude that patients bear the burden of finding additional healthcare services outside the hospital.

Assessment of Healthcare to PLWHA at the HUB

The result of ACIC questionnaire at HUB yielded an overall score of 4 (in the 2–5 range), assigning level C (basic) to the hospital's capacity of care delivery to PLWHA. The outpatient pharmacy scored lowest (2, level D: limited capacity) (**Figure 2**).

When analyzing the mean scores of ACIC for each component (**Figure 3**) it was observed that the capacity to employ community resources and policies was rated as basic (mean score 4) by healthcare professionals. The management board acknowledged the importance of the District Healthcare Plan in the care delivery practiced in the HUB. Overall, the coordination between hospital

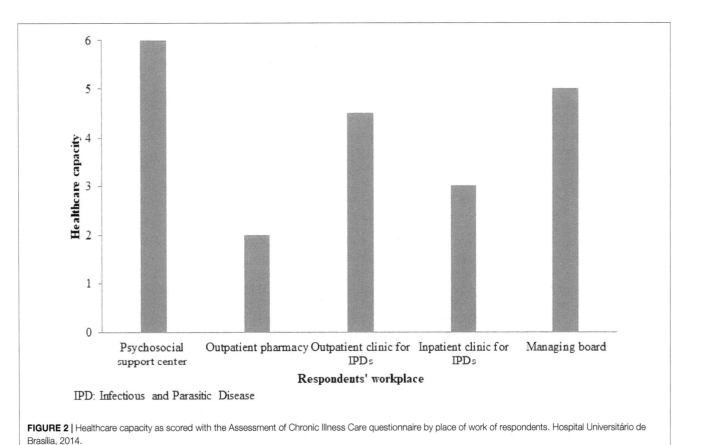

FIGURE 2 | Healthcare capacity as scored with the Assessment of Chronic Illness Care questionnaire by place of work of respondents. Hospital Universitário de Brasília, 2014.

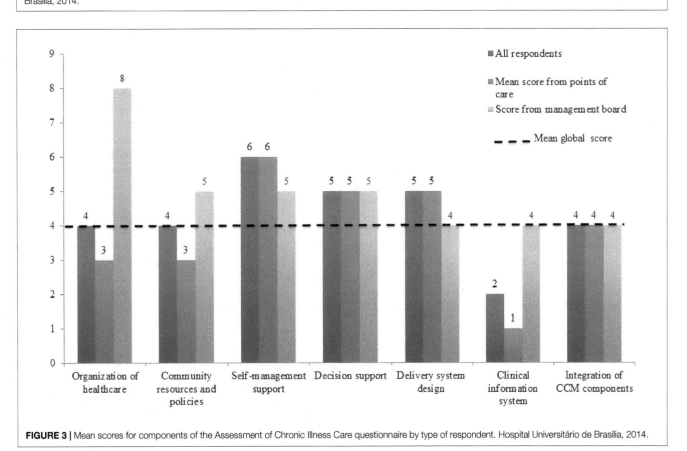

FIGURE 3 | Mean scores for components of the Assessment of Chronic Illness Care questionnaire by type of respondent. Hospital Universitário de Brasília, 2014.

and community resources was regarded as limited. In the view of respondents, the care delivery was not shared between the HUB and community organizations.

A pronounced contrast was observed in the component "Organization of healthcare," rated as basic (mean, 3) by the point of care staff, but as good (mean, 8) by the managing board (**Figure 3**). Health professionals acknowledged the role of organizational leadership in effecting changes in PLWHA care. However, they viewed the organizational goals as unclear and the strategies for improvement as restricted to emergency solutions, which are devised and implemented on a case-by-case basis as problems arise. Incentives and regulations for professionals were not employed for PLWHA management purposes.

Next, the components mean scores were analyzed individually to assess how each indicator contributed to the mentioned results. The capacity for self-management support was deemed good (mean score 6) by health professionals. Particularly, they acknowledged the role played by the psychosocial support center in assisting the healthcare team to empower and provide psychosocial support to PLWHA. In general, all the points of care showed engagement with contexts related to treatment adherence, and commitment to seeking suitable solutions for each individual user.

The capacity for clinical decision support was rated as basic (mean score 5) by health professionals who viewed the involvement of other specialists in PLWHA care as limited. Among the healthcare team, continuing education was pursued either by holding weekly meetings to discuss clinical cases and scientific papers or at the personal initiative of staff members, often without acknowledgment from the managing board. The Ministry of Health rarely provided updates or refresher courses on national clinical guidelines. PLWHA had access to information on clinical guidelines (verbally or in the form of educational materials) only upon request. The Com-Vivência center continually added this information to the strategies for self-management support.

Delivery system design was rated as basic (mean score 5) by health professionals. The *Com-Vivência* and emergency service were described as the principal entry points. Although PLWHA can use the entire range of services available from the hospital, their delivery system design takes place primarily at the points of care identified, which, however, are not coordinated for multiprofessional teamwork. There is a chief of staff who heads each of these services, but leadership was not clearly perceived by respondents. A medical appointment management system is currently in operation, and periodic appointments with a single specialist are given priority. PLWHA monitoring complies with clinical guidelines or is tailored to the patient's needs, being mostly performed by the outpatient clinic for IPDs and the *Com-Vivência* center. Programmed care was only available for complications or when requested by users. Because neither referral nor return-referral system is in operation, it has been dealt with in a non-standardized, case-by-case manner. Communication between points of care was poor.

Health professionals assigned the lowest score to the clinical information system, evaluated as limited (mean score 1), since the HUB has no electronic outpatient registry or outpatient medical record system. In fact, each point of care has its own record system—paper-based, except at the inpatient unit for IPDs. The outpatient pharmacy employs an electronic system for drug dispensing control, managed by the Ministry of Health, but does not keep clinical records. Pharmacy staff has access only to data retrievable from medical records or directly informed by users. The healthcare team has standardized a care delivery plan for PLWHA.

The indicators rated as limited (ACIC mean score ≤ 2) are shown in **Figure 4**, based on a stratified analysis of all 35 ACIC indicators.

DISCUSSION

The ACIC is a comprehensive tool designed to represent poor to optimal healthcare management and support, assessing technical and interpersonal processes which may influence the quality of care (Donabedian, 1988). It may be applied to all chronic conditions or constellations of conditions (Bonomi et al., 2002; Hibbard and Greene, 2013). The proposal of ACIC being applied for HIV/AIDS care in Brazil is innovative and it fulfills an important gap in the assessment of quality of care. Despite of being an external tool for assessment of quality of care, Qualiaids is not able to measure the nuances of interpersonal processes. For this, both questionnaires, ACIC and Qualiaids, could support the improvement of quality of care for PLWHA, as the ACIC tool complements the Qualiaids as a self-assessment tool in the perspective of improving results.

Moreover, the application of ACIC is fast and each indicator facilitates discussion, converging to a consensus. The highest score describes the optimal practice, situating the best position that an organization could reach during the diagnoses, the intervention or the assessment (Bonomi et al., 2002; Moysés et al., 2012). Therefore, this questionnaire quickly highlights which areas of the healthcare need to be improved, delivers guidance along this process and monitors progress over time in order to promote a comprehensive care (Bonomi et al., 2002; Drabo et al., 2010; Schwab et al., 2014).

The ACIC proved useful as a soft technology for the situational diagnosis of healthcare delivered to PLWHA at the teaching hospital in the Brazilian setting. The questionnaire fostered discussions within the healthcare team, encouraging its members to actively seek approaches for improvement.

The self-assessment of the hospital's capacity of care delivery to PLWHA, rated as basic (mean score 4), was the main finding emerging from the ACIC instrument, revealing that several aspects need to be improved for a proper management addressing chronic conditions. A literature survey retrieved a single study that applied the complete ACIC to HIV/AIDS care. The study, by Drabo et al. (2010), comprised three hospitals and eight healthcare centers randomly selected from three districts in Burkina Faso and yielded a mean score of 4, assigning basic capacity to PLWHA care (Drabo et al., 2010). In both studies, healthcare system

Organization of healthcare

- Organizational goals for PLWHA care
- Regulation and incentives for PLWHA management

Resources from the community

- Partnerships with community-based organizations

Clinical information system

- Electronic clinical records
- Patient registry (organized by specific condition)
- Alerts to health professionals about situations of risk
- Feedback to healthcare teams
- Relevant information on subgroups of users requiring specialized services

Integration of CCM components

- Community programs
- Formulation and monitoring of goals in PLWHA care plans

FIGURE 4 | Assessment of Chronic Illness Care indicators rated as having limited healthcare capacity. Hospital Universitário de Brasília, 2014.

organization was rated as basic. In the present study, the organizational goals, strategies to improve healthcare delivery, and regulation and incentives to professionals, all of which were rated lowest, were the indicators that most influenced the global result.

The differences observed in the perceptions held by health professionals and managing board indicate the need for greater transparency in leadership responsibilities and organizational strategies for PLWHA care. Institutional goals and plans were viewed as poorly defined, a feature that can undermine the motivation of health professionals (Wagner et al., 2001). Proactive leaderships, capable of establishing rapport with team members, are associated with a more positive stance in the workplace and greater commitment of staff, translating to consistent, effective changes in care delivery (Wagner et al., 2001; Benzer et al., 2011). Lack of interest and poor commitment of team leaders, absence of committed professionals, and the unavailability of updated information technologies seem to negatively impact CCM implementation. Having contradictory results is intrinsic of ACIC questionnaire, that is why it should be applied periodically (at least once every 6 months), from the perspective that with each new assessment the results will come closer to reality in order to improve quality of care (Improving Chronic Illness Care [ICIC], 2018). Further studies to clarify conditions predictive of CCM success are warranted (Coleman et al., 2009; Davy et al., 2015).

Both studies highlighted low or ineffective use of community resources. In our study an interaction of the health service with the community resources and non-governmental organizations were highly limited. However, Drabo et al. (2010) reported

that, despite the absence of formal partnership arrangements, the institutions investigated worked with community-based organizations, promoting joint efforts, with gains for PLWHA.

Using community resources minimizes duplication of effort, reduces healthcare system costs, and raises the quality of care delivered (Wagner et al., 2005; Mendes, 2011).

On the other hand, in both studies the best rating was assigned to self-management support, for its emphasis on providing advice at treatment outset, combined with individual appointments and peer group support. Studies have shown promising results of interventions designed to promote self-management and user empowerment, even when support is provided via telephone calls (Wagner et al., 2001; Damush et al., 2010). Interventions should be user-centered, provide support and health education to enhance the user's ability in the management of their condition. Additionally, psychosocial support to users and their families should be offered (Damush et al., 2010; Malta and Merhy, 2010; Tu et al., 2013).

Both clinical decision support and delivery system design were rated as basic by Drabo et al. (2010) and likewise in the present study. Poor communication between specialists and other professionals, including primary care physicians, characteristic of the current referral and return-referral system, was perceived as a hurdle to be overcome. A comprehensive care requires smoother communication among all providers to accomplish an individualized therapeutic plan (Barceló et al., 2010; Mendes, 2011).

At the teaching hospital, clinical decision support to PLWHA followed the *Clinical protocol and therapeutic guidelines for management of HIV infection*, in compliance with recommendations of the Ministry of Health (Ministério da

Saúde, 2015a). In contrast with the obstacles to the provision of antiretroviral therapy reported for Burkina Faso (Drabo et al., 2010), Brazil ensures free access to antiretroviral therapy to all PLWHA, managed through the National Medication Logistics Control System. This contrast reveals a weakness of the ACIC instrument in the evaluation of a crucial measure, the access of PLWHA to drug therapy, since the questionnaire assigned the same score to the two very different policies adopted by each respective country.

While Drabo et al. (2010) reported a lack of health professionals, the present study revealed obstacles in multidisciplinary training and in communication across points of care. The aggregation of pharmacists, nurses, and social workers to the service network and the promotion of communication across points of care as routine are expected to decrease teamwork fragmentation, ultimately allowing the monitoring of users, to meet the needs of this population. Multiprofessional teamwork has been associated with positive functional outcomes in users with chronic conditions (Bodenheimer et al., 2009; Carter et al., 2009).

The clinical information system was critical in both studies. Incomplete and paper-based records not only have a detrimental effect on the management of interventions, but also preclude reliable evaluation of the quality of care delivered, increasing the likelihood of medical error (Hillestad et al., 2005; Chaudhry et al., 2006; Kalogriopoulos et al., 2009). Safety can be increased with the use of electronic clinical records, as well as by employing more low-tech resources such as reminders, alerts, brochures, and letters tailored for users. Electronic prescriptions, combined with ready access to clinical information from different services and points of care, contribute toward comprehensiveness in care delivery. The benefits of clinical information systems have been observed in health promotion efforts and in the prevention of complications and risk factors (Hillestad et al., 2005; Chaudhry et al., 2006; Carter et al., 2009; Kalogriopoulos et al., 2009). However, these systems typically require large investments in material and human resources to become efficient and can often be met with resistance by health professionals. Nonetheless, clinical information systems can be convenient facilitating tools, although insufficient to transform the healthcare system by themselves (Tomasi et al., 2004; Hillestad et al., 2005; Kalogriopoulos et al., 2009).

Some of observed limitations about the ACIC questionnaire should be considered. It is a technology that qualifies but does not describe all the pieces of evidence related to care – as structure, process and outcomes at Donabedian evaluation; in this sense, it must be analyzed according to the local context and other supportive data. Importantly, this tool is not a "step-by-step," detailed evaluation about the care process, but it provides the pillars to reach high quality of care (Bonomi et al., 2002; Drabo et al., 2010). The consensus method is important to gather every opinion and summarize them in only one. However, it could conceal biases because of the opinion coming from a person in leadership role during the process. For this, we stratified datareal to board manager and health professionals.

Besides, in the first assessment, we could observe that the teams frequently over- or underestimate the quality of care as a result from the misperception of the care they are providing. However, during the CCM Framework implementation process the teams notice what effective care is and their scores could decrease or increase depending on their recently acquired knowledge. When the capability of comprehensive care increases and teams continue implementing effective changes, these scores tend to be improved. Of note, most studies that applied CCM Framework and ACIC addressed a variety of chronic conditions other than HIV/AIDS (Mendes, 2011; Schwab et al., 2014). Therefore, there is a scarce evidence for HIV assessment with this technology, allowing mild consistency about the strengths and limitations in the tool application.

CONCLUSION

Despite the limitations, we considered that the ACIC succeeds to evaluate the key components for a comprehensive healthcare, encourages reflection from the healthcare team at the HUB, generates helpful discussions, raises awareness among the professionals overwhelmed with service routines, and indicates goals to be pursued to improve the quality of healthcare for PLWHA.

In summary, the ACIC technology proved useful for the situational diagnosis of healthcare delivery to PLWHA at a teaching hospital in Brazil. ACIC concomitant application with Qualiaids provides interpersonal processes indicators, often disregarded in most assessments, which would improve the PLWHA quality of care. Additional aspects to be explored include the ACIC use in other settings, interventions evaluations and monitoring and the CCM implementation at institutions that provide healthcare improvement to PLWHA.

AUTHOR CONTRIBUTIONS

AS and MM designed this work, drafted, and reviewed the manuscript. MT and EN reviewed the draft. All authors approved the manuscript for publication and agreed to be accountable for all aspects of this work.

FUNDING

The investigation was part of the subproject entitled Evaluation of care delivery to and pharmacotherapeutic follow-up of people living with HIV/AIDS treated at the Hospital Universitário de Brasília, funded with resources from the project Improving management, surveillance, prevention, and control of STDs, AIDS, and viral hepatites among drug users, sex workers, inmates, and people living with HIV/AIDS, run by the Brazilian Ministry of Health (Grant No. 01/2013).

REFERENCES

Barceló, A., Cafiero, E., de Boer, M., Mesa, A. E., Lopez, M. G., Jiménez, R. A., et al. (2010). Using collaborative learning to improve diabetes care and outcomes: the VIDA project. *Prim. Care Diabetes* 4, 145–153. doi: 10.1016/j.pcd.2010.04.005

Benzer, J. K., Young, G., Stolzmann, K., Osatuke, K., Meterko, M., Caso, A., et al. (2011). The relationship between organizational climate and quality of chronic disease management. *Health Serv. Res.* 46, 691–711. doi: 10.1111/j.1475-6773.2010.01227.x

Berenguer, J., Álvarez, D., Dodero, J., and Azcoaga, A. (2018). Modelo de seguimiento, organización y gestión de la infección por VIH. *Enferm. Infecc. Microbiol. Clín.* 36, 45–49. doi: 10.1016/S0213-005X(18)30247-7

Bodenheimer, T., Chen, E., and Bennett, H. D. (2009). Confronting the growing burden of chronic disease: can the U.S. health care workforce do the job? *Health Affairs* 28, 64–74. doi: 10.1377/hlthaff.28.1.64

Bonomi, A. E., Wagner, E. H., Glasgow, R. E., and Vonkorff, M. (2002). Assessment of Chronic Illness Care (ACIC): a practical tool to measure quality improvement. *Health Serv. Res.* 37, 791–820. doi: 10.1111/1475-6773.00049

BRASIL (1999). *Ministério Da Saúde. Política Nacional De DST/Aids - Princípios E Diretrizes.* Available at: http://bvsms.saude.gov.br/bvs/publicacoes/cd03_17.pdf

Carter, B. L., Ardery, G., Dawson, J. D., James, P. A., Bergus, G. R., Doucette, W. R., et al. (2009). Physician and pharmacist collaboration to improve blood pressure control. *Arch. Intern. Med.* 169, 1996–2002. doi: 10.1001/archinternmed.2009.358

Chaudhry, B., Wang, J., Wu, S., Maglione, M., Mojica, W., Roth, E., et al. (2006). Systematic review: impact of health information technology on quality, efficiency, and costs of medical care. *Ann. Intern. Med.* 144, 742–752. doi: 10.7326/0003-4819-144-10-200605160-00125

Clarke, C. M., Cheng, T., Reims, K. G., Steinbock, C. M., Thumath, M., Milligan, R. S., et al. (2015). Implementation of HIV treatment as prevention strategy in 17 Canadian sites: immediate and sustained outcomes from a 35-month Quality Improvement Collaborative. *BMJ Qual. Saf.* 25, 345–354. doi: 10.1136/bmjqs-2015-004269

Coleman, K., Austin, B. T., Brach, C., and Wagner, E. H. (2009). Evidence on the Chronic Care Model in the new millennium. *Health Affairs* 28, 75–85. doi: 10.1377/hlthaff.28.1.75

Damush, T. M., Jackson, G. L., Powers, B. J., Bosworth, H. B., Cheng, E., Anderson, J., et al. (2010). Implementing evidence-based patient self-management programs in the veterans health administration: perspectives on delivery system design considerations. *J. Gen. Intern. Med.* 25, 68–71. doi: 10.1007/s11606-009-1123-5

Davy, C., Bleasel, J., Liu, H., Tchan, M., Ponniah, S., and Brown, A. (2015). Factors influencing the implementation of chronic care models: a systematic literature review. *BMC Family Pract.* 16:102. doi: 10.1186/s12875-015-0319-5

Donabedian, A. (1988). The quality of care: how can it be assessed? *JAMA* 260, 1743–1748. doi: 10.1001/jama.1988.03410120089033

Drabo, K. M., Konfe, S., and Macq, J. (2010). Assessment of the health system to support tuberculosis and AIDS care. A study of three rural health districts of burkina faso. *J. Public Health Africa* 1, 11–16. doi: 10.4081/jphia.2010.e4

Epping-Jordan, J. E., Pruitt, S. D., Bengoa, R., and Wagner, E. H. (2004). Improving the quality of health care for chronic conditions. *Qual. Saf. Health Care* 13, 299–305. doi: 10.1136/qshc.2004.010744

Goetz, M. B., Bowman, C., Hoang, T., Anaya, H., Osborn, T., Gifford, A. L., et al. (2008). Implementing and evaluating a regional strategy to improve testing rates in VA patients at risk for HIV, utilizing the QUERI process as a guiding framework?: QUERI series. *Implement. Sci.* 3, 1–13. doi: 10.1186/1748-59 08-3-16

Hibbard, J. H., and Greene, J. (2013). What the evidence shows about patient activation: better health outcomes and care experiences; fewer data on costs. *Health Affairs* 32, 207–214. doi: 10.1377/hlthaff.2012.1061

Hillestad, R., Bigelow, J., Bower, A., Girosi, F., Meili, R., Scoville, R., et al. (2005). Can electronic medical record systems transform health care? Potential health benefits, savings, and costs. *Health Affairs* 24, 1103–1117. doi: 10.1377/hlthaff.24.5.1103

Improving Chronic Illness Care [ICIC] (2018). *The Chronic Care Model.* Available at: http://www.improvingchroniccare.org

Kalogriopoulos, N. A., Baran, J., Nimunkar, A. J., and Webster, J. G. (2009). "Electronic medical record systems for developing countries: review," in *Proceedings of the 2009 Annual International Conference of the IEEE Engineering in Medicine and Biology Society,* (Piscataway, NJ), 1730–1733. doi: 10.1109/IEMBS.2009.5333561

Mahomed, O. H., and Asmall, S. (2015). Development and implementation of an integrated chronic disease model in South Africa: lessons in the management of change through improving the quality of clinical practice. *Int. J. Integr. Care* 15:e038. doi: 10.5334/ijic.1454

Malta, D. C., and Merhy, E. E. (2010). O percurso da linha do cuidado sob a perspectiva das doenças crônicas não transmissíveis. *Interface Commun. Health Educ.* 14, 593–605. doi: 10.1590/S1414-32832010005000010

Massoud, M. R., Shakir, F., Livesley, N., Muhire, M., Nabwire, J., Ottosson, A., et al. (2015). Improving care for patients on antiretroviral therapy through a gap analysis framework. *AIDS* 29, S187–S194. doi: 10.1097/QAD.0000000000000742

Mendes, E. V. (2011). *As Redes De Atenção À Saúde,* 2nd Edn. Brasília: Organização Pan-Americana da Saúde, 549.

Ministério da Saúde (2015a). *Protocolo Clínico E Diretrizes Terapêuticas Para Manejo Da Infecção Pelo HIV Em Adultos.* Brasília: Ministério da Saúde, 227.

Ministério da Saúde (2015b). *The Brazilian Response to HIV and AIDS: Global AIDS Response Progress Reporting.* Brasília: Ministério da Saúde, 67.

Ministério da Saúde [MS] (2017). *Boletim Epidemiológico HIV/Aids.* 5:1–64. Brazil: Ministério da Saúde.

Moysés, S. T., Filho, S. A. D., and Moysés, S. J. (2012). *Laboratório De Inovações No Cuidado Das Condições Crônicas Na APS: A Implantação Do Modelo De Atenção Às Condições Crônicas Na UBS Alvorada Em Curitiba, Paraná.* Brasília: Organização Pan-Americana da Saúde/Conselho Nacional de Secretarios de Saude, 193.

Pasricha, A., Deinstadt, R. T., Moher, D., Killoran, A., Rourke, S. B., and Kendall, C. E. (2013). Chronic care model decision support and clinical information systems interventions for people living with HIV: a systematic review. *J. Gen. Intern. Med.* 28, 127–135. doi: 10.1007/s11606-012-2145-y

Schwab, G. L., Moysés, S. T., Kusma, S. Z., Ignácio, S. A., and Moysés, S. J. (2014). Percepção de inovações na atenção às doenças/condições crônicas: uma pesquisa avaliativa em Curitiba. *Saúde Em Debate* 38, 307–318. doi: 10.5935/0103-1104.2014S023

Tomasi, E., Facchini, L. A., Maia, M., and de, F. S. (2004). Health information technology in primary health care in developing countries: a literature review. *Bull. World Health Organ.* 82, 867–874.

Tu, D., Pedersen, J. S., Belda, P., Littlejohn, D., Valle-Rivera, J., and Tyndall, M. (2013). Adoption of the chronic care model to improve HIV care in a marginalized, largely aboriginal population. *Cana. Family Phys.* 59, 650–657.

United Nations Programme on HIV/AIDS [UNAIDS] (2018). *2018 PROGRESS Reports Submitted by Countries: Brazil.* Genebra: UNAIDS.

Universidade de São Paulo [USP] (2018). *QualiAids.* Available at: http://www.qualiaids.fm.usp.br/index.html

Wagner, E. H., Austin, B. T., Davis, C., Hindmarsh, M., Schaefer, J., and Bonomi, A. (2001). Improving chronic illness care: translating evidence into action. *Health Affairs* 20, 64–78. doi: 10.1377/hlthaff.20.6.64

Wagner, E. H., Bennett, S. M., Austin, B. T., Greene, S. M., Schaefer, J. K., and Vonkorff, M. (2005). Finding common ground: patient-centeredness and evidence-based chronic illness care. *J. Altern. Complement. Med.* 11, S7–S15. doi: 10.1089/acm.2005.11.s-7

Wagner, E. H. (1998). Chronic disease management: what will take to improve care for chronic illness? *Eff. Clin. Pract.* 1, 2–4.

World Health Organization [WHO] (2013). *Global Action Plan for the Prevention and Control of Noncommunicable Diseases 2013-2020.* Geneva: World Health Organization, 55.

World Health Organization [WHO] (2018). *Data and Statistics, HIV.* Available at: http://www.who.int/hiv/data/en/

6

Ensuring Privacy when Integrating Patient-Based Datasets: New Methods and Developments in Record Linkage

Adrian P. Brown, Anna M. Ferrante*, Sean M. Randall, James H. Boyd and James B. Semmens

Centre for Population Health Research, Curtin University, Bentley, WA, Australia

*Correspondence:
Anna M. Ferrante
a.ferrante@curtin.edu.au

In an era where the volume of structured and unstructured digital data has exploded, there has been an enormous growth in the creation of data about individuals that can be used for understanding and treating disease. Joining these records together at an individual level provides a complete picture of a patient's interaction with health services and allows better assessment of patient outcomes and effectiveness of treatment and services. Record linkage techniques provide an efficient and cost-effective method to bring individual records together as patient profiles. These linkage procedures bring their own challenges, especially relating to the protection of privacy. The development and implementation of record linkage systems that do not require the release of personal information can reduce the risks associated with record linkage and overcome legal barriers to data sharing. Current conceptual and experimental privacy-preserving record linkage (PPRL) models show promise in addressing data integration challenges. Enhancing and operationalizing PPRL protocols can help address the dilemma faced by some custodians between using data to improve quality of life and dealing with the ethical, legal, and administrative issues associated with protecting an individual's privacy. These methods can reduce the risk to privacy, as they do not require personally identifying information to be shared. PPRL methods can improve the delivery of record linkage services to the health and broader research community.

Keywords: record linkage, data integration, privacy, encryption, data quality, linkage quality

INTRODUCTION

Unabating growth in the creation of data, coupled with advances in information technology and Internet connectivity, provides tremendous potential for data-driven breakthroughs in the understanding, treatment, and prevention of disease. These health research innovations are being complemented by data from non-traditional sources (i.e., from sources other than administrative health and survey records). Opportunities include the use of mobile phone records (1) and Google search histories (2) for disease surveillance, patient collected data from wearable devices (3), and manual journaling through mobile phone applications (4). Data from the private health sector and government administrative datasets that lie outside the health sector (5) are also of interest, as is spatial information that has direct application for understanding exposures and inequalities (6).

Genetic information unavailable a generation ago is already used in clinical decision making (7), and its importance is only likely to increase. The key to unlocking these data is in relating details at an individual patient level to provide an understanding of risk factors and appropriate interventions (8).

A key methodology that has supported health research is record linkage, a process of accurately bringing together records from multiple datasets that belong to the same person. Through record linkage, it has been possible to construct and analyze population-wide datasets comprising "linked" administrative records pertaining to each individual. Health-based record linkage frameworks have been established, which routinely integrate data from hospital admissions, emergency departments, primary care facilities, birth, death, and disease registries (1, 2), creating a rich analytic resource to support evidence-based decision making (9–11).

Present models of record linkage use trusted third parties (TTPs) or data linkage units (DLUs) to accurately match records using personal identifiers (12). Incorporating information from new and diverse data sources into these linkage frameworks are likely to have significant benefits to research; however, the operational and administrative overheads are substantial. Technical issues (i.e., scalability, efficiency) and effects on linkage quality (accuracy) will also be impacted and need to be assessed.

Sharing of public and private datasets also presents privacy and confidentiality challenges. Protecting the privacy of individuals is paramount in the record linkage process and essential to maintain community support and trust. There are serious ethical implications in combining information on individuals (generally without direct consent) from government and other sources; essentially a form of surveillance of an entire population. For some privacy advocates, this is a bridge too far, conjuring up images of an Orwellian dystopia or the excesses of totalitarian regimes (13, 14). Health researchers argue that privacy risks can be minimized and that the public benefit of utilizing these rich datasets outweighs the risk to privacy; that is, there is an ethical imperative to conduct record linkage for research (15). The public's view on this issue is not always clear; numerous surveys have been conducted in Australia, which sometimes return contradictory results regarding Australian views on the use of personal health information [see Ref. (16). for a review]. Similar contradictions have been observed in results from Canadian surveys (14).

While a number of existing processes and techniques are used to maintain patient privacy during record linkage (17), the development of new and improved linkage methods may provide an opportunity for alternative approaches that further reduce privacy risks without compromising on linkage quality.

This article discusses the emergence and potential benefit of record linkage techniques that limit the release of personal identifiers for linkage. These methods, collectively referred to as privacy-preserving record linkage (PPRL), operate in such a way that they do *not* require the release of personally identifying information by data custodians. PPRL methods work on information that has been permanently encoded, encrypted, or transformed before releasing the data for linkage. Through PPRL methods, the benefits of linkage can be realized without the risks associated with disclosure of personal information.

EXISTING RECORD LINKAGE FRAMEWORKS

There is a long history in Australia of record linkage supporting both jurisdictional level and national research and health decision making (10, 12, 18). Record linkage capabilities in all jurisdictions (19–21) have recently been strengthened, and in many cases expanded, through strategic national investment: through the National Collaborative Research Infrastructure Strategy in Australia; the Canadian Institutes of Health Research in Canada; and through the Farr Institute initiative in the United Kingdom (22).

The record linkage framework adopted by most of these jurisdictions is a TTP model, whereby dedicated linkage units undertake record linkage to service and support research. Administrative data collections (such as hospital discharges, emergency presentations, mortality, and cancer registers) have typically formed the backbone of enduring record linkage systems (18, 23). Such collections are highly confidential, containing sensitive personal information that is protected by law.

RECORD LINKAGE AND PRIVACY

Linkage of person-level records through the use of personally identifying information, and generally without consent, has significant ethical and legal implications that have been at the forefront of issues confronted and addressed by DLUs (12, 24).

The extent to which data can be used in record linkage depends on the applicable legislation in each jurisdiction. Some administrative collections are bound by specific laws which either prohibit or severely curtail the release of personal information from these systems.[1] It has been claimed that more than 500 secrecy and privacy provisions exist in Australian Commonwealth laws, imposing considerable limits on the availability and use of identifiable data (25). At Commonwealth level, privacy laws permit some level of disclosure of personal information by authorities for human research (*Commonwealth Privacy Act 1988 s 95*). The release of personal data for linkage can be authorized if public benefit outweighs the privacy of individuals (26).

Working within these legal frameworks, data custodians, DLUs, and the research community in Australia have developed secure data access and usage models that provide important safeguards to privacy. DLUs have also implemented best practice data governance policies and practices to minimize further the privacy risks posed by their operations (12, 18, 19, 27–29).

This includes utilizing the "separation principle" (30), a simple method for restricting the type of data received by each organization in the linkage process. Under this principle, the DLU receives only the personally identifying information required for linkage, but not the content data. The researcher, on the other

---

[1] In Western Australia, for example, both the WA Children's Court Act 1988 and the Young Offenders Act 1994 curtail the release of information for research in relation to juvenile offenders. In South Australia, state-based regulations restrict the release of information from the SA Perinatal Statistics Collection (SA Health Care Variation Regulations 2010, Reg 4). Similar legal barriers exist in other jurisdictions, both locally and internationally.

hand, receives only the content but not personal identifying information. Only the data custodian has access to both personal identifying information and clinical content data.

The use of the separation principle greatly enhances privacy. However, in many instances, the risk to privacy can be still large. For instance, knowledge that a particular individual has a record within a data collection is itself revealing, especially for specific data collections such as mental health inpatient datasets or cancer registries. This information will be still provided to the linkage unit under the separation principle.

The release of personally identifying information always carries some additional risk, as more individuals have access to this information. While rare, attempting to determine whether a person of interest is contained within a dataset does occur; for instance, US intelligence agents have used their surveillance capabilities to spy on romantic interests (31), as have Australian telecommunications workers (32).

Some custodians remain averse to the release of personal information for reasons that extend beyond privacy risks, such as discrimination, reputational damage and/or embarrassment, criminal misuse of the data, and commercial harm (25).

Legislative barriers and risk aversion by data custodians are currently being challenged by open data policies and a growing need by and for government to work with private industry to more effectively service community needs. A recent Productivity Commission Inquiry into the benefits and costs of increasing the availability and use of public and private sector data recognizes the barriers and risks associated with working with named data (25). The Inquiry outlines a framework for data sharing underpinned by legislative change, governance structures (to remove blocks and increase data access), and the development of "systems and processes […] to identify, assess, manage and mitigate risks related not just to data release and sharing, but also data collection and storage" [(25), p.9].

The issues being encountered in Australia are shared internationally. DLUs in the United States, Canada, and Europe face similar legal and risk-related hurdles (e.g., the United States: *Health Insurance Portability and Accountability Act 1996*, Canada: *Personal Health Information Protection Act 2004*, and Europe: *Data Protection Directive 95/46/EC*). German laws in relation to the disclosure of personal information are particularly restrictive (*Bundesdatenschutzgesetz—Federal Data Protection Act of Germany*) and, in some cases, only a single data item can be used for anonymous linkage (33).

PRIVACY-PRESERVING SOLUTIONS

Privacy-preserving record linkage protocols utilize algorithms and techniques to conduct linkage on encrypted or masked information; these methods do not require data custodians to release personal identifiers to third parties. This reduces the risks associated with the release of personal data. Three important attributes characterize all PPRL protocols: accuracy, efficiency, and privacy.

Different classes of privacy-preserving linkage methods provide differing levels of privacy protection. These range from techniques such as the statistical linkage key that simply amalgamates parts of a person's identifiers into a single variable (34) to methods

that encrypt or encode the data so that those with access cannot learn any information directly from the encrypted values. The exact level of privacy required will always depend on context, but all things being equal, a protocol with higher privacy is preferred.

An important difference in PPRL protocols is the method of matching which impacts on linkage quality (accuracy). Protocols may perform matching on a particular set of identifiers, using either exact or similarity comparisons. Similarity matching enables records with slight differences to come together, which is vital for obtaining high-quality linkage results (accuracy). For this reason, PPRL protocols that utilize approximate matching are favored.

Efficiency can be often a concern for record linkage and will continue to present challenges to DLUs as the volume of data continues to grow. Although there are no established performance standards, record linkage is computationally slow, and for any PPRL protocol to be practical, it must complete within a reasonable time frame.

The extent to which these protocols are used in practice varies. To date, most PPRL implementations use exact matching on particular attributes of a dataset (35), which are typically irreversibly encoded to ensure privacy (36). Though efficient, these methods have reduced linkage quality and, therefore, are operationally unsuitable in DLUs.

Of all PPRL methods, the Bloom filter method appears to be the most promising for operational use (37). An advantage of the Bloom method over other PPRL methods is that it utilizes approximate matching while providing similar or superior privacy protection. The method has been evaluated on large-scale, real world health datasets, with results returning equal linkage quality and similar efficiency to traditional linkage methods (which use personal identifiers in the matching process) (38). No record linkage method, privacy preserving or not, achieves perfect accuracy—to be able to achieve equal accuracy to the standard non-privacy-preserving approach is a considerable accomplishment. The security of the protocol has been rigorously investigated (39–41). Cryptographic attacks on the algorithm found ways to reveal some identifiers (40). However, modifications to the protocol have rendered these attacks fruitless (42); there are currently no known security vulnerabilities with the protocol.

The introduction of the Bloom filter method brings new challenges (17). As well as operational requirements around designing optimal linkage strategies, new ways of validating record linkage results need to be developed. In traditional record linkage, linkage results are validated through clerical inspection (or "manual review") of personal identifiers; however, in a privacy-preserved context where all data are encoded, there is no way to manually review the data or correct possible data or linkage errors. New methods for validating linkage results under privacy-preserved linkage model are emerging, however (43).

PPRL: AN EXAMPLE

Consider the (hypothetical) scenario: to attempt to reduce the rate of youth suicide, the government of the day has invested in a comprehensive mental health care package for those who have attempted suicide. The government wishes to see whether their program has worked in reducing the rate of suicide and attempted suicide.

To answer this question, two datasets will be required: a hospital admissions dataset and a mortality register. From the hospital admissions dataset, records will be required to be sent to the linkage unit for all those persons who have attempted suicide before and after the start of the health intervention; all records from the mortality register will be required by the linkage unit. The linkage unit will receive only the personal identifying information required for linkage (i.e., name, date of birth, gender, address). The linkage unit identifies which records from the supplied hospital dataset have associated mortality records. The linkage unit passes this information back to the data custodians, who then provide the content data (i.e., not personally identifying information) to the researcher for the hospital records, and any linked mortality records, along with a key that identifies which records belong to which individual. The researcher can then use this information to determine whether the intervention reduced suicide and attempted suicide rates.

The privacy risk in the aforementioned scenario is the delivery to the linkage unit of personal identifying information from hospital records of those who have attempted suicide. This extremely sensitive information has been made available to a third party. The use of privacy-preserving linkage methods would remove this risk; instead, the linkage unit would receive encrypted personal identifiers; they would have no means of identifying any of these individuals, but would still have the ability to determine which records belong to the same individual between datasets.

GROWING INTERNATIONAL INTEREST IN PPRL

With a growing demand for linked data from government and the university sector, interest in PPRL, particularly the Bloom filter method, is flourishing. Interest stems from two principal sources: at a technical level, by computer scientists and cryptographers with interests in information and data security, and at an operational level, by groups with interest in and responsibility for delivering record linkage services.

Several groups are actively developing and refining PPRL methods at the scientific level including the German Record Linkage Center (University of Duisburg-Essen) (44, 45), the Research School of Computer Science (Australian National University) (46–48), and the Health Information Privacy Laboratory (Vanderbilt University) (39, 49). Researchers from these groups and others recently participated in a 2016 Data Linkage and Anonymisation programme at the Isaac Newton Institute for Mathematical Sciences (Cambridge University, supported by EPSRC grant no EP/K032208/1)[2]; this 6-month international programme included seminars and workshops on linkage and privacy protection to share and advance knowledge in the mathematical sciences and related disciplines. A key goal of the forum was to "enhance opportunities for the analysis of data,

especially obtained through linkage, whilst protecting privacy and taking account of related practical constraints."

At an operational level, PPRL featured prominently in the 2016 International Population Data Linkage Network Conference (Swansea University), with several presentations on the topic including a keynote session that described a collaboration between international research institutions in Canada, Australia, and Wales (44, 46, 50–53).

OPPORTUNITY AND CHANGE MANAGEMENT

In addition to reducing the privacy risks associated with record linkage, the advent of PPRL protocols potentially heralds a new era of population-focused research using linked data, bridging gaps, and opening up opportunities for new and different forms of linkage-based research. PPRL methods may provide an avenue to access previously "hard to get" datasets (i.e., those with significant legal or regulatory constraints). PPRL methods may also provide a mechanism for accessing and integrating data from new and emerging sources. As well as data from new technologies (e.g., wearable devices, smartphone apps), these new sources may include the private health sector that has, to date, had limited exposure to, and engagement with, data linkage frameworks (54, 55).

New methods may require new or adjusted models of operation. Some custodians have expressed a desire to have flexibility in record linkage models to accommodate the features of different data collections (50). However, different or altered data linkage operating models can have significant implications for end-user timeframes, operational efficiency, and linkage quality (50), and these need to be carefully managed and monitored. It is important that the strengths and limitations of the PPRL methods are understood. This will require conversations with stakeholders (i.e., data custodians, linkage units, researchers, and the community) around the risk–benefit of these new models and the expected realization of public benefit.

CONCLUSION

The implementation of PPRL methods that do not require the release of personal information but protect privacy through other mechanisms (e.g., encryption methods) represents a breakthrough in record linkage, substantially reducing privacy risks without negatively impacting on linkage quality. By utilizing methods that do not require the release of personally identifying information, concerns regarding personal surveillance and government overreach can be allayed. Supplementing traditional linkage methods with PPRL methods will increase the number and type of datasets that can be included in record linkage studies.

The advent of PPRL methods to protect patient privacy expands the toolkit of techniques that are available to DLUs. Used in conjunction with traditional linkage methods, PPRL widens the net of record linkage without compromising privacy or linkage quality. These methods will hopefully allow more diverse, patient-centered data sources to be utilized for health research,

---

[2]https://www.newton.ac.uk/event/dla.

bringing enormous opportunities to increase our understanding of disease and to tailor interventions and treatment to each individual.

AUTHOR CONTRIBUTIONS

AB and AF accept immediate responsibility for the manuscript. AF, AB, SR, JB, and JS each contributed to the conception and design of the paper. AF and AB drafted the first version of the

article, with SR, JB, and JS providing important additional input and intellectual content. All authors were involved in revising the manuscript and approving its final form.

FUNDING

This work was discussed at the Isaac Newton Institute for Mathematical Sciences, Cambridge, supported by EPSRC grant no EP/K032208/1.

REFERENCES

1. Ebola and big data – call for help. *The Economist*. London: The Economist Group (2014).

2. Ginsberg J, Mohebbi MH, Patel RS, Brammer L, Smolinski MS, Brilliant L. Detecting influenza epidemics using search engine query data. *Nature* (2009) 457(7232):1012–4. doi:10.1038/nature07634

3. Pantelopoulos A, Bourbakis NG. A survey on wearable sensor-based systems for health monitoring and prognosis. *IEEE Trans Syst Man Cybern C Appl Rev* (2010) 40(1):1–12. doi:10.1109/TSMCC.2009.2032660

4. Klasnja P, Pratt W. Healthcare in the pocket: mapping the space of mobile-phone health interventions. *J Biomed Inform* (2012) 45(1):184–98. doi:10.1016/j.jbi.2011.08.017

5. Stanley PF. *Developmental Pathways in WA Children Project*. Perth, WA: Chief Investigator and Director, Telethon Institute for Child Health Research (2006–2007).

6. Waller LA, Gotway CA. *Applied Spatial Statistics for Public Health Data*. Hoboken, NJ: John Wiley and Sons (2004).

7. Aronson SJ, Rehm HL. Building the foundation for genomics in precision medicine. *Nature* (2015) 526(7573):336–42. doi:10.1038/nature15816

8. Khoury MJ, Iademarco MF, Riley WT. Precision public health for the era of precision medicine. *Am J Prev Med* (2015) 50(3):398–401. doi:10.1016/j.amepre.2015.08.031

9. Brook EL, Rosman DL, Holman CDAJ. Public good through data linkage: measuring research outputs from the Western Australian Data Linkage System. *Aust N Z J Public Health* (2008) 32(1):19–23. doi:10.1111/j.1753-6405.2008.00160.x

10. Holman CDAJ, Bass AJ, Rosman DL, Smith MB, Semmens JB, Glasson EJ, et al. A decade of data linkage in Western Australia: strategic design, applications and benefits of the WA data linkage system. *Aust Health Rev* (2008) 32(4):766–77. doi:10.1071/AH080766

11. Lyons RA, Ford DV, Moore L, Rodgers SE. Use of data linkage to measure the population health effect of non-health-care interventions. *Lancet* (2014) 383(9927):1517–9. doi:10.1016/S0140-6736(13)61750-X

12. Boyd JH, Ferrante AM, O'Keefe CM, Bass AJ, Randall SM, Semmens JB. Data linkage infrastructure for cross-jurisdictional health-related research in Australia. *BMC Health Serv Res* (2012) 12(1):480. doi:10.1186/1472-6963-12-480

13. Green E, Ritchie F, Mytton J, Webber DJ, Deave T, Montgomery A, et al. *Enabling Data Linkage to Maximise the Value of Public Health Research Data*. London: Wellcome Trust (2015).

14. Upshur RE, Morin B, Goel V. The privacy paradox: laying Orwell's ghost to rest. *Can Med Assoc J* (2001) 165(3):307–9.

15. Hetzel D. Data linkage research – can we reap benefits for society without compromising public confidence? *Aust Health Consum* (2005) 2:27–8.

16. Holman CDAJ. *Anonymity and Research: Health Data and Biospecimen Law in Australia*. Perth: Uniprint, UWA (2012).

17. Boyd JH, Randall SM, Ferrante AM. *Application of Privacy-Preserving Techniques in Operational Record Linkage Centres. Medical Data Privacy Handbook*. Berlin: Springer (2015). p. 267–87.

18. Lawrence G, Dinh I, Taylor L. The centre for health record linkage: a new resource for health services research and evaluation. *Health Inf Manag* (2008) 37(2):60–2. doi:10.1177/183335830803700208

19. Ford DV, Jones KH, Verplancke J-P, Lyons RA, John G, Brown G, et al. The SAIL databank: building a national architecture for e-health research and evaluation. *BMC Health Serv Res* (2009) 9(1):157. doi:10.1186/1472-6963-9-157

20. Martens PJ. Using the repository housed at the Manitoba centre for health policy: learning from the past, planning for the future. In: *Conference Proceedings of the Statistics Canada Conference: Longitudinal Social and Health Surveys in an International Perspective*. Montreal, Quebec (2006).

21. Gill LE. *OX-LINK: The Oxford Medical Record Linkage System. Record Linkage Techniques*. Oxford: University of Oxford (1997). 19 p.

22. Farr Institute. (2016). Available from: http://www.farrinstitute.org/

23. Rosman D, Garfield C, Fuller S, Stoney A, Owen T, Gawthorne G. Measuring data and link quality in a dynamic multi-set linkage system. In: *Symposium on Health Data Linkage*. Sydney (2002). Available from: http://www.phidu.torrens.edu.au/pdf/1999-2004/symposium-proceedings-2003/rosman_a.pdf

24. Hobbs M, McCall M. Health statistics and record linkage in Australia. *J Chronic Dis* (1970) 23(5):375–81. doi:10.1016/0021-9681(70)90020-2

25. Productivity Commission. *Data Availability and Use, Draft Report*. Canberra: Australian Government (2016).

26. Allen J, Holman CDJ, Meslin E, Stanley F. Privacy protectionism and health information: is there any redress for harms to health? *J Law Med* (2013) 21(2):473–85.

27. Harris J. Next generation linkage management system. In: *Sixth Australasian Workshop on Health Informations and Knowledge Management*. Adelaide: Australian Computer Society (2013).

28. Trutwein B, Holman D, Rosman D. Health data linkage conserves privacy in a research-rich environment. *Ann Epidemiol* (2006) 16(4):279–80. doi:10.1016/j.annepidem.2005.05.003

29. Roos LL, Brownell M, Lix L, Roos NP, Walld R, MacWilliam L. From health research to social research: privacy, methods, approaches. *Soc Sci Med* (2008) 66(1):117–29. doi:10.1016/j.socscimed.2007.08.017

30. Kelman CW, Bass AJ, Holman CDJ. Research use of linked health data – a best practice protocol. *Aust N Z J Public Health* (2002) 26(3):251–5. doi:10.1111/j.1467-842X.2002.tb00682.x

31. NSA officers spy on love interests. *Wall Street J* (2013). Available from: http://blogs.wsj.com/washwire/2013/08/23/nsa-officers-sometimes-spy-on-love-interests/

32. Vodafone sacks staff over alleged security breach. *IT News* (2011). Available from: http://www.itnews.com.au/News/244672,vodafone-sacks-staff-over-alleged-security-breach.aspx

33. Bundestag D. Gesetz ueber Krebsregister (Krebsregistergesetz KRG). *Bundesgesetzblatt* (1994) 79:994.

34. Karmel R. *Data Linkage Protocols Using a Statistical Linkage Key*. Canberra: Australian Institute of Health and Welfare (2005).

35. Karmel R, Anderson P, Gibson D, Peut A, Duckett S, Wells Y. Empirical aspects of record linkage across multiple data sets using statistical linkage keys: the experience of the PIAC cohort study. *BMC Health Serv Res* (2010) 10(41):1–13.

36. Quantin C, Bouzelat H, Allaert F, Benhamiche A-M, Faivre J, Dusserre L. How to ensure data security of an epidemiological follow-up: quality assessment of an anonymous record linkage procedure. *Int J Med Inform* (1998) 49(1):117–22. doi:10.1016/S1386-5056(98)00019-7

37. Schnell R, Bachteler T, Reiher J. Privacy-preserving record linkage using Bloom filters. *BMC Med Inform Decis Mak* (2009) 9:41. doi:10.1186/1472-6947-9-41

38. Randall SM, Ferrante AM, Boyd JH, Semmens JB. Privacy-preserving record linkage on large real world datasets. *J Biomed Inform* (2014) 50:205–12. doi:10.1016/j.jbi.2013.12.003

39. A constraint satisfaction cryptanalysis of Bloom filters in private record linkage. In: Kuzu M, Kantarcioglu M, Durham E, Malin B, editors. *Privacy Enhancing Technologies*. Springer (2011).

40. Niedermeyer F, Steinmetzer S, Kroll M, Schnell R. Cryptanalysis of basic Bloom filters used for privacy preserving record linkage. *J Pri Confidentiality* (2014) 6(2):59–79.

41. Kroll M, Steinmetzer S. Automated cryptanalysis of bloom filter encryptions of health records. (2014). arXiv preprint arXiv:14106739.

42. Schnell R, Bachteler T, Reiher J. *A Novel Error-Tolerant Anonymous Linking Code. Working Paper Series No. WP-GRLC-2011-02.* Nürnberg, Germany: German Record Linkage Center (2011).

43. Randall SM, Boyd JH, Ferrante AM, Bauer JK, Semmens JB. Use of graph theory measures to identify errors in record linkage. *Comput Methods Programs Biomed* (2014) 115(2):55–63. doi:10.1016/j.cmpb.2014. 03.008

44. Schnell R, Borgs C. Secure privacy preserving record linkage of large databases by modified Bloom filter encodings. *2016 International Population Data Linkage Conference.* Swansea, Wales: Swansea University (2016).

45. Schnell R, Borgs C. Randomized response and balanced Bloom filters for privacy preserving record linkage. In: *Data Mining Workshops (ICDMW), 2016 IEEE 16th International Conference on.* IEEE (2016). p. 218–24. doi:10.1109/ICDMW.2016.0038

46. Christen P. Advanced computational and privacy methods for data linkage. *2016 International Population Data Linkage Conference.* Swansea, Wales: Swansea University (2016).

47. Vatsalan D, Christen P, O'Keefe C, Verykios V. An evaluation framework for privacy-preserving record linkage. *J Pri Confidentiality* (2014) 6(1):35–75.

48. Vatsalan D, Christen P, Verykios VS. A taxonomy of privacy-preserving record linkage techniques. *Inf Syst* (2013) 38(6):946–69. doi:10.1016/j.is.2012. 11.005

49. Durham EA, Kantarcioglu M, Xue Y, Toth C, Kuzu M, Malin B. Composite bloom filters for secure record linkage. *IEEE Trans Knowl Data Eng* (2014) 26:2956–68. doi:10.1109/TKDE.2013.91

50. Irvine K, Hollis S. Multiple operating models for data linkage: a privacy positive. *2016 International Population Data Linkage Conference.* Swansea, Wales: Swansea University (2016).

51. Pow C, Iron K, Boyd J, Brown A, Thompson S, Chong N, et al. Privacy-preserving record linkage: an international collaboration between Canada, Australia and Wales. *2016 International Population Data Linkage Conference.* Swansea, Wales: Swansea University (2016).

52. Adrian Brown CB, Randall S, Schnell R. High quality linkage using multibit trees for privacy-preserving blocking. *2016 International Population Data Linkage Conference.* Swansea, Wales: Swansea University (2016).

53. Boyd J, Ferrante A, Brown A, Randall S, Semmens J. Implementing privacy-preserving record linkage: welcome to the real world. *2016 International Population Data Linkage Conference.* Swansea, Wales: Swansea University (2016).

54. Holman D, Bass A, Rouse I, Hobbs M. Population-based linkage of health records in Western Australia: development of a health services research linked database. *Aust N Z J Public Health* (1999) 23(5):453–59. doi:10.1111/j.1467-842X.1999.tb01297.x

55. Magnusson RS. Data linkage, health research and privacy: regulating data flows in Australia's health information system. *Syd Law Rev* (2002) 24(1):5–55.

7

Physico-Chemical Characterization and Biopharmaceutical Evaluation of Lipid-Poloxamer-Based Organogels for Curcumin Skin Delivery

Aryane Alves Vigato[1], Samyr Machado Querobino[2], Naially Cardoso de Faria[1], Ana Carolina Bolela Bovo Candido[3], Lizandra Guidi Magalhães[3], Cíntia Maria Saia Cereda[4], Giovana Radomille Tófoli[4], Estefânia Vangelie Ramos Campos[1,5], Ian Pompermayer Machado[6], Leonardo Fernandes Fraceto[5], Mirela Inês de Sairre[1] and Daniele Ribeiro de Araujo[1]*

[1] Human and Natural Sciences Center, ABC Federal University, Santo André, Brazil, [2] Department of Biomedical Sciences, State University of Minas Gerais, Passos, Brazil, [3] Research Group on Natural Products, Center for Research in Sciences and Technology, University of Franca, Franca, Brazil, [4] São Leopoldo Mandic Research Unit, São Leopoldo Mandic Faculty, Campinas, Brazil, [5] Department of Environmental Engineering, State University "Júlio de Mesquita Filho", Sorocaba, Brazil, [6] Department of Fundamental Chemistry, Institute of Chemistry, University of São Paulo, São Paulo, Brazil

*Correspondence:
Daniele Ribeiro de Araujo
daniele.araujo@ufabc.edu.br;
draraujo2008@gmail.com

Organogels (ORGs) are semi-solid materials, in which an organic phase is immobilized by a three-dimensional network composed of self-organized system, forming the aqueous phase. In this context, lipid–Pluronics (PLs) ORGs form a two-phase system which can be effectively used as skin delivery systems, favoring their permeation across the skin. In this study, we presented the development of ORG skin drug-delivery systems for curcumin (CUR), a liposoluble phenolic pigment extracted from the turmeric rhizome. In special, we designed the formulation compositions in order to carry high amounts of CUR soluble in oleic acid (OA), as organic phase, entrapped into an aqueous phase composed of micellar PL-based hydrogels by associating two polymers with different hydrophilic–lipophilic balances, Pluronic F-127 (PL F-127), and Pluronic L-81 (PL L-81), to enhance the permeation across the skin. Results revealed that the incorporation of PL L-81 favored the CUR incorporation into micelle–micelle interface. CUR insertion into OA-PL F-127/L-81 reduced both G'/G" relationship (~16 x) and viscosity values (η^* ~ 54 mPa.s, at 32.5°C), disturbing the ORG network structural organization. *In vitro* permeation assays through Strat-M® skin-model membranes showed that higher CUR-permeated amounts were obtained for OA-PL F-127/L-81 (4.83 µg.cm^{-2}) compared to OA-PL F-127 (3.51 µg.cm^{-2}) and OA (2.25 µg.cm^{-2}) or hydrogels (~1.2 µg.cm^{-2}, p < 0.001). Additionally, ORG formulations presented low cytotoxic effects and evoked pronounced antileishmanial activity (IC_{50} < 1.25 µg.ml^{-1}), suggesting their potential use as skin delivery systems against *Leishmania amazonensis*. Results from this study pointed out OA-PL-based ORGs as promising new formulations for possible CUR topical administration.

Keywords: organogel, pluronic, skin-delivery, curcumin, oleic acid

INTRODUCTION

Curcumin (CUR) and its derivatives have shown a wide variety of biological activities, such as anti-oxidant (Dall'Acqua et al., 2016), anti-inflammatory (Zhu et al., 2016), anti-tumor (Han et al., 2011), antimicrobial (Cetin-Karaca and Newman, 2015), and antiparasitic effects (Morais et al., 2013), as well as for the treatment of ulcers (Magalhaes et al., 2009) and skin diseases (Patel et al., 2009; Rachmawati et al., 2015), among others (Aggarwal and Harikumar, 2009). Despite its efficacy and safety, CUR has not yet been approved as a therapeutic agent (Anand et al., 2008). In addition, due to its physico-chemical limitations such as low aqueous solubility and low bioavailability (Priyadarsini, 2014), several studies have been devoted to developing new pharmaceutical formulations to overcome those limitations. In fact, CUR extensive first-pass biotransformation and low aqueous solubility became an interesting molecule for skin delivery (Anand et al., 2008).

In this context, skin delivery is an important strategy for drug administration, since this procedure is non-invasive and avoids first-pass biotransformation and enables the use of self-administered pharmaceutical forms, improving patient compliance. However, the clinical efficacy of this type of administration depends on the drug physico-chemical and pharmacological properties, as well as its bioavailability at the site of action, which is limited by the low permeability of the stratum corneum (Godin and Touitou, 2007; Prausnit and Langer, 2008). Considering that most skin pathological processes occur locally, CUR topical application may offer the advantage for delivering the molecule into the site of action. Nanocarrier systems such as gels and nanoemulsions can therefore provide the chemical stabilization and permeation of the CUR molecule (Rachmawati et al., 2015).

Among the various nanostructured systems are those formed by the poloxamers or Pluronics® (PL), copolymers used in preformulations such as hydrogels and as aqueous phase of organogels (ORGs). Particularly, as recent hybrid systems, ORGs stand out as semi-solid colloidal systems that has an oil phase dispersed in an aqueous phase, being used as reservoirs for lipophilic molecules. Those systems present advantages over conventional formulations (creams, ointments, hydrogels) due to their ability to incorporate higher concentrations of lipophilic molecules (Patel et al., 2009; Esposito et al., 2018) such as CUR, being capable to modulate the time and rate of skin permeation according to their composition. In fact, lipid (oil or organic phase) and PL (aqueous phase) gels form a two-phase system which can be effectively used as skin delivery promoters for hydrophilic and lipophilic drugs, favoring their permeation across the stratum corneum. Additionally, ORGs present other advantages such as (i) adhesion to the skin due to the formation of a homogeneous film on the stratum corneum surface, (ii) increases the contact area with the application site, (iii) improves the chemical stability of incorporated molecules, and (iv) absence of organic solvents in formulation preparation, which increases the ORG biocompatibility (Vintiloiu and Leroux, 2008; Iwanaga et al., 2012; Esposito et al., 2018).

In this study, we have developed ORGs with organic phase (OP) composed of oleic acid (OA), a free fatty acid ($C_{18}H_{34}O_2$) well-described as permeation enhancer, incorporated into an aqueous phase (AP) containing Pluronic F-127 (PL F-127) isolated or in association with Pluronic L81 (PL L-81). The PL physico-chemical features such as molecular weight (PL F-127 = 12,400 g.mol^{-1} and PL L-81 = 2,800 g.mol^{-1}), hydrophilic–lipophilic balances (HLB, PL F-127 = 22 and PL L-81 = 2), and polypropylene oxide (PPO):polyethylene oxide (PEO) relationships (PL F-127 = ~1:3 PPO:PEO and for PL L-81 = ~7:1 PPO:PEO) provide a differential structural organization (Oshiro et al., 2014) to modulate the CUR permeation. Then, we have studied those ORG systems regarding to their physico-chemical, structural, and biopharmaceutical properties e.g., the micellization process, the sol–gel transition, rheological features, structural organization and–, especially, the influence of OA-PL F-127/L-81 association on CUR permeation profile, photostability, citotoxicty, and its biological activity.

MATERIALS AND METHODS

Chemicals and Reagents

Pluronic® F-127 (PL F-127), Pluronic® L-81 (PL L-81), OA, and CUR were purchased from Sigma–Aldrich (St. Louis, MO, USA). All chemicals and solvents were analytical grade.

High-Performance Liquid Chromatography (HPLC) Analysis

CUR analysis was performed using an HPLC system (Ultimate 3000, Chromeleon 7.2 software, Thermo Fisher Scientific, Waltham, USA) with a gradient pump, DAD detector, and C18 column (150 x 4.6 mm, 5 μm; Phenomenex). Drug samples were analyzed at 425 nm, 0.8 ml/min flow rate at 25°C. The mobile phase was composed by a mixture of acetonitrile and water with acetic acid (0.05%) solution (70:30). The drug retention time was 3.4 min. All results represent three experiments, in 3 days, performed in triplicate. The limits of detection (LD) and quantification (LQ) were determined from a standard curve of CUR at 10, 20, 40, 60, 80, and 100 μg/ml. The LD and LQ values were 0.31 and 0.94 μg/ml, respectively. CUR concentration was determined using the equation y = 2.616x ± 0.003 with correlation coefficient (R^2) value of 0.998.

ORG Preparation

Initially, the AP was prepared by mixing appropriate amounts of PL F-127 (20% wt) isolated or in association with PL L-81 (0.6%) in HPLC-grade water under ice bath with continuous stirring (350 rpm, for at least 12 h) until the solution became transparent. The hydrogels formulations, used in this study as AP, were previously designed and characterized (Oshiro et al., 2014). For OP preparation, CUR (2 mg) was added to 2 ml of OA under magnetic stirring (350 rpm, at 25°C) until the complete drug dissolution. Then, OP was added to the AP (1:4 v/v) and magnetically stirred (350 rpm) until the formation of an homogeneous gel (Boddu et al., 2014; Vigato et al., 2019). Finally, sodium benzoate (0.25% wt) was added to all formulations as a preservative. For comparisons regarding to morphology and permeation profiles, hydrogels were prepared at the same composition from ORG AP. All formulation compositions are presented on **Table 1**.

TABLE 1 | Formulations components for different ORG containing curcumin (CUR).

Formulations	Organic phase (OP)	Aqueous phase (AP)	
	Oleic acid (OA) organic solvent	Pluronic F-127 (F-127, %wt)	Pluronic L-81 (L-81, %wt)
OA-F-127		20	–
OA-F-127–CUR	OA	20	–
OA-F-127/L-81		20	0.6
OA-F-127/L-81–CUR		20	0.6
F-127-H	–	20	–
F-127-CUR-H	–	20	–
F-127/L-81-H	–	20	0.6
F-127/L-81-CUR-H	–	20	0.6

Organic: aqueous phase ratio of 1:4 (OP : AP, v/v); CUR final concentration was 0.1%. H—indicates hydrogels formulations (without oleic acid); OA, oleic acid; PL F-127, Pluronic® F-127; PL L-81, Pluronic® L-81; CUR, curcumin.

Organoleptic Characterization, Drug Content, and pH Determination

The ORG formulations were evaluated by color, odor, and phase separation. The pH measurements were performed for all ORG formulations inserting the probe into the ORGs until the equilibrium determination. For drug content determination, samples of ORGs (0.05 g) were weighted, mixed with 10 ml of acetonitrile:water (70:30 v/v) and sonicated for ~ 20 min. Samples of 1 ml were filtered (nylon syringe filter, 0.22-μm pore) and analyzed by HPLC for determining CUR concentration. Drug content was expressed as a percentage.

Structural and Morphological Analysis

ORG formulations were analyzed by atomic force microscopy (AFM). For samples preparation, a thin film of each formulation was disposed in a glass slide and dried and dripped on a silicon plate. Samples were analyzed in a Nanosurf easyScan 2 Basic microscope (Nanosurf, Switzerland) in non-contact mode in an instrument equipped with a TapAl-G cantilever (BudgetSensors, Bulgaria) operated at a scan rate of 90Hz. Images (256×256 pixels, TIFF format) were captured in time mode and were analyzed using Gwyddion software. In addition, the formulation structural properties were analyzed by X-ray diffraction (XRD) technique, using a Rigaku Miniflex II instrument with CuKα1 radiation (λ = 1.5406 Å). ORG samples were pressed against a glass sample holder to obtain a homogeneous surface and analyzed over the 5–70° 2θ range, employing a 0.05° step with 1 s of integration time.

Differential Scanning Calorimetry (DSC) and Rheological Analysis

Differential scanning calorimetry (DSC) experiments were carried out by a Netzsch DSC Polyma Calorimeter (NETZSCH, Selb, Germany). ORG samples (20 mg) were placed in a sealed aluminum pan and analyzed by three cycles (heating-cooling-heating) from 0 to 50°C at 5°C/min rate. Thermograms were presented as heat flux (J/g) against temperature (°C). For all analyzes, an empty pan was used as the reference.

For rheological analyses, an oscillatory Kinexus rheometer (Malvern Instruments Ltd., UK) with cone-plate geometry was employed. In order to determine the sol–gel transition temperature ($T_{sol–gel}$), the frequency was set at 1 Hz, and a temperature range from 10 to 50°C was used. Additionally, for frequency sweep mode, the temperature was kept at 32.5°C, and formulations were analyzed from 0.1 to 10 Hz. For both measurements, the oscillatory mode was used to obtain the elastic (G') and viscous modulii (G"), as well as viscosity (η^*) values for each formulation. Data were analyzed with the RSpace for Kinexus® software.

In Vitro Permeation Studies

For *in vitro* permeation assays, vertical Franz-type diffusion cells (Vision Microette Plus; Hanson Research, Chatsworth, CA, USA) were used. The cells presented two compartments, donor (1.72 cm² permeation area) and receptor (7 ml), separated by an artificial skin-model membrane (Strat-M® membranes, 25-mm discs, Millipore Co., USA, ultrafiltration membrane, 325 μm thick) (Uchida et al., 2015; Kaur et al., 2018). Each formulation (0.3 g/cm²) was applied to the donor compartment (in contact with the upper surface of the artificial membrane). The receptor compartment was filled with 7 ml of pH 7.4 sodium phosphate (5 mM) with sodium chloride (154 mM) buffer and magnetically stirred (350 rpm) at 32.5 ± 0.5°C for 48 h. During the time interval from 15 min to 48 h, aliquots (1 ml) from the receptor compartment were collected and analyzed by HPLC. All experiments were performed in triplicate. The cumulative amounts of permeated CUR were expressed as μg.cm⁻², and the results were plotted as a function of time (h). For data analyzes, flux values were obtained from the slope of the curve over the 8-h period. Data were analyzed according to the equation (eq. 1):

$$J = P.Cd \tag{1}$$

where J (μg.cm⁻².h⁻¹) is the drug flux across the membrane, P (cm.h⁻¹) is the permeability coefficient, and Cd (μg.cm⁻³) is the drug concentration in the donor compartment. The lag time was calculated by extrapolating a straight line to time axis (de Araujo et al., 2010).

In Vitro Cytotoxicity and Antileishmanial Activity

Epidermal keratinocytes (HaCaT cell line, Thermo Fisher Scientific, Waltham, Massachusetts, USA) were used for the cytotoxicity experiments. Cells were seeded for 48 h in 96-well plates (2.104 cells/well), in Dubelcco's Modified Eagle Medium (DMEM; Gibco Laboratories, Grand Island, NY, USA) with 10% (v/v) fetal bovine serum (pH 7.2–7.4), humidified atmosphere at 37°C and 5% CO₂) and 100 μg.ml⁻¹ of penicillin/streptomycin. For experiment design, ORG formulations were previously diluted in DMEM medium on concentration range from 10 to 100 mg.ml^{-1}, and 200 μl from each solution were used for cell treatment during 24 h. Then, 100 μl of MTT solution (5 mg/ml, in phosphate buffered saline) was added to each well and incubated with cells for 4 h. After that, MTT solution was removed and 50 μl of DMSO added to the wells for 10 min. Absorbance was measured at 570 nm. For comparisons with non-toxicity, cells were treated only with DMEM at the same volume used for ORGs.

For pharmacological assays, in order to evaluate the antileishmanial activity, *Leishmania amazonensis* promastigote forms (MHOM/BR/PH8) were maintained in RPMI 1640 (Gibco) culture medium supplemented with 10% fetal bovine serum, penicillin (100 UI/ml), and streptomycin (100 μg/ml). Subsequently, about 1 x 10^6 parasites were seemed in 96-well plates, and ORGs dissolved in culture medium were added at concentrations from 1.25 to 10 μg.ml^{-1} to the cultures. Amphotericin B (Sigma Aldrich Chem. Co., 97% purity) was added to cultures at concentrations ranging from 0.05 to 0.40 μg/ml and used as positive control. CUR was dissolved in dimethyl sulfoxide (DMSO) and added at same concentrations described before. Cultures were incubated at 25°C for 24 h, and the antileishmanial activity was determined by verifying the growth of the promastigote forms was inhibited, as revealed by counting the total number of live promastigotes using a Neubauer chamber according to the flagellar motility. The results were expressed as the mean of the percentage of growth inhibition relative to the negative control (RPMI 1640 medium+0.1% DMSO or RPMI 1640 medium). Two experiments were performed in triplicate. The 50% inhibitory concentration (IC$_{50}$) values were determined by means of non-linear regression curves using GraphPad Prism version 5.0 software for Windows (GraphPad software, USA) (Bezerra et al., 2006).

Statistical Analysis

Results were presented as mean ± standard deviation. For statistical comparisons, one-way analysis of variance (ANOVA) with Tukey–Kramer *post hoc* test was used. Statistical significance was defined as $p < 0.05$.

RESULTS

Structural and Morphological Characterization, pH, and Drug Content Determination

Before CUR incorporation, ORGs presented white-opaque aspect while hydrogels were colorless and transparent, as observed on **Figures 1 A**, **C**. After CUR incorporation, all formulations became yellow (opaque or clear, **Figures 1 B, D**), and neither particulate materials nor any phase separation were observed. For morphological characterization, AFM images revealed smooth surfaces with small and sparse protuberances for hydrogels (control formulations), as a result of the dry process before analysis. On the other hand, ORG morphology was characterized by wrinkles distributed for all surface, which can be attributed to the incorporation of the OP into the hydrogels forming a system with low water content resulting in a different morphology from hydrogels. Morphological differences between hydrogels and ORGs were also previously described using scanning electron microscopy (SEM) (Vigato et al., 2019). The ORGs were also characterized by X-ray diffraction (XRD), as shown in **Figure 2**. All formulations exhibited the same pattern, with two diffraction peaks at 19 and 23°, which are correspondent to the PL F-127 and crystalline structure (Shin et al., 2000; Saxena et al., 2012). The very broad diffraction peak observed in the diffractograms indicates that the ORGs also exhibit an amorphous character. This feature can be attributed to the presence of OA as OP,

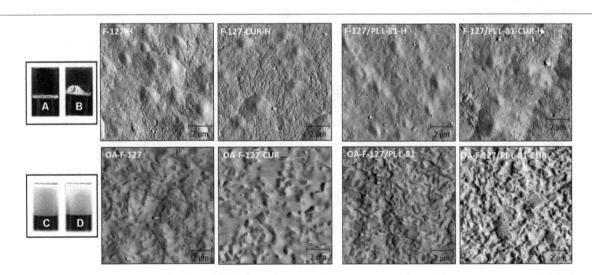

FIGURE 1 | Micrographs for organogels and hydrogel formulations obtained from atomic force microscopy (AFM). **(A)** F-127/L-81-H, **(B)** F-127/L-81-CUR-H, **(C)** OA-F-127/L-81, and **(D)** OA-F-127/L-81-CUR. H—indicates hydrogel formulations (without oleic acid). OA, oleic acid; F-127, Pluronic® F-127; L-81, Pluronic® L-81; CUR, curcumin.

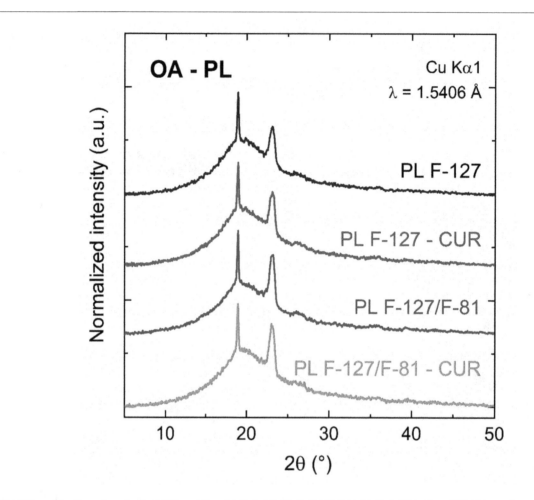

FIGURE 2 | X-ray diffraction patterns for the ORG formulations OA-PL F-127, OA-PL F-127-CUR, OA-PL F-127/L-81, and OA-PL F-127/L-81-CUR (OA, oleic acid; PL F-127, Pluronic® F-127; PL L-81, Pluronic® L-81; and CUR, curcumin.

which disturbs the well-known crystalline nature of PL after incorporation into the formulations.

The pH values for ORG formulations were from 5.5 to 5.9, for OA-PL F-127 and OA-PL F-127/L-81, even after CUR incorporation. Those results are in agreement with previous reports about other ORG compositions such as lanolin-PL F-127 (Vigato et al., 2019), ricinoleic acid-PL F-127 (Boddu et al., 2015), and lecithin-PL F-127 (Agrawal et al., 2010), reflecting no possible risk of skin irritation. For all formulations, the CUR content was ~ 95.2%, confirming the homogeneous drug distribution throughout the ORGs.

Differential Scanning Calorimetry (DSC) and Rheological Analysis

All ORG formulations were analyzed regarding to micellization and sol–gel transition processes considering their initial (T_{onset}), peak (T_{peak}), final (T_{endset}) phase transition temperatures; enthalpy change (ΔH); and rheological parameters such as elastic (G') and viscous (G") moduli, as well as viscosity (η^*). All results are presented on **Table 2** and **Figure 3**.

DSC analysis revealed that, in general, T_{onset} and T_{peak} values were similar for all formulations, but small shifts were observed on phase transition temperatures in response to CUR and/or PL L-81, since T_{endset} values were reduced from 14.2 to 12.8°C after PL L-81 incorporation, while CUR insertion increased the T_{endset} value for 15.3°C, being observed only for OA-PL F-127/L-81. Regarding to enthalpy variation, a more pronounced CUR interference was observed for the systems composed of OA-PL F-127, since similar ΔH values were obtained before and after CUR incorporation into the OA-PL F-127/L-81. Those results reflect the CUR influence on the phase transition process, considering the possible drug dispersion into the ORG oil phase and the potential hydrophobic interactions between the OA carbon backbone (C18) and CUR.

The rheological parameters elastic (G') and viscous (G") moduli, as well as apparent viscosity (η^*), were determined for all ORG formulations. Additionally, the sol–gel transition temperature was also obtained in order to predict the possible influence of CUR incorporation and both PL on ORG AP composition, their compatibility and structural organization. In this context, ORG formulations were also analyzed specially

TABLE 2 | Temperatures (T), enthalpy variation (ΔH), and rheological parameters relative to the organogels phase transition before and after curcumin incorporation.

Formulations	DSC				Rheology				
	T_{onset} (°C)	T_{peak} (°C)	T_{endset} (°C)	ΔH_m (J.g⁻¹)	G'(Pa)	G" (Pa)	G'/G"	η*(32.5°C)(x 10³, mPas.s)	Tsol–gel(°C)
OA-F-127	10.2	12.0	14.2	0.44	5,666	94.1	60.2	84.6	14.8
OA-F-127-CUR	10.1	12.9	15.3	3.34	4,960	111.3	44.6	85.5	15.9
OA-F-127/L-81	10.1	11.7	12.8	0.36	3,481	63.7	54.6	85.9	15.3
OA-F-127/L-81-CUR	10.5	12.3	12.7	0.52	1,984	124.3	15.9	53.8	15.2

T_{onset}, T_{peak}, and T_{endset} represent the initial, peak, and final temperatures for phase transitions. G' (elastic) and G" (viscous) moduli, apparent viscosity (η*), and sol–gel transition temperatures (Tsol-gel). OA, oleic acid; F-127, Pluronic® F-127; L-81, Pluronic® L-81; CUR, curcumin.

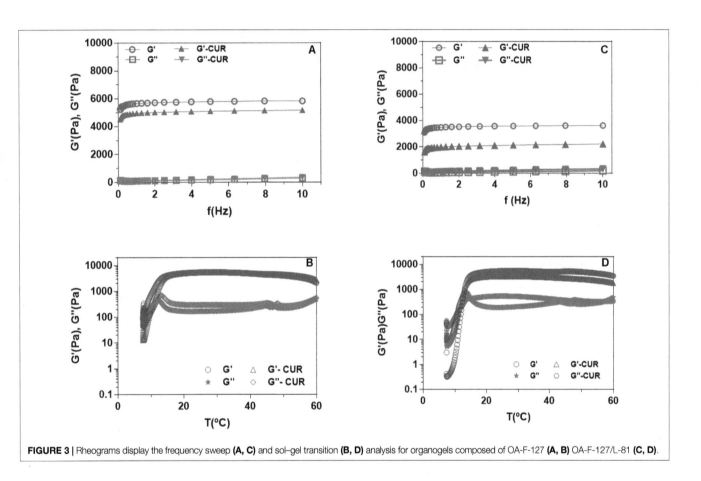

FIGURE 3 | Rheograms display the frequency sweep **(A, C)** and sol–gel transition **(B, D)** analysis for organogels composed of OA-F-127 **(A, B)** OA-F-127/L-81 **(C, D)**.

according to the PL types forming binary systems into the AP (**Table 2** and **Figure 3**).

Rheological analysis revealed similar $T_{sol-gel}$ values ranging from 14.8 to 15.9°C for isolated PL F-127 and its binary system with PL L-81, as well as after CUR incorporation. All ORG formulations presented viscoelastic behavior, being stable under temperature variation, since G' > G" values. However, the presence of CUR reduced the G'/G" relationships (from ~ 60 to 16), specially for the system OA-PL F-127/L-81. Similar effects were also observed on η* parameter (**Table 2**), which can be attributed to the influence of CUR molecules into the gels

three-dimensional network formed by the AP, disturbing their structural organization (Mady et al., 2016).

Regarding to the frequency sweep analysis, results revealed that the parameters G' and G" were not significantly affected by the applied frequency range, since G' > G" were observed for all formulations. After CUR incorporation, the system OA-PL F-127/L-81 presented the lowest G'/G" relationship value, compared to OA-PL F-127, showing the drug influence on ORG structural organization in addition to the presence of L-81 into the AP, as described before for other parameters such as viscosity and $T_{sol-gel}$.

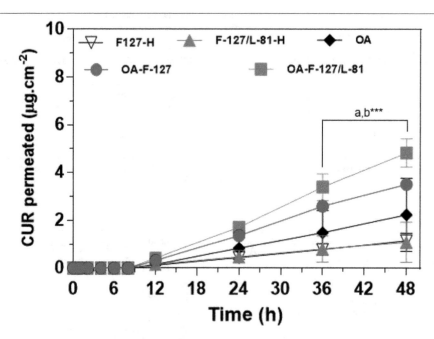

FIGURE 4 | Curcumin (CUR) permeation profiles from formulations across Strat-M® artificial membranes (mean ± standard deviation, n = 4–6). Organogels formulations containing 0.1% CUR. OA, oleic acid; PL F-127, Pluronic® F-127; PL L-81, Pluronic® L-81; CUR, curcumin. H—indicates hydrogels formulations (without oleic acid). a- OA-F-127/L-81 vs. F-127/L-81-H (PL-F-127-H; b- OA-F-127/L-81 vs. OA-F-127. ***p < 0.001.

TABLE 3 | Curcumin permeation parameters across Strat-M® membranes from organogel formulations.

Formulations	Flux (µg.cm⁻².h⁻¹)	Permeability coefficient (cm.h⁻¹)	Lag time (h)
OA	0.047 ± 0.003	0.028 ± 0.002	3.66 ± 0.21
OA-F-127	0.076 ± 0.005	0.107 ± 0.001	3.49 ± 0.18
OA-F-127/L-81	0.102 ± 0.006ᵃ***,ᵇ**	0.170 ± 0.003 ᵃ***,ᵇ**	3.61 ± 0.22
F-127-H	0.024 ± 0.001	0.040 ± 0.002	3.14 ± 0.12
F-127/L-81-H	0.025 ± 0.001	0.041 ± 0.004	3.44 ± 0.19

*F-127, Pluronic® F-127; L-81, Pluronic® L-81; OA, oleic acid; H—indicates hydrogel formulations (without oleic acid). Data presented as mean ± SD, Statistical differences are expressed as: a- OA-PL F-127/L-81 vs. hydrogels (F-127/L-81-H and F-127-H); b- OA-F-127/L-81 vs. OA or OA-F-127. ***p < 0.001 and **p < 0.01.*

In Vitro Permeation Studies

In order to characterize the CUR permeation from ORG formulations, experiments were performed using Strat-M® artificial membranes as barrier. In addition, hydrogels composed of each AP used for preparing the ORGs were also included as formulations, for evaluating the influence of OA- and PL-type on CUR permeation profiles. Results from those assays are summarized on **Figure 4** and **Table 3**.

Results from permeation experiments across Strat-M® presented different profiles according to the presence of OA and the AP composition. All formulations showed CUR gradual permeation during the experiment (48 h), and no different profiles were observed until 12 h. However, from this time point, formulations were segregated in different profiles where higher CUR-permeated concentrations were obtained for the systems OA-PL F-127 and OA-PL F-127/L-81 than those

determined for OA, PL F-127-H, and PL F-127/L-81-H. In fact, CUR permeation rate was significantly enhanced (p < 0.001) by OA-PL F-127/L-81 (4.83 µg.cm⁻²) compared with OA-PL F-127 (3.51 µg.cm⁻²), OA (2.25 µg.cm⁻²), PL F-127-H (1.16 µg.cm⁻²), and PL F-127/L-81-H (1.21 µg.cm⁻²) (**Figure 4**). Similar results were also observed after comparisons among the parameters drug flux and permeability coefficient for OA-PL F-127/L-81, which were significantly lower in relation to hydrogels (PL F-127-H and PL F-127/L-81-H) and OA-PL F-127, with p < 0.001 and p < 0.01, respectively (**Table 3**). On the other hand, latency times were very close for all formulations (from 3.14 to 3.66 h), and no statistical differences were observed, indicating a possible drug retention into the formulation.

In Vitro Cytotoxicity and Antileishmanial Activity

In vitro cytotoxicity assays were carried out in order to assess the effects of the vehicle OA, and the formulations (OA-PF F-127 and OA-PL F-127/L-81) in keratinocytes from HaCat cell line, evaluated by the MTT reduction test. All results are presented on **Figure 5**.

The increase on OA concentrations evoked toxic effects to the cells. However, the cell treatment with both ORG formulations did not induce pronounced cell toxicity. In addition, OA-PF F-127 presented the lowest cytotoxic effects (p < 0.001), with percentages ranging from 100 to 73.6%, compared to OA-PL F-127/L-81 (from 87.1 to 45.5%) and OA (from 87.4 to 10.1%), since the incorporation of OA into the PL-based AP reduced its cytotoxicity, being associated to the highest cell viability percentages. In addition, the reduced cell viability percentage after PL L-81 incorporation can be due to its lower HLB value

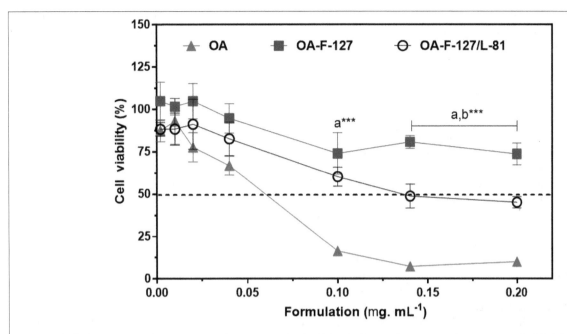

FIGURE 5 | Effects of organogels formulations on HaCat cells determined by MTT reduction test. Data expressed as mean ± standard deviation with n = 6 replicates/concentration). F-127, Pluronic® F-127; L-81, Pluronic® L-81; OA, oleic acid. a- OA-F-127 and OA-F-127/L-81 vs. OA; b- OA-F-127 vs. OA-F-127/L-81. *** p < 0.001.

TABLE 4 | Percentage of inhibition of growth L. amazonensis promastigote forms/concentrations (µg.ml⁻¹).

Treatments	Concentrations (µg/ml)					
	20	10	5.0	2.5	1.25	IC_{50}
OA						
OA-F-127						
OA-F-127/L-81	100 ± 0.00	100 ± 0.00	100 ± 0.00	100 ± 0.00	100 ± 0.00	<1.25
OA-F-127-CUR						
OA-F-127/L-81-CUR						
CUR	74.00 ± 5.65	57.50 ± 3.53	19.50 ± 0.70	14.70 ± 3.53	8.20 ± 0.56	9.45 (8.00–11.24)#
	0.40	0. 20	0.10	0.05		IC_{50}
Amph. B	66.57 ± 3.06	56.79 ± 2.99	40.50 ± 0.70	31.90÷0.14		0.15 (0.13–0.21)#

Results were expressed as the mean percentage of growth inhibition relative to the negative control. Two experiments were performed in triplicate. The 50% inhibitory concentration values (IC_{50}) and 95% confidence limits (in parenthesis) were determined by non-linear regression curves. Positive control: amphotericin B, Amph. B; negative control: medium RPMI +0.1% dimethylsulfoxide. F-127, Pluronic® F-127; L-81, Pluronic® L-81; OA, oleic acid.

compared to PL F-127, which possibly enhanced the PL cell membrane partitioning.

Additionally, the potential leishmanicidal activity was also investigated. All ORGs were incubated with *L. amazonensis* promastigote forms during 24h and their effects compared with amphotericin B, as positive control. In general, all ORG formulations OA, OA-PL F-127, and OA-PL F-127/L-81 evoked pronounced antileishmanial activity (IC_{50} < 1.25 µg.ml⁻¹) before and after CUR incorporation. Additionally, it is necessary to highlight that all formulations presented lower IC values compared with isolated CUR (IC_{50} = 9.45 µg.ml⁻¹), as observed on **Table 4**. Even considering that low CUR concentration can be

permeated from ORGs, all formulations exhibited leishmanicidal effects suggesting their potential use as skin delivery systems against *L. amazonensis*.

DISCUSSION

Natural products have been reported as a source of medicines for thousands of years. Since the discovery of pure compounds as bioactive molecules, the art of exploring natural products has become part of the molecular sciences. Many drugs used to treat different pathologies have been extracted from plants, and CUR has a long application for the treatment of several pathological processes including inflammatory, immunogenic, wound healing, and infectious conditions (Priyadarsini, 2014; de Moraes, 2015; Vaughn et al., 2016).

Despite its extensive pharmacological activities, CUR presents physico-chemical limitations, such as low aqueous solubility and bioavailability, reducing its permeation across the skin, since the clinical efficacy of bioactive molecules administered by topical route depends mainly on their physico-chemical and pharmacological properties, as well as their bioavailability at the site of action, which is limited by the low permeability of the stratum corneum. Then, due to the special structure and skin properties, novel formulations, such as lipid-based ORGs, have been developed in attempt to overcome those limitations.

In this study, we have presented the development, physico-chemical characterization, and biopharmaceutical evaluation of ORGs for CUR skin-delivery. In special, we designed the formulation compositions in order to carry high amounts of CUR soluble in OA (OP) and, then, entrapped into a tridimensional PL-based micellar AP, associating two polymers with different HLB values (PL F-127 and PL L-81) for promoting the permeation enhancement across the skin.

In this context, comparisons between the systems OA-PL F-127 and OA-PL F-127/L-81 suggest that the differences on thermodynamics parameters can be attributed to the presence of L-81 on AP. Since, PL L-81 is more hydrophobic (HLB = 8) compared to PL F-127 (HLB = 22), this feature can favor the possible CUR incorporation into micelle–micelle interface, as previously described by other hydrophobic drugs (Sharma et al, 2008; Esposito et al., 2018; Vigato et al., 2019). Additionally, those observations can suggest that different endothermic processes are capable to promote changes on ORG structural organization, particularly considering variations on aqueous and/or OP compositions.

As expected for hydrophobic molecules, such as CUR (log P = 3.62), there is a high partition on OP, but is possible that these molecules could be interacting with micellar central propylene glycol hydrophobic blocks from PL molecules, especially for the system composed by the association PL F-127/L-81. Additionally, it is necessary to point out CUR reduced both G'/G" relationship and η* values, as an indicative of a disturbance on the ORG network structural organization caused by the CUR molecule insertion into the system. Those results are also in agreement with previous reports describing the structural organization of PL-based systems for delivering hydrophobic molecules (Sharma et al., 2008; Sharma et al., 2018; Nascimento et al., 2018; Vigato et al., 2019), also corroborating the calorimetric results. Although this effect has been observed, ORG formulations maintained the high G'/G" ratio, an important feature to obtain adequate spreadability, forming a thin film on skin, but without loss of the formulation structural organization and potentially prolonging the contact time with the skin.

Despite the differences between *in vitro* (using artificial membranes) and *ex vivo* skin permeation profiles, Strat-M® has been used as skin model for evaluating the drug diffusion profiles from new delivery systems during the early stages of the development. In fact, its lipid matrix composition (ceramides, free fatty acids, cholesterol, and phospholipids) can simulate the skin barrier, being useful for determining permeation parameters for different types of pharmaceutical formulations such as hydrogels, nanoparticulate systems, emulsions, and ORGs (Uchida et al., 2015; Simon et al., 2016; Haq et al., 2018; Grillo et al., 2019; Vigato et al., 2019).

Several studies have been reported regarding the development of new skin delivery systems for CUR such as monoolein aqueous dispersion and lecithin ORGs (Esposito et al., 2014), liquid crystalline systems composed of OA, polyoxypropylene/polyoxyethylene cetyl alcohol (Fonseca-Santos et al., 2016), Pluronic F-127/P-123 micelles (Akbar et al., 2018), Pluronic F-127 hydrogel (Yen et al., 2018), and methoxy poly (ethylene glycol)-block-poly (ε-caprolactone) (MPEG-PCL) hydrogels (Zhou et al., 2019) for antioxidant, anti-inflammatory, antileishmanial, and wound-healing purposes. However, the influence of structural parameters on drug permeation, the presence of OA, and association of polymers on AP have been not discussed. In this context, we can postulate that the high permeated CUR amounts from the system OA-PL F-127/L-81 can be attributed to some structural factors: (i) the hydrophobic interactions between CUR and OA, into the OP, promoting the drug solubilization and acting as a permeation enhancer; (ii) the association of L-81 into the AP that, possibly, allowed the CUR interaction with its PPO hydrophobic units on organic-AP interface and also promoted CUR incorporation into Strat-M® lipid matrix; and (iii) the formation of a more fluid ORG system, OA-PL F-127/L-81, presenting lower viscosity and G'/G" relationship, compared to OA-PL F-127, but capable to maintain the formulation in contact with the skin-membrane model and enhance the drug permeation. Additionally, different PL-based systems have been used as new therapeutic strategies for several purposes, such as leishmaniosis treatment. Recent reports described formulations based on PL F-127 micelles encapsulating a naphthoquinone derivative (Mendonça et al., 2019), clioquinol (Tavares et al., 2019), amphotericin B (Mendonça et al., 2016), and PL F-68 micellar systems for amphotericin B (Espuelas et al., 2000). In this study, we present the development of lipid-PL formulations containing CUR; in particular, OA has been described as an important component of skin formulations for enhanced efficacy on leishmaniosis treatment (Pinheiro et al., 2016), as well as due to its involvement on transition from promastigotes to amastigotes (Bouazizi-Ben et al., 2017). In this context, further experiments will be necessary in order to evaluate the performance of each formulation and its isolated components on proliferation process for both promastigote and amastigote host-cell stages as well as on different *Leishmania* strains. In summary, results from this study pointed out OA-PL-based ORGs as promising new formulations for CUR skin delivery with potential pharmacological activity against *L. amazonensis*.

AUTHOR CONTRIBUTIONS

AV, NF, SQ and IM were responsible for physico-chemical characterization experiments, summarized the data and wrote the manuscript. EC and LF performed microscopy analysis. CC and GT were responsible for cell culture assays. AC and LC carried out antileishmanial activity assays. MS and DA contributed to the design, review and wrote the manuscript.

FUNDING

This research work was supported by Coordenação de Aperfeiçoamento de Pessoal de Nível Superior (CAPES), Fundação de Amparo à Pesquisa do Estado de São Paulo (FAPESP 2014/14457-5, 2018/04036-3, 2018/02482-6, 2016/18045-9, 2016/24456-1), Conselho Nacional de Desenvolvimento Científico e Tecnológico (CNPq 309207/2016-9, 402838/2016-5, 303946/2018-0) and UFABC Multiuser Central Facilities (CEM-UFABC).

ACKNOWLEDGMENTS

The authors are grateful to Prof. Hermi Felinto de Brito (Institute of Chemistry, University of São Paulo) and Maria Claudia França da Cunha Felinto (Nuclear and Energy Research Institute, São Paulo, SP, Brazil) for their support on X-ray diffraction experiments.

REFERENCES

Aggarwal, B. B., and Harikumar, K. B. (2009). Potential therapeutic effects of curcumin, the anti-inflammatory agent, against neurodegenerative, cardiovascular, pulmonary, metabolic, autoimmune and neoplastic diseases. *Int. J. Biochem. Cell. Biol.* 41, 40–59. doi: 10.1016/j.biocel.2008.06.010

Agrawal, V., Gupta, V., Ramteke, S., and Trivedi, P. (2010). Preparation and evaluation of tubular micelles of pluronic lecithin organogel for transdermal delivery of sumatriptan. *AAPS Pharm. Sci. Tech.* 11, 1718–1725. doi: 10.1208/s12249-010-9540-7

Akbar, M. U., Zia, K. M., Nazir, A., Iqbal, J., Ejaz, S. A., and Akash, M. S. H. (2018). Pluronic-based mixed polymeric micelles enhance the therapeutic potential of curcumin. *AAPS Pharm. Sci. Tech.* 19, 2719–2739. doi: 10.1208/s12249-018-1098-9

Anand, P., Thomas, S. G., Kunnumakkara, A. B., Sundaram, C. H., Kumar, K. B., Sung, B., et al. (2008). Biological activities of curcumin and its analogues (Congeners) made by man and Mother Nature. *Biochem. Pharmacol.* 76, 1590–1611. doi: 10.1016/j.bcp.2008.08.008

Bezerra, J. L., Costa, G. C., Lopes, T. C., Carvalho, I. C. D. S., Patrício, F. J., Sousa, S. M., et al. (2006). Avaliação da atividade leishmanicida *in vitro* de plantas medicinais. *Rev. Bras. Farmacogn.* 16, 631–637. doi: 10.1590/S0102-695X2006000500008

Boddu, S., Bonam, S., Wei, Y., and Alexander, K. (2014). Preparation and *in vitro* evaluation of a pluronic lecithin organogel containing ricinoleic acid for transdermal delivery. *Int. J. Pharm. Compd.* 18, 256–261.

Boddu, S. H., Bonam, S. P., and Jung, R. (2015). Development and characterization of a ricinoleic acid poloxamer gel system for transdermal eyelid delivery. *Drug Dev. Ind. Pharm.* 41, 605–612. doi: 10.3109/03639045.2014.886696

Bouazizi-Ben, M. H., Guichard, M., Lawton, P., Delton, I., and Azzouz-Maache, S. (2017). Changes in lipid and fatty acid composition during intramacrophagic transformation of leishmania donovani complex promastigotes into amastigotes. *Lipids* 52, 433–441. doi: 10.1007/s11745-017-4233-6

Cetin-Karaca, H., and Newman, M. C. (2015). Antimicrobial efficacy of plant phenolic compounds against Salmonella and Escherichia Coli. *Food Biosci.* 11, 8–16. doi: 10.1016/j.fbio.2015.03.002

Dall'Acqua, S., Stocchero, M., Boschiero, I., Schiavon, M., Golob, S., Uddin, J., et al. (2016). New findings on the *in vivo* antioxidant activity of Curcuma longa extract from an integrated 1H NMR and HPLC–MS metabolomic approach. *Fitoterapia* 109, 125–131. doi: 10.1016/j.fitote.2015.12.013

de Araujo, D. R., Padula, C., Cereda, C. M., Tófoli, G. R., Brito, R. B., Jr., de Paula, E., et al. (2010). Bioadhesive films containing benzocaine: correlation between *in vitro* permeation and in vivo local anesthetic effect. *Pharm. Res.* 27, 1677–1686. doi: 10.1007/s11095-010-0151-5

de Moraes, J. (2015). Natural products with antischistosomal activity. *Future Med. Chem.* 7, 801–820. doi: 10.4155/fmc.15.23

Esposito, C. L., Kirilov, P., and Roullin, V. G. (2018). Organogels, promising drug delivery systems: an update of state-of-the-art and recent applications. *J. Control Rel.* 271, 1–20. doi: 10.1016/j.jconrel.2017.12.019

Esposito, E., Ravani, L., Mariani, P., Huang, N., Boldrini, P., Drechsler, M., et al. (2014). Effect of nanostructured lipid vehicles on percutaneous absorption of curcumin. *Eur. J. Pharm. Biopharm.* 86, 121–132. doi: 10.1016/j.ejpb.2013.12.011

Espuelas, S., Legrand, P., Loiseau, P. M., Bories, C., Barratt, G., and Irache, J. M. (2000). *In vitro* reversion of amphotericin B resistance in Leishmania donovani by poloxamer 188. *Antimicrob. Agents Chemother.* 44, 2190–2192. doi: 10.1128/AAC.44.8.2190-2192.2000

Fonseca-Santos, B., Dos Santos, A. M., Rodero, C. F., Gremião, M. P., and Chorilli, M. (2016). Design, characterization, and biological evaluation of curcumin-loaded surfactant-based systems for topical drug delivery. *Int. J. Nanomed.* 11, 4553–4562. doi: 10.2147/IJN.S108675

Godin, B., and Touitou, E. (2007). Transdermal skin delivery: predictions for humans from *in vivo, ex vivo* and animal models. *Adv. Drug Deliv. Rev.* 59, 1152–1161. doi: 10.1038/nbt.1504

Grillo, R., Dias, F. V., Querobino, S. M., Alberto-Silva, C., Fraceto, L. F., de Paula, E., et al. (2019). Influence of hybrid polymeric nanoparticle/thermosensitive hydrogels systems on formulation tracking and *in vitro* artificial membrane permeation: a promising system for skin drug-delivery. *Coll. Surf. B Biointerfaces.* 174, 56–62. doi: 10.1016/j.colsurfb.2018.10.063

Han, Y.-M., Shin, D.-S., Lee, Y.-J., Ismail, I. A., Hong, S.-H., Han, D. C., et al. (2011). 2-Hydroxycurcuminoid induces apoptosis of human tumor cells through the reactive oxygen species–mitochondria pathway. *Bioorg. Med. Chem. Lett.* 21, 747–751. doi: 10.1016/j.bmcl.2010.11.114

Haq, A., Dorrani, M., Goodyear, B., Joshi, V., and Michniak-Kohn, B. (2018). Membrane properties for permeability testing: skin versus synthetic membranes. *Int. J. Pharm.* 539, 58–64. doi: 10.1016/j.ijpharm.2018.01.029

Iwanaga, K., Kawai, M., Miyazaki, M., and Kakemi, M. (2012). Application of organogels as oral controlled release formulations of hydrophilic drugs. *Int. J. Pharm.* 436, 869–872. doi: 10.1016/j.ijpharm.2012.06.041

Kaur, L., Singh, K., Paul, S., Singh, S., Singh, S., and Jain, S. K. (2018). A mechanistic study to determine the structural similarities between artificial membrane Strat-M™ and biological membranes and its application to carry out skin permeation study of amphotericin B nanoformulations. *AAPS Pharm. Sci. Tech.* 19, 1606–1624. doi: 10.1208/s12249-018-0959-6

Mady, F. M., Essa, H., El-Ammawi, T., Abdelkader, H., and Hussein, A. K. (2016). Formulation and clinical evaluation of silymarin pluronic-lecithin organogels for treatment of atopic dermatitis. *Drug Des. Devel. Ther.* 10, 1101–1110. doi: 10.2147/DDDT.S103423

Magalhaes, L. G., Machado, C. B., Morais, E. R., Moreira, E. B., Soares, C. S., da Silva, S. H., et al. (2009). *In vitro* schistosomicidal activity of curcumin against Schistosoma mansoni adult worms. *Parasitol. Res.* 104, 1197–1201. doi: 10.1007/s00436-008-1311-y

Mendonça, D. V., Lage, L. M., Lage, D. P., Chávez-Fumagalli, M. A., Ludolf, F., Roatt, B. M., et al. (2016). Poloxamer 407 (Pluronic(®) F127)-based polymeric micelles for amphotericin B: *in vitro* biological activity, toxicity and in vivo therapeutic efficacy against murine tegumentary leishmaniasis. *Exp. Parasitol.* 169, 34–42. doi: 10.1016/j.exppara.2016.07.005

Mendonça, D. V. C., Tavares, G. S. V., Lage, D. P., Soyer, T. G., Carvalho, L. M., Dias, D. S., et al. (2019). In vivo antileishmanial efficacy of a naphthoquinone derivate incorporated into a Pluronic® F127-based polymeric micelle system against Leishmania amazonensis infection. *Biomed. Pharmacother.* 109, 779–787. doi: 10.1016/j.biopha.2018.10.143

Morais, E. R., Oliveira, K. C., Magalhaes, L. G., Moreira, E. B., and Verjovski-Almeida, S. (2013). Effects of curcumin on the parasite Schistosoma mansoni:

a transcriptomic approach. *Mol. Biochem. Parasitol.* 187, 91–97. doi: 10.1016/j.molbiopara.2012.11.006

Nascimento, M. H. M., Franco, M. K. K. D., Yokaichyia, F., de Paula, E., Lombello, C. B., and de Araujo, D. R. (2018). Hyaluronic acid in Pluronic F-127/F-108 hydrogels for postoperative pain in arthroplasties: influence on physico-chemical properties and structural requirements for sustained drug-release. *Int. J. Biol. Macromol.* 111, 1245–1254. doi: 10.1016/j.ijbiomac.2018.01.064

Oshiro, A., da Silva, D. C., de Mello, J. C., de Moraes, V. W., Cavalcanti, L. P., Franco, M. K., et al. (2014). Pluronics f-127/l-81 binary hydrogels as drug-delivery systems: influence of physicochemical aspects on release kinetics and cytotoxicity. *Langmuir* 30, 13689–13698. doi: 10.1021/la503021c

Patel, N. A., Patel, N. J., and Patel, R. P. (2009). Design and evaluation of transdermal drug delivery system for curcumin as an anti-inflammatory drug. *Drug Dev. Ind. Pharm.* 35, 234–242. doi: 10.1080/03639040802266782

Pinheiro, I. M., Carvalho, I. P., de Carvalho, C. E., Brito, L. M., da Silva, A. B., Conde Júnior, A. M., et al. (2016). Evaluation of the in vivo leishmanicidal activity of amphotericin B emulgel: an alternative for the treatment of skin leishmaniasis. *Exp. Parasitol.* 164, 49–55. doi: 10.1016/j.exppara.2016.02.010

Prausnit, M. R., and Langer, R. (2008). Transdermal drug delivery. *Nat. Biotechnol.* 26, 1261–1268. doi: 10.1038/nbt.1504

Priyadarsini, K. Y. (2014). The chemistry of curcumin: from extraction to therapeutic agent. *Molecules.* 19, 20091–20112. doi: 10.3390/molecules191220091

Rachmawati, H., Budiputra, D. K., and Mauludin, R. (2015). Curcumin nanoemulsion for transdermal application: formulation and evaluation. *Drug Dev. Ind. Pharm.* 41, 560–566. doi: 10.3109/03639045.2014.884127

Shin, S.-C., Kim, J.-Y., and Oh, I.-J. (2000). Mucoadhesive and physicochemical characterization of carbopol-poloxamer gels containing triamcinolone acetonide. *Drug Dev. Ind. Pharm.* 26, 307–312. doi: 10.1081/DDC-100100358

Saxena, V., and Hussain, M. D. (2012). Poloxamer 407/TPGS mixed micelles for delivery of gambogic acid to breast and multidrug-resistant cancer. *Int. J. Nanomed.* 7, 713–721. doi: 10.2147/IJN.S28745

Sharma, G., Devi, N., Thakur, K., Jain, A., and Katare, O. P. (2018). Lanolin-based organogel of salicylic acid: evidences of better dermatokinetic profile in imiquimod-induced keratolytic therapy in BALB/c mice model. *Drug Deliv. Transl. Res.* 8, 398–413. doi: 10.1007/s13346-017-0364-9

Sharma, P. K., Reilly, M. J., Bhatia, S. K., Sakhitab, N., Archambault, J. D., and Bhatia, S. R. (2008). Effect of pharmaceuticals on thermoreversible gelation of PEO–PPO–PEO copolymers. *Coll. Surf. B Biointerfaces* 63, 229–235. doi: 10.1016/j.colsurfb.2007.12.009

Simon, A., Amaro, M. I., Healy, A. M., Cabral, L. M., and de Sousa, V. P. (2016). Comparative evaluation of rivastigmine permeation from a transdermal system in the Franz cell using synthetic membranes and pig ear skin with *in vivo-in vitro* correlation. *Int. J. Pharm.* 512, 234–241. doi: 10.1016/j.ijpharm.2016.08.052

Tavares, G. S. V., Mendonça, D. V. C., Miyazaki, C. K., Lage, D. P., Soyer, T. G., Carvalho, L. M., et al. (2019). A Pluronic® F127-based polymeric micelle system containing an antileishmanial molecule is immunotherapeutic and effective in the treatment against Leishmania amazonensis infection. *Parasitol. Int.* 68, 63–72. doi: 10.1016/j.parint.2018.10.005

Uchida, T., Kadhum, W. R., Kanai, S., Todo, H., Oshizaka, T., and Sugibayashi, K. (2015). Prediction of skin permeation by chemical compounds using the artificial membrane, Strat-M. *Eur. J. Pharm. Sci.* 67, 113–118. doi: 10.1016/j.ejps.2014.11.002

Vaughn, A. R., Branum, A., and Sivamani, R. K. (2016). Effects of turmeric (Curcuma longa) on skin health: a systematic review of the clinical evidence. *Phytother. Res.* 30, 1243–1264. doi: 10.1002/ptr.5640

Vigato, A. A., Querobino, S. M., de Faria, N. C., de Freitas, A. C. P., Leonardi, G. R., de Paula, E., et al. (2019). Synthesis and characterization of nanostructured lipid-poloxamer organogels for enhanced skin local anesthesia. *Eur. J. Pharm. Sci.* 128, 270–278. doi: 10.1016/j.ejps.2018.12.009

Vintiloiu, A., and Leroux, J. C. (2008). Organogels and their use in drug delivery—a review. *J. Control Rel.* 125, 179–192. doi: 10.1016/j.jconrel.2007.09.014

Yen, Y. H., Pu, C. M., Liu, C. W., Chen, Y. C., Chen, Y. C., Liang, C. J., et al. (2018). Curcumin accelerates cutaneous wound healing via multiple biological actions: the involvement of TNF-α, MMP-9, α-SMA, and collagen. *Int. Wound J.* 15, 605–617. doi: 10.1111/iwj.12904

Zhou, F., Song, Z., Wen, Y., Xu, H., Zhu, L., and Feng, R. (2019). Transdermal delivery of curcumin-loaded supramolecular hydrogels for dermatitis treatment. *J. Mater. Sci. Mater Med.* 30, 11. doi: 10.1007/s10856-018-6215-5

Zhu, H., Xu, T., Qiu, C., Wu, B., Zhang, Y., Chen, L., et al. (2016). Synthesis and optimization of novel allylated mono-carbonyl analogs of curcumin (MACs) act as potent anti-inflammatory agents against LPS-induced acute lung injury (ALI) in rats. *Eur. J. Med. Chem.* 121, 181–193. doi: 10.1016/j.ejmech.2016.05.041

8

Improving the Estimation of Risk-Adjusted Grouped Hospital Standardized Mortality Ratios Using Cross-Jurisdictional Linked Administrative Data

Katrina Spilsbury[1]*, Diana Rosman[1,2], Janine Alan[1], Anna M. Ferrante[3], James H. Boyd[3] and James B. Semmens[1]

[1] Centre for Population Health Research, Curtin University, Perth, WA, Australia, [2] Data Linkage, Department of Health WA, Perth, WA, Australia, [3] PHRN Centre for Data Linkage, Centre for Population Health Research, Curtin University, Perth, WA, Australia

*Correspondence:
Katrina Spilsbury
katrina.spilsbury@curtin.edu.au

Background: Hospitals and death registries in Australia are operated under individual state government jurisdictions. Some state borders are located in heavily populated areas or are located near to major capital cities. Mortality indicators for hospital located near state borders may not be estimated accurately if patients are lost as they cross state borders. The aim of this study was to evaluate how cross-jurisdictional linkage of state hospital and death records across state borders may improve estimation of the hospital standardized mortality ratio (HSMR), a tool used in Australia as a hospital performance indicator.

Method: Retrospective cohort study of 7.7 million hospital patients from July 2004 to June 2009. Inhospital deaths and deaths within 30 days of hospital discharge from four state jurisdictions were used to estimate the standardized mortality ratio of hospital groups defined by geography and type of hospital (grouped HSMR) under three record linkage scenarios, as follows: (1) cross-jurisdictional person-level linkage, (2) within-jurisdictional (state-based) person-level linkage, and (3) unlinked records. All public and private hospitals in New South Wales, Queensland, Western Australia, and public hospitals in South Australia were included in this study. Death registrations from all four states were obtained from state-based registries of births, deaths, and marriages.

Results: Cross-jurisdictional linkage identified 11,116 cross-border hospital transfers of which 170 resulted in a cross-border inhospital death. An additional 496 cross-border deaths occurred within 30 days of hospital discharge. The inclusion of cross-jurisdictional person-level links to unlinked hospital records reduced the coefficient of variation among the grouped HSMRs from 0.19 to 0.15; the inclusion of 30-day deaths reduced the coefficient of variation further to 0.11. There were minor changes in grouped HSMRs between cross-jurisdictional and within-jurisdictional linkages, although the impact of cross-jurisdictional linkage increased when restricted to regions with high cross-border hospital use.

Conclusion: Cross-jurisdictional linkage modified estimates of grouped HSMRs in hospital groups likely to receive a high proportion of cross-border users. Hospital identifiers will be required to confirm whether individual hospital performance indicators change.

Keywords: cross-jurisdictional record linkage, hospital standardized mortality ratios, risk adjustment, epidemiology, cohort studies

INTRODUCTION

Advances in information technology are changing the research environment in public health with increasing access to affordable, large, and complex administrative and surveillance health datasets. The potential of such data to improve population health outcomes is undisputed as whole populations can be followed more precisely in time and space. It has been proposed that precision public health could have particular benefit in preventative health with earlier detection and more precise risk estimates (1). However, the ethical and legal responsibility of protecting individual confidentiality must be balanced against the health benefits as these large amounts of data are brought together.

Following a $20 million government investment strategy, the Population Health Research Network (PHRN) was established to develop an accurate, reliable, and load-bearing national capability for data linkage in Australia. In 2009, the Centre for Data Linkage (CDL) was established within Curtin University and it provides the secure data linkage infrastructure necessary for cross-jurisdictional linkage of health-related data in Australia (2). The PHRN commissioned several proof of concept projects to demonstrate the feasibility and benefit of linking large datasets from across the country; the findings presented are from the first of these projects with the aim of demonstrating how estimation of the hospital standardized mortality ratio (HSMR) can be improved through cross-jurisdictional linkage.

Deaths in hospitals have long been of interest as an indicator of the quality of hospital care. The HSMR is an attempt to measure whether a hospital has a higher (or lower) number of hospital-related deaths relative to the overall mortality experience. HSMR is calculated by dividing the observed number of deaths by the expected number of deaths in that hospital. The expected number of deaths is estimated as the average of all deaths in all hospitals after accounting for case-mix variation by a range of possible risk-adjustment methodologies.

Hospital standardized mortality ratios as a measure of hospital quality of care have been the subject of considerable debate as to their value and how they should be used. It has been argued that HSMRs are a poor indicator of quality of care for several reasons. First, risk adjustment usually relies on variables collected from administrative data and not all may have been identified and reported accurately (3); second, a non-constant association of case-mix variables with death across hospitals could result in biases referred to as the constant risk fallacy (4), third, the statistical phenomenon that smaller hospitals

are more likely to occur at the top and bottom of league tables (5), fourth, the fact that most hospital deaths are not avoidable means there is low signal to noise ratio in trying to assess the rarer preventable deaths (6); fifth, concerns have been raised that hospitals may modify their coding practices or policies, such as refusing to accept very ill patients in an attempt to modify their HSMR (7); and finally, there is very little consistent or reliable evidence that hospitals with higher HSMRs actually provide poorer quality of care (8, 9).

Proponents of the HSMR argue that they should be used as a screening tool that alerts institutions to a possible problem rather than being a definitive measure of quality of care (10). Moreover, they counter that HSMRs are computed from data already existing in hospital databases and therefore are practical and cost-efficient to estimate (11), the constant risk fallacy is unlikely to be an issue for most hospitals (12), they are only used as a small part of an overall system for monitoring quality of care (10) and they can be used to monitor hospital changes over time (11).

In Australia, the Australian Commission on Safety and Quality in Health Care (ACSQHC) developed a toolkit that contains a set of risk-adjusted coefficients constructed from national inhospital mortality data (13). This enables hospitals to compare their HSMR against the Australian average. While practical to implement, a limitation of the current Australian approach for estimating HSMRs is that they are based on unlinked hospital records. This means that (i) multiple hospital records belonging to the same individual may not be brought together even if they are part of the same hospital admission that will fail to describe the patient pathways accurately or account for patient transfer policies, (ii) any deaths that occur soon after hospital discharge are not captured and therefore the HSMR is subject to discharge biases, and (iii) important historical or longitudinal patient characteristics are not available for use in the case-mix risk-adjustment process.

In the absence of a unique person identifier in Australia, some of these limitations can be overcome by using person-level linkage methods. Until recently, person-level linkage of administrative hospital and death records has been limited to only two standalone state-based data linkage centers; the Western Australia (WA) Data Linkage System and the Centre for Health Record Linkage in New South Wales (NSW). A constraint of state based or within-jurisdictional person-linkage is that it cannot follow patients if they cross state borders to attend hospital, a problematic issue when major urban areas such as Brisbane (QLD) are located close to a heavily populated region across a state border (NSW). Cross-jurisdictional linkage can overcome this limitation.

Cross-jurisdictional linkages of hospital and death records from NSW, WA, SA, and Queensland (QLD) were generated by the CDL, the first study in Australia to combine hospital and death data from multiple jurisdictions at the person level (14). This allowed an understanding of the patterns of cross-border hospital use not previously attempted (15). It further enabled assessment of the impact of cross-jurisdictional person-level linkage on the estimation of HSMRs. Due to hospital confidentiality concerns, identification of individual hospitals was not possible for this proof of concept study; therefore, estimated standardized mortality ratios were limited to groups of hospitals based on peer group and geographical location instead, that is, a grouped hospital SMR (GHSMR).

MATERIALS AND METHODS

Study Design

A retrospective cohort of all persons who were discharged (separated) from a NSW, WA, SA, or QLD participating hospital during the period 1st July 2004 to 30th June 2009 was identified. An additional 5 years of prior hospital separation records back to 1st July 1999 (where available) were used to identify past history of inpatient hospital use and preexisting comorbid medical conditions.

The main outcome measure was hospital-related deaths: both inhospital deaths and deaths that occurred within 30 days of separating from the last hospital stay. These deaths were used to estimate SMRs under three different record linkage scenarios, as follows: (1) cross-jurisdictional linkage, (2) jurisdictional (state-based) linkage, and (3) unlinked records. Ethical approval for this study was obtained from Human Research Ethics Committees in WA Health, QLD Health, SA Health Departments, the Cancer Institute NSW, and Curtin University (WA).

A detailed description of the hospital and death records used in this study have been published elsewhere (15). Briefly, inpatient records from public, psychiatric, and private hospitals, and private day surgery centers were available from NSW, WA, and QLD. SA provided public hospital inpatient records only. Death registration data were obtained from state-based registries of births, deaths, and marriages. The CDL created a set of person-level national linkage keys that linked all the hospital and death registration records across the four jurisdictions. These keys allowed the data custodians from each jurisdiction to provide relevant de-identified extractions of clinical and death data for analysis. The details of the cross-jurisdictional linkage process involved in this study are presented elsewhere (16).

Data Cleaning and Standardization

Hospital records from the four jurisdictions underwent extensive cleaning and standardization to maximize analytical comparability. A standard set of exclusions included hospital boarders, organ procurements, aged care residents, funding hospital (duplicate) cases, canceled procedure admissions, unqualified newborns, and healthy qualified newborns. Records with missing age, sex, principal diagnosis or mode of separation were also excluded. Consensus categorical variables were constructed based on the

variables from the jurisdictions that provided the least number of categories compared to other jurisdictions.

A number of jurisdictional coding differences were observed. For example, admissions for chemotherapy (ICD-10-AM code Z51.1) in public hospitals in NSW are mostly coded as outpatient events and were not included in the data, whereas they were coded as inpatient events and included in the data from the other three jurisdictions. Jurisdictional variations were identified by systematic cross-checking and with reference to the published metadata and local expertise.

Variable Definitions

Eligible hospital stays had (i) acute care or, for multiple episodes of care, the first episode of care was acute care, (ii) a final discharge date that fell from 1st July 2004 to 30th June 2009, (iii) a total length of stay less than 1 year, and (iv) an Australian postcode of residence.

For this study, a hospital transfer was defined as a compilation of hospital records that indicated either a subsequent transfer to another acute hospital or a statistical discharge within the same hospital had occurred. A maximum of 48 h was allowed for a patient to transfer from one acute hospital to another.

The principal reasons for admission to hospital (principal diagnosis codes) were aggregated into broader diagnostic groups by recoding the ICD-10-AM code into one of 256 Clinical Classification System (CCS) groups (17). These 256 CCS groups were further aggregated into 150 CCS group classifications similar to that reported by Campbell et al. (18) when constructing the summary hospital mortality index (SHMI) with some modification. For example, there were sufficient numbers of hospital stays to create a separate category for melanoma and non-melanoma skin cancers.

The Quan ICD-10 coding algorithm for the Deyo/Charlson index was used to create a Charlson comorbidity score (19) with a 5-year look back period for person-level-linked records and no look back period for unlinked hospital records. An average depth of coding weighting was estimated to account for the extent to which preexisting medical conditions were coded in each calendar year and within each hospital group. Variation in the comprehensiveness of hospital coding practice has been shown to impact estimation of HSMRs (20).

Risk Adjustment and GHSMR Estimation

Estimation of GHSMRs was restricted to (A) principal referral and specialist women's and children's hospitals, (B) large hospitals, (C) medium hospitals, and (D) small acute hospitals peer groups as defined by the Australian Institute of Health and Welfare (21). Hospital groups were created by splitting the four peer groups A, B, C, and D into smaller categories defined by geographical location and state jurisdiction; this created 43 different hospital groupings. Hospital geographic classifications were major city, inner regional, outer regional, and remote as assigned by the providing jurisdiction. Hospital-related deaths were attributed to the hospital associated with the first episode of care in a multicare episode hospital stay involving transfers.

The method for risk adjustment was based on that reported for the SHMI (18) with modification. The probability of a hospital-related death was estimated by fitting separate logistic regression models for each of the 48 most frequent CCS diagnostic groups that accounted for 80% of hospital-related deaths for each of the three different linkage scenarios. The dependent variables in these models were either (a) all hospital-related deaths (inhospital and 30-day deaths) or (b) inhospital deaths only. The independent variables used in these models were those factors likely to be associated with patient mortality outcomes and included patient age as quadratic term, gender, year, average depth of ICD coding weighting, length of stay, raw Charlson comorbidity score (5-year look back period), urgency of the hospital admission, accessibility to services (ARIA+), socioeconomc status (Index of Relative Social Disadvantage), marital status, aboriginality, number of times hospitalized in previous 5 years, whether the hospital stay involved intensive care or a ventilator, and whether the hospital stay involved a hospital transfer. Hospitalization history was excluded from the unlinked regression models. The discriminatory ability of each of these regression models to correctly classify hospital-related deaths was quantified using the area under the curve (c-statistic) from receiver-operating characteristic (ROC) analysis.

The expected number of hospital-related deaths was calculated by summing the probability of a hospital-related death for each hospital stay over each of the 43 different hospital groups. The GHSMRs were calculated as the ratio of actual observed number of hospital-related deaths in a hospital grouping to the expected number of deaths in that hospital grouping × 100. The 95% confidence intervals for the GHSMR estimates were calculated using Byar's approximation to the exact results based on the Poisson distribution (22). To increase the sensitivity of detecting differences in GHSMRS between those estimated using cross-jurisdictional links and those estimated using jurisdictional links in the absence of unique hospital identifiers, a subset analysis was performed. This involved conducting the risk adjustment and GHSMR estimation on the subset of patients who lived in statistical local areas (SLAs) where more than 1,200 patients crossed a state border to attend hospital over the 5-year study, an effective sample size of 302,191 (2.7%) hospital stays. GHSMRs are presented only for the hospital groups with more than 10 observed deaths within this population subset.

RESULTS

There were 19.7 million hospital records from July 2004 to June 2009 that met the inclusion criteria. After applying jurisdictional person-level linkages that allowed multiple records pertaining to the same individual and admission to be bought together into a single hospital stay, the total number of records reduced 4% to 18.9 million hospital stays, which represented 7.8 million unique individuals (**Table 1**).

The further addition of cross-jurisdictional linkages brought together both episodes of care that involved hospital transfers across a state border ($n = 11,116$) into a single hospital stay and allowed patients who had hospital stays in more than one jurisdiction to be merged into a single patient. Cross-jurisdictional linkage reduced the number of unique hospital stays by 0.6% and reduced the total number of individual patients by a further 1.4% compared with jurisdictional linkages.

TABLE 1 | The number and percentage of hospital stays, episodes of care, individual patients, and hospital-related deaths in the four participating jurisdictions under the three different data linkage scenarios.

	NSW[d]		WA		QLD		SA[c]		Total
	N	**%**	**N**	**%**	**N**	**%**	**N**	**%**	
1. Cross-jurisdictional linkage									
Hospital stays	8,723,879	46.2	2,799,646	14.8	5,919,025	31.4	1,427,780	7.6	18,870,330
Individuals	3,660,991	47.9	1,094,303	14.3	2,286,449	30.0	608,921	8.0	7,650,664
Inhospital deaths[a]	104,439	2.9	23,725	2.2	58,484	2.6	20,073	3.3	206,721
30-day deaths[b]	33,868	1.0	8,038	0.8	16,496	0.7	7,922	1.4	66,324
Hospital stays by non-residents[e]	157,851	1.8	11,834	0.4	155,620	2.6	27,664	1.9	352,969
Cross-border transfers sent	9,442	84.9	65	0.6	1,278	11.5	331	3.0	11,116
Cross-border transfers received	1,584	14.2	28	0.3	8,164	73.4	1,340	12.1	11,116
Cross-border deaths	239	48.2	12	2.4	205	41.3	40	8.1	496
2. Within-jurisdictional linkage									
Hospital stays	8,725,254	46.2	2,799,122	14.8	5,927,122	31.4	1,429,133	7.6	18,881,226
Individuals	3,699,822	47.7	1,104,067	14.2	2,331,133	30.2	617,175	8.0	7,762,197
Inhospital deaths[a]	103,958	2.81	23,719	2.15	58,760	2.51	20,113	3.26	206,550
30-day deaths[b]	33,666	0.9	8,030	0.7	16,292	0.7	7,903	1.3	65,891
3. Unlinked separation-level data									
Hospital records	9,130,886	46.4	2,881,774	14.7	6,165,476	31.4	1,479,786	7.5	19,657,922
Inhospital deaths	96,556	1.1	19,446	0.7	50,041	0.8	19,157	1.3	185,200

[a]Percentage represents proportion of deaths in individuals who had a hospital stay in the 5-year period.
[b]Percentage represents proportion of 30-day deaths in individuals who were discharged alive from their last hospital stay (i.e., excluded individuals who died in hospital).
[c]SA data included public hospitals only.
[d]NSW inpatient data include deaths in emergency departments.
[e]Proportion of hospital stays by non-state residents (cross-border users) relative to all hospital stays in the jurisdiction.

The number and proportions of hospital-related deaths also varied depending on the data linkage scenario used (**Table 1**). When cross-jurisdictional linkage was used, there were 207,000 inhospital deaths identified, of which 48,380 (23%) occurred during hospital stays involving multiple episodes of care (transfers). Around 22,000 of these inhospital deaths were identified only in the person-linked data scenarios compared with unlinked data because the primary acute care episode of care in a hospital stay involving a transfer was linked to a subsequent non-acute episode of care in which the death occurred.

A further 170 inhospital deaths were identified using cross-jurisdictional linkage compared with jurisdictional links because it detected patients who had a hospital transfer across a state border to receive non-acute care and who then died in hospital. Additionally, there were 496 patients who died within 30 days of discharge and their death was registered in a different jurisdiction; 433 deaths in a different jurisdiction and 53 patients who had dual death registrations (all were dual registered in QLD and NSW).

The logistic regression models used to estimate the probability of hospital-related death in each of the 48 most frequent diagnostic groups had areas under the ROC curve (c-statistics) that ranged from 0.95 for the cardiac arrest and ventricular fibrillation to 0.70 for non-hypertensive congestive heart failure; a consistent finding for both the cross-jurisdictional and single-jurisdictional linked data. The ability of the logistic regression models to correctly classify inhospital deaths in the unlinked separation-level data varied from the person-linked hospital data with a maximum c-statistic of 0.95 for biliary tract disease and a lower 0.82 for cardiac arrest and ventricular fibrillation. The average c-statistic for the unlinked separation-level data for inhospital deaths was 0.84, slightly less than the average for person-linked data models at 0.85.

Grouped hospital SMRs estimated using inhospital deaths only were compared for cross-jurisdictional and unlinked hospital records (**Figure 1A**). The addition of the person-level links allowed episodes of care for an individual to be bought together into a single admission and resulted in a change of GHSMR toward the group average GHSMR of 100 in most cases.

For example, Hospital Group 1 with a SMR of 118 (95% CI: 116–119) using unlinked data dropped to 109 (95% CI: 108–110) with person-level cross-jurisdictional linked records. For some hospital groups with relatively low numbers of observed deaths, the observed changes in GHSMR were not always statistically significant. For example, Hospital Group 7 with around 50 observed deaths had an unlinked GHSMR of 118 (95% CI: 83–162) that increased to 136 (95% CI: 101–180) with person-level cross-jurisdictional linkage.

The inclusion of deaths within 30 days of hospital discharge into the GHSMR estimates for the cross-jurisdictional linkage scenario resulted in GHSMR changes more consistently toward the group average (**Figure 1B**). In some cases, the addition of 30-day deaths reversed the change in GHSMR observed when person-level cross-jurisdictional links were first added to unlinked data (see Hospital Group 7 in **Figures 1A,B** for example). Overall, the inclusion of cross-jurisdictional person-level

links to unlinked separation data reduced the coefficient of variation among the hospital groups from 0.19 to 0.15; the inclusion of 30-day deaths reduced the coefficient of variation further to 0.11.

There were only minor changes to the GHSMR estimates when cross-jurisdictional linkages were compared to jurisdictional linkages (**Figure 2A**). Hospital groups in remote areas tended to show the greatest difference as a result of cross-jurisdictional linkage. To increase the sensitivity of this comparison due to the limitation of not having individual hospital identifiers, the GHSMR estimation was restricted to the subset of patients residing in SLAs with high proportions of cross-border hospital users (**Figure 2B**). This restriction demonstrated increased variation in GHSMRs estimated using cross-jurisdictional links compared with jurisdictional links for several of the 11 hospital groups that had more than 10 observed deaths.

DISCUSSION

We have demonstrated that using cross-jurisdictional linked hospital and death records can modify estimates of SMRs based on broad hospital groupings compared with both unlinked and jurisdictional linked records. For this study, the largest changes in GHSMRs for inhospital deaths were between unlinked records and person-level linked data. Person-level data allowed multiple episodes of care to be bought together into a single hospital stay. This allowed more accurate estimation of the number of patients, and their care pathways, and improved the identification of hospital-related deaths during non-acute care that were linked to an acute care admission. Additionally, the more complete ascertainment of patient comorbidity and hospital stay history improved the GHSMR estimation.

Including all 30-day deaths into the GHSMR estimation reduced the overall spread of GHSMRs and tended to bring outlying hospital groups toward the group average. This is consistent with previous work for NSW hospital data that showed that including 30-day deaths reduced the variation in HSMRs (23). It is likely that this overall reduction in variation occurs because including 30-day deaths into GHSMR estimation reduces the hospital-related death variation associated with early-discharge practices and varying hospital transfer processes.

Estimation of GHSMRs for hospital-related deaths using cross-jurisdictional links compared with jurisdictional links included additional deaths associated with the 11,116 cross-jurisdictional hospital transfers and the 496 cross-border hospital deaths. These additional deaths made only minor changes to the GHSMRs in this study because of the reduced sensitivity of using hospital groups rather than individual hospitals. In this study, individual hospital identifiers were not available and SMR estimation was restricted to broad geographical and peer group categories. It is expected that significant changes in mortality rates could result for hospitals located close to jurisdictional borders when cross-jurisdictional linkages are included at an individual hospital level. This hypothesis is supported by the larger effect observed for cross-jurisdictional linked GHSMRs when restricted to patients living in high cross-border hospital use regions.

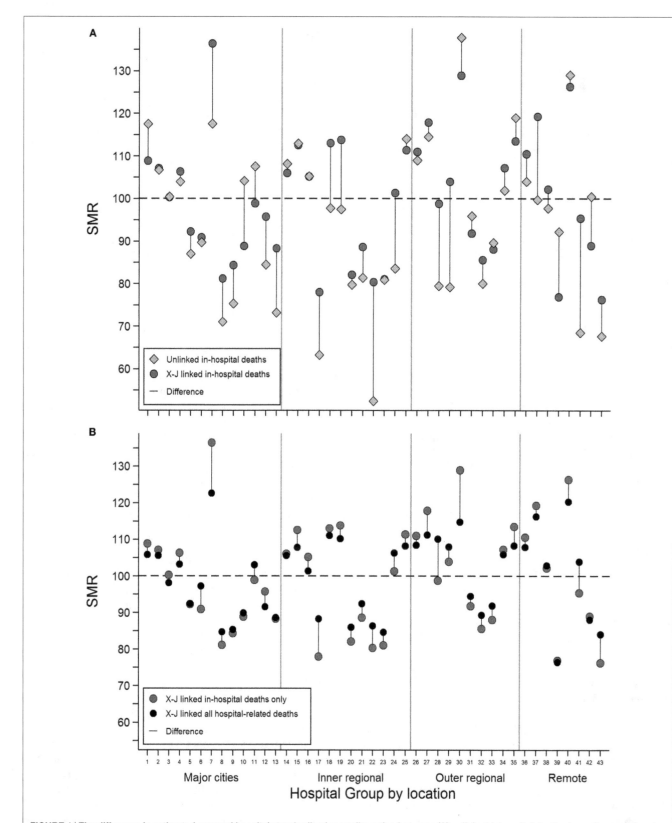

FIGURE 1 | The difference in estimated grouped hospital standardized mortality ratios between **(A)** unlinked inhospital deaths (gray diamonds) and cross-jurisdictional linked inhospital deaths (dark gray circles) and **(B)** cross-jurisdictional linked inhospital deaths (dark gray circles) and cross-jurisdictional linked all hospital-related deaths, inhospital, and 30-day deaths (black circles) for each of the 43 hospital groups defined by broad geographical areas and peer groups.

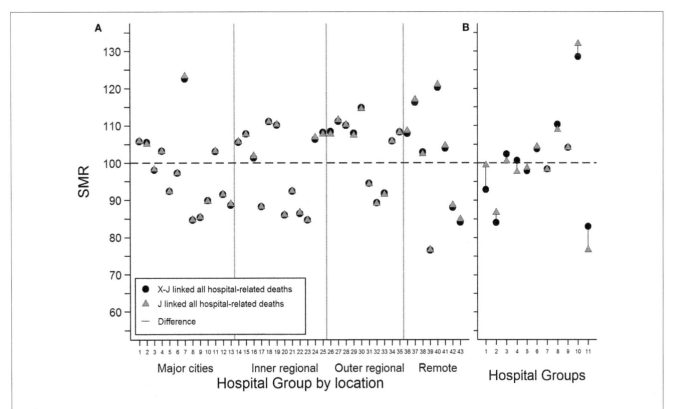

FIGURE 2 | The difference in estimated grouped hospital standardized mortality ratios for all hospital-related deaths between cross-jurisdictional linked (black circles) and jurisdictional linked (gray triangles) hospital records for (A) all hospital stays and (B) a subset of hospital stays restricted to patients living in statistical local areas with relatively high proportions of cross-border hospital users. Only hospital groups with more than 10 observed deaths were included.

The risk-adjustment method used in this report were designed to make full use of the linked data available and thus differs from the method presented in the toolkit developed by the ACSQHC for hospitals to estimate their HSMR core hospital-based outcome indicators (13). While the regression models used to estimate the expected number of hospital-related deaths had high c-statistics, the approach used here would be impractical to implement on a real-time basis for monitoring hospital performance unless timely access to death registration data to identify deaths within 30 days of discharge can be contrived.

A condition of data release for this study prevented identification of individual hospitals, which was a major limitation. This restriction was primarily the result of privacy concerns and prevented the comparison of individual hospitals with similar characteristics. As a result, the GHSMRs reported here cannot, nor are meant to be, interpreted in any clinically meaningful way. This limitation highlights that there are still ethical, legal, and social barriers to overcome before cross-jurisdictional linkage is implemented regularly in Australia. Ensuring public confidence in the technology of data linkage to maintain individual confidentiality, advocating for changes to out-dated legislation and providing a strong ethical base to research training undertaken by organization such as the PHRN and the Centre for Big Data Research in Health will contribute to positive change. Other innovations such as secure remote-access computer environments

and the development and use of privacy-preserving record linkage techniques will continue to play a role in the future of data linkage.

CONCLUSION

We have shown that linking individuals and their hospital stays across jurisdictional borders can modify estimates of standardized mortality ratios. Hospital identifiers will be required to confirm these findings. Improving the precision of the HSMR as a hospital performance indicator is particularly relevant for hospitals that are located close to borders or that have relatively high numbers of interstate travelers.

AUTHOR CONTRIBUTIONS

KS carried out the data manipulation, data analysis, and drafted the manuscript. DR conceived the design of the study, negotiated data acquisition, and contributed to manuscript preparation. JA conceived the design of the study, negotiated data acquisition, and contributed to manuscript preparation. AF contributed to data acquisition, data analysis, and manuscript preparation. JB contributed to data acquisition, data analysis, and manuscript preparation. JS contributed to overall study concept and critically reviewed the manuscript.

ACKNOWLEDGMENTS

This study would not have been possible without the collaboration, assistance, and expertise provided by a large number of people including Lee Taylor, Kim Lim, Baohui Yang, and Zoran Bolevich from the NSW Ministry of Health; Almond Sparrow and Stacy Vasquez from SA-NT DataLink; Paul Basso, Tina Hardin, and Tomi Adejoro at SA Department of Health and Ageing; Helen Paues from SA Registry of Births Deaths and Marriages; Darren Shaw at Promadis; Jessica Lee, Alexandra Godfrey, Carol Garfield, and Paul Stevens from WA Department of Health; WA Registry of Births, Deaths and Marriages; the Health Statistics Branch, QLD Department of Health; Julie Hall and Erica Finlay at QLD Registry of Births Deaths and Marriages; Sean Randall and Jacqui Bauer at the Centre for Data Linkage; Merran Smith, Felicity Flack, Angela Rate, Natalie Wray, Emma Fuller, and Tony Woollacott at the PHRN Program Office; James E. Harrison, Flinders University; Bruce Armstrong, University of Sydney; and Neville Board, Australian Commission on Safety and Quality in Health. Part of this manuscript was presented at the International Population Data Linkage Conference 2016, Swansea, UK.

FUNDING

This work was funded by the PHRN, an initiative of the Australian Government being conducted as part of the National Collaborative Research Infrastructure Strategy.

REFERENCES

1. Khoury MJ, Iademarco MF, Riley WT. Precision public health for the era of precision medicine. *Am J Prev Med* (2016) 50:398–401. doi:10.1016/j.amepre.2015.08.031

2. Boyd JH, Ferrante AM, O'Keefe CM, Bass AJ, Randall SM, Semmens JB. Data linkage infrastructure for cross-jurisdictional health-related research in Australia. *BMC Health Serv Res* (2012) 12:480. doi:10.1186/1472-6963-12-480

3. Lilford R, Pronovost P. Using hospital mortality rates to judge hospital performance: a bad idea that just won't go away. *BMJ* (2010) 340:c2016. doi:10.1136/bmj.c2016

4. Mohammed MA, Deeks JJ, Girling A, Rudge G, Carmalt M, Stevens AJ, et al. Evidence of methodological bias in hospital standardised mortality ratios: retrospective database study of English hospitals. *BMJ* (2009) 338:b780. doi:10.1136/bmj.b780

5. Tu YK, Gilthorpe MS. The most dangerous hospital or the most dangerous equation? *BMC Health Serv Res* (2007) 7:185. doi:10.1186/1472-6963-7-185

6. Scott IA, Brand CA, Phelps GE, Barker AL, Cameron PA. Using hospital standardised mortality ratios to assess quality of care – proceed with extreme caution. *Med J Aust* (2011) 194:645–8.

7. Kahn JM, Kramer AA, Rubenfeld GD. Transferring critically ill patients out of hospital improves the standardized mortality ratio: a simulation study. *Chest* (2007) 131:68–75. doi:10.1378/chest.06-0741

8. Pitches DW, Mohammed MA, Lilford RJ. What is the empirical evidence that hospitals with higher-risk adjusted mortality rates provide poorer quality care? A systematic review of the literature. *BMC Health Serv Res* (2007) 7:91. doi:10.1186/1472-6963-7-91

9. Thomas JW, Hofer TP. Research evidence on the validity of risk-adjusted mortality rate as a measure of hospital quality of care. *Med Care Res Rev* (1998) 55:371–404. doi:10.1177/107755879805500401

10. Bottle A, Jarman B, Aylin P. Strengths and weaknesses of hospital standardised mortality ratios. *BMJ* (2011) 342:c7116. doi:10.1136/bmj.c7116

11. Ben-Tovim DI, Pointer SC, Woodman R, Hakendorf PH, Harrison JE. Routine use of administrative data for safety and quality purposes – hospital mortality. *Med J Aust* (2010) 193:S100–3.

12. Ben-Tovim DI, Woodman RJ, Hakendorf P, Harrison J. Standardised mortality ratios. Neither constant nor a fallacy. *BMJ* (2009) 338:b1748. doi:10.1136/bmj.b1748

13. Australian Commission on Safety and Quality in Health Care. *National Core, Hospital-Based Outcome Indicator Specification*. Sydney: ACSQHC (2012).

14. Rosman D, Spilsbury K, Alan J, Ferrante A, Young A, Fuller E, et al. Multi-jurisdictional linkage in Australia: proving a concept. *Aust N Z J Public Health* (2016) 40:96–96. doi:10.1111/1753-6405.12420

15. Spilsbury K, Rosman D, Alan J, Boyd JH, Ferrante AM, Semmens JB. Cross-border hospital use: analysis using data linkage across four Australian states. *Med J Aust* (2015) 202:582–6. doi:10.5694/mja14.01414

16. Boyd JH, Randall SM, Ferrante AM, Bauer JK, McInneny K, Brown AP, et al. Accuracy and completeness of patient pathways – the benefits of national data linkage in Australia. *BMC Health Serv Res* (2015) 15:312. doi:10.1186/s12913-015-0981-2

17. Healthcare Cost and Utilization Project (HCUP). *Clinical Classifications Software (CCS) for ICD-10*. Rockville, MD: Agency for Healthcare Research and Quality (2012).

18. Campbell MJ, Jacques RM, Fotheringham J, Maheswaran R, Nicholl J. Developing a summary hospital mortality index: retrospective analysis in English hospitals over five years. *BMJ* (2012) 344:e1001. doi:10.1136/bmj.e1001

19. Quan H, Sundararajan V, Halfon P, Fong A, Burnand B, Luthi JC, et al. Coding algorithms for defining comorbidities in ICD-9-CM and ICD-10 administrative data. *Med Care* (2005) 43:1130–9. doi:10.1097/01.mlr.0000182534.19832.83

20. Bottle A, Jarman B, Aylin P. Hospital standardized mortality ratios: sensitivity analyses on the impact of coding. *Health Serv Res* (2011) 46:1741–61. doi:10.1111/j.1475-6773.2011.01295.x

21. Australian Institute of Health and Welfare (AIHW). *Australian Hospital Statistics 1998-99*. Canberra: AIHW (2000).

22. Itskovich I, Roudebush B. Using re-sampling methods in mortality studies. *PLoS One* (2010) 5(8):e12340. doi:10.1371/journal.pone.0012340

23. Lujic S, Jorm L, Randall D. *Deaths After Admission to Hospital: A NSW Population-Based Data Linkage Study*. Parramatta, NSW: The SAX Institute and School of Medicine, University of Western Sydney (2012).

9

Post-Marketing Study of Linagliptin

Gabrielle Kéfrem Alves Gomes, Mariana Linhares Pereira, Cristina Sanches and André Oliveira Baldoni*

Grupo de Pesquisa em Epidemiologia e Avaliação de Novas Tecnologias em Saúde, Universidade Federal de São João del-Rei, Divinópolis, Brazil

*Correspondence:
André Oliveira Baldoni
andrebaldoni@ufsj.edu.br

Introduction: Linagliptin is a high-cost oral antidiabetic that has been widely used, and studies on its effectiveness and safety for the treatment of type 2 diabetes mellitus (DM2) in the real world is rare and necessary.

Objective: To analyze the values of glycated hemoglobin (HbA1c) and adverse events before and after the use of linagliptin in the post-marketing context of a pilot study.

Methods: This is a descriptive observational and exploratory study with a retrospective longitudinal approach, conducted between January 2014 and December 2016. All patients who participated in the study were over 18 years of age, with DM2, assisted by the Brazilian Public Health System (*Sistema Único de Saúde* – SUS) and had been indicated for use of linagliptin. The users were followed up and the variables of interest were collected from a computerized health information system (*sistema informatizado de saúde* – SIS) and patient records. For effectiveness analysis, HbA1c before (T_0) and after (T_1) the use of linagliptin was considered in patients registered as having collected linagliptin at the pharmacy for at least three consecutive months. For safety analysis, registered adverse events (AE) were verified in patients' records. The sample was stratified according to the pharmacotherapeutic scheme of the users. To compare the means before (T_0) and after (T_1), a paired *t*-test (data with normal distribution) and Wilcoxon Signed Rank Sum test (non-normal distribution data) were performed.

Results: Considering the total population of the study, in a different pharmacotherapeutic regimen, a median reduction in HbA1c of −0.86% ($p < 0.05$) was observed. After stratification by pharmacotherapeutic regimen, the most significant reduction of HbA1c was −1.07% ($p = 0.014$) for the linagliptin group associated with insulins and oral antidiabetic agents ($n = 13$). On the other hand, patients taking linagliptin in monotherapy had the lowest HbA1c reduction, −0.48% ($p > 0.05$). AE occurred in 12 (36.4%) patients, and 16.7% were in monotherapy.

Conclusion: Linagliptin did not presented, in real world, the desired performance as showed in randomized premarketing clinical trials and it should be carefully evaluated in public health services.

Keywords: linagliptin, Dipeptidyl peptidase 4 inhibitors, diabetes mellitus type 2, effectiveness, safety, pharmacovigilance, pharmacoepidemiology

INTRODUCTION

Diabetes mellitus type 2 (DM2) is a chronic disease highly prevalent in the adult population. The main objectives of DM2 treatment are metabolic control, the reduction of microvascular and macrovascular complications associated with the disease, as well as the reduction of its acute manifestations. To meet these goals it is necessary that blood glucose reach normal levels, both in fasting and in the postprandial period. Regarding the choice of pharmacological therapy, this should take into consideration the mechanisms of insulin resistance, secretory capacity of the pancreas, metabolic disorders involved, and the complications of DM2 present (American Diabetes Association [ADA], 2018). In healthy individuals, glucagon-like peptide 1 (GLP-1) and glucose-dependent insulinotropic polypeptide (GIP), which are intestinal hormones or incretins, account for up to 70% of the insulin response, as they contribute to the modulation of pancreatic beta-cell activity, stimulating insulin secretion (Morris et al., 2013; American Diabetes Association [ADA], 2018).

In DM2 there is a reduced response of the insulin effect, which alters the regulation of the amount of glucose present in the blood, contributing to a lack of glycemic control of the sick individual. In this sense, incretin analogs and inhibitors of the enzyme Dipeptidyl peptidase-4 (DPP-4) have been developed in order to potentiate the function of these endogenous hormones. Incretin-based therapy has been increasingly prominent among treatment options for type 2 diabetes (DM2) (Websky et al., 2013). Studies demonstrate the efficacy of these substances in glycemic control as well as in the weight reduction of these patients (International Diabetes Federation [IDF], 2017; American Diabetes Association [ADA], 2018).

As members of the incretin class, gliptins are the inhibitors of the DPP-4 enzyme. Linagliptin, a representative of this class, has a peculiar pharmacological profile: pharmacokinetics allowing only one daily administration and no dose adjustment requirement for patients with renal and hepatic dysfunction (Richard, 2014; American Diabetes Association [ADA], 2018). Linagliptin can be used both in monotherapy and in combination with other antidiabetic agents (Chen et al., 2015; Marx et al., 2015; Mikhael, 2016; Thrasher, 2016). Studies have demonstrated that this association of other antidiabetic agents with linagliptin has been shown to be effective and widely used in clinical practice in order to optimize treatment of DM2 (Defronzo et al., 2015; Haak, 2015).

Several clinical trials have shown that incretins, such as linagliptin, have been considered a great therapeutic promise in terms of effectiveness and safety (Chen et al., 2015; Defronzo et al., 2015; Haak, 2015; Marx et al., 2015; Mikhael, 2016; Thrasher, 2016). However, data on the use of this class in the real world in monotherapy or in combination are scarce (Barnett et al., 2013; Sortino et al., 2013; Richard, 2014). In addition, linagliptin, and other representatives of the class of gliptins, are on the list of medications to be avoided, according to data published in the journal "Prescrire" and there is concern about an unfavorable profile of adverse effects including urinary tract infections and upper respiratory tract infections (Prescrire International, 2017).

In addition, studies on the effectiveness and adverse event profile of linagliptin in the post-marketing context is rare and necessary. In this context, this study, considered a pilot, aims to reduce this gap between the use of linagliptin by patients in the "real world" and the evidence from randomized clinical trials in developed countries. This study aims is to analyze the values of glycated hemoglobin and adverse events before and after the use of linagliptin in the post-marketing context of a pilot study.

MATERIALS AND METHODS

Study Design

This is a descriptive observational and exploratory study with a retrospective longitudinal approach (Elseviers et al., 2016). The study was outlined and described following the recommendations of Kempen (2011).

Setting

The city where the study was conducted has 21,3016 inhabitants, Human Development Index (HDI) of 0.764, and 43 primary health care units, and only one center of endocrinology.

Participants

All patients served at health units of the Brazilian Public Health System (SUS) of the city of Divinópolis, in the state of Minas Gerais (MG) who received a medical indication for the use of linagliptin during the period from January 2014 to December 2016 were identified and considered eligible for the study. Identification was made through a computerized health information system (SIS) that records the medication dispensed to the patients.

All participants who took linagliptin for at least three consecutive months were considered. The 3-month period was established so that it was possible to analyze the effectiveness of linagliptin according to the time required for variation of HbA1c levels (Malta et al., 2010). Participants in concomitant use of other medicinal products of the DPP-4 inhibitor class were excluded. This information was collected together with the patient's medical record and dispensing record.

Variables and Data Source

The outcome variables considered were the effectiveness and safety of linagliptin. The analysis of the effectiveness of linagliptin was performed by comparing patients' HbA1c values shortly before linagliptin (T_0) and after the first 3 months of consecutive use of the medication (T_1).

Safety was analyzed from the active search for adverse events (AE) registered in patients' medical records during the period of linagliptin use. A list of adverse events related to linagliptin was developed to direct and systematize the search for AE reported in patients' records. This list was constructed after a systematized search in the literature on adverse medication events (Andriolo and Vieira, 2005; Food And Drug Administration [FDA], 2013; ANVISA, 2017; Gomes et al., 2018). To investigate possible laboratory abnormalities, the results of microalbuminuria, urea, aspartate transaminase (AST), alanine aminotransferase (ALT), and gamma-glutamyltransferase (GAMA-GT) were investigated. Only the AE that were recorded in the patients' records during the period of linagliptin use were considered for this analysis.

In addition to the outcome variables, the following variables were analyzed: (I) demographic data: gender, self-reported race; (II) clinical data: pharmacotherapy used for DM2, family history, presence of comorbidities, and time of diagnosis of DM2; (III) biochemical data: fasting glycemia, glycated hemoglobin, postprandial glucose, creatinine, and urea. Medical records were used to define the presence of alcoholism, degree of obesity, renal failure, and other diagnoses.

Statistics

Data analysis was performed with STATA software – Data Analysis and Statistical Software, version 12.0. To compare the biochemical tests before (T_0) and after (T_1) the use of linagliptin, the normality of the data of each variable was analyzed through the value of skewness and kurtosis, after which comparative analyses were performed between groups. For the data with normal distribution the paired t-test was performed and for the data with non-normal distribution the Wilcoxon Signed Rank Sum test was used. For the variable DM2 diagnosis time, the data were classified into groups according to the interquartile ranges observed ($<25\%$, between 25 and 50%, $>50\%$). To analyses differences in the values of HbA1c before (T_0) and after (T_1) the treatment with linagliptin, and stratification by pharmacotherapy of the medications of the patients was used paired t-test. All analyses were performed considering the level of significance of 5% and confidence level of 95%.

Ethics Statement

This research was approved by Ethics in Research Committee of the Federal University of São João del-Rei (UFSJ), whose approval protocol is 1,827,849.

RESULTS

It was observed that 108 participants had access to linagliptin for at least 1 month, however, only 33 (30.6%) had access for at least three consecutive months (inclusion criteria of the study). **Table 1** shows the profile of the 33 patients. It was observed that the majority of the patients were female (72.7%), evenly distributed among the age groups. The majority of patients were mixed race (36.3%), non-alcoholic (75.8%) and non-smokers (72.7%), and 48.5% reported a sedentary lifestyle. Regarding baseline glycated hemoglobin values (T_0), it was observed that the majority of the patients (63.7%) had values above 9%. However, a significant number of patients (33%) presented HbA1c values within the normal range before starting treatment.

About the clinical characteristics of the patients, concerning the time of diagnosis for DM2, a higher prevalence of diagnostic times of 7–15 years (48.5%) was observed in this population. Regarding the observed comorbidities, 78.8% of the patients had systemic arterial hypertension, 36.4% dyslipidemia, and 27.3% cardiovascular disease. As for family history, the most prevalent

TABLE 1 | Sociodemographic characteristics; lifestyle and glycated hemoglobin (HbA1c) in patients with linagliptin use in the period 2014–2016 ($n = 33$).

Variable	n (%)
Gender	
Female	24 (72.7)
Male	9 (27.3)
Age range (years)	
30–49	6 (18.1)
50–59	9 (27.3)
60–69	9 (27.3)
Over 70	9 (27.3)
Self-reported race	
Black	2 (6.1)
Mixed	12 (36.3)
White	7 (21.2)
Oriental	2 (6.1)
Not informed	10 (30.3)
Alcoholism	
Yes	2 (6.1)
No	25 (75.8)
Not informed	6 (18.1)
Smoker	
Yes	2 (6.1)
No	24 (72.7)
Not informed	7 (21.2)
Sedentary	
Yes	16 (48.5)
No	11 (33.3)
Not informed	6 (18.2)
Range of HbA1c values prior to linagliptin use	
<6%	11 (33.3)
6–8%	1 (3.0)
>9%	21 (63.7)

Data collected at T_0 – prior to the use of linagliptin.

diseases were cardiovascular disease (30.3%), diabetes mellitus (21.2%), and systemic arterial hypertension (15.2%) (**Table 2**).

Regarding the laboratory parameters, there was no statistical difference before and after the use of linagliptin (T_0 and T_1) (**Table 3**). In the results of microalbuminuria, AST, ALT, and GAMA-GT, which were investigated to analyze the safety associated with the use of linagliptin, no altered values were observed. However, it was not possible to carry out the statistical analyses due to the scarce recording of these data.

In relation to pharmacotherapy, the association of "linagliptin with other oral antidiabetics and insulin" was the most used pharmacotherapeutic scheme among patients (45.4%). Data observed at baseline showed patients with microvascular complications such as chronic kidney disease (21.2%), diabetic retinopathy (12.1%), diabetic neuropathy (6.1%), amputation (3.1%), and glaucoma (3.1%).

Regarding the effectiveness of linagliptin, it was observed that the mean HbA1c of the patients reduced from 8.94% (± 2.2) to 8.08% (± 1.7). These data correspond to an absolute reduction of -0.86% ($p < 0.05$) in HbA1c values. After stratification of the sample according to the pharmacotherapeutic scheme for DM2

TABLE 2 | Clinical characteristics of patients in continuous use of linagliptin attended by the Brazilian Public Health System (SUS) from 2014 to 2016 (n = 33).

Observed characteristics	n (%)
Time of diagnosis in years (n = 29)	
Less than 7	8 (24.2)
From 7 to 15	16 (48.5)
More than 15	6 (27.3)
Comorbidities (n = 31)	
Systemic arterial hypertension	26 (78.8)
Dyslipidemia	12 (36.4)
Cardio vascular disease[1]	10 (27.3)
Obesity[2]	8 (24.2)
Chronic kidney disease[3]	7 (21.2)
Hypothyroidism	6 (18.2)
Depression	5 (15.2)
Cataract	2 (6.1)
Fibromyalgia	2 (6.1)
Family history (n = 29)	
Cardiovascular disease	10 (30.3)
Diabetes mellitus (unspecified)	7 (21.2)
Systemic arterial hypertension	5 (15.2)
Hypothyroidism	2 (6.7)
Others[4]	4 (12.2)

Data collected at T_0 – prior to the use of linagliptin. [1]Cardiovascular diseases considered for this analysis were: cerebrovascular accident (CVA), congestive heart failure (CHF), unstable angina. [2]Patients with degrees of obesity type I and type II were grouped in this class of clinical condition. [3]Patients with degrees of renal failure III and III were grouped in this class of clinical condition. [4]Other family histories found less frequently: throat cancer, bowel cancer, breast cancer, and hearing loss.

used by the patients, the reduction of HbA1c was lower when linagliptin was used as monotherapy (**Table 4**).

Among the 12 (36.4%) patients who presented AE records during the use of linagliptin, 16.7% were on monotherapy with linagliptin and 83.3% in association with other antidiabetics. Occurrences of 25 types of AE were observed and hypoglycemia corresponded to 20.0% of the total; 60.0% of the complaints about hypoglycemia occurred in the association of "linagliptin with insulin and other oral antidiabetics" (**Table 5**).

DISCUSSION

In the effectiveness analysis of linagliptin in the present study, a difference of −0.86% (p < 0.05) of the mean values of HbA1c was observed, when considering the total population in use of the medication. However, when analyzing the effectiveness of linagliptin in monotherapy, the difference in HbA1c values was −0.48% (p > 0.05). Results of a phase III study that demonstrated its efficacy in monotherapy are close to the results here presented, with a difference in HbA1c of −0.67% after 24 weeks of study (Nogueira et al., 2014) and −0.87% after 12 weeks of study (Tang et al., 2015). In addition, according to the consensus algorithm for initiation and adjustment of therapy for DM2, the expected difference in HbA1c with iDPP-4 in monotherapy is −0.50 to −0.80%. It is also worth noting that treatment with this class has

a neutral effect on weight, has long-term safety, but is expensive pharmacotherapy (Kawamori et al., 2012).

Therefore, it is important to note that this pilot study has limitations that limit the generalization of results, such as, the study has a small sample size and it is not a randomized clinical trial with control group. In addition, it was not possible to control confounders. Another point concerns the follow-up time of patients taking linagliptin, which was relatively short, so that it was not possible to observe probable AE associated with the chronic use of the medication. Also, it is important to note that it was not possible to evaluate adherence to treatment by primary and direct methods. This study also presents limitations inherent in observational studies, such as the lack of control of the researcher on the scenario investigated. In addition, information biases can be attributed to data collection performed with secondary sources of information.

The study by Nathan et al. (2009) and Lauand et al. (2014) suggests that the effect of linagliptin on the reduction of HbA1c appears to be moderate when compared to other oral agents such as metformin and sulphonylurea, reducing from 1.0 to 2.0%, and thiazolidinedione of 0.5–1.4%. The authors consider that linagliptin has a relatively low occurrence of hypoglycemia. Therefore, this medication has been proposed to be used as a second line therapy associated with metformin in the treatment of adult patients with DM2, or even as a first line therapy in those patients intolerant to metformin. The study also points to linagliptin as an option to be used in a triple pharmacotherapeutic scheme, as observed in this investigation, which would be in combination with oral antidiabetics and insulin.

Regarding the pharmacotherapy for DM2 used by patients included in the effectiveness analysis of the present study, it was found that linagliptin was indicated as monotherapy or associated with other antidiabetics and insulins. Regarding the treatment of DM2, in the current protocols there is no specific and clear information about which stage of the disease linagliptin is indicated (American Diabetes Association [ADA], 2018). However, there are premarketing studies that demonstrate the efficacy and safety of associating linagliptin with insulin receptor sensitizers, such as biguanides and glitazones (Haak, 2015) or with other medicinal products that act to stimulate insulin production and secretion (Ross et al., 2016) and also with insulin (Haak et al., 2013; Lauand et al., 2014; Defronzo et al., 2015).

Among the four pharmacotherapeutic groups used in conjunction with linagliptin, the insulin group in combination with oral antidiabetics was the most used among patients (45.4%). Although linagliptin was not approved in Brazil by the National Agency of Sanitary Surveillance (ANVISA) for use with insulin, an off-label use of this medication was observed in this study. However, linagliptin-specific warnings and precautions given by the Food and Drug Administration (FDA) indicate that when this medication is being used with an insulin secretagogue (e.g., sulphonylurea) or insulin, we should consider reducing the dose of the insulin or insulin secretagogue to reduce the risk of hypoglycemia. Despite the divergences of indication for the association of linagliptin and insulins between regulatory agencies, phase III studies demonstrate that the association of basal insulin and other DPP-4 inhibitors significantly improves

TABLE 3 | Comparison of laboratory parameters before (T_0) and after (T_1) the continued use of linagliptin by patients attended by the Brazilian Public Health System (SUS) from 2014 to 2016 ($n = 33$).

Laboratory parameter	Reference value	Before (T_0)*	After (T_1)*	p-value*
Fasting glycemia ($n = 32$)	<130 mg/dL	171.8 (114 − 190)	139.4 (101.5 − 156.5)	0.1299
Postprandial glucose ($n = 23$)	<180 mg/dL	205.7 (143 − 252)	189.3 (120 − 237)	0.7320
Serum creatinine ($n = 28$)	From 0.4 to 1.3 mg/dL	1.4 (0.93 − 1.48)	1.1 (0.9 − 1.3)	0.7208
Serum urea ($n = 25$)	From 10 to 45 mg/dL	49.1 (26 − 63)	47 (27 − 62)	0.9256

*Non-parametric data presented in median (interquartile range: 25–75%) and statistical analyzes performed by the Wilcoxon Signed Rank Sum Test. Source: ADA, 2018 and VII Brazilian Guidelines on Hypertension. HbA1c, glycated hemoglobin.

TABLE 4 | Differences in the values of HbA1c before (T_0) and after (T_1) the treatment with linagliptin, and stratification by pharmacotherapy of the medications of the patients served by the Brazilian Public Health System (SUS) from 2014 to 2016 ($n = 33$).

Pharmacotherapeutic scheme	% HbA1c T_0 (DP)*	% HbA1c T_1 (DP)*	Effectiveness (HbA1c: T_1–T_0)	p-value of effectiveness	Frequency of adverse events (%)
Linagliptin ($n = 6$)	8.62 (1.3)	8.14 (1.5)	−0.48	0.177	16.70
Linagliptin + oral antidiabetics ($n = 11$)	7.80 (1.3)	7.36 (1.0)	−0.44	0.15	16.70
Linagliptin + insulins ($n = 3$)	11.53 (4.4)	9.23 (2.8)	−2.3	0.095	8.30
Linagliptin + insulin + oral antidiabetics ($n = 13$)	9.47 (2.0)	8.40 (1.9)	−1.07	0.014*	58.30
All patients ($n = 33$)	8.94 (2.2)	8.08 (1.7)	−0.86	0.001*	36.40

*Parametric data presented on average (standard deviation) and statistical analyses performed by the paired t-test. HbA1c, glycated hemoglobin. Pharmacotherapeutic groups: LINA, linagliptin monotherapy; LINA + AO, linagliptin associated with oral antidiabetics; LINA + INS, linagliptin associated with insulins; LINA + INS + AO, linagliptin associated with insulin and oral antidiabetic agents.

glycemic control over placebo (Rosenstock et al., 2009; Barnett et al., 2013; Yki-Järvinen et al., 2013; Marra et al., 2017).

However, in spite of the investigations demonstrating efficacy and safety in the use of linagliptin associated with insulin, in none of them was justified the rationale of this association, since the progression of DM2 reflects in the reduction of the production of insulin by the organism, a consequence of the reduction of the functioning beta cells (International Diabetes Federation [IDF], 2017). Another important factor is that the studies do not define the time of diagnosis of the patients included, or an evaluation of the tests that prove the secretory capacity of the pancreas. In the study by Yki-Järvinen et al. (2013) and Lauand et al. (2014) they observed that the type of insulin used, basal or bolus, did not interfere with the efficacy and safety of the combination with linagliptin. The literature suggests that the use of iDPP-4 should be a co-adjuvant in the treatment of DM2 (Vilsbøl et al., 2010), but it is not yet clear what are the therapeutic regimens in which it is most effective.

Studies have shown the efficacy of linagliptin associated with other pharmacotherapeutic regimens such as with metformin, suggesting a 2.72% HbA1c difference (Haak, 2015). In the results found in this study, a difference of HbA1c of −0.44% ($p = 0.150$) was observed for the association of linagliptin and oral antidiabetics, which included metformin 850 mg, metformin XR 500 mg, glibenclamide 5 mg, and gliclazide 30 mg. The differences in the values found may be related to two main factors at T_0 of the study, being (a) the difference of clinical parameters (diagnosis time, comorbidities, etc.), and (b) mean HbA1c. In the study by Ross et al., HbA1c at T_0 was 9.80 (1.1)%, being higher than in this study's population, which was 8.94 (2.2)%. According to the ADA, in patients with HbA1c values greater than 9%, gliptins may be more effective (American Diabetes Association [ADA], 2018). A meta-analysis involving 98 observational studies with 24,163 patients using iDPP-4 in different associations, attributed the cause of HbA1c reduction of 36.0% at the baseline level of HbA1c in patients. The study also found that variables such as prior oral treatment, age, gender, and body mass index (BMI), and the treatment time of the participants had no significant additional effect on the HbA1c reduction variance (Esposito et al., 2014b).

In the present study, a greater prevalence of diagnostic times of 7–15 years was observed, suggesting a population with a reduced secretory capacity of insulin by beta cells of the pancreas. In the analysis between the time of diagnosis of DM2 and the reduction in HbA1c values it was not possible to establish a correlation between the two variables. Even if these variables did correlate, it is admitted that this is a heterogeneous population with different pharmacotherapeutic regimens associated with linagliptin. Therefore, the reduction of observed HbA1c could not be attributed in a restricted way to the effectiveness of linagliptin, since insulin behaves as a powerful agent for the reduction of glucose (Esposito et al., 2015).

The literature indicates that the HbA1c reduction profile of iDPP-4 reduces with the treatment time, showing greater effectiveness in the first weeks (Vilsbøl et al., 2010). However, the time of accomplishment of the present study did not allow for the observation of this effectiveness profile, which suggests the importance of additional investigations with longer follow-up times.

Regarding the safety results of linagliptin, it was observed that more than one third of the 33 patients who used the medication continuously had some adverse event described in the literature related to linagliptin. The pharmacotherapeutic regimen that presented the most adverse events (58.3%) was that of triple pharmacotherapy (linagliptin + oral antidiabetic + insulin), with hypoglycemia being the most reported AE in this group. In this sense, considering the pharmacodynamics of these medications,

TABLE 5 | Adverse events using linagliptin described in the records of patients served by the Brazilian Public Health System (SUS), from 2014 to 2016 (*n* = 33).

Profile of recorded adverse events (AE)	*n* (%)
Total number of patients with adverse events	12(36.4%)
Number of registered AE	25
Types of adverse events	
Hypoglycemia[1]	5 (20.0)
Muscular pain[2]	3 (12.5)
Gastrointestinal[3]	3 (12.5)
Others[4]	14 (56.0)

[1]Unspecified hypoglycemia (4); hypoglycemia at night (1). [2]Pain in lower limbs (2); lower back pain (1). [3]Gastrointestinal events: intestinal constipation (1); vomiting (1); diarrhea (1). [4]Other: hepatomegaly, polydipsia, polyuria, polyphagia, weight loss, nocturia, altered sleep-wake cycle, edema, fever, fetid urine, weight gain, decreased visual acuity, dizziness, and otitis.

it is valid to consider that this event may be related more strictly to the use of insulin than to linagliptin. However, the study design and the co-medications used do not allow to infer the causality of the AE. In addition, information on the insulin doses used was not available. It is important to note that in this study only those AE that occurred after starting treatment with linagliptin were considered.

The total frequency of hypoglycemia in the 33 patients was approximately 15.0%. In the study by Gomis et al. (2012) and Esposito et al. (2014a), a similar frequency of hypoglycemia of 14.6% was observed in patients using linagliptin with other antidiabetics over a period of 24 weeks, twice the time of the present study (Esposito et al., 2014a).

In monotherapy with linagliptin the observed frequency of hypoglycemia was 16.7%, being a higher frequency when compared to studies by Haak et al. (2013), Defronzo et al. (2015), and Ross et al. (2016) whose incidence of this adverse event was lower than 8.0%. The present study differs from the clinical trials regarding the follow-up time of the participants, which ranged from 24 to 52 weeks in these studies, and also the characteristics of the population, since the clinical trials were controlled and since they excluded from the study any participants presenting comorbidities and who were inserted into the real world of polypharmacy.

Gomis et al. (2012) and Inagaki et al. (2013) evaluated hypoglycemia in the linagliptin-associated groups of biguanide, glinid, glitazone, sulfonylurea, and α-glucosidase inhibitors. In that study, only in the groups treated with linagliptin associated with sulphonylurea did hypoglycemia occur (9.5 and 5.9%). The incidence of hypoglycemia was significantly lower (<4.0%) in other studies using this AE as one of the outcomes (Kawamori et al., 2012; Inagaki et al., 2013; Tang et al., 2015).

The literature reports that hypoglycemic events are rare because of the glucose-ingestion dependent action (Haak et al., 2013), but they occur predominantly when a DPP-4 inhibitor is associated with sulfonylureas (American Diabetes Association [ADA], 2018). In the present study six patients (18.2%) were using glibenclamide or gliclazide, which are representatives of sulfonylureas associated with hypoglycemia.

It is important to note that in most premarketing studies, patients with these clinical conditions were not eligible for the

study because of exclusion criteria, or family history data were not assessed (Haak et al., 2013; Inagaki et al., 2013; Lauand et al., 2014; Defronzo et al., 2015; Tang et al., 2015). In view of this, the importance of the post-marketing studies that accompany, record, and analyze data on the use of the medication in the real world stands out. All these factors can justify the differences found in this study, both in the effectiveness results and those related to medication safety.

Although the laboratory parameters analyzed did not present statistically significant differences between T_1 and T_0, a reduction was observed in fasting glucose, postprandial glucose, serum creatinine and serum urea levels. The fact that these parameters did not show significant improvement in their values can be explained by the small sample size and the short follow-up period. In addition, it is important to note that the scarcity of recording in the patient's medical record of safety parameters such as microalbuminuria, AST, ALT, and GAMA-GT suggests absence of clinical monitoring or non-occurrence of an adverse event.

A systematic review by Gomes et al. (2018) presented results from 16 randomized clinical trials, evaluating the effectiveness and safety of linagliptin. The study identified that 93.8% of the studies were funded by the pharmaceutical industry, which evidences the need for studies free of conflicts of interest (Andriolo and Vieira, 2005).

Regarding the strengths of the study, it should be considered that this is the first real-world investigation conducted with Brazilian patients who used linagliptin, free from the influence of the pharmaceutical industry, in which the pharmacotherapy studied is immersed in a complex scenario which is related to the existing comorbidities and the presence of other factors extrinsic to the participants. In this sense, it is valid to consider that 93.8% of the studies evaluating the safety of linagliptin are financed by the pharmaceutical industry, and most of them had a comparison with placebo rather than with conventional pharmacotherapies (Andriolo and Vieira, 2005). On the other hand, the results of this study cannot be generalized, given the small sample size and the specificity of the participants.

In summary, the relevance of post-marketing studies as a tool for decision makers is recognized, especially in the face of unfavorable economic scenarios. Pharmacoeconomic studies and with a greater number of patients are needed to subsidize information for more assertive choices, maximizing the benefits of investments, without compromising the sustainability of the public health system.

CONCLUSION

In the real world, linagliptin presented lower performance than in randomized premarketing clinical trials. These results reinforce the relevance of post-marketing studies as a tool for decision, especially in the face of unfavorable economic scenarios. In addition, it is important that further research be conducted through pragmatic clinical trials to be performed to assess possible confounding variables of real-world, such as adherence and access to medications. Because in public health system is not feasible that the therapeutic alternative has only efficacy. It needs to be effective and efficient.

AUTHOR CONTRIBUTIONS

GG, MP, CS, and AB contributed to conception and design of the study. GG organized the database and performed the statistical analysis. MP, CS, and AB wrote the first draft of the manuscript. All authors contributed to manuscript revision, and read and approved the submitted version.

FUNDING

The present work was carried out with the support of the Coordination of Improvement of Higher Education Personnel – Brazil (CAPES) – Financing Code 001.

ACKNOWLEDGMENTS

We thank the Federal University of São João del-Rei (UFSJ), Dona Lindu Center – West Campus (CCO) for infrastructure and institutional support. We also thank the editors of Frontiers Pharmacology for their support, especially Dr. Brian Boyle and Dra. Luciane Cruz Lopes.

REFERENCES

American Diabetes Association [ADA] (2018). *ADA: Standards of Medical Care.* Arlington, VA: American Diabetes Association.

Andriolo, A., and Vieira, J. G. H. (2005). "Diagnóstico e acompanhamento laboratorial do diabetes mellitus," in *Guias De Medicina Ambulatorial e Hospitalar Unifesp/Escola Paulista de Medicina*, ed. A. Andriolo (Sao. Paulo: Manole).

ANVISA (2017). *Agência Nacional de Vigilância Sanitária. Trayenta – linagliptina. Bula professional.* Ingelheim: Boehringer Ingelheim.

Barnett, A. H., Huisman, H., Jones, R., Eynatten, M. V., Patel, S., Woerle, H. J., et al. (2013). Linagliptin for patients aged 70 years or older with type 2 diabetes inadequately controlled with common antidiabetes treatments: a randomised, double-blind, placebo-controlled trial. *Lancet* 382, 1413–1423

Chen, Y., Ning, G., Wang, C., Gong, Y., Patel, S., Zhang, C., et al. (2015). Efficacy and safety of linagliptin monotherapy 24-week, randomized, clinical trial. *J. Diabetes Investig.* 6, 692–698. doi: 10.1111/jdi.12346

Defronzo, R. A., Lewin, A., Patel, S., Liu, D., Kaste, R., Woerle, H. J., et al. (2015). Combination of empagliflozin and linagliptin as second-line therapy in subjects with type 2 diabetes inadequately controlled on metformin. *Diabetes Care* 38, 384–393. doi: 10.2337/dc14-2364

Elseviers, M., Wettermark, B., Almarsdóttir, A. B., Andersen, M., Benko, R., Bennie, M., et al. (2016). *Drug Utilization Research.* Hoboken, NY: ED Wiley-Blackwell.

Esposito, K., Chiodini, P., Capuano, A., Maiorino, M. I., Bellastella, G., Giugliano, D., et al. (2014a). Baseline glycemic parameters predict the hemoglobin A1c response to DPP-4 inhibitors. Meta-regression analysis of 78 randomized controlled trials with 20,053 patients. *Endocrine* 46, 43–51. doi: 10.1007/s12020-013-0090-0

Esposito, K., Chiodini, P., Maiorino, M. I., Bellastella, G., and Capuano, A. (2014b). Glycaemic durability with dipeptidyl peptidase-4 inhibitors in type 2 diabetes: a systematic review and meta-analysis of long-term randomized controlled trials. *BMJ Open* 4:e005442. doi: 10.1136/bmjopen-2014-005442

Esposito, K., Chiodini, P., Maiorino, M. I., Capuano, A., Cozzolino, D., Petrizzo, M., et al. (2015). A nomogram to estimate the HbA1c response to different DPP-4 inhibitors in type 2 diabetes: a systematic review and meta-analysis of 98 trials with 24 163 patients. *BMJ Open* 5:e005892. doi: 10.1136/bmjopen-2014-005892

Food And Drug Administration [FDA] (2013). *Incretin Mimetic Drugs for Type 2 Diabetes: Early Communication - Reports of Possible Increased Risk of Pancreatitis and Precancerous Findings of the Pancreas.* Available at: https://www.fda.gov/drugs/drug-safety-and-availability/fda-drug-safety-communication-fda-investigating-reports-possible-increased-risk-pancreatitis-and-pre (accessed December 5, 2018).

Gomes, G. K. A., Ramos, A. I. C., Sousa, C. T., Sanches, C., Pereira, M. L., and Baldoni, A. O. (2018). Linagliptin safety profile: a systematic review. *Primary Care Diabetes* 12, 477–490. doi: 10.1016/j.pcd.2018.04.006

Gomis, R., Owens, D. R., Taskinen, M. R., Del Prato, S., Patel, S., Pivovarova, A., et al. (2012). Long-term safety and efficacy of linagliptin as monotherapy or in combination with other oral glucose-lowering agents in 2121 subjects with type 2 diabetes: up to 2 years exposure in 24-week phase III trials followed by a 78-week open-label extension. *Int. J. Clin. Pract.* 66, 731–740. doi: 10.1111/j.1742-1241.2012.02975.x

Haak, T. (2015). Combination of linagliptin and metformin for the treatment of patients with type 2 diabetes. *Clin. Med. Insights Endocrinol. Diabetes* 8, 1–6. doi: 10.4137/CMED.S10360

Haak, T., Meinicke, T., Jones, R., Weber, S., Eynatten, M. V., and Woerle, H. J. (2013). Initial combination of linagliptin and metformin in patients with type 2 diabetes: efficacy and safety in a randomised, double-blind 1-year extension study. *Int. J. Clin. Pract.* 67, 1283–1293. doi: 10.1111/j.1463-1326.2012.01590.x

Inagaki, N., Watada, H., Murai, M., Kagimura, T., Gong, Y., Pate, L. S., et al. (2013). Linagliptin provides effective, well-tolerated add-on therapy to preexisting oral antidiabetic therapy over 1 year in Japanese patients with type 2 diabetes. *Diabetes Obes. Metab.* 15, 833–843. doi: 10.1111/dom.12110

International Diabetes Federation [IDF] (2017). *Diabetes Atlas – Executive Summary*, 8th Edn. Belgium: International Diabetes Federation.

Kawamori, R., Inagaki, N., Araki, E., Watada, H., Hayashi, N., Horie, Y., et al. (2012). Linagliptin monotherapy provides superior glycaemic control versus placebo or voglibose with comparable safety in japanese patients with type 2 diabetes: a randomized, placebo and active comparator-controlled, double-blind study. *Diabetes Obes. Metab.* 14, 348–357. doi: 10.1111/j.1463-1326.2011.01545.x

Kempen, J. H. (2011). Appropriate use and reporting of uncontrolled case series in the medical literature. *Am. J. Ophthalmol.* 151, 7–10. doi: 10.1016/j.ajo.2010.08.047

Lauand, F., Hohl, A., Ronsoni, M. F., Guedes, E. P., and Melo, T. G. (2014). Linagliptin: DDP-4 inhibition in the treatment of type 2 diabetes mellitus. *J. Diabetes Metab. Disord. Control* 1, 13–19. doi: 10.15406/jdmdc.2014.01.00005

Malta, M., Magnanini, M., Cardoso, L. O., and Silva, C. M. F. (2010). Iniciativa STROBE: subsídios para a comunicação de estudos observacionais Strobe initiative: guidelines on reporting observational studies. *Revista de Saúde Pública* 44, 559–565. doi: 10.1590/S0034-89102010000300021

Marra, L. P., Araújo, V., Oliveira, O. C. C., Diniz, L. M., Junior, A. G., Acurcio, F. A., et al. (2017). The clinical effectiveness of insulin glargine in patients with Type I diabetes in Brazil: findings and implications. *J. Comp. Eff. Res.* 6, 519–527. doi: 10.2217/cer-2016-0099

Marx, N., Rosenstock, J., Kahn, S., Zinman, B., Kastelein, J., Lachin, J., et al. (2015). Design and baseline characteristics of the cardiovascular outcome trial of linagliptin versus glimepiride in type 2 diabetes (CAROLINA®). *Diab. Vasc. Dis. Res.* 12, 164–174. doi: 10.1177/1479164115570301

Mikhael, E. M. (2016). Effectiveness and safety of newer antidiabetic medications for ramadan fasting diabetic patients. *J. Diabetes Res.* 2016:6962574. doi: 10.1155/2016/6962574

Morris, D. H., Khunti, K., Achana, F., Srinivasan, B., Gray, L. J., Davies, M. J., et al. (2013). Progression rates from HbA1c 6.0–6.4% and other prediabetes definitions to type 2 diabetes: a meta-analysis. *Diabetologia* 56, 1489–1493. doi: 10.1007/s00125-013-2902-4

Nathan, D. M., Buse, J. B., Davidson, M. B., Ferrannini, E., Holman, R. R., Sherwin, R., et al. (2009). medical management of hyperglycemia in type 2 diabetes: a consensus algorithm for the initiation and adjustment of therapy. *Diabetes Care* 32, 193–203. doi: 10.2337/dc08-9025

Nogueira, T. A. S., Aquino, J. A., Giraud, C. S., and Baldoni, A. O. (2014). Perfil de segurança e efetividade dos Inibidores da dipeptidil peptidase-4. *Rev. Bras. Farm. Hosp. Serv. Saúde* 5, 6–12.

Prescrire International (2017). Towards better patient care: drugs to avoid in 2017. *Rev. Prescrire* 37, 137–148.

Richard, E. P. (2014). Linagliptin use in older individuals with diabets. *Clin. Interv. Aging* 9, 1109–1114. doi: 10.2147/CIA.S62877

Rosenstock, J., Rendell, M. S., Gross, J. L., Fleck, P. R., Wilson, C. A., and Mekki, Q. (2009). Alogliptin added to insulin therapy in patients with type 2 diabetes reduces HbA1c without causing weight gain or increased hypoglycaemia. *Diabetes Obes. Metab.* 11, 1145–1152. doi: 10.1111/j.1463-1326.2009.01124.x

Ross, S. A., Caballero, A. E., Del Prato, S., Gallwitz, B., Lewis, D., Bailes, Z., et al. (2016). Initial combination of linagliptin and metformin compared with linagliptin monotherapy in patients with newly diagnosed type 2 diabetes and marked hyperglycaemia: a randomized, double-blind, active-controlled, parallel group, multinational clinical trial. *Diabetes Obes. Metab.* 17, 136–144. doi: 10.1111/dom.12399

Sortino, M. A., Sinagra, T., and Canonico, P. L. (2013). Linagliptin: a thorough characterization beyond its clinical efficacy. *Front. Endocrinol.* 4:16. doi: 10.3389/fendo.2013.00016

Tang, Y., Wang, G., Jiang, Z., Yan, T., Chen, Y., Yang, M., et al. (2015). Efficacy and safety of vildagliptin, sitagliptin, and linagliptin as add-on therapy in Chinese patients with T2DM inadequately controlled with dual combination of insulin and traditional oral hypoglycemic agent. *Diabetol. Metab. Syndr.* 7:91. doi: 10.1186/s13098-015-0087-3

Thrasher, L. (2016). Pharmacologic management of type 2 diabetes mellitus: available therapies. *Am. J. Med.* 130, S4–S17. doi: 10.1016/j.amjcard.2017.05.009

Vilsbøl, T., Rosenstock, L. J., Yki-Järvinen, H., Cefalu, W. T., Chen, Y., Luo, E., et al. (2010). Efficacy and safety of sitagliptin when added to insulin therapy in patients with type 2 diabetes. *Diabetes Obes. Metab.* 12, 167–177. doi: 10.1111/j.1463-1326.2009.01173.x

Websky, K., Reichetzeder, C., and Hocher, B. (2013). Linagliptin as add-on therapy to insulin for patients with type 2 diabetes. *Vasc. Health Risk Manag.* 9, 681–694. doi: 10.2147/VHRM.S40035

Yki-Järvinen, H., Rosenstock, J., Durán-Garcia, S., Pinnetti, S., Bhattacharya, S., Thiemann, S., et al. (2013). Effects of adding linagliptin to basal insulin regimen for inadequately controlled type 2 diabetes: a 52-week randomized, double-blind study. *Diabetes Care* 36, 3875–3881. doi: 10.2337/dc12-2718

10

Spatially Enabling the Health Sector

Tarun Stephen Weeramanthri[1,2]* and Peter Woodgate[2,3]

[1] Department of Health, Government of Western Australia, Perth, WA, Australia, [2] Cooperative Research Centre for Spatial Information, Carlton, VIC, Australia, [3] Global Spatial Network Board, Cooperative Research Centre for Spatial Information, Carlton, VIC, Australia

*Correspondence:
Tarun Stephen Weeramanthri
tarun.weeramanthri@health.wa.gov.au

Spatial information describes the physical location of either people or objects, and the measured relationships between them. In this article, we offer the view that greater utilization of spatial information and its related technology, as part of a broader redesign of the architecture of health information at local and national levels, could assist and speed up the process of health reform, which is taking place across the globe in richer and poorer countries alike. In making this point, we describe the impetus for health sector reform, recent developments in spatial information and analytics, and current Australasian spatial health research. We highlight examples of uptake of spatial information by the health sector, as well as missed opportunities. Our recommendations to spatially enable the health sector are applicable to high- and low-resource settings.

Keywords: spatial information, health sector, health reform, health information, innovation, technology, end-user development

THE IMPETUS FOR HEALTH SECTOR REFORM

Spatial information describes the physical location of either people or objects, and the measured relationships between them. We argue in this article that well-established geographic information systems (GIS), as well as more recent advances in spatial technologies, analytics, and visualization, have the potential to enrich our understanding of health systems and drive strategies for health sector reform.

In defining "health systems," the World Health Organization (WHO) includes "all the activities whose primary purpose is to promote, restore and/or maintain health" as well as associated "people, institutions and resources."[1] The use of the word "sector" emphasizes the industry aspects, including its organization (public and private), financing, and performance dimensions. Health sector reforms have been defined as "sustained, purposeful changes to improve the efficiency, equity and effectiveness of the health sector" (1).

There are a number of pressures on health systems that are present in many countries, regardless of their level of development. These include an aging population, with an increasing burden of chronic disease; introduction of new technologies (services, drugs, and medical devices); and increased consumer expectations (which tend to rise with increasing wealth). In short, demand for health services is increasingly outstripping supply, and as a result, costs are rising in an unsustainable way. In the five decades to 2008, spending on health care grew by 2% points in excess of GDP growth across all Organisation for Economic Cooperation and Development (OECD) countries. From 2005 to 2009, average annual health spending growth across the OECD was 3.4%, though this slowed to 0.6% in the period from 2009 to 2013, in the aftermath of the global financial crisis (2).

---

[1] http://www.who.int/healthsystems/hss_glossary/en/.

Senkubuge and colleagues (3) argue that there is no single global or regional policy formula for health sector reform and that it will depend on a country's history, values, and culture. On the one hand, many developed countries are approaching health reform from a cost-efficiency perspective, aiming to reduce costs while maintaining quality of care and improvements in longevity. On the other hand, there is a strong agenda for change in less wealthy countries, which emphasizes universal health insurance, equity, strengthening of primary care, and addressing of social and environmental determinants of health.

The WHO describes how a well-functioning health information system allows for reliable and timely decision making at different levels of the health system (4). It outlines three domains of health information: health status; determinants of health; and health system performance. These three domains have been used by many countries, including Australia, to develop performance frameworks,[2] which can also then serve as ways to measure the success or otherwise of health reform efforts.

Having made the argument that information is a key pillar for health reform, we now turn to the value of spatial information in particular.

THE FUTURE IS SPATIAL, BUT HEALTH SECTOR UPTAKE IS PATCHY

Spatial information is a broad term that describes the connection between data on positioning and location with that of people, objects (both built and natural), and activities. It includes tools such as aerial and satellite remote sensors, Global Navigation Satellite Systems (e.g., GPS), and computerized GIS software. Traditionally spatial data have been uniquely characterized as geographic (e.g., longitude and latitude) or map-based coordinates. In more recent years, the concepts of location and place ("the railway station" and "my home," respectively) have gained broader attention. For example, "what3words"[3] has divided the world into a 3 m-by-3 m grid and assigned a unique combination of three words to each grid cell to enable a fine granularity of positioning using language, not coordinates. So "spatial" is not "just maps."

Spatial analytics is also changing. Traditional approaches using GIS software have typically undertaken distance and proximity analyses on single and multiple datasets that are co-registered and "stacked" in a single database. More recently, there has been a trend for spatial analytics to become increasingly web-based, accessing both data and tools from multiple sources.

Adoption of spatial technology by the public *via* Internet-enabled and mobile devices is now commonplace, and health professionals are no exception in terms of their use for personal purposes. Case studies of potential uses in the health sector include mapping and matching of needs and services, and evaluation of outcomes (including adverse events and medical errors), depending on location of residence or work (5). For example, a recent study looked at the variation in common hospital procedures (such as arthroscopies, cesarean sections, and cardiac procedures) across regions in Australia and found that much of the variation was unwarranted, unrelated to demonstrable need, and hence not a good use of scarce resources (6).

Spatial tools have also been used for many years to explore environmental determinants of cancer, describe risk factors for chronic disease, investigate disease transmission, and plan for and respond to natural disasters, including in low-resource settings, where application to infectious disease surveillance and outbreak response predominates (7). Indeed, modern public health, in the English-speaking world, was founded in the work of John Snow and his carefully drawn cholera maps in the London of the 1850s (8).

Our argument is that despite all of the above, there is little evidence that such technologies are being used in a comprehensive or planned way across the health sector to drive health reform. Certainly, in developed economies, the hospital and acute care sector has seen the benefits of precision location technology through sophisticated *within the body* imaging techniques (CT, MRI, etc.). But this has not translated into a consistent desire for location precision *outside the body*.

As a result, good spatial health practice remains the exception rather than the rule, GIS practitioners remain relatively isolated from other information analysts, the role of location or spatial information is rarely discussed at an executive level in health organizations, and it is often neglected in strategic planning. We miss many opportunities to utilize spatial technology in the health sector, and its potential remains significantly under-utilized.

AUSTRALASIAN SPATIAL HEALTH RESEARCH

The geoservices market is dynamic and expanding faster than the global economy (9). Many sectors, including defense, engineering, transport, energy, agriculture, environment, and mining and resources, have been utilizing spatial technology in a systematized way for many decades, and several were instrumental in a successful bid in 2003 for a Cooperative Research Centre in Spatial Information (CRC-SI).[4] The Australian Government's Cooperative Research Centre's Programme[5] supports industry-led collaborations between researchers, industry, and the community, and forms part of the National Innovation and Science Agenda.[6] In 2010, a Health Program was included in a successful second-phase funding bid of the CRC-SI.

The CRC-SI aims for end-user-driven research, and this same principle underpins the Health Program, which has major programs on visualization and privacy protection (based in Western Australia), spatial statistical modeling (based in Queensland), and healthy cities and recovery from natural disasters (based in New Zealand).[7]

---

[2]http://meteor.aihw.gov.au/content/index.phtml/itemId/435314.
[3]http://what3words.com/.

[4]http://www.crcsi.com.au/.
[5]http://www.industry.gov.au/industry/IndustryInitiatives/IndustryResearch Collaboration/CRC/Pages/default.aspx.
[6]http://www.innovation.gov.au/page/agenda.
[7]http://www.crcsi.com.au/research/4-4-health/.

It is helpful for end-users if spatial tools are available and accessible to more than a few GIS specialists. Therefore, the Department of Health in Western Australia (DoHWA) has developed an online geovisualisation tool called *HealthTracks*, with both interactive mapping and reporting functions, that makes a broad range of demographic, health, and environmental data available *via* a web interface to all employees (10). Non-expert users, including clinicians, program managers, policy makers, and planners, can generate their own local area reports, tables, and maps.

HealthTracks has successfully extended the number of users of GIS information in DoHWA. Prior to its development, around six epidemiologists and GIS analysts were regular users of spatial technologies. The semi-automation of analytics, coupled with a largely plain language interface, has seen 150 users generate over 7000 maps and reports in the last year. However, this number remains a fraction of the total workforce of over 40,000.

A related project called *Epiphanee* has focused on generating dynamic privacy protections, based on a complex algorithm that takes into account small number analysis and reporting – a particularly important issue for health data, and of particular concern to data custodians charged with protecting health privacy (11). The program allows the user, when making a single data request from multiple datasets, to trade-off competing dimensions of area size, disease specificity, and demographic composition, and generate a report that falls within probabilistic privacy limits set by the data custodians. This project highlights the distinctive and highly sensitive nature of health information.

A good spatial analytics program for health relies on fundamental spatial concepts, including scale, accuracy, and geocoding uncertainty (12), as well as a critical approach to spatial thinking, reasoning, and language (13). Data analysis also requires specialized statistical expertise to deal with the heterogeneity of spatial data, and its tendency to exhibit autocorrelation. Using the release of the Atlas of Cancer in Queensland (14) as a foundation, Queensland researchers have developed new spatiotemporal modeling techniques to examine cancer incidence and survival within small areas, important for understanding and reducing population-level inequities. Analysis based on the Atlas led the Queensland government to double its rural travel subsidy for patients to attend screening and treatment facilities.

Epidemiological studies have traditionally looked at the aggregate relationship between geographic areas and disease risk factors or outcomes (e.g., a certain neighborhood may have an elevated level of obesity or diabetes). Longitudinal spatial studies are much less frequent. In New Zealand, University of Canterbury researchers have used fine-grained spatial tools and modeling, to examine the medium to long-term health and mental health impacts of the 2010/2011 earthquakes, particularly as they relate to place of exposure and subsequent mobility (15). The New Zealand research builds on a joint Ministry of Health-University of Canterbury venture, called the GeoHealth Laboratory (16), a partnership that helps ensure research results inform the targeting and ongoing design of social support and health services.

Even less frequently explored is how geocoded social determinants can be used to improve patient care at the community health center level (17). Research has identified the spatial clustering of older patients with poorly controlled diabetes within a large Australian general practice using individual-level data (18). Such analyses have the potential to promote new preventive strategies and stimulate better targeted approaches to patient management at a community level.

Australia has also focused on building capacity through international partnerships and is a member of the Global Spatial Network (GSN),[8] which has identified the health sector as a priority sector for growth and application of spatial technology. The GSN is made up of research organizations that specialize in collaborative research. Member organizations must have partners drawn from the research sector, the private sector, and the government sector. Partnering organizations have come from Sweden, the EU, the US, Canada, Mexico, Korea, New Zealand, and Australia. The GSN seeks to promote international collaboration in complex, multi-organization spatial research and facilitate information sharing. As a result of the Network's activities, Sweden now hosts an annual workshop of spatial and health researchers as part of their "Geolife Region program."[9]

Training is central to building capacity, and the teaching of spatial skills encompasses much more than the use of GIS software. Specially commissioned special "GIS Awareness for Health Professionals" training courses that use case studies and scenarios to promote the intelligent application of spatial data and analysis within the health sector have now begun to be developed.[10]

These projects and products have not yet, however, been game changers in the health sector in Australia. There are a number of factors, including the relatively modest size of the program (less than one million Australian dollars per year), and its positioning as a "research" rather than a "services" program within a very large industry. But there may be other factors. In thinking through this issue, we adopted a model of technology use as the product of "context, tool and user," and a "spatial maturity" model as a *set of capabilities* required for the effective use of spatial technology (19).

The CRC-SI has developed and trialed this model in a health sector setting, in order to benchmark performance and drive organizational improvement. The messages were clear: there is more to technology adoption than just "cool tools"; use of a generic framework can help assess and improve "capacity to use"; and mixed methods analysis (combining quantitative and qualitative approaches) can generate critical organizational insights (20).

CHALLENGES AND FUTURE DIRECTIONS

Spatial technology encompasses much more than static maps. The global public are already familiar with an array of new dynamic location tools from GPS-enabled mobile phones to Google Earth. Newer trends in data sharing made possible through wearable sensors, crowdsourcing, and interactive social media platforms are developing quickly and will stimulate debate about the social

---

[8]http://www.globalspatial.org/.
[9]http://geoliferegion.com/about-geo-life-region/about-geo-life-region-2/.
[10]http://ngis.com.au/gis-awareness-for-health-professionals/.

and contextual dimensions of *place*, to complement the technical considerations of *space* and *location* (21).

Developments in remote sensing and positioning technology will provide more precise environmental data, wearable sensors will provide a wealth of individual data, and informatics will allow the analysis of such big and complex datasets in much closer to real time. Importantly, computing power has increased, and technology costs have fallen, leading to potential applications even in low-resource settings.

There is likely to be increasing public demand for more tailored risk communication and personalized medicine, which will depend, in part, on more accurate and accessible spatial data. But there is no guarantee that advances in the use of spatial technology for individuals will aggregate neatly into improvements at a population level. In other words, precision medicine or precision "wellness" that is available only to a minority, and does not give consideration to other determinants of health, can aggravate inequity in a population (22). Hence, there is need for a broader performance framework for successful health reform.

In the health sector, uptake of spatial technology will also be affected by parallel developments in e-Health, telehealth, business intelligence, "Big Data," and the web (3.0 and beyond). Over time, more datasets will be linked, more health information will be available online, and more use made of off-the-shelf software and automated processing. As governments make more of their data open and freely available, the potential to combine such data with open analytic tools and personal data from other sources will also increase, leading to potentially greater insights but also foreseeable dangers. Privacy, data sharing, and data security concerns will need to be continuously addressed. In this new environment, the semantic web[11] has the potential to empower users to access sophisticated programs through plain language queries. For example, it may be feasible to perform a geographic search for all cancer screening facilities within a radius of a chosen location and combine this with patient screening behavior, sociodemographic information, and cancer outcomes, so as to better target interventions to increase screening rates – all from a web browser.

MISSED OPPORTUNITIES

The public, clinicians, health system planners, and policy makers each have a stake in improving both the spatial specificity of the information that underpins advanced analytics and our ability to visually communicate that information for a variety of purposes, including risk communication, service delivery, and planning, and policy.

However, we think that much more needs to be done to catalyze a transformation of what is a massive and complex industry sector, so that spatial information can become integral to evidence-based, data-rich, and patient-centered health reform. Supporting spatial data infrastructures (such as the European Union INSPIRE[12] initiative) are well established in some regions, but it is the culture and capabilities within the health sector that are poorly developed.

As a result, the health community misses clear opportunities to add value to information from a spatial perspective. Two recent Australian examples are the Personally Controlled Electronic Health Record[13] and the National Disability Insurance Scheme.[14] Neither of these large potentially transformative national programs, critical to health sector reform, considered or built detailed spatial specifications into their initial roll out plans.

We would like to see such initiatives, and indeed all large agencies that handle health data, undertake a "spatial maturity" review to identify their existing operational capabilities, and any measures that could be readily adopted or adapted to improve information handling and analysis in a systematic way and in a strategic context. This would transform the potential of spatial information – from an optional extra to an essential ingredient of a strong information strategy underpinning health reform. Spatial maturity reviews also serve as a form of future due diligence, setting up a pathway that links agencies to both the activities of the spatial analytics research community and the proprietary tools of the private sector.

RECOMMENDATIONS

In summary, based on our experience in health delivery and spatial health research, we believe that the core technology is present and developing rapidly for spatial information to contribute to health sector reform. No major technological breakthrough is needed. What is missing is an attitude change to see the potential and make the most of spatial data and analytics, as well as to incorporate spatial thinking into strategic thinking.

We therefore make the following recommendations to spatially enable the health sector:

(a) continue to communicate strong case studies of where spatial technology has led to improved decision making and value for end-users, mapped against key health performance areas;

(b) formally evaluate the use, costs, and benefits that the technology provides in the health sector and test its applicability in high- and low-resource settings;

(c) use spatial data to describe patient pathways, particularly for common chronic conditions, across an integrated health system from community to primary care to hospital and back;

(d) explicitly consider the "spatial maturity" model as a tool to drive organizational change;

(e) commission national-level studies that focus on pathways to adoption of spatial technology that includes major health industry stakeholders;

(f) learn the lessons from other major industry sectors, which are more advanced in their use of spatial information;

(g) include spatial information and supporting technologies when developing broader information, digital health, and "big data" strategies; and

(h) build training, capacity, and new stakeholder partnerships, nationally and internationally.

---

[11] https://www.w3.org/standards/semanticweb/.
[12] http://inspire.ec.europa.eu/.

[13] http://www.health.gov.au/internet/main/publishing.nsf/content/ehealth-record.
[14] https://myplace.ndis.gov.au/ndisstorefront/index.html.

AUTHOR CONTRIBUTIONS

TW created the first draft of this article, based on a set of discussions with PW over many years. Both TW and PW have contributed ideas, text, and references to subsequent and final versions.

ACKNOWLEDGMENTS

The authors would like to gratefully acknowledge the contribution of all members of the CRC-SI Health Program since its inception – program managers, researchers, science directors, board members, administrators, and partners – as well as the support of the broader CRC-SI administration and board.

FUNDING

The Cooperative Research Centre for Spatial Information (CRC-SI) is funded through the Australian Government Cooperative Research Centre Programme that supports industry-led collaborations between researchers, industry, and the community. PW is the salaried Chief Executive Officer of the CRC-SI, and TW acts as the Chair of the Health Program Board in an unpaid capacity.

REFERENCES

1. Cassels A. Health sector reform: key issues in less developed countries. *J Int Dev* (1995) 7:329–47. doi:10.1002/jid.3380070303
2. OECD. *Fiscal Sustainability of Health Systems: Bridging Health and Finance Perspectives*. Paris: OECD Publishing (2015).
3. Senkubuge F, Modisenyane M, Bishaw T. Strengthening health systems by health sector reforms. *Glob Health Action* (2014) 7:23568. doi:10.3402/gha.v7.23568
4. WHO. *Everybody's Business: Strengthening Health Systems to Improve Health Outcomes*. Geneva: World Health Organisation (2015). 46 p.
5. Lang L. *GIS for Health Organisations*. California: ESRI Press (2000). 100 p.
6. Australian Commission on Safety and Quality in Health Care, Australian Institute of Health and Welfare. *Exploring Healthcare Variation in Australia: Analyses Resulting from an OECD Study*. Sydney: ACSQHC (2014).
7. Lyseen AK, Nohr C, Sorensen EM, Gudes O, Geraghty EM, Shaw NT, et al. A review and framework for categorizing current research and development in health related geographical information systems (GIS) studies. *Yearb Med Inform* (2014) 9:110–24. doi:10.15265/IY-2014-0008
8. Snow J. *On the Mode of Communication of Cholera*. London: John Churchill (1855). 162 p.
9. Woodgate P, Coppa I, Hart N. *Global Outlook 2014: Spatial Information Industry*. (Vol. 102). Australia and New Zealand Cooperative Research Centre for Spatial Information (2014). Available from: http://www.crcsi.com.au/assets/Resources/Global-Outlook-Report-November-2014.pdf
10. Jardine A, Mullan N, Gudes O, Moncrieff S, West G, Cosford J, et al. Web-based geovisualisation of spatial information to support evidence-based health policy: a case study of the development process of *HealthTracks*. *HIM J* (2014) 43:7–16. doi:10.12826/18333575.2014.0004.Jardine
11. Moncrieff S, West G, Cosford J, Mullan N, Jardine A. An open source, server-side framework for analytical web mapping and its application to health. *Int J Digit Earth* (2013) 7:294–315. doi:10.1080/17538947.2013.786143
12. Goldberg DW, Ballard M, Boyd JH, Mullan N, Garfield C, Rosman D, et al. An evaluation framework for comparing geocoding systems. *Int J Health Geogr* (2013) 12:50. doi:10.1186/1476-072X-12-50
13. Goodchild MF, Janelle DG. Towards critical spatial thinking in the social sciences and humanities. *GeoJournal* (2010) 75:3–13. doi:10.1007/s10708-010-9340-3
14. Cramb SM, Mengersen KL, Baade PD. Developing the atlas of cancer in Queensland: methodological issues. *Int J Health Geogr* (2011) 10:9. doi:10.1186/1476-072X-10-9
15. Hogg D, Kingham S, Wilson T, Ardagh M. The effects of relocation and level of affectedness on mood and anxiety symptom treatments after the 2011 Christchurch earthquake. *Soc Sci Med* (2016) 152:18–26. doi:10.1016/j.socscimed.2016.01.025
16. Bowie C, Beere P, Griffin E, Campbell M, Kingham S. Variation in health and social equity in the spaces where we live: a review of previous literature from the GeoHealth Laboratory. *NZ Sociol* (2013) 28:164–91.
17. Bazemore AW, Cottrell EK, Gold R, Hughes LS, Phillips RL, Angier H, et al. "Community vital signs": incorporating geocoded social determinants into electronic records to promote patient and population health. *J Am Med Inform Assoc* (2016) 23:407–12. doi:10.1093/jamia/ocv088
18. Jiwa M, Gudes O, Varhol R, Mullan N. Impact of geography on the control of type 2 diabetes mellitus: a review of geocoded clinical data from general practice. *BMJ Open* (2015) 5:e009504. doi:10.1136/bmjopen-2015-009504
19. Makela J. *Model for Assessing GIS Maturity of an Organisation [Doctoral Dissertation]*. Helsinki: Department of Real Estate, Planning and Geoinformatics, Aalto University (2012).
20. Gudes O, Mullan N, Weeramanthri TS. *Spatial Maturity in a Health Agency: A Pilot Study*. Australia and New Zealand Cooperative Research Centre for Spatial Information (2014). 22 p. Available from: http://www.crcsi.com.au/assets/Resources/CRCSI-Spatial-Maturity-in-a-Health-Agency-Report-June2015.pdf
21. Goodchild MF. Formalising place in geographic information systems. In: Burton L, Kemp S, Leung M, Matthews S, Takeuchi D, editors. *Communities, Neighborhoods, and Health*. New York: Springer (2011). p. 21–33.
22. Khoury MJ, Galea S. Will precision medicine improve population health? *JAMA* (2016) 316(13):1357–8. doi:10.1001/jama.2016.12260

11

Comparative Efficacy and Safety of Neuroprotective Therapies for Neonates with Hypoxic Ischemic Encephalopathy

Clare Yuen Zen Lee[1], Pairote Chakranon[2] and Shaun Wen Huey Lee[1,3,4]*

[1] School of Pharmacy, Monash University Malaysia, Bandar Sunway, Malaysia, [2] Faculty of Pharmacy, Silapakorn University, Pathom, Thailand, [3] Asian Centre for Evidence Synthesis in Population, Implementation and Clinical Outcomes (PICO), Health and Well-being Cluster, Global Asia in the 21st Century (GA21) Platform, Monash University Malaysia, Selangor, Malaysia, [4] School of Pharmacy, Taylor's University, Subang Jaya, Malaysia

*Correspondence:
Shaun Wen Huey Lee
shaun.lee@monash.edu

PROSPERO Registration:
CRD42016053390

Context: Several interventions are available for the management of hypoxic ischemic encephalopathy (HIE), but no studies have compared their relative efficacy in a single analysis. This study aims to compare and determine the effectiveness of available interventions for HIE using direct and indirect data.

Methods: Large randomized trials were identified from PubMed, EMBASE, CINAHL Plus, AMED, and Cochrane Library of Clinical Trials database from inception until June 30, 2018. Two independent reviewers extracted study data and performed quality assessment. Direct and network meta-analysis of randomized controlled trials was performed to obtained pooled results comparing the effectiveness of different therapies used in HIE on mortality, neurodevelopmental delay at 18 months, as well as adverse events. Their probability of having the highest efficacy and safety was estimated and ranked. The certainty of evidence for the primary outcomes of mortality and mortality or neurodevelopmental delay at 18 months was evaluated using GRADE criteria.

Results: Fifteen studies comparing five interventions were included in the network meta-analysis. Whole body cooling [Odds ratio: 0.62 (95% credible interval: 0.46–0.83); 8 trials, high certainty of evidence] was the most effective treatment in reducing the risk of mortality, followed by selective head cooling (0.73; 0.48–1.11; 2 trials, moderate certainty of evidence) and use of magnesium sulfate (0.79; 0.20–3.06; 2 trials, low certainty of evidence). Whole body hypothermia (0.48; 0.33–0.71; 5 trials), selective head hypothermia (0.54; 0.32–0.89; 2 trials), and erythropoietin (0.36; 0.19–0.66; 2 trials) were more effective for reducing the risk of mortality and neurodevelopmental delay at 18 months (moderate to high certainty). Among neonates treated for HIE, the use of erythropoietin (0.36; 0.18–0.74, 2 trials) and whole body hypothermia (0.61; 0.45–0.83; 7 trials) were associated with lower rates of cerebral palsy. Similarly, there were lower rates of seizures among neonates treated with erythropoietin (0.35; 0.13–0.94; 1 trial) and whole body hypothermia (0.64; 0.46–0.87, 7 trials).

Conclusion: The findings support current guidelines using therapeutic hypothermia in neonates with HIE. However, more trials are needed to determine the role of adjuvant therapy to hypothermia in reducing the risk of mortality and/or neurodevelopmental delay.

Keywords: hypoxic ischemic encephalopathy, neonatal, systematic review, meta-analysis, neuroprotective, perinatal

INTRODUCTION

Neonatal hypoxic ischemic encephalopathy (HIE) is one of the most common causes of severe neurological deficit in children, affecting an estimated 15 per 10,000 live births (Graham et al., 2008; American College of Obstetricians and Gynecologists, and American Academy of Pediatrics, 2014). Several reviews have suggested that therapeutic hypothermia (both whole body and selective head) reduces mortality and improves survival with normal neurological outcome and is now a standard treatment protocol for most neonatal centers in developed countries (Edwards et al., 2010; Jacobs et al., 2013; Martinello et al., 2017). Despite this, their effectiveness is still limited, with mortality rates of approximately 10% –20% in several large trials (Jacobs et al., 2013). As a result, alternative strategies, including the use of adjuvant therapies such as xenon, allopurinol, erythropoietin, magnesium sulfate, and melatonin, have been suggested (Perrone et al., 2012). Other strategies suggested include cooling for longer periods of time, cooling at lower temperature or both (Shankaran et al., 2017).

Recently, several randomized controlled trials have examined the effects of such adjuvant therapy in neonates with HIE, yielding a complex evidence base that requires careful examination across different strategies (Bhat et al., 2009; Aly et al., 2015; Azzopardi et al., 2016; Filippi et al., 2017). However, most of these studies are relatively small and the results remains inconclusive and mixed. There are no reviews that attempted to summarize these data from large studies.

Furthermore, previous meta-analyses have often compared the efficacy of treatment within pairs of active treatment, which provides limited insights into the overall treatment hierarchy as treatment effects are estimated from two different treatment comparison only (Jacobs et al., 2013; Pauliah et al., 2013). Over the past few years, the use of network meta-analyses which allows for the simultaneous comparison of two or more interventions has increasingly been used (Lee et al., 2015; Lee et al., 2017; Bukhsh et al., 2018; Teoh et al., 2019). Network meta-analysis includes both direct and indirect comparison within a single analysis, thereby providing an integrated and more holistic conclusion, providing decision makers with a more complete evidence matrix (Watt et al., 2019). In this study, we aimed to estimate the efficacy and safety of available neuroprotective interventions for HIE who participated in randomized controlled studies.

MATERIALS AND METHODS

Search Strategy

A literature search was performed to identify for studies from inception to June 30, 2018, on the following databases: PubMed,

EMBASE, CINAHL Plus, Allied and Complementary Medicines (AMED), and the Cochrane Central Register of Controlled Trials without any language restriction. We also obtained additional records by reviewing the reference list of the retrieved articles and other resources including Google Scholar, NDLTD database, and ClinicalTrials.gov. A full list of search terms can be found in **eText** in **Supplementary Material**.

Study Selection

Studies were considered eligible for inclusion if they (1) were randomized controlled studies (RCT), (2) recruited term or preterm infants (gestational age ≥35 weeks) diagnosed with HIE (3) had a control group or comparison group, (4) sufficiently powered to detect differences in the outcome of death and/or disability, and (5) the infants were given any of the following as intervention: magnesium sulfate, deferoxamine, cannabinoids, melatonin, statin, topiramate, xenon, allopurinol, erythropoietin, N-acetylcysteine, or therapeutic hypothermia; either as single intervention or adjunct therapy. Studies which had significant methodological limitations such as poor description of inclusion/exclusion criteria were excluded.

Data Collection and Extraction

All identified records were screened independently by titles and abstracts by two reviewers (CL and PC) and validated by another reviewer (SL). The full texts of relevant articles were retrieved for further eligibility assessment, extracted, and any discrepancies were resolved through discussion. The information extracted included the author, study design and population, outcomes, and quality of the study using a standardized data extraction form. We subsequently assessed the study quality using the Cochrane risk of bias assessment tool (Higgins et al., 2011).

Outcome Measures

The co-primary outcomes of interest were the composite of mortality or major neurodevelopmental disability and/or mortality assessed at least 18 months of age. Secondary outcomes include cerebral palsy, development delay based upon the mental development and psychomotor indices of the Bayley II scales of infant development (Bayley, 1993), seizures, quality of vision and hearing, and potential adverse effects caused by the treatment.

Statistical Analyses

We used a stepwise approach whereby traditional meta-analysis was performed using the Mantel-Haenszel random-effects model since we expect the presence of heterogeneity. We calculated the risk ratio and risk difference for dichotomous outcomes, and its 95% confidence interval. To determine whether the benefit of treatment on outcomes was affected by the severity of encephalopathy, we examined subgroups for which the severity of encephalopathy was graded as moderate or severe on the basis of clinical examination and/or amplitude integrated electroencephalography. The consistency of the treatment effect across subgroups was explored by calculating the ratio of relative risks with 95% confidence interval. Potential small study publication bias was assessed using visual inspection of the funnel plot and Eggers test. Between studies heterogeneity was assessed using I^2 and Cochran's Q method.

We subsequently performed a network meta-analysis which combines the direct and indirect effects of treatment, allowing for simultaneous comparison of multiple treatments. These were ranked using the surface under the curve ranking (SUCRA). Inconsistency checks were performed for closed loop in the network (Higgins et al., 2012; Veroniki et al., 2013). Subsequently, we calculated the number needed to treat (NNT) or number needed to harm (NNH) to better understand the potential benefits of different treatments examined. We used the odds ratios (OR) derived from the usual care comparison in network meta-analysis for mortality outcome to estimate the absolute benefits (Dulai et al., 2016).

Preplanned sensitivity analyses include comparison between high versus low-middle income countries as well as severity of encephalopathy. All analyses were conducted using Stata version 13.0 (StataCorp, College TX). This study is registered with PROSPERO, number CRD42016053390.

RESULTS

Study Selection and Characteristics
The literature search identified a total of 1,731 studies and 71 full-text articles were assessed for eligibility (**Figure 1** and **eTables 1** and **2**). Fifteen studies enrolling 2,313 newborns were included in the review (Gluckman et al., 2005; Shankaran et al., 2005; Li et al., 2009; Zhu et al., 2009; Simbruner et al., 2010; Zhou et al., 2010; Joy et al., 2013; Azzopardi et al., 2016; Savitha and Prakash, 2016; Malla et al., 2017; Sreenivasa et al., 2017). Most of the included studies had a similar enrollment criteria and included infants with evidence of birth asphyxia as defined by the American College of Obstetrician and Gynecologists (American College of Obstetricians and Gynecologists, and American Academy of Pediatrics, 2014) with moderate to severe HIE. These studies had recruited newborns which were at least 35 weeks in 1 study, at least 36 weeks in 3 studies, and gestation weeks of more than or equal to 37 weeks in 9 studies. Interventions examined by studies were therapeutic hypothermia examined in 10 studies (8 whole body cooling and 2 selective head cooling), magnesium sulfate in 2 studies, erythropoietin in 2 studies, and use of xenon with therapeutic hypothermia in 1 study (**Table 1**). Eight studies (53.3%) were published in 2011 or later, and the studies were conducted in

India (40%), China (20%), or were multicentered studies (20%). Nine studies (60%) had a duration (from recruitment to end of follow-up) of at least 18 months or more.

Methodological Quality of Included Studies
Twelve (80.0%) studies had adequate reporting on sequence generation, 12 (80.0%) studies described the loss to follow-up, 10 (66.7%) studies described the selection concealment adequately, and 6 (40.0%) studies described the blinding of participants and outcome assessment. However, a high proportion [10 (66.7%)] had unclear risk of bias for blinding of outcome assessors (**eFigure 1**).

Primary Outcomes
Mortality
Fifteen RCTs reported the effectiveness of intervention in reducing the risk of mortality. Pairwise meta-analysis showed that whole body hypothermia was effective in reducing the risk of mortality (OR: 0.71; 0.52–0.92, $I^2 = 0\%$) compared to usual care (**eTable 3**).

Mortality and/or Neurodevelopmental Delay at 18 Months
Nine studies reported the long term effects of pharmacotherapy or hypothermia on mortality and neurodevelopmental delay at 18 months (Gluckman et al., 2005; Shankaran et al., 2005; Azzopardi et al., 2009; Li et al., 2009; Zhu et al., 2009; Simbruner et al., 2010; Zhou et al., 2010; Jacobs et al., 2011; Malla et al., 2017). Pooled analysis of studies suggest that both erythropoietin (OR: 0.57; 0.36–0.91, $I^2 = 0\%$) and whole body hypothermia (0.74; 0.59–0.92, $I^2 = 0\%$) were effective in reducing the risk of mortality and neurodevelopmental delay at 18 months.

Secondary Outcomes
Among infants who survived, 12 trials including 1,951 infants reported on cerebral palsy outcome. Whole body hypothermia was found to be statistically superior in reducing the odds developing cerebral palsy (0.70; 0.54–0.92, $I^2 = 0\%$) compared to usual care. With respect to seizures, 10 trials including 1,703 infants were included. Whole body hypothermia was superior in reducing the rates of seizure compared to usual care (0.73; 0.56–0.96, $I^2 = 0\%$).

Five studies reported the neuromotor delay and neurodevelopmental delay among neonates using the Bayley II index, but results were not significant. For the other outcomes of renal failure, sepsis, hypotension, hypoglycemia, bradycardia, hearing loss, and blindness, the evidence base were sparse (**eTable 4**). Meta-analysis suggests that therapeutic hypothermia (both whole body and selective head cooling) were associated with an increased rate of normal survival, defined as survival without cerebral palsy, seizures, normal vision, and hearing.

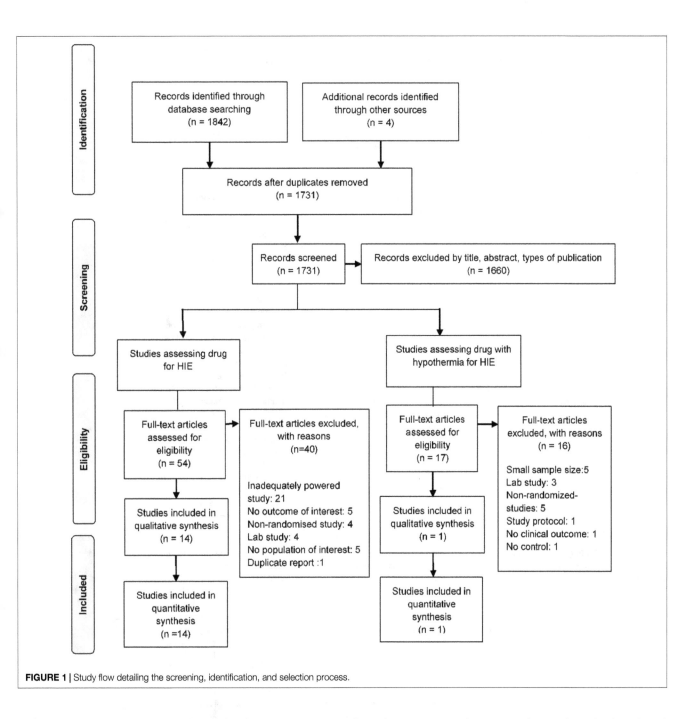

FIGURE 1 | Study flow detailing the screening, identification, and selection process.

Effect of Severity of Encephalopathy

Most studies assessed the severity of encephalopathy by clinical assessment using Sarnat's criteria (Sarnat and Sarnat, 1976), which classifies the degree of encephalopathy to either stages I, II or III, correlating with mild, moderate or severe encephalopathy. Pooled analysis suggests that the relative odds of mortality or neurodevelopmental disability were lower among infants with moderate encephalopathy when treated with erythropoietin (0.27; 0.11–0.63, I^2 = 0%) or whole body hypothermia (0.63; 0.44–0.89, I^2 = 0%). Among infants with severe encephalopathy, all interventions including erythropoietin, whole body hypothermia or selective head hypothermia was ineffective in reducing the risk of combined outcomes of mortality or neurodevelopmental disability (**eTable 5**).

Network Meta-Analysis
Mortality or Mortality and Neurodevelopmental Disability at 18 Months

Overall, of the 15 unique pairwise comparisons that could be made, only 5 were studied head to head. The network meta-analysis gave an adequate fit to the data and design-by-treatment model showed no evidence of inconsistency (**eFigure 2**).

TABLE 1 | Characteristics of included studies.

		First Author, Year (Study)	Study Population	Interventions	Number of Patients Enrolled	Mean gestational age or age range, weeks
Drug Intervention as Single Treatment	Erythropoietin	Malla et al., 2017	Neonates (≥37 weeks) with moderate or severe HIE (10 min Apgar score <5) evidence of fetal distress, need for resuscitation at 10 mins after birth	**I:** 500 U/kg rhEPO intravenously on alternate dose for a total of 5 doses with the 1st dose within 6 hours after birth **C:** 2mL of normal saline	100	39.5
		Zhu et al., 2009	Term neonates (≥37 weeks), body weights >2500 g with evidence of perinatal HIE (5-min Apgar score ≤5, need for resuscitation at 10 mins after birth)	**I:** 300 U/kg or 500 U/kg rhEPO subcutaneously for 1st dose and intravenously every other day for 2 weeks **C:** Conventional treatment	167	37.5
	Magnesium	Savitha and Prakash, 2016	Term neonates with perinatal asphyxia, 1-min Apgar score < 7, need for resuscitation at birth, failure to initiate breath at birth	**I:** 250 mg/kg $MgSO_4$ intravenous infusion over 1 h within 6 h of birth, with additional doses repeated at 24 h and 48 h **C:** Supportive care	120	38.5
		Sreenivasa et al., 2017	Term neonates with perinatal asphyxia, 1-min Apgar score <3 or 5-min Apgar score <6	**I:** 250 mg/kg $MgSO_4$ intravenous infusion over 1 h within 6 h of birth, with additional doses repeated at 24 h and 48 h **C:** Supportive care	100	38.7
	Cooling (Whole body)	Azzopardi et al., 2009 (TOBY)	Term neonates (≥36 gestation weeks) with moderate to severe HIE, Apgar score <6, seizure on aEEG	**I:** Manually adjusted cooling blanket to target rectal temperature of 33.0°C–34.0°C for 72hr **C:** Conventional care with overhead radiant heater to target rectal temperature of 36.8°C–37.2°C	325	38.8–41.3†
		Bharadwaj, 2012	Term neonates (>37 gestation weeks) with perinatal asphyxia (10-min Apgar score ≤6), and encephalopathy	**I:** Whole body cooling with gel packs to target rectal temperature of 33.0 °C–34.0°C **C:** Conventional care with servo-controlled overhead radiant heater to target rectal temperature of 36.5°C	130	40.0
Drug Intervention as Single Treatment	Cooling (Whole body)	Gane, 2013	Term neonates (≥37 weeks) with evidence of encephalopathy (10-min Apgar <5)	**I:** Cloth covered gel packs to target rectal temperature of 33°C–34°C for 72 h **C:** Conventional care for HIE to target of 36.5°C	122	40.1
		Jacobs et al., 2011 (ICE)	Term or near term neonates (≥35 gestation weeks) with moderate to severe HIE, perinatal asphyxia, 10-min Apgar score <6	**I:** Refrigerated gel pack across chest and/or under head and shoulders to target rectal temperature of 33.0°C–34.0°C for 6–72 h **C:** Conventional care with overhead radiant heater to target rectal temperature of 36.8°C –37.2°C	221	39.1
		Joy et al., 2013	Term neonates (≥37 weeks) with evidence of encephalopathy (10-min Apgar ≤5)	**I:** Cloth covered gel packs to target rectal temperature of 33–34 °C for 72 h **C:** Conventional care for HIE to target rectal temperature of 36.5°C	160	-
		Li et al., 2009	Term neonates (≥37 weeks), weight > 2500 g, with moderate to severe encephalopathy (5-min Apgar ≤5)	**I:** Whole body cooling with cooling mattress to target rectal temperature of 33 °C–34 °C for 72 h **C:** Conventional care for HIE to target rectal temperature of 36.5°C–37.5 °C	93	39.1

(Continued)

TABLE 1 | Continued

		First Author, Year (Study)	Study Population	Interventions	Number of Patients Enrolled	Mean gestational age or age range, weeks
		Shankaran et al., 2005 (NICHD study)	Term neonates (≥37 gestation weeks) with moderate to severe HIE, perinatal asphyxia (10 min Apgar score ≤5))	**I:** Two servo-controlled cooling blanket to target oesophageal temperature of 34.5 °C for 72 h **C:** Conventional care with overhead radiant heater to target skin temperature of 36.5 °C–37.0 °C	208	4.3 h*
		Simbruner et al., 2010 (neo,nEURO)	Term neonates (≥36 gestation weeks) with moderate to severe HIE, perinatal asphyxia (10 min Apgar score <5) and encephalopathy as evidence by abnormal standard EEG or aEEG findings	**I:** Cooling blanket to target rectal temperature of 33.0°C–34.0°C for 72 h **C:** Conventional care to target rectal temperature of 36.5°C–37.5°C	129	39.3
	Cooling (Selective head)	Gluckman et al., 2005 (CoolCap)	Term neonates (≥37 gestation weeks) with moderate to severe HIE, perinatal asphyxia, 10-min Apgar score ≤5, severe acidosis (pH < 7) or a base deficit of 16 mmol/L	**I:** Manual controlled cooling cap to target temperature of 34.0°C–35.0°C for 72 h **C:** Conventional care with overhead radiant heater to target of 36.5°C–37.5°C	234	39.0
		Zhou et al., 2010	Term neonates (≥37 gestation weeks) with perinatal asphyxia (5-min Apgar score ≤5 or 1-min Apgar score ≤3), birth weight ≥2500 g, and encephalopathy	**I:** Manually controlled cooling cap to rectal target temperature of 34.5°C–35.0°C for 72 h **C:** Conventional care whereby infants are cared on radiant warmers servo-controlled to rectal target of 36.0°C–37.5°C	194	4.0 h*
Drug Intervention as Adjuvant	Xenon	Azzopardi et al., 2016 (TOBY-Xe)	Gestation weeks (36–43 weeks), had signs of moderate to severe encephalopathy, moderately or severely abnormal background activity for ≥30 min or seizures shown by aEEG, 10-min Apgar score ≤5, continued need for resuscitation for ≥10 min	**I:** Whole body hypothermia to target rectal temperature of 33.5°C plus 30% inhaled xenon for 24 h **C:** Whole body hypothermia alone to target rectal temperature of 33.5°C	92	39.8

AAP, American Association of Pediatrics; ACOG, American College of Obstetricians and Gynecologists; aEEG, amplitude-integrated continuous electroencephalopathy; C, control group; CBV, cerebral blood volume; EAA, excitatory amino acids; EPO, erythropoietin; 1st, first; I, intervention group; h, hours; HIE, hypoxic-ischemic encephalopathy; MgSO4, magnesium sulfate; min, minutes; m, months; NaCl, normal saline; NO, nitric oxide; rhEPO, recombinant human erythropoietin; subcut, subcutaneously.
* Age at randomization; †Interquartile range.

TABLE 2 | Network meta-analysis for primary outcomes mortality.

Whole body hypothermia	1.11 (0.59, 2.08)	0.66 (0.26, 1.67)	0.78 (0.20, 3.14)	0.77 (0.29, 2.09)	<u>0.62 (0.46, 0.83)</u>
	Selective head hypothermia	0.78 (0.30, 2.07)	0.92 (0.22, 3.83)	0.91 (0.30, 2.79)	0.73 (0.48, 1.11)
		Erythropoietin	1.18 (0.24, 5.96)	1.17 (0.30, 4.55)	0.93 (0.39, 2.25)
			Magnesium sulfate	0.99 (0.18, 5.45)	0.79 (0.20, 3.06)
				Whole body hypothermia with xenon	0.80 (0.28, 2.26)
					Usual care

Comparisons should be read from left to right. The estimate is located at the intersection of the column-defining treatment and the row-defining treatment. An OR value below 1 favors the column-defining treatment. To obtain ORs for comparisons in the opposing direction, reciprocals should be taken. Any significant results are in bold and underlined.

All interventions examined showed a reduction in risk of mortality compared to usual care (**Figure 2**, **Table 2** and **eTable 6**). However, only whole body hypothermia was significantly better than usual care (0.62; 0.46–0.83), with an NNT of 11 (95% CI: 7–26) in reducing the risk of mortality (**eTable 7**). With respect to the composite mortality or neurodevelopmental disability outcome at 18 months or longer, erythropoietin was significantly better than usual care in patients with moderate encephalopathy (0.36; 0.19–0.66; **eFigure 3**). Therapeutic hypothermia (both whole body and selective head cooling) was the only treatment statistically superior to usual care in patients with moderate (whole body: 0.45; 0.31–0.66 and selective head: 0.51; 0.29–0.89) or severe encephalopathy (whole body: 0.32; 0.12–0.86).

Secondary Outcomes

Network meta-analysis suggest that, compared to usual care, treatment with either erythropoietin or whole body hypothermia were associated with lower rates of cerebral palsy (0.36; 0.18–0.74 and 0.61; 0.45–0.83, respectively) and seizures (0.35; 0.13– 0.94 and 0.64; 0.46–0.87, **Figure 3**).

Sensitivity Analyses

Comparison-adjusted funnel plots of the network meta-analysis for primary outcomes did not suggest any publication bias (**eFigure 4**). Ranking of treatment based upon cumulative probability plots (**eFigure 5**) and SUCRA showed that the most effective treatment for primary outcome mortality was whole body hypothermia (77.8%) and the least effective was usual care (24.5%). In terms of the composite outcome of mortality or neurodevelopmental disability at 18 months, the most effective treatment was erythropoietin (88.8%) and the least effective was usual care (0.2%). Using GRADE, the quality of evidence for primary outcomes were moderate to very low for most comparison (**Table 3** and **eTable 8**).

In the preplanned sensitivity analyses, we excluded studies which were conducted in low-middle income countries since previous meta-analysis have suggested that these study setting could influence the results (Pauliah et al., 2013). When studies from high-income countries were only included, only three comparisons were possible for the outcome of mortality. Results from the network meta-analysis was largely unchanged, and whole body cooling was found to reduce the risk of mortality by 36% (0.64; 0.46–0.90) as well as mortality or major neurodevelopmental disability at 18 months by 49% (0.51; 0.33–0.78) compared to usual care. These results were largely unchanged when we included studies which had examined full term neonates (≥37 weeks), where whole body cooling reduced the risk of mortality (0.50; 0.31–0.81) as well as mortality or major neurodevelopmental disability at 18 months (0.44; 0.27–0.71) compared to usual care (**eTable 9**). In addition, selective

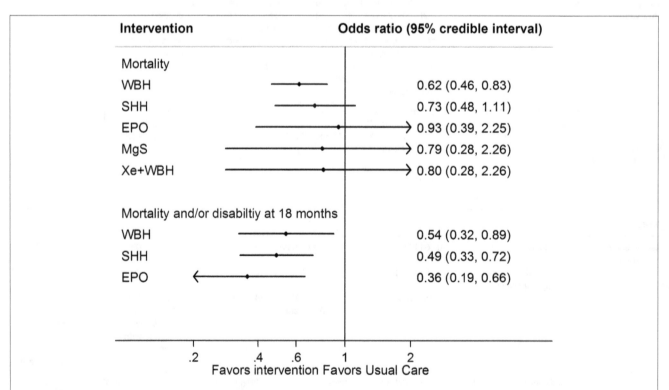

FIGURE 2 | Network meta-analysis forest plots for each treatment versus usual care on mortality or mortality and neurodevelopmental delay at 18 months outcome. Each rhombus represents the summary treatment effect estimated in the network meta-analysis on the odds ratio (OR) scale. The black horizontal lines represent the credible intervals (CrI) for the summary treatment effects; an OR > 1 suggests that usual care is more effective to reduce the risk of mortality, whereas an OR < 1 suggests that the comparable treatment is better. The vertical blue line corresponds to an OR = 1.

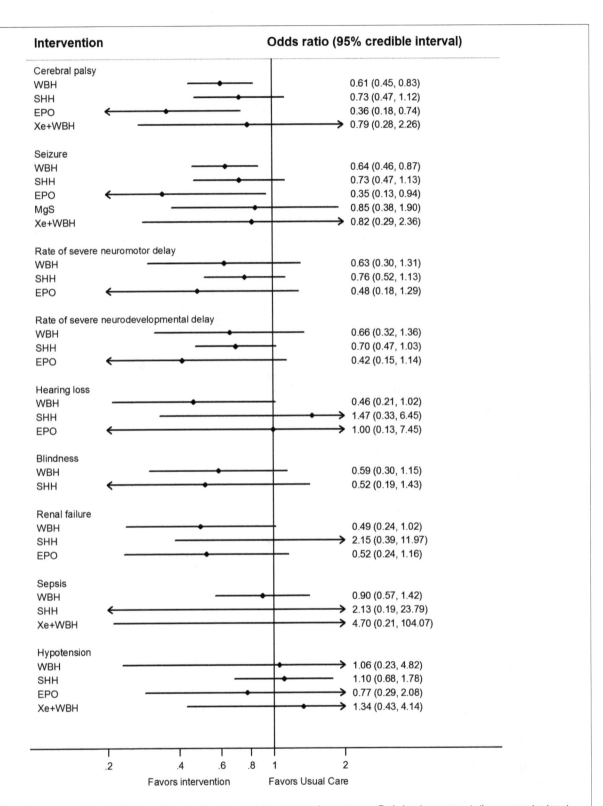

FIGURE 3 | Network meta-analysis forest plots for each treatment versus usual care on secondary outcomes. Each rhombus represents the summary treatment effect estimated in the network meta-analysis on the odds ratio (OR) scale. The black horizontal lines represent the credible intervals (CrI) for the summary treatment effects; an odds ratio > 1 suggests that usual care is more effective to reduce the risk of mortality, whereas an OR < 1 suggests that the comparable treatment is better. The vertical blue line corresponds to an OR = 1.

TABLE 3 | Summary of findings table for the primary outcomes assessed in this study.

Estimates of effects, credible intervals, and certainty of the evidence for comparison of neuroprotective therapies for neonates with hypoxic ischemic encephalopathy

Patient or population: Neonates with hypoxic ischemic encephalopathy
Interventions: Whole body cooling, selective head cooling, magnesium sulfate, erythropoietin, whole body cooling with xenon
Comparator (reference): Usual care
Outcome: Mortality; mortality or neurodevelopmental disability at 18 months or later
Setting(s): Inpatient and outpatient

Geometry of the Network

Total studies:15 RCT Total Participants: 2,103	Odds ratio (95% CrI)	Anticipated absolute effect(95% CrI)			Certainty of the evidence	Interpretation of Findings
		With placebo	With intervention	Difference		
Mortality						
Whole body cooling (Direct evidence; 8 RCT; 1324 participants)	**0.62** (0.46 to 0.83)	261 per 1,000	180 per 1,000	81 fewer per 1,000 (from 121 fewer to 34 fewer)	⊕⊕⊕⊕ **High**	Whole body cooling improves survival in newborns with HIE
Selective head cooling (Direct evidence; 2 RCT; 428 participants)	**0.73** (0.48 to 1.11)	259 per 1,000	204 per 1,000	56 fewer per 1,000 (from 115 fewer to 21 more)	⊕⊕⊕○ **Moderate**[1]	Selective head cooling probably improves survival in newborns with HIE
Magnesium sulfate (Direct evidence; 2 RCT; 220 participants)	**0.79** (0.20 to 3.06)	36 per 1,000	29 per 1,000	7 fewer per 1,000 (from 29 fewer to 67 more)	⊕⊕○○ **Low**[1,2]	Use of magnesium sulfate has limited effect on survival in newborns with HIE
Erythropoietin (Direct evidence; 2 RCT; 253 participants)	**0.93** (0.39 to 2.25)	89 per 1,000	84 per 1,000	6 fewer per 1,000 (from 53 fewer to 92 more)	⊕⊕○○ **Low**[1,2]	Use of erythropoietin has limited effect on survival in newborns with HIE
Whole body cooling with xenon (Indirect evidence; 1 RCT; 92 participants)	**0.80** (0.28 to 2.26)	196 per 1,000	163 per 1,000	33 fewer per 1,000 (from 132 fewer to 159 more)	⊕○○○ **Very low**[1,2,3]	Use of xenon as an adjuvant with whole body cooling has limited effect on survival in newborns with HIE
Mortality or neurodevelopmental delay at 18 months						
Whole body cooling (Direct evidence; 5 RCT; 934 participants)	0.54 (0.32 to 0.89)	607 per 1,000	455 per 1,000	152 fewer per 1,000 (from 276 fewer to 28 fewer)	⊕⊕⊕⊕ **High**	Whole body cooling improves survival and neurodevelopment in newborns with HIE
Selective head cooling (Direct evidence; 2 RCT; 412 participants)	**0.49** (0.33 to 0.72)	583 per 1,000	407 per 1,000	176 fewer per 1,000 (from 267 fewer to 81 fewer)	⊕⊕⊕○ **Moderate**[1]	Selective head cooling probably improves survival and neurodevelopment in newborns with HIE
Erythropoietin (Direct evidence; 2 RCT; 253 participants)	**0.36** (0.29 to 0.67)	538 per 1,000	296 per 1,000	243 fewer per 1,000 (from 286 fewer to 100 fewer)	⊕⊕⊕○ **Moderate**[1]	Use of erythropoietin probably improves survival and neurodevelopment in newborns with HIE

[1]Study was downgraded due to imprecision and lack of direct RCTs contributing to direct evidence; [2]Few event rates with wide confidence intervals leading to imprecision; [3]Serious indirectness; [4]Contributing direct evidence of moderate quality with inadequate concealment of allocation and blinding.

head cooling was also noted to lower the risk of mortality or major neurodevelopmental disability at 18 months compared to usual care (0.54; 0.36–0.81).

DISCUSSION

In this study, direct and indirect evidence from 15 RCTs was combined to compare the association of each therapy used for neuroprotection in HIE. The study has several key findings. Firstly, therapeutic hypothermia was significantly associated with lower odds of mortality and neurodevelopmental delays compared to usual care, with high confidence estimates and a number to treat of between 11 and 16. Secondly, whole body hypothermia should be offered to all infants with HIE, irrespective of the severity as it was effective in reducing the risk of morbidity as well as neurodevelopmental delays when compared to usual care.

Over the past decade, numerous drugs have been proven useful to be beneficial in animal models for neonates with HIE, but how these can be translated into clinical use remains unknown (Nair and Kumar, 2018). Our study provides novel insights into how different neuroprotective agents could be useful in patients with HIE especially when used in combination with hypothermia (Martinello et al., 2017). Although there is much progress, further studies are needed to determine the effectiveness of these adjuvant therapies. Several large clinical studies are underway to examine the benefits of these neuroprotective agents.

A previous review suggested that key differences exists in terms of efficacy between high-income and low-middle income countries, due to the use of low-technology devices, degree of encephalopathy, maternal pre-existing diseases, malnutrition status, infections, as well as study inclusion criteria (Pauliah et al., 2013). In this study, we showed that therapeutic hypothermia especially whole body hypothermia was the most effective intervention irrespective of study setting as well as device used. As HIE is the major cause of up to 23% of 2.8 million neonatal deaths especially in low-resource setting, our findings provide a further impetus for therapeutic hypothermia to be part of standard of care especially in low-middle income countries.

Our findings support the Cochrane review on hypothermia in patients with HIE for the primary outcome, where we found that cooling was beneficial in reducing the risk of mortality and disability (Jacobs et al., 2013). This has similarly been reported by other authors which concluded that hypothermia improves survival and neurodevelopmental delays in newborns (Tagin et al., 2012; Douglas-Escobar and Weiss, 2015). The current review was larger (an additional 4 RCTs and 808 infants) and includes information on the effectiveness of different neuroprotective agents. While the authors of a recent systematic review on hypothermia did not conduct network meta-analysis, the results presented were similar to those reported here and suggest that therapeutic hypothermia is effective.

Study Strength

Strengths of our review are that we conducted a comprehensive search as well as the identification of new additional studies. We also used multiple approaches to assess the relationship of effects and performed a network meta-analysis, which provides added information on effects of different combination of interventions (drugs and non-drugs). The quality of the evidence generated were rated using the GRADE criterion (Puhan et al., 2014). We used a comprehensive search strategy and searched all pertinent sources for eligible studies, which reduces the possibility of missing any relevant studies. This study also included preterm infants ≥35 weeks as part of the inclusion criteria and provides a more holistic overview on the clinical safety and efficacy of therapeutic hypothermia in this group of infants where data on outcomes are sparse. Nevertheless, these results need to be confirmed from larger randomized controlled trials such as the Premmie Hypothermia for Neonatal Encephalopathy study which is currently in progress (NCT01793129). Until then, clinicians should take precaution especially when treating preterm neonates since evidence from a recent retrospective cohort analysis have suggested that a high incidence of complication and composite outcome of death and neurodevelopmental impairment (Herrera et al., 2018).

Study Limitations

The limitations of our review are the inherent heterogeneity in terms of study design, intervention, as well as outcome assessment of included studies. We attempted to minimize this by using rigorous selection criteria and performing several sensitivity analyses to ensure the robustness of our results. Secondly, analysis for other outcomes such as neurodevelopmental outcomes, blindness, as well as adverse events should be interpreted with caution, owing to the few data points available. However, a recent high quality long-term study on effects of depth and duration of cooling showed that there is little to no effect of different hypothermia therapy or duration of therapy on outcome (Shankaran et al., 2014; Laptook et al., 2017). This independent analysis reinforces the case that hypothermia should be standard therapy, and additional policy options may be needed in low resource settings to improve outcomes. As with most network meta-analyses, there were only sparse data for some of the treatment comparison especially those related to erythropoietin, and thus, it is recommended that these treatment effect estimates be interpreted together with their precision.

Our study also revealed that additional studies are needed to further optimize cooling therapy as well as rewarming methods, such as the recently concluded NICHD funded study which examined the impact of different cooling depth and duration in neonates with HIE (Shankaran et al., 2014; Laptook et al., 2017). In addition, sufficiently powered studies which examine the use of adjuvant therapies in addition to hypothermia are needed. Another research goal is to reliably identify for subgroups of newborns who will go on to develop worsening encephalopathy and significant brain injury, possibly through the use of electroencephalography, or other biomarker to ensure that they benefit most from hypothermia. In summary, results of our analysis generally support current guidelines using hypothermia for neonates with HIE irrespective of setting. Our findings further support whole body hypothermia as first line, due to its ease of use, improving mortality and neurodevelopmental outcomes. However, further research is needed to determine if the use of additional adjuvant therapies could further improve outcomes of HIE.

AUTHOR CONTRIBUTIONS

SL conceptualized the study, designed the data collection instrument, carried out the statistical analysis, drafted the initial manuscript, and reviewed and revised the manuscript. CL and PC carried out the data acquisition and helped drafted out the initial manuscript. All authors approved the final manuscript as submitted and agree to be accountable for all aspects of the work.

ACNOWLEDGMENTS

We wish to thank Dr. Nai Ming Lai of Taylor's University for helping edit the manuscript for clarity, Dr. Mohamed Tagin of University of Toronto, and Dr. Seetha Shankaran of Wayne State University School of Medicine for providing input and advice on this article.

REFERENCES

Aly, H., Elmahdy, H., El-Dib, M., Rowisha, M., Awny, M., El-Gohary, T., et al. (2015). Melatonin use for neuroprotection in perinatal asphyxia: a randomized controlled pilot study. *J. Perinatol.* 35, 186. doi: 10.1038/jp.2014.186

American College of Obstetricians and Gynecologists, and American Academy of Pediatrics. (2014). Neonatal encephalopathy and neurologic outcome, second edition. *Obstet. Gynecol.* 123, 896–901. doi: 10.1097/01. AOG.0000445580.65983.d2

Azzopardi, D., Robertson, N. J., Bainbridge, A., Cady, E., Charles-Edwards, G., Deierl, A., et al. (2016). Moderate hypothermia within 6 h of birth plus inhaled xenon versus moderate hypothermia alone after birth asphyxia (TOBY-Xe): a proof-of-concept, open-label, randomised controlled trial. *Lancet Neurol.* 15, 145–153. doi: 10.1016/S1474-4422(15)00347-6

Azzopardi, D. V., Strohm, B., Edwards, A. D., Dyet, L., Halliday, H. L., Juszczak, E., et al. (2009). Moderate hypothermia to treat perinatal asphyxial encephalopathy. *N. Engl. J. Med.* 361, 1349–1358. doi: 10.1056/NEJMoa0900854

Bayley, N. (1993). *Bayley scales of infant and development- second edition.* San Antonio, TX: Psychological Corporation.

Bharadwaj, S. K., and Vishnu Bhat, B. (2012). Therapeutic hypothermia using gel packs for term neonates with hypoxic ischaemic encephalopathy in resource-limited settings: a randomized controlled trial. *J. Trop. Pediatr.* 58(5), 382–388.

Bhat, M. A., Charoo, B. A., Bhat, J. I., Ahmad, S. M., Ali, S. W., and Mufti, M.-U.-H. (2009). Magnesium sulfate in severe perinatal asphyxia: a randomized, placebo-controlled trial. *Pediatrics* 123, e764–e769. doi: 10.1542/peds.2007-3642

Bukhsh, A., Khan, T. M., Lee, S. W. H., Lee, L.-H., Chan, K.-G., and Goh, B.-H. (2018). Efficacy of pharmacist based diabetes educational interventions on clinical outcomes of adults with type 2 diabetes mellitus: a network meta-analysis. *Front. Pharmacol.* 9. doi: 10.3389/fphar.2018.00339

Douglas-Escobar, M., and Weiss, M. D. (2015). Hypoxic-ischemic encephalopathy: a review for the clinician. *JAMA Pediatr.* 169, 397–403. doi: 10.1001/jamapediatrics.2014.3269

Dulai, P. S., Singh, S., Marquez, E., Khera, R., Prokop, L. J., Limburg, P. J., et al. (2016). Chemoprevention of colorectal cancer in individuals with previous colorectal neoplasia: systematic review and network meta-analysis. *BMJ* 355, i6188. doi: 10.1136/bmj.i6188

Edwards, A. D., Brocklehurst, P., Gunn, A. J., Halliday, H., Juszczak, E., Levene, M., et al. (2010). Neurological outcomes at 18 months of age after moderate hypothermia for perinatal hypoxic ischaemic encephalopathy: synthesis and meta-analysis of trial data. *BMJ* 340. doi: 10.1136/bmj.c363

Filippi, L., Fiorini, P., Catarzi, S., Berti, E., Padrini, L., Landucci, E., et al. (2017). Safety and efficacy of topiramate in neonates with hypoxic ischemic encephalopathy treated with hypothermia (NeoNATI): a feasibility study. *J. Matern. Fetal. Neonatal. Med.* 31(8), 973–80.

Gane, B. D., Bhat, V., Rao, R., Nandhakumar, S., Harichandrakumar, K. T. and Adhisivam, B. (2013). Effect of therapeutic hypothermia on DNA damage and neurodevelopmental outcome among term neonates with perinatal asphyxia: a randomized controlled trial. *J. Trop. Pediatr.* 60(2), 134–140.

Gluckman, P. D., Wyatt, J. S., Azzopardi, D., Ballard, R., Edwards, A. D., Ferriero, D. M., et al. (2005). Selective head cooling with mild systemic hypothermia after neonatal encephalopathy: multicentre randomised trial. *Lancet* 365, 663–670. doi: 10.1016/S0140-6736(05)17946-X

Graham, E. M., Ruis, K. A., Hartman, A. L., Northington, F. J., and Fox, H. E. (2008). A systematic review of the role of intrapartum hypoxia-ischemia in the causation of neonatal encephalopathy. *Am. J. Obstet. Gynecol.* 199, 587–595. doi: 10.1016/j.ajog.2008.06.094

Herrera, T. I., Edwards, L., Malcolm, W. F., Smith, P. B., Fisher, K. A., Pizoli, C., et al. (2018). Outcomes of preterm infants treated with hypothermia for hypoxic-ischemic encephalopathy. *Early Hum. Dev.* 125, 1–7. doi: 10.1016/j.earlhumdev.2018.08.003

Higgins, J. P. T., Altman, D. G., Gøtzsche, P. C., Jüni, P., Moher, D., Oxman, A. D., et al. (2011). The Cochrane Collaboration's tool for assessing risk of bias in randomised trials. *BMJ* 343, d5928. doi: 10.1136/bmj.d5928

Higgins, J. P. T., Jackson, D., Barrett, J. K., Lu, G., Ades, A. E., and White, I. R. (2012). Consistency and inconsistency in network meta-analysis: concepts and models for multi-arm studies. *Res Synth Methods* 3, 98–110. doi: 10.1002/jrsm.1044

Jacobs, S. E., Berg, M., Hunt, R., Tarnow-Mordi, W. O., Inder, T. E., and Davis, P. G. (2013). Cooling for newborns with hypoxic ischaemic encephalopathy. *Cochrane Database Syst Rev.* 165 (8). doi: 10.1002/14651858.CD003311.pub3

Jacobs, S. E., Morley, C. J., Inder, T. E., Stewart, M. J., Smith, K. R., Mcnamara, P. J., et al. (2011). Whole-body hypothermia for term and near-term newborns with hypoxic-ischemic encephalopathy: a randomized controlled trial. *Arch. Pediatr. Adolesc. Med.* 165, 692–700. doi: 10.1001/archpediatrics.2011.43

Joy, R., Pournami, F., Bethou, A., Bhat, V. B., and Bobby, Z. (2013). Effect of therapeutic hypothermia on oxidative stress and outcome in term neonates with perinatal asphyxia: a randomized controlled trial. *J. Trop. Pediatr.* 59, 17–22. doi: 10.1093/tropej/fms036

Laptook, A. R., Shankaran, S., Tyson, J. E., Munoz, B., Bell E. F., Goldberg, R. N., et al. (2017). Effect of therapeutic hypothermia initiated after 6 hours of age on death or disability among newborns with hypoxic-ischemic encephalopathy: a randomized clinical trial. *JAMA* 318, 1550–1560. doi: 10.1001/jama.2017.14972

Lee, S. W.-H., Chaiyakunapruk, N., Chong, H.-Y., and Liong, M.-L. (2015). Comparative effectiveness and safety of various treatment procedures for lower pole renal calculi: a systematic review and network meta-analysis. *BJU Int.* 116, 252–264. doi: 10.1111/bju.12983

Lee, S. W. H., Chan, C. K. Y., Chua, S. S., and Chaiyakunapruk, N. (2017). Comparative effectiveness of telemedicine strategies on type 2 diabetes management: a systematic review and network meta-analysis. *Sci. Rep.* 7, 12680. doi: 10.1038/s41598-017-12987-z

Li, T., Xu, F., Cheng, X., Guo, X., Ji, L., Zhang, Z., et al. (2009). Systemic hypothermia induced within 10 hours after birth improved neurological outcome in newborns with hypoxic-ischemic encephalopathy. *Hosp. Pract.* 37, 147–152. doi: 10.3810/hp.2009.12.269

Malla, R., Asimi, R., Teli, M., Shaheen, F., and Bhat, M. (2017). Erythropoietin monotherapy in perinatal asphyxia with moderate to severe encephalopathy: a randomized placebo-controlled trial. *J. Perinatol.* 37, 596–601. doi: 10.1038/jp.2017.17

Martinello, K., Hart, A. R., Yap, S., Mitra, S., and Robertson, N. J. (2017). Management and investigation of neonatal encephalopathy: 2017 update. *Arch. Dis. Child. Fetal Neonatal Ed.* fetalneonatal-2015-309639. 102(4) doi: 10.1136/archdischild-2015-309639

Nair, J., and Kumar, V. H. S. (2018). Current and emerging therapies in the management of hypoxic ischemic encephalopathy in neonates. *Children (Basel, Switzerland)* 5, 99. doi: 10.3390/children5070099

Comparative Efficacy and Safety of Neuroprotective Therapies for Neonates With Hypoxic Ischemic...

95

Pauliah, S. S., Shankaran, S., Wade, A., Cady, E. B., and Thayyil, S. (2013). Therapeutic hypothermia for neonatal encephalopathy in low- and middle-income countries: a systematic review and meta-analysis. *PLoS One* 8, e58834. doi: 10.1371/journal.pone.0058834

Perrone, S., Stazzoni, G., Tataranno, M. L., and Buonocore, G. (2012). New pharmacologic and therapeutic approaches for hypoxic-ischemic encephalopathy in the newborn. *J. Matern. Fetal. Neonatal. Med.* 25, 83–88. doi: 10.3109/14767058.2012.663168

Puhan, M. A., Schünemann, H. J., Murad, M. H., Li, T., Brignardello-Petersen, R., Singh, J. A., et al. (2014). A GRADE Working Group approach for rating the quality of treatment effect estimates from network meta-analysis. *Br. Med. J.* 349. doi: 10.1136/bmj.g5630

Sarnat, H. B., and Sarnat, M. S. (1976). Neonatal encephalopathy following fetal distress: a clinical and electroencephalographic study. *Arch. Neurol.* 33, 696–705. doi: 10.1001/archneur.1976.00500100030012

Savitha, M. R., and Prakash, R. (2016). Beneficial effect of intravenous magnesium sulphate in term neonates with perinatal asphyxia. *Int. J. Contemp. Pediatr.* 3, 150–154. doi: 10.18203/2349-3291.ijcp20160149

Shankaran, S., Laptook, A. R., Ehrenkranz, R. A., Tyson, J. E., Mcdonald, S. A., Donovan, E. F., et al. (2005). Whole-body hypothermia for neonates with hypoxic–ischemic encephalopathy. *N. Engl. J. Med.* 353, 1574–1584. doi: 10.1056/NEJMcps050929

Shankaran, S., Laptook, A. R., Pappas, A., Mcdonald, S. A., Das, A., Tyson, J. E., et al. (2014). Effect of depth and duration of cooling on deaths in the NICU among neonates with hypoxic ischemic encephalopathy: a randomized clinical trial. *JAMA* 312, 2629–2639. doi: 10.1001/jama.2014.16058

Shankaran, S., Laptook, A. R., Pappas, A., Mcdonald, S. A., Das, A., Tyson, J. E., et al. (2017). Effect of depth and duration of cooling on death or disability at age 18 months among neonates with hypoxic-ischemic encephalopathy: a randomized clinical trial. *JAMA* 318, 57–67. doi: 10.1001/jama.2017.7218

Simbruner, G., Mittal, R. A., Rohlmann, F., and Muche, R. (2010). Systemic hypothermia after neonatal encephalopathy: outcomes of neo. nEURO. network RCT. *Pediatrics*, 2009–2441. doi: 10.1542/peds.2009-2441d

Sreenivasa, B., Lokeshwari, K., and Joseph, N. (2017). Role of magnesium sulphate in management and prevention of short term complications of birth asphyxia. *Sri Lanka J. Child Health* 46, 148–151. doi: 10.4038/sljch.v46i2.8271

Tagin, M. A., Woolcott, C. G., Vincer, M. J., Whyte, R. K., and Stinson, D. A. (2012). Hypothermia for neonatal hypoxic ischemic encephalopathy: an updated systematic review and meta-analysis. *Arch. Pediatr. Adolesc. Med.* 166, 558–566. doi: 10.1001/archpediatrics.2011.1772

Teoh, K. W., Khan, T. M., Chaiyakunapruk, N., and Lee, S. W. H. (2019). Examining the use of network meta-analysis in pharmacy services research: a systematic review. *J. Am. Pharm. Assoc.* doi: 10.1016/j.japh.2019.06.015

Veroniki, A. A., Vasiliadis, H. S., Higgins, J. P., and Salanti, G. (2013). Evaluation of inconsistency in networks of interventions. *Int. J. Epidemiol.* 42, 332–345. doi: 10.1093/ije/dys222

Watt, J., Tricco, A. C., Straus, S., Veroniki, A. A., Naglie, G., and Drucker, A. M. (2019). Research techniques made simple: network meta-analysis. *J. Investig. Dermatol.* 139, 4–12.e11. doi: 10.1016/j.jid.2018.10.028

Zhou, W.-H., Cheng, G.-Q., Shao, X.-M., Liu, X.-Z., Shan, R.-B., Zhuang, D.-Y., et al. (2010). Selective head cooling with mild systemic hypothermia after neonatal hypoxic-ischemic encephalopathy: a multicenter randomized controlled trial in China. *J. Pediatr.* 157, 367–372. e363. doi: 10.1016/j.jpeds.2010.03.030

Zhu, C., Kang, W., Xu, F., Cheng, X., Zhang, Z., Jia, L., et al. (2009). Erythropoietin improved neurologic outcomes in newborns with hypoxic-ischemic encephalopathy. *Pediatrics* 124, e218–e226. doi: 10.1542/peds.2008-3553

12

How to Prevent or Reduce Prescribing Errors: An Evidence Brief for Policy

Bruna Carolina de Araújo, Roberta Crevelário de Melo, Maritsa Carla de Bortoli, José Ruben de Alcântara Bonfim and Tereza Setsuko Toma*

Department of Health, Institute of Health, Government of the State of São Paulo, São Paulo, Brazil

Correspondence:
Tereza Setsuko Toma
ttoma@isaude.sp.gov.br

- Preventing prescribing errors is critical to improving patient safety.
- We developed an evidence brief for policy to identify effective interventions to avoid or reduce prescribing errors.
- Four options were raised: promoting educational actions on prudent prescribing directed to prescribers; incorporating computerized alert systems into clinical practice; implementing the use of tools for guiding medication prescribing; and, encouraging patient care by a multidisciplinary team, with the participation of a pharmacist.
- These options can be incorporated into health systems either alone or together, and for that, it is necessary that the context be considered.
- Aiming to inform decision makers, we included considerations on the implementation of these options regarding upper-middle income countries, like the Brazilian, and we also present considerations regarding equity.

Keywords: inappropriate prescribing (MeSH term), prescription errors, pharmaceutical services (MeSH), evidence brief for policy, patient safety

PRESCRIBING ERRORS: A WORLDWIDE PROBLEM

Patient safety became the focus of attention of the World Health Organization (WHO), which in 2004 launched the World Alliance for Patient Safety (World Health Organization (WHO), 2017). During the second Global Ministerial Summit on Patient Safety in 2017, the WHO Director-General announced a third challenge to be faced: drug safety.

Medication errors are a relevant problem to face, in terms of patient damage and health systems sustainability, since worldwide their costs are estimated to reach 42 billion US dollars per year. The goal proposed by WHO is to reduce the level of serious and preventable drug-related harm by 50% within a 5-year period. One of the recommendations is the development of specific action programs to improve safety in situations where a drug can cause unintended harm, including health professionals' behavior and medication practices and systems (Donaldson et al., 2017).

In this context, it is important to distinguish "medication error" and "prescribing error," often used interchangeably in the literature. A medication error can be characterized as "a failure in the treatment process that leads to, or has the potential to lead to, harm to the patient," which encompasses prescribing errors (**Table 1**), dispensing errors and administration errors (Ferner and Aronson, 2006; Ferner, 2014). Nevertheless, medication errors are difficult to assess because of the variety of terms that are misused for this purpose. Several types of errors can be influenced by different factors and result in a variety of outcomes that may require specific courses of action

TABLE 1 | Classification of prescribing errors.

Prescribing errors	
Omission error	Suppression of a drug previously used
Commission error	Addition of a drug not previously used
Dosing error	Incorrect dose
Frequency error	Incorrect dose frequency
Pharmaceutical form error	Incorrect pharmaceutical form
Substitution error	A drug from one class is substituted for another drug from the same class not previously used
Duplication error	Two drugs from the same class are prescribed

Adapted from Lavan et al. (2016).

(Rosa et al., 2009; Ferner, 2014; Lavan et al., 2016). It is worth noting that the errors committed by prescribers are the major factor behind the occurrence of medication errors (Qureshi et al., 2011; Porter and Grills, 2016).

Prescribed drugs are considered to rank as the third leading cause of death in the United States and Europe, surpassed only by heart disease and cancer. While about 100,000 deaths each year in the United States could be related to people taking drugs correctly, another equivalent number of deaths would occur due to errors like the use of contraindicated drugs or in very large doses. Impotent drug regulation, corruption of scientific evidence, drug marketing, and bribery of physicians are pointed out as factors that contribute to this situation (Gøtzsche, 2014).

In India, drug misuse is also common, and the major determinants of the problem include the lack of effective regulation and education on the appropriate use of these products. It is estimated that ∼50% of the average family spending on medicines is unreasonable or unnecessary (Porter and Grills, 2016).

In Brazil, Martins et al. (2011) analyzed medical records of 103 patients from three different hospitals and found that the occurrence of avoidable adverse events was 2.3%, whereas the mortality rate related to adverse events was about 8.5%. Among the elderly individuals, a use prevalence of 11.5–62.5% of potentially inappropriate drugs was associated with adverse effects, hospitalization, morbidity, mortality, and a higher cost of health services (Lucchetti and Lucchetti, 2017).

In this context, this study was aimed at identifying evidence in the scientific literature of effective interventions to avoid or reduce prescribing errors.

SUPPORT TOOLS FOR DRAWING UP EVIDENCE BRIEFS FOR POLICY

This is an evidence brief for policy that followed the methodological guidelines proposed by the SUPPORT collaboration group—Supporting Policy Relevant Reviews and Trials (Lavis et al., 2009).

Evidence briefs for policy are documents that identify, through the most reliable scientific evidences, interventions to deal with a policy-related issue. They are tailored to inform decision makers on the best available and efficient actions to handle with health policy problems, without posing a recommendation, since the process of decision making depends on a variety of factors, including the local context. Within this structure, it is usually found a problem and its relevance for health policies, options to deal with the problem, considerations regarding implementation and equity (Bortoli et al., 2017).

The search for studies was carried out in December 2017, in nine databases: BVS Regional Portal; PubMed, Health Systems Evidence; Health Evidence, PDQ-Evidence; Center for Reviews and Dissemination; Embase; Cochrane Database of Systematic Reviews; and Epistemonikos. In our search strategy, we used the terms "Inappropriate Prescribing" and "Prescription Errors." Search filters were used for identifying systematic reviews published in English, Spanish, and Portuguese. This process was performed by a researcher from our team, and no limits were placed on the publication date.

Article selection and data extraction were carried out independently by two investigators, and disagreements were resolved by a third investigator. The studies thus identified that did not fit our inclusion criteria (systematic reviews, strategies/interventions to enhance prescribing, strategies that involved not only physicians) were excluded after reading their titles, abstracts and full texts (**Supplementary Table S1**). Data from the selected systematic reviews were extracted into a spreadsheet containing information related to the study population, interventions administered, outcomes, and countries according to their income (**Supplementary Table S2**). From this extraction, we came up with a range of interventions, which were arranged in groups according to their similarity, resulting in options for dealing with the problem.

The methodological quality of the selected systematic reviews was assessed independently by two investigators who used the Assessing Methodological Quality of Systematic Reviews tool—AMSTAR (Shea et al., 2007). Any divergences were settled by consensus.

In order to implement health policies, it is necessary to reflect on their implications so as not to cause or increase health iniquities. In this study, we used the tool PROGRESS—an acronym standing for Place of residence; Race/ethnicity/culture/language; Occupation; Gender/sex; Religion; Education; Socioeconomics status; Social capital (Evans and Brown, 2003)—for making considerations on equity in the policy options.

Most systematic reviews included in the options were developed in HIC (high-income countries), thus, in order to best address considerations about the process of implementation, for each one of the options we searched qualitative articles at the BVS Regional Portal. This step aimed to identify, preferably, strategies performed in Brazil, our context, and that could be relatable to other UMIC (Upper-Middle-Income Countries).

POLICY OPTIONS FOR PREVENTING OR REDUCING PRESCRIBING ERRORS

Of the 1,191 systematic reviews identified, 40 were selected and analyzed in order to draw up the options provided (**Figure 1**). From the set of interventions extracted from the

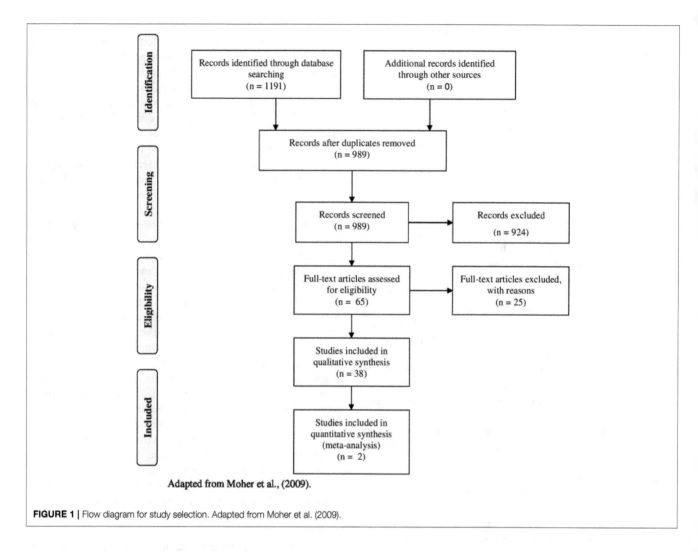

Adapted from Moher et al., (2009).

FIGURE 1 | Flow diagram for study selection. Adapted from Moher et al. (2009).

systematic reviews, we devised four options for dealing with prescribing errors, which we present below: (1) Promoting educational actions on prudent prescribing directed to prescribers; (2) Incorporating computerized alert systems into clinical practice; (3) Implementing the use of tools for guiding medication prescribing; and (4) Encouraging patient care by a multidisciplinary team, with the participation of a pharmacist.

Option 1. Promoting Educational Actions on Prudent Prescribing Directed to Prescribers

Thirteen systematic reviews addressed the effectiveness of educational actions in preventing or reducing prescribing errors, of which six were deemed as having high methodological quality, three as moderate, and four of low quality.

The following studies highlighted the positive effects produced by educational actions through different approaches: educational performance of pharmacists (Ross and Loke, 2009; Tesfaye et al., 2017); actions that improve the transfer

of information among prescribers and discussion of cases in the multidisciplinary team in long–term care facilities for the elderly (Alldred et al., 2016); educational actions with multidisciplinary teams (Chiatti et al., 2012); distribution of clinical protocols and therapeutic guidelines, educational meetings, audit and feedback (Arnold and Straus, 2005); small group workshops, use of decision trees, sharing of quarterly reports, and annual educational actions (Kaur et al., 2009); educational initiatives dissemination, targeted studies and meetings with the participation of professionals (Forsetlund et al., 2011); use of web-based education program, use of performance feedback, along with patient and clinician education, direct and individualized education actions (Brennan and Mattick, 2013); multifaceted interventions (Brennan and Mattick, 2013; Ivanovska and Holloway, 2013; Roque et al., 2014; Coxeter et al., 2015); educational actions that promote behavior change (Tonkin-Crine et al., 2011) tailored to antimicrobial stewardship teams (Davey et al., 2017); interactive educational workshops with reinforcement by a local opinion leader (Fleming et al., 2013).

All reviews concluded that different educational interventions can be effective in reducing inappropriate prescriptions.

Option 2. Incorporating Computerized Alert Systems Into Clinical Practice

Eighteen systematic reviews, of which eleven were classified as high methodological quality, three of moderate one and four as low quality, addressed the use of electronic systems and showed the effectiveness of using different systems in reducing prescribing errors.

The studies emphasized a positive effect on improving prescription writing or reducing prescribing errors by using: alert systems (Schedlbauer et al., 2009; Davey et al., 2017); drug dose adjustment supported by information technology (Mekonnen et al., 2016); electronic archives in hospitals (Sánchez et al., 2014); electronic prescribing resources for undergraduate students (Ross and Loke, 2009); medical reminders, information provided at the time of prescription writing on an online prescription editor (Arnold and Straus, 2005); a Clinical Decision Support System (Kaushal et al., 2003; Yourman et al., 2008; Kaur et al., 2009; Pearson et al., 2009; Reckmann et al., 2009; Lainer et al., 2013; Maaskant et al., 2015; Clyne et al., 2016); a Medical Order Entry System (Kaur et al., 2009) at an intensive care unit (Kaushal et al., 2003; Hodgkinson et al., 2006; Van Rosse et al., 2009; Khajouei and Jaspers, 2010); a Prescription Automatic Screening System (Yang et al., 2012).

Nevertheless, some studies have shown increased medication and prescribing errors when using complex Physician Order Entry Systems (Khajouei and Jaspers, 2010), due to excessive available information (Lainer et al., 2013).

Option 3. Implementing the Use of Tools for Guiding Medication Prescribing

Nine systematic reviews, four of which were considered to be of high methodological quality, four of moderate and three of low quality, provided information on the use of medication prescribing tools.

The findings showed that the tools that may be useful for improving prescribing quality and reducing inadequate prescription are: STOPP/START (Cooper et al., 2015; Santos et al., 2015; Hill-Taylor et al., 2016; Hyttinen et al., 2016) and Beers criteria (Garcia, 2006; Jano and Aparasu, 2007; Soares et al., 2011; Cooper et al., 2015; Santos et al., 2015; Hyttinen et al., 2016). In addition, these tools can be combined with other actions, such as educational ones (Alldred et al., 2016; Valencia et al., 2016).

STOPP - Screening Tool of Older Persons' Prescriptions and START - Screening Tool to Alert to Right Treatment are prescribing screening tools for older people (Mahony et al., 2010).

Beers criteria are lists of potentially inappropriate drugs for the elderly (DeSevo and Klootwyk, 2012).

Option 4. Encouraging Patient Care by a Multidisciplinary Team, With the Participation of a Pharmacist

Nine systematic reviews, of which four were regarded as being of high methodological quality, three of moderate and three of low quality, showed that working as a multidisciplinary team reduces prescribing errors, especially when there is a pharmacist in the team (Chiatti et al., 2012; Sánchez et al., 2014; Alldred et al., 2016; Clyne et al., 2016).

These studies indicated that, as far as patient care is concerned, a multidisciplinary team is better indicated to reduce inappropriate or multiple prescribing (Garcia, 2006; Kaur et al., 2009), decrease inappropriate prescribing in elderly patients (Riordan et al., 2016; Walsh et al., 2016), and antibiotic inappropriate prescribing (Fleming et al., 2013; Maaskant et al., 2015).

CONSIDERATIONS ABOUT IMPLEMENTING POLICY OPTIONS AND THEIR EQUITY

Although the options presented, do not necessarily have to be implemented together nor in a comprehensive way, their practical implementation should consider local feasibility and whether they can be integrated into the governability of decision making, irrespective of a health system's size (whether national, regional, or local). When implementing health policy options, managers usually need to tackle several types of obstacles. Not only it is necessary to consider them, but also to find ways to overcome them, especially those related to cultural and social representations of health care users and workers. The following are some difficulties that may be encountered when implementing each of the options and issues that may give rise to iniquities, especially in Upper-Middle Income Countries.

Option 1. Promoting Educational Actions on Prudent Prescribing Directed to Prescribers

Implementing these interventions may aggravate iniquities when the prescriber does not participate in those activities, whatever the reasons, which may be a consequence of institutional disorganization, lack of personal motivation, or overvaluation of the knowledge they already have.

In the literature, the barriers that must be overcome may be encountered both at the individual level (courses and training of their interest and a belief that empirical knowledge is enough on its own), and at the collective level (communication difficulties among teams, infrastructure, a lack of available time to perform those activities, and punitive management, all of which can have a negative impact on professionals). In addition, difficulties may arise due to insufficient human resources or in complying with previously established guidelines (Carvalho et al., 2011; Bonadiman et al., 2013; Marchon and Mendes, 2014; Ugarte and Acioly, 2014; Santos, 2016; Silva, 2016).

Option 2. Incorporating Computerized Alert Systems Into Clinical Practice

It should be highlighted that the implementation of these electronic resources requests some infrastructure (for example, computer or Internet access, human resources for support), as well as actions to raise awareness about and encourage the use of these technologies by prescribers.

The obstacles observed include a lack of rapid and simplified access to information by means of electronic systems in emergency situations (Cassiani et al., 2003; Gimenes et al., 2006), a lack of culture regarding the adequate inputting of information into the system (Cassiani et al., 2003; Marchon and Mendes, 2014), and a lack of participation in trainings aimed at enhancing the understanding of how the electronic system actually works. It is also important to note that these systems require financial resources, which can make them difficult to deploy (Freire et al., 2004).

Option 3. Implementing the Use of Tools for Guiding Medication Prescribing

These tools are tailored for use mostly in the elderly population, which therefore limits their use in the entire population. Furthermore, the difficulty of access or even the lack of knowledge about these resources precludes them from being used in the clinical practice (Jano and Aparasu, 2007; Soares et al., 2011; Hill-Taylor et al., 2016; Hyttinen et al., 2016; Valencia et al., 2016).

Based on the tools, it can be noted that the lack of knowledge about the resources (Miasso et al., 2006), not considering specific characteristics of the patient (Hyttinen et al., 2016) and the constant updates (Soares et al., 2011) are all obstacles to their incorporation and use.

Option 4. Encouraging Patient Care by a Multidisciplinary Team, With the Participation of a Pharmacist

Among the barriers that we found, there are a reduced number of professionals, work overload, a lack of communication among team members (Silva et al., 2007), not to mention resistance to incorporating the pharmacist into the care management staff.

In addition, we have also observed that verbal interaction among professionals (pharmacists and doctors) alone, does not produce significant results (Silva, 2016). Not sharing the patients' clinical data (medical records, for example) with all professionals that exert an influence over the therapeutic conduct, hamper prescription validation (Cardinal and Fernandes, 2014). It should also be emphasized that inadequate resources may prevent professionals from being employed or replaced.

EVIDENCE GAPS

Further studies should be conducted on factors influencing prescribing and evaluating specific strategies (Davey et al., 2017). High-quality studies assessing the effectiveness of educational actions are still scarce in the literature (Alldred et al., 2016).

Pearson et al. (2009) reported that further studies should analyze the benefits of automated prescribing screening systems, since there is a lack of studies on the impact of the system on drug-related adverse events, safety, quality, cost, and patient outcomes (Yang et al., 2012). Evidence of effective interventions based on computerized systems to prevent medication errors in the pediatric inpatient population is also incipient (Maaskant et al., 2015). Further research is also needed to check the effectiveness of the strategies found in the implementation of computerized alert tools (Kaushal et al., 2003; Hodgkinson et al., 2006), as well as to assess the impact of interventions on legibility and completeness of electronic prescriptions (Reckmann et al., 2009).

The use of the STOPP/START criteria remains incipient in health services, except in emergency services, and further studies are thus needed to assess this tool's efficacy in detecting potentially inappropriate prescriptions (Hill-Taylor et al., 2016).

CONCLUSION

There are several options indicated in the scientific literature that are effective and safe to assist professionals in order to avoid or reduce medication prescribing errors in health services. Our evidence brief for policy present four options that may be useful to deal with this problem, although there is no recommendation on which one is the best. The decision to implement one or more options depends on the context where the decision makers are inserted.

The options are not exclusive and can be used together, according to the local reality of implementation.

When implementing these options, however, it should be taken into account that the number of studies is still incipient and confidence in the results could be improved with further research with high methodological quality.

AUTHOR CONTRIBUTIONS

BA, RM, JB, and TT contributed with the design and conception of the study. BA and RM wrote the first draft of the manuscript. BA, RM, and TT participated in the study selection process. MB and TT contributed to the revision of the manuscript, read and approved the submitted version.

ACKNOWLEDGMENTS

The authors are grateful to the Librarians of the Library of the Faculty of Medicine of the University of São Paulo, for providing articles of restricted access.

REFERENCES

Alldred, D. P., Kennedy, M., Hughes, C., Chen, T. F., and Miller, P. (2016). Interventions to optimise prescribing for older people in care homes. *Cochrane Database Syst. Ver.* 2:CD009095. doi: 10.1002/14651858.CD009095.pub3

Arnold, S. R., and Straus, S. E. (2005). Interventions to improve antibiotic prescribing practices in ambulatory care. *Cochrane Database Syst. Rev.* 4:CD003539. doi: 10.1002/14651858.CD003539.pub2

Bonadiman, R. L., Bonadiman, R. L., Bonadiman, S. L., and Silva, D. A. (2013). Estudo das prescrições medicamentosas em uma farmácia básica de Itapemirim, Espírito Santo - Brasil. *Acta Biomed. Bras.* 4, 114–123.

Bortoli, M. C., Freire, L. M., and Tesser, T. R. (2017) "Políticas de saúde informadas por evidências: propósitos e desenvolvimento no mundo e no país" em *Avaliação de Tecnologias de Saúde e Políticas Informadas por Evidências*, ed T. S. Toma (São Paulo, FCL: Instituto de Saúde), 29–50.

Brennan, N., and Mattick, K. (2013). A systematic review of educational interventions to change behaviour of prescribers in hospital settings, with a particular emphasis on new prescribers. *Br. J. Clin. Pharmacol.* 75, 359–372. doi: 10.1111/j.1365-2125.2012.04397.x

Cardinal, L., and Fernandes, C. (2014). Intervenção farmacêutica no processo da validação da prescrição médica. *Rev. Bras. Farm. Hosp. Serv. Saúde São Paulo* 5, 14–19.

Carvalho, B. G., Turini, B., Nunes, E. F. P. A., Bandeira, I. F., Barbosa, P. F. A., and Takao, T. S. (2011). Percepção dos médicos sobre o curso facilitadores de educação permanente em saúde. *Rev. Bras. Educ. Med.* 35, 132–141. doi: 10.1590/S0100-55022011000100018

Cassiani, S. H. B., Freire, C. C., and Gimenes, F. R. (2003). A prescrição médica eletrônica em um hospital universitário: falhas de redação e opiniões de usuários. *Rev. Esc. Enferm. USP.* 37, 51–60. doi: 10.1590/S0080-62342003000400006

Chiatti, C., Bustacchini, S., Furneri, G., Mantovani, L., Cristiani, M., Misuraca, C., et al. (2012). The economic burden of inappropriate drug prescribing, lack of adherence and compliance, adverse drug events in older people: a systematic review. *Drug Saf.* 35, 73–87. doi: 10.1007/BF03319105

Clyne, B., Fitzgerald, C., Quinlan, A., Hardy, C., Galvin, R., Fahey, T., et al. (2016). Interventions to address potentially inappropriate prescribing in community-dwelling older adults: a systematic review of randomized controlled trials. *J. Am. Geriatr. Soc.* 64, 1210–1222. doi: 10.1111/jgs.14133

Cooper, J. A., Cadogan, C. A., Patterson, S. M., Kerse N., Bradley, M. C., Ryan C., et al. (2015). Interventions to improve the appropriate use of polypharmacy in older people: a Cochrane systematic review. *BMJ Open* 5:e009235. doi: 10.1136/bmjopen-2015-009235

Coxeter, P., Del Mar, C. B., McGregor, L., Beller, E. M., and Hoffmann, T. C. (2015). Interventions to facilitate shared decision making to address antibiotic use for acute respiratory infections in primary care. *Cochrane Database Syst. Ver.* 12:11. doi: 10.1002/14651858.CD010907.pub2

Davey, P., Marwick, C. A., Scott, C. L., Charani, E., McNeil, K., Brown, E., et al. (2017). Interventions to improve antibiotic prescribing practices for hospital inpatients. *Cochrane Database Syst. Ver.* 2:CD003543. doi: 10.1002/14651858.CD003543.pub4

DeSevo, G., and Klootwyk, J. (2012). Pharmacologic issues in management of chronic disease. *Prim. Care Clin. Off. Pract.* 39, 345–362. doi: 10.1016/j.pop.2012.03.007

Donaldson, L. J., Kelley, E. T., Dhingra-Kumar, N., Kieny, M. P., and Sheik, A. (2017). Medication without harm: WHO's third global patient safety challenge. *Lancet* 389, 1680–1681. doi: 10.1016/S0140-6736(17)31047-4.

Evans, T., and Brown, H. (2003). Road traffic crashes: operationalizing equity in the context of health sector reform. *Inj. Control Saf. Promot.* 10, 11–12. doi: 10.1076/icsp.10.1.11.14117

Ferner, R. E. (2014). Harms from medicines: inevitable, in error or intentional. *Br. J. Clin. Pharmacol.* 77, 403–409. doi: 10.1111/bcp.12156

Ferner, R. E., and Aronson, J. K. (2006). Clarification of terminology in medication errors: definitions and classification. *Drug Saf.* 29, 1011–1022. doi: 10.2165/00002018-200629110-00001

Fleming, A., Browne, J., and Byrne, S. (2013). The effect of interventions to reduce potentially inappropriate antibiotic prescribing in long-term care facilities: a systematic review of randomised controlled trials. *Drugs Aging* 30, 401–408. doi: 10.1007/s40266-013-0066-z

Forsetlund, L., Eike, M. C., Gjerberg, E., and Vist, G. E. (2011). Effect of interventions to reduce potentially inappropriate use of drugs in nursing homes: a systematic review of randomised controlled trials. *BMC Geriatr.* 11:16. doi: 10.1186/1471-2318-11-16

Freire, C. C., Gimenes, F. R. E., and Cassiani, S. H. B. (2004). Análise da prescrição informatizada, em duas clínicas de um hospital universitário. *RMRP.* 37, 91–96.

Garcia, R. M. (2006). Five ways you can reduce inappropriate prescribing in the elderly: a systematic review. *J. Fam. Pract.* 55, 305–312.

Gimenes, F. R. E., Miasso, A. I., Lyra D. P. Jr., and Grou, C. R. (2006). Prescrição Eletrônica como fator contribuinte para segurança de pacientes hospitalizados. *Pharm. Pract. (Granada).* 4, 13–17. doi: 10.4321/S1885-642X2006000100003

Gøtzsche, P. C. (2014). Our prescription drugs kill us in large numbers. *Pol. Arch. Med. Wewn.* 124, 628–634. doi: 10.20452/pamw.2503

Hill-Taylor, B., Walsh, K. A., Stewart, S., Hayden, J., Byrne, S., and Sketris, I. S. (2016). Effectiveness of the STOPP/START (screening tool of older persons' potentially inappropriate prescriptions/screening tool to alert doctors to the right treatment) criteria: systematic review and meta-analysis of randomized controlled studies. *J. Clin. Pharm. Ther.* 41, 158–169. doi: 10.1111/jcpt.12372

Hodgkinson, B., Koch, S., Nay, R., and Nichols, K. (2006). Strategies to reduce medication errors with reference to older adults. *Int. J. Evid. Based Healthc.* 4, 2–41. doi: 10.1111/j.1479-6988.2006.00029.x

Hyttinen, V., Jyrkka, J., and Valtonen, H. (2016). A systematic review of the impact of potentially inappropriate medication on health care utilization and costs among older adults. *Med. Care* 54, 950–964. doi: 10.1097/MLR.0000000000000587

Ivanovska, V., and Holloway, K. A. (2013). Interventions to improve antibiotic prescribing in upper middle income countries: a systematic review of the literature 1990–2009. *Maced. J. Med. Sci.* 6, 84–91. doi: 10.3889/mjms.1857-5773.2012.0268

Jano, E., and Aparasu, R. (2007). Healthcare outcomes associated with beers' criteria: a systematic review. *Ann. Pharmacother.* 41, 438–447. doi: 10.1345/aph.1H473

Kaur, S., Mitchell, G., Vitetta, L., and Roberts, M. (2009). Interventions that can reduce inappropriate prescribing in the elderly: a systematic review. *Drugs Aging* 26, 1013–1028. doi: 10.2165/11318890-000000000-00000

Kaushal, R., Shojania, K. G., and Bates, D. W. (2003). Effects of computerized physician order entry and clinical decision support systems on medication safety: a systematic review. *Arch. Intern. Med.* 163, 1410–1416. doi: 10.1001/archinte.163.12.1409

Khajouei, R., and Jaspers, M. W. (2010). The impact of CPOE medication systems' design aspects on usability, workflow and medication orders: a systematic review. *Methods Inf. Med.* 49, 3–19. doi: 10.3414/ME0630

Lainer, M., Mann, E., and Sönnichsen, A. (2013). Information technology interventions to improve medication safety in primary care: a systematic review. *Int. J. Qual. Health Care* 25, 590–598. doi: 10.1093/intqhc/mzt043

Lavan, A. H., Gallagher, P. F., and O'Mahony, D. (2016). Methods to reduce prescribing errors in elderly patients with multimorbidity. *Clin. Interv. Aging* 23, 857–866. doi: 10.2147/CIA.S80280

Lavis, J. N., Oxman, A. D., Lewin, S., and Fretheim, A. (2009). Ferramenta SUPPORT para elaboração de políticas de saúde baseadas em evidências. *Health Res. Policy Syst.* 7, 1–16. doi: 10.1186/1478-4505-7-S1-I1

Lucchetti, G., and Lucchetti, A. L. (2017). Inappropriate prescribing in older persons: a systematic review of medications available in different criteria. *Arch. Gerontol. Geriatr.* 68, 55–61. doi: 10.1016/j.archger.2016.09.003

Maaskant, J. M., Vermeulen, H., Apampa, B., Fernando, B., Ghaleb, M. A., Neubert, A., et al. (2015). Interventions for reducing medication errors in children in hospital. *Cochrane Database Syst. Rev.* 3, 1–64, doi: 10.1002/14651858.CD006208.pub3

Mahony, D. O., Gallagher, P., Ryan, C., Byrne, S., Hamilton, H., Barry, P., et al. (2010). STOPP and START criteria: a new approach to detecting potentially inappropriate prescribing in old age. *Eur. Geriatr. Med.* 1, 45–51. doi: 10.1016/j.eurger.2010.01.007

Marchon, S. G., and Mendes W. V. Jr. (2014). Segurança do paciente na atenção primária à saúde: revisão sistemática. *Cad. Saúde Pública* 30, 1–21. doi: 10.1590/0102-311X00114113

Martins, M., Travassos, C., Mendes, W., and Pavão, A. L. B. (2011). Hospital deaths and adverse events in Brazil. *BMC Health Serv. Res.* 11:223. doi: 10.1186/1472-6963-11-223

Mekonnen, A. B., Abebe, T. B., McLachlan, A. J., and Brien, J. E. (2016). Impact of electronic medication reconciliation interventions on medication discrepancies at hospital transitions: a systematic review and meta-analysis. *BMC Med. Inf. Decis. Mak.* 16, 1–14. doi: 10.1186/s12911-016-0353-9

Miasso, A. I., Grou, C. R., Cassiani, S. H. B., Silva, A. E. B. C., and Fakih, F. T. (2006). Erros de medicação: tipos, fatores causais e providências tomadas em quatro hospitais brasileiros. *Rev. Esc. Enferm. USP.* 40, 524–532. doi: 10.1590/S0080-62342006000400011

Moher, D., Liberati, A., Tetzlaff, J., Altman, D. G., and The PRISMA Group (2009). Preferred reporting items for systematic reviews and meta-analyses: the PRISMA statement. *PLoS Med.* 6:e1000097. doi: 10.1371/journal.pmed.1000097

Pearson, S., Moxey, A., Robertson, J., Hains, I., Williamson, M., Reeve, J., et al. (2009). Do computerised clinical decision support systems for prescribing change practice? A systematic review of the literature (1990-2007). *BMC Heal. Serv. Res.* 9:154. doi: 10.1186/1472-6963-9-154

Porter, G., and Grills, N. (2016). Medication misuse in India: a major public health issue in India. *J. Public Health* 38, 150–7. doi: 10.1093/pubmed/fdv072

Qureshi, N. A., Neyaz, Y., Khoja, T., Magzoub, M. A., Haycox, A., and Walley, T. (2011). Physicians' medication prescribing in primary care in Riyadh city, Saudi Arabia. Literature review, part 3: prescribing errors. *East Mediterr. Health J.* 2, 140–148.

Reckmann, M. H., Westbrook, J. I., Koh, Y., Lo, C., and Day, R. O. (2009). Does computerized provider order entry reduce prescribing errors for hospital inpatients? A systematic review. *J. Am. Med. Inf. Assoc.* 16, 613–623. doi: 10.1197/jamia.M3050

Riordan, D. O., Walsh, K. A., Galvin, R., Sinnott, C., Kearney, P. M., and Byrne, S. (2016). The effect of pharmacist-led interventions in optimising prescribing in older adults in primary care: a systematic review. *SAGE Open Med.* 4: 2050312116652568. doi: 10.1177/2050312116652568

Roque, F., Herdeiro, M. T., Soares, S., Rodrigues, A. T., Breitenfeld, L., and Figueiras, A. (2014). Educational interventions to improve prescription and dispensing of antibiotics: a systematic review. *BMC Public Health* 14:1276. doi: 10.1186/1471-2458-14-1276

Rosa, M. B., Perini, E., Anacleto, T. A., Neiva, H. M., and Bogutchi, T. (2009). Erros na prescrição hospitalar de medicamentos potencialmente perigosos. *Rev. Saúde Pública* 43, 490–498. doi: 10.1590/S0034-89102009005000028

Ross, S., and Loke, Y. K. (2009). Do educational interventions improve prescribing by medical students and junior doctors? A systematic review. *Br. J. Clin. Pharmacol.* 67, 662–670. doi: 10.1111/j.1365-2125.2009.03395.x

Sánchez, A. N., Bravo, J. M. C., and Morales, M. E. P. (2014). Evaluación de estudios prospectivos sobre errores de medicación en la prescripción: revisión sistemática. *Rev. Mex. Cienc. Farm.* 45, 7–14.

Santos, A. P., Silva, D. T., Alves-Conceição, V., Antoniolli, A. R., and Lyra, D. P. Jr. (2015). Conceptualizing and measuring potentially inappropriate drug therapy. *J. Clin. Pharm. Ther.* 40, 167–176. doi: 10.1111/jcpt.12246

Santos, T. D. D. (2016). *O Consentimento Informado na Prática Médica: Revisão Sistemática*. Thesis. Federal University of Bahia, Salvador.

Schedlbauer, A., Prasad, V., Mulvaney, C., Phansalkar, S., Stanton, W., Bates, D. W., et al. (2009). What evidence supports the use of computerized alerts and prompts to improve clinicians' prescribing behavior?. *J. Am. Med. Inf. Assoc.* 16, 531–538. doi: 10.1197/jamia.M2910

Shea, B. J., Grimshaw, J. M., Wells, G. A., Boers, M., Andersson, N., Hamel, C., et al. (2007). Development of AMSTAR: a measurement tool to assess the methodological quality of systematic reviews. *BMC Med. Res. Methodol.* 15, 7–10. doi: 10.1186/1471-2288-7-10

Silva, A. E. B. C., Cassiani, S. H. B., Miasso, A. I., and Opitz, S. P. (2007). Problemas na comunicação: uma possível causa de erros de medicação. *Acta Paul Enferm.* 20, 272–276. doi: 10.1590/S0103-21002007000300005

Silva, N. M. O. (2016). *Erros de Prescrição e Intervenção Farmacêutica em uma Unidade de Internação Obstétrica de Alto Risco: Uma Questão de Segurança no Uso de Medicamentos*. Thesis. Campinas State University, Campinas.

Soares, M. A., Fernandez-Llimos, F., Cabrita, J., and Morais, J. (2011). Critérios de avaliação de prescrição de medicamentos potencialmente inapropriados Uma Revisão Sistemática. *Acta Med. Port.* 24, 775–784.

Tesfaye, W. H., Castelino, R. L., Wimmer, B. C., and Zaidi, S. T. R. (2017). Inappropriate prescribing in chronic kidney disease: a systematic review of prevalence, associated clinical outcomes and impact of interventions. *Int. J. Clin. Pr.* 71, 1–16. doi: 10.1111/ijcp.12960

Tonkin-Crine, S., Yardley, L., and Little, P. (2011). Antibiotic prescribing for acute respiratory tract infections in primary care: a systematic review and meta-ethnography. *J. Antimicrob. Chemother.* 66, 2215–2223. doi: 10.1093/jac/dkr279

Ugarte, O. N., and Acioly, M. A. (2014). O princípio da autonomia no Brasil: discutir é preciso. *Rev. Col. Bras. Cir.* 41, 274–277. doi: 10.1590/0100-69912014005013

Valencia, M. G., Velilla, N. M., Fabo, E. L., Telleria, I. B., and Sola, B. L. (2016). Intervenciones para optimizar el tratamiento farmacológico en ancianos hospitalizados: una revisión sistemáticaInterventions to optimize pharmacologic treatment in hospitalized older adults: a systematic review. *Rev. Clín. Española* 216, 205–221. doi: 10.1016/j.rce.2016.01.005

Van Rosse, F., Maat, B., Rademaker, C. M., Van Vught, A. J., Egberts, A. C., Bollen, C. W., et al. (2009). The effect of computerized physician order entry on medication prescription errors and clinical outcome in pediatric and intensive care: a systematic review. *Pediatrics* 123, 1184–1190. doi: 10.1542/peds.2008-1494

Walsh, K. A., O'Riordan, D., Kearney, P. M., Timmons, S., and Byrne, S. (2016). Improving the appropriateness of prescribing in older patients: a systematic review and meta-analysis of pharmacists' interventions in secondary care. *Age Aging* 45, 201–209. doi: 10.1093/ageing/afv190

World Health Organization (WHO) (2017). *Patient Safety Making Health Care Safer*. Geneva World Health Organization.

Yang, C., Yang, L., and Xiang, X. (2012). Interventions assessment of prescription automatic screening system in Chinese hospitals: a systematic review. *Drug Inf. J.* 46, 669–676. doi: 10.1177/0092861512454417

Yourman, L., Concato, J., and Agostini, J. V. (2008). Use of computer decision support interventions to improve medication prescribing in older adults: a systematic review. *Am. J. Geriatr. Pharmacother.* 6, 119–129. doi: 10.1016/j.amjopharm.2008.06.001

13

SimAlba: A Spatial Microsimulation Approach to the Analysis of Health Inequalities

Malcolm Campbell[1]* and Dimitris Ballas[2,3]

[1] GeoHealth Laboratory, Department of Geography, University of Canterbury, Christchurch, New Zealand, [2] Department of Geography, University of Sheffield, Sheffield, UK, [3] Department of Geography, University of the Aegean, Mytilene, Greece

*Correspondence:
Malcolm Campbell
malcolm.campbell@canterbury.ac.nz

This paper presents applied geographical research based on a spatial microsimulation model, *SimAlba*, aimed at estimating geographically sensitive health variables in Scotland. *SimAlba* has been developed in order to answer a variety of "what-if" policy questions pertaining to health policy in Scotland. Using the *SimAlba* model, it is possible to simulate the distributions of previously unknown variables at the small area level such as smoking, alcohol consumption, mental well-being, and obesity. The *SimAlba* micro-dataset has been created by combining Scottish Health Survey and Census data using a deterministic reweighting spatial microsimulation algorithm developed for this purpose. The paper presents *SimAlba* outputs for Scotland's largest city, Glasgow, and examines the spatial distribution of the simulated variables for small geographical areas in Glasgow as well as the effects on individuals of different policy scenario outcomes. In simulating previously unknown spatial data, a wealth of new perspectives can be examined and explored. This paper explores a small set of those potential avenues of research and shows the power of spatial microsimulation modeling in an urban context.

Keywords: spatial microsimulation, urban health inequalities, health policy, Scotland, geographic information systems, small area microdata

INTRODUCTION

SimAlba is a spatial microsimulation model, which has been used to estimate geographically sensitive health variables for Scotland's largest city, Glasgow. Spatial microsimulation is now a well-established method in geography for public policy analysis in a wide range of domains (1, 2). Building on these efforts, *SimAlba*[1] has been developed in order to answer a variety of "what-if" policy questions pertaining to health policy in Scotland. We aim to show how this data could be (and have been) used to create "what-if" policy scenarios. A "what-if" policy scenario is an estimation of what may happen to health outcomes as a result of a hypothetical change in policy using modeled data.

There is a significant body of literature describing the uses of complex statistical models to analyze social and spatial inequalities in a variety of contexts. Specifically, the use of spatial microsimulation models (3–8) provide a new perspective on existing data sources and contribute to the relevant academic literature as well as applied health policy analysis efforts offering an opportunity to estimate previously unknown data as well as to analyze both individuals and areas simultaneously.

---

[1] The model is named *SimAlba* as Alba is the Scots Gaelic name for Scotland, and it is a Spatial Microsimulation model of Scotland.

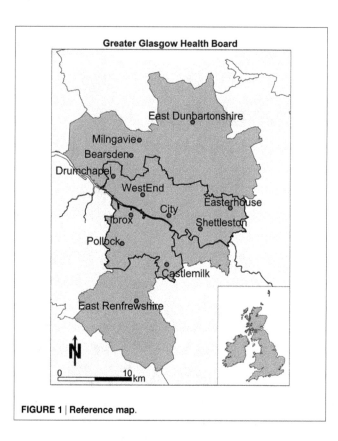

FIGURE 1 | Reference map.

This paper aims to further demonstrate how spatial micro-simulation can be used to estimate previously unavailable data and then to show how this data can be analyzed and visualized, using geographic information systems (GISs), to illuminate both the social and the spatial patterns in health-related behavior and outcomes in Glasgow, Scotland (see **Figure 1**). This paper forwards a new small area perspective on health-related variables in Scotland, showing how Scottish Health Survey (SHS) and Census data for Scotland can be combined to create a powerful policy modeling and visualization framework.

The paper is organized as follows: it begins by painting the health landscape of the study area; then giving an introduction to the microsimulation literature and explaining how spatial microsimulation can be operationalized in simple terms. Some outputs of the *SimAlba* model are then presented and explored, particularly focusing on the health-related variables created. A discussion of the relevance of the results simulated follows; concluding with directions for future research and the policy implications of the analysis presented.

A BACKGROUND TO THE HEALTH LANDSCAPE IN SCOTLAND

The recent past has been marked by a series of deteriorations in Scottish health relative to the rest of Europe, which has led to Scotland being labeled as "the sick man of Europe." This label has been applied to Scottish health more recently, signifying the noticeable divergence from the 1950s onward in terms of health compared with the rest of Europe. Glasgow, in particular, exhibited

the highest levels of self-reported bad or very bad general health and psychological distress for both men and women compared across 32 other Europe metropolitan areas (9). The "Scottish Effect" (10) or the "Glasgow Effect" (11) details the excess mortality in Scotland and Glasgow, in particular, even after accounting for socioeconomic circumstances. This suggests that Scotland is peculiar in regards to population health, and that this effect may be even stronger in Glasgow; hence the focus in this paper on the urban area of this city. In other words, after taking account of deprivation, there is still an excess of mortality in Scotland compared to England and Wales (12). This issue is well-studied. For example, a report on Scottish health (13), identified "risk factors" in Scotland as tobacco, alcohol, low fruit and vegetable intake, physical activity levels, and obesity. More broadly, within the UK, there has long been ample evidence on the existence of health inequalities, especially, since the highly influential Black Report (14) that highlighted health inequalities by both place and socioeconomic status that continue to exist and persist over time (15) in the UK. Furthermore, when compared to the rest of Great Britain (GB) or the UK (16, 17) or its western European neighbors (18), Scotland does not do well. There have been many studies examining these broader country level differences over time between Scotland and the rest of GB [for a recent example comparing mortality patterns, see Ref. (12)].

Looking in more depth at Glasgow, the evidence of a specific "Glasgow Effect" as discussed above is a particular concern for this paper. A specific cause of concern is that premature mortality is 30% higher in Glasgow compared to similarly deprived UK cities (11). This paper adds to the understandings of why this may be the case by estimating previously unknown data. For example, discussion around the importance of alcohol consumption or drug use as contributing to half of the excess observed (19), with much of the deprivation potentially unmeasured, points to the usefulness of small area estimates to fill this gap. The specific spatial patterning of deprivation in Glasgow has been examined as a possible cause of the "Glasgow Effect"; evidence suggests that there is a strong impact of deprivation of surrounding areas on health outcomes (20) but not quite as originally hypothesized by McCartney et al. (21) as a concentrated monoculture. As McCartney et al. (21) explains, there are 17 possible explanations for the unique situation in Glasgow, concluding that understanding of the Scottish mortality patterning requires, as well as a clear focus on behaviors, an understanding of the most "upstream" determinants of health, to which spatial microsimulation can add some important value. Previous analysis of poverty and benefit take-up show that there are some geographical patterns, but only at unitary authority level (22), noting that the "worst" areas are concentrated around Glasgow combined with relative affluence nearby. Other work examining the geography of disadvantage in Glasgow (23) notes the persistence of disadvantage in areas in the east end (Shettleston, Easterhouse) as well as to the northwest (Drumchapel) and to the South (Castlemilk) and southwest of the center (Pollok) in the 1970s, 1980s, and 1990s. Of particular note is that Glasgow performs worse on all the deprivation-related variables compared to the Scottish average and the persistence of disadvantage, in particular, small areas of Glasgow. This pattern of higher deprivation in Glasgow continues, linking it with mortality rates, showing a strong bivariate relationship across Scotland; in other words, spatial proximity to deprivation is important for mortality outcomes (24). Qualitative evidence from Glasgow also points to the importance of area on health behaviors, that poorly resourced, stressful environments with strong community norms may foster smoking as well as undermining attempts to increase cessation rates (25). Moreover, the perceptions, as well as the health outcomes in neighborhoods in Glasgow have a social gradient, as outlined by Sooman and Macintyre (26), such that perceptions of an area can influence health outcomes. Overall, we can see the pattern of evidence pointing to the importance of area influence on health outcomes in Glasgow.

The role of smoking, alcohol consumption, diet, and physical activity in explaining socioeconomic differentials in mortality in the west of Scotland noted the importance of these behaviors for longer-term outcomes (27). Thus, having estimates of such behaviors at small area level can help increase understanding of the broader forces of health inequality associated with health behaviors. A Scottish specific issue is the role that alcohol plays in contributing to poor health outcomes linked to the minimum pricing of alcohol as a policy response (28). Scotland has among the highest alcohol-related deaths in Western Europe (29), although this has been falling since the 1990s. Scotland also embarked on a smoke-free policy, designed to reduce exposure to secondhand smoke. Evidence has shown that it has been a success (30) as well as having none of the hypothesizing negative outcome, such as more smoking in the home or economic impacts on businesses. Of particular relevance is the debate around the independence question for Scotland. Although the outcome was a "no," there is still significant potential for further departure with respect to health policy compared to the rest of the UK (31).

Therefore, we can see that Glasgow has been the subject of much research into health inequalities as well as economic and social inequality. We add estimated health variables to this body of work at a small area level to further enhance knowledge and to highlight relevant social and spatial patterns and inequalities.

A BRIEF BACKGROUND TO SPATIAL MICROSIMULATION MODELING IN HEALTH

Spatial microsimulation is an established methodology in the social sciences with a long successful history in Economics since the late 1950s and with more recent significant developments in other disciplines, including geography in the last three decades (1, 2). In particular, there have been significant advances in spatial microsimulation models, in other words, adding geography to models (32). This adds to the potential uses of microsimulation, for example, by allowing assessment of area-based policies relating to social and health policy (3, 7, 33). Additionally, the geographic distribution of health-related variables can be simulated (3–6, 34), not just the socioeconomic or demographic patterns aspatially. This allows previously unknown small area spatial patterns to be investigated, and the spatial effects to be considered in concert with the socioeconomic and demographic factors. Building on these efforts, SimAlba has been developed in order to answer a variety of "what-if" policy questions pertaining to health policy in Scotland, with geography included as a

key element. The SimAlba model has previously been used to estimate and model in the economic sphere (35, 36). We add to this literature by focusing on health.

DATA AND METHODS: SIMALBA – A SPATIAL MICROSIMULATION MODEL

The SimAlba model was developed with the use of data from the Census of Population 2001 and the SHS 2003. The Census of Population is carried out decennially, while the SHS 2003 was the third survey of Scottish health (after 1995 and 1998) and included all ages. Each SHS samples a new set of addresses and has both an adult and child component with a total of 8,148 adults and 3,324 children interviewed on a variety of health conditions and behaviors as well as socioeconomic and demographic information. The health variables include: smoking and alcohol consumption, physical activity, dental health, general health, and many others.

It is important to point out that the time periods of data collection (2001 and 2003) do not match precisely, but in the absence of any other temporally consistent health data, for Scotland, this is a pragmatic compromise. Spatial microsimulation uses the data contained in the SHS and "upscales" it to reflect the populations of census areas as closely as possible. This can be achieved using a process called deterministic reweighting (3, 8, 37). Deterministic reweighting has become an established method for estimating health variables in multiple contexts such as area smoking prevalence (4, 6) or obesity prevalence (38). Spatial microsimulation works by using a series of constraints that are used to construct the model, and which must be present in both datasets; this limits the potential constraint options available. A constraint variable is chosen by either using the literature or a more formal regression approach to see which variables in the datasets are most correlated with the variable to be predicted. Therefore, the choice of the constraints, though informed by the literature and other empirical research, must be pragmatic. Constraints are keys to the model set up (39) and, therefore, an important part of the spatial microsimulation modeling process.

SimAlba uses age, sex, marital status, illness, qualifications, economic activity, tenure, and an employment classification (National Socioeconomic Classification, NSSEC) as constraints. Note that the deterministic reweighting process is not explained in depth in this paper for reasons of brevity [for more details, see Ref. (36)]. The method is deterministic as it produces the same output for the same input data, which were an important consideration for policy end users. The stylized formula that can be applied to create microdata is $NW_i = W_i \times CEN_{ij}/SHS_{ij}$.

The equation is constructed as follows: a new weight (NW) for individual i is calculated by multiplying the weight (W) for individual i by element ij of the Census table divided by element ij of the SHS table. This process is completed iteratively until a suitable level of convergence is reached, and NW_i is the number of a particular individual created for a specific small area in Scotland. The process was followed to adjust the weights of individuals in the SHS to match census output areas (OAs) populations, which have a minimum population of around 40 households or 100 individuals. The end result is a spatially simulated dataset, which previously did not exist and which can now be used as the basis for further analysis.

Microsimulation has been used to estimate many different types of data in multiple contexts as discussed above. One of the key points of concern in the literature pertains to the reliability and accuracy of the microsimulated data. There is now a growing body of evidence showing that the technique provides robust estimates of health-related variables in particular (6, 38, 40). *SimAlba* has been internally and externally validated (see **Figure 8**) and has demonstrated that it provides robust data (35, 36). From **Figure 8**, it can be seen that the model produces estimates within 10% error, with most of the data falling close to the 45° line, signifying an exact match.

SPATIAL MICROSIMULATION MODEL OUTPUTS: ESTIMATING HEALTH BEHAVIORS AND OUTCOMES

This section shows some of the microsimulated data tabulated and mapped so as to give a small snapshot of the type of data that can be produced by *SimAlba* and its policy relevance. Several of the variables simulated are now visualized using a quintile distribution, which can help us to better highlight the extremes of the spatially simulated data. Q1 refers to the highest

values, Q5 the lowest in the distribution of variables. Only a small fraction of the data that can be mapped is, as any variable in the SHS can, potentially be simulated using the *SimAlba* algorithms.

In this paper, we demonstrate the relevance of the outputs of models like *SimAlba* to policy debates briefly discussed above by focusing on smoking prevalence, subjective well-being, alcohol consumption, and obesity. We therefore pose five policy relevant research questions that are readily applicable to spatially microsimulated data. Specifically, we demonstrate how models like *SimAlba* can be used to address research questions such as:

1. Which OAs in Glasgow have the greatest proportions of "unhappy" people?
2. Which areas have the greatest proportions of obese people?
3. Where do those men drinking over the daily limits reside?
4. What is the distribution of smokers in Greater Glasgow and to what extent is this altered by income?
5. Which OAs do those people who exhibit several simultaneous "unhealthy" characteristics reside in the greatest proportions?

General health questionnaire (GHQ) scores are a measure of subjective well-being based on a series of questions resulting in a single number summary of mental health, where a higher score denotes increased mental distress. First, the simulated

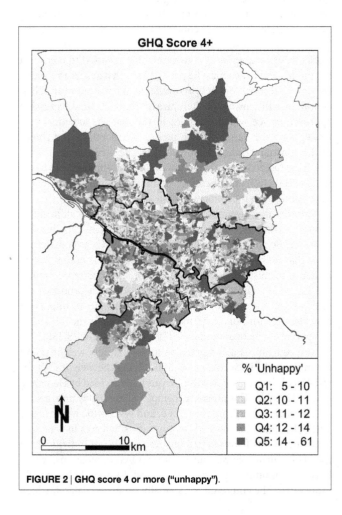

FIGURE 2 | GHQ score 4 or more ("unhappy").

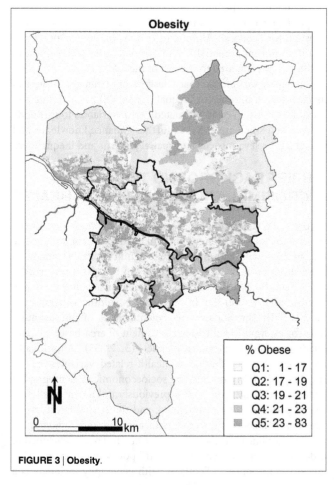

FIGURE 3 | Obesity.

spatial pattern of subjective well-being is visualized as shown in **Figure 2**. There is a notable series of clusters in the east end of Glasgow. The areas with the lower percentages of individuals (lighter colors) appear to be spread around the west end and to the northern edges of Glasgow, which is what is likely to be expected *a priori* from the socioeconomic geography of Glasgow. In other words, the most deprived areas have worse mental health outcomes. Elsewhere, the pattern of mental well-being appears sporadic in Glasgow with smaller scattered clusters toward Drumchapel for example.

Second, the geography of Glasgow in terms of BMI is looked at briefly in this paragraph. Those areas colored darkest (Q5) with large numbers of obese people are in the east of Glasgow in **Figure 3**, Easterhouse, and Shettleston. Areas with higher proportions of obesity are also concentrated in the Castlemilk area of Glasgow to the south east. There are similar small enclaves of areas in the areas bordering the river Clyde to the western edge on the south side of Glasgow city. The pattern would appear to follow an explanation of poor socioeconomic conditions correlating with obesity in the Glasgow area.

Third, the focus moves to the spatial patterns of alcohol consumption in Greater Glasgow. Overall, the summary is that there is little in the way of a clear pattern (**Figure 4**). The pattern of east end doing "poorly" is not as apparent for this variable. The message overall is that there are few "pockets" of problem drinking, so it is more difficult to conclude that this is linked to the area.

Fourth, the geography of smoking in Glasgow in **Figure 5** shows smokers using over 20 cigarettes a day. Focusing on the spatial pattern, areas toward Castlemilk in the south east, the east end around Easterhouse, and the parts of the central areas bordering the river Clyde have the highest proportions of heavy smokers.

The spatial patterns demonstrated in each of the estimated health outcomes and behaviors, to a greater or lesser extent, mimic the aforementioned patterns of deprivation. The particular social geography within the Greater Glasgow area is therefore important context to the estimates produced here.

A STYLISED POLICY SCENARIO: IDENTIFYING AREAS OF HIGH NEED

This section explores the power of spatial microsimulation in more depth by again demonstrating some of the consideration advantages over more "traditional approaches." Imagine a policy scenario where the aim is to identify the areas with the most "unhealthy" persons, and the areas in which they reside. This can be achieved in spatial microsimulation modeling. Data can be combined, such that the people who are smoking 20 or more cigarettes a day, drinking more alcohol than the guidelines suggest, have low subjective well-being and also obese simultaneously are selected, then mapped. This combination of factors

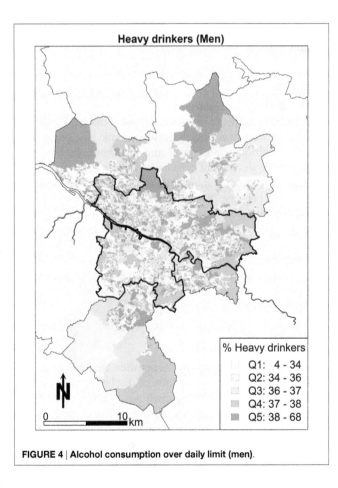

FIGURE 4 | Alcohol consumption over daily limit (men).

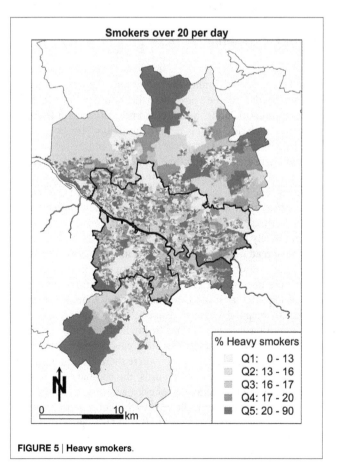

FIGURE 5 | Heavy smokers.

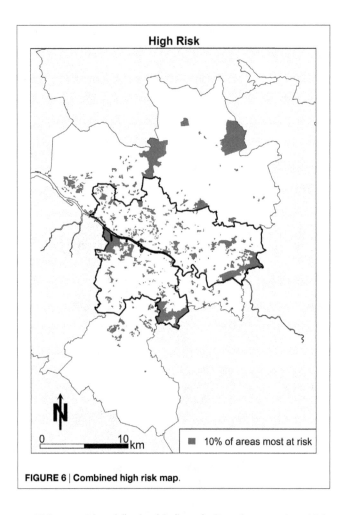

FIGURE 6 | Combined high risk map.

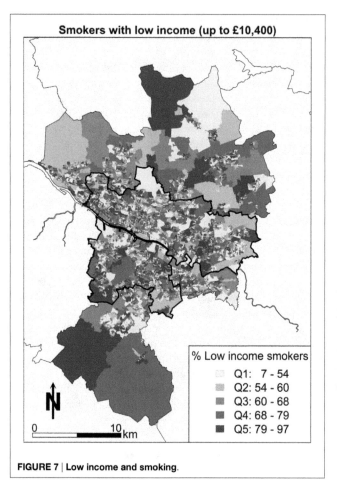

FIGURE 7 | Low income and smoking.

could be considered "unhealthy," so finding the areas in which these people live may be a priority so that health policy can target concentrations of "poor" health outcomes. The map in **Figure 6** shows the "high risk" areas in terms of health for Greater Glasgow. The spatial pattern in Glasgow shows that some areas stand out visually. There are areas of clustering in places that are expected to feature in the "poor" health end of the distribution, such as areas in the east end of Glasgow, around Easterhouse, and Castlemilk. Other areas, such as Drumchapel, have pockets of "high risk" health features. On balance, the pattern is concentrated more within the city boundary than outside it, punctuated by smaller clusters spread across the city with notable "gaps" (i.e., white space) in the more affluent areas of the city, such as the west end. The pattern does show elements of the other health maps, which is to be expected as it is a combination of all four of the previous health maps of Glasgow. The concentration of "high risk" areas could have important health implications and additional effects on health that smaller isolated clusters may not exhibit would have a much greater effect where there are combinations of "high risk" health. In other words, the combination of high alcohol consumption, smoking, obesity, and poor mental health may well have longer-term effects as well as compounding effects on individual and area-level health. It could be argued that area-based policies, i.e., targeting a specific neighborhood, would work by targeting these "high risk" areas, and this may well have an

impact at the national or city level in terms of an improvement to health outcomes more generally.

A further example of the power of spatial microsimulation is to combine and cross tabulate socioeconomic and health variables geographically. In **Figure 7**, the map shows the areas with the highest proportions of people who have low income and are smokers. What the map shows is those areas with the darkest reds (Q5) contain between 78 and 96% of people in that category as a proportion of all people in each area. In other words, almost all of the people in some areas of Glasgow are low-income smokers. There is an advantage to know which of those areas are worth focusing resources in terms of stopping smoking services. Areas to the south, such as Shettleston and areas to the East, such as Easterhouse, are highlighted with respect to smoking behaviors and low income.

DISCUSSION

In 2006, Scotland introduced a nationwide ban on smoking in public places and plans to end tobacco displays in shops as well as to ban sales from vending machines. Scottish studies (41) report that reductions in exposure to secondhand smoke of the order observed in Scotland may generate immediate health gains in the Scottish population as well as longer-term reductions in morbidity and mortality related to secondhand smoke due to the smoking ban. Haw and Gruer (41) argue that quitting smoking is probably the most effective way of reducing secondhand smoke exposure in the home; and that smoking cessation services must continue to be promoted. Additional evidence (30) again supports the thesis that smoke-free legislation has been a success. An option would be to model smokers to better target this group of the population if desired. The use of microsimulation to model smoking rates is not new, as the geography of smoking in Leeds (4) has previously been estimated. The microsimulation of smoking rates in *SimAlba* builds on this type of work and brings it to a Scottish context, which does not appear to have been modeled before. There are also arguments about broader macroeconomic forces, such as income inequality (42), being the cause of a plethora of health and social ills. The debates around greater income inequality leading to higher rates of not just smoking but also poorer mental health outcomes and higher rates of obesity are well rehearsed in the literature.

Another aspect of health that is relevant in Scotland is mental health outcomes. Scotland has high rates of suicide (43) compared to England and Wales. Spatial microsimulation could be used to specifically target "at risk" groups, geographically. Previous modeling has been completed in England (44) showing the spatial patterning of small-area prevalence of psychological distress and alcohol consumption. Also, there have been attempts to estimate happiness in Scotland with the use of spatial microsimulation (34) by combing the British Household Panel Survey (BHPS) with census data. What the analysis in this paper adds is a more complete picture of other health variables, also using a health-specific survey data set (SHS instead of the BHPS), and building on the existing work from elsewhere in the UK.

Alcohol policy is also of particular policy relevance due to the debates on the introduction of a minimum price per unit of alcohol (45). The Scottish government previously introduced an alcohol bill to try and begin the process of legislating for the changes needed, such as the minimum price per unit of alcohol. In the background of alcohol consumption debates is the framework of the recommended daily limits for alcohol consumption of no more than 3 or 4 U (2 or 3 U) of alcohol per day for men or women, respectively. The analysis presented here shows the estimated geographic location and the characteristics of people who drink over the guideline limits adding extra depth to the existing data. As noted by Katikireddi and McLean (28), there is a lack of empirical evidence in this regard which, it could be argued, can be addressed by spatial microsimulation models (e.g., *SimAlba*).

Obesity is a growing problem worldwide. It is also a costly problem with between 0.7 and 2.8% of a country's total healthcare expenditures being spent on this health issue (46). There are complex pathways and dynamics behind the determinants of obesity (47) that explain the doubling of the rate, since 1980 worldwide, to a rate of around 20% in most developed economies, such as the context explored here (48). More concerning is that patterns among children and adolescents continue to show growth in rates of obesity (49). Interestingly, when looking at the relationship between play areas and deprivation and subsequent links to childhood obesity (50), it was found that

more deprived areas are better provided for, but, the quality has not been accounted for, neither has the lack of private green space relative to more affluent areas, so causal pathways in some instances are unclear. Moreover, in Glasgow, there is evidence to suggest that more deprived neighborhoods are no more likely to be exposed to energy dense out-of-home eating outlets (51). So, simple explanations relating to providing more play areas and reducing exposure to out-of-home eating outlets are not sufficient explanation for increasing obesity rates, The *SimAlba* model adds to a literature on simulated obesity rates for small areas seen elsewhere in the UK (38). More recent literature (52) has continued in a similar vein, emphasizing the importance of designing policies targeted at the small area level, but also that account for population group differences simultaneously.

CONCLUSION

A comprehensive dataset, such as that generated by *SimAlba* that provides data on health-related behaviors for individuals and small areas in Scotland, has previously not been available. Although the data simulated are now updated, it provides an important addition to understanding the health behaviors at small area geographies. The missing piece of the puzzle has always been that reliable small area data on all these types of behaviors and conditions are not collected, except, for very broadly, by the Census, which exists for self-reported health for example. What spatial microsimulation adds is the lower level, small area

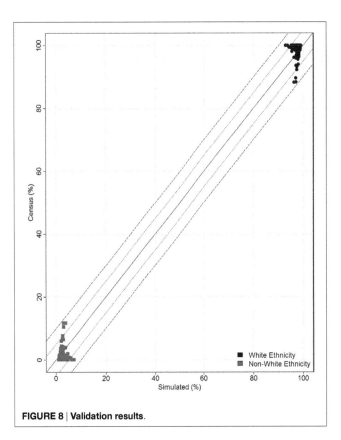

FIGURE 8 | Validation results.

geography, the ability to examine both composition, and context simultaneously.

Nevertheless, it should be noted that one concern with spatial microsimulation is the issue of validation – how accurate simulated data are – and how to assess quality of outputs. This concern has been addressed or discussed in papers looking at deterministic reweighting models (6), and there are ongoing debates (53) on this specific issue. Therefore, the main limitation of microsimulation is that it is difficult to verify that the outputs against what the real population data may be. The paradox of this approach is that the reason the data are simulated in the first instance is that it is difficult or too expensive to collect. On balance, the *SimAlba* model appears to produce reasonably accurate microsimulated data where validation or use of a proxy variable to test results have been possible as demonstrated elsewhere (35, 36), as well as seen in **Figure 8**.

The analysis presented provides policy makers with an indication of those areas where individuals with a variety of health outcomes (smoking, alcohol consumption, obesity, and mental well-being) are potentially living within Glasgow, and this information could potentially be used to target smaller area interventions compared to a universal intervention. Subjective well-being (measured by GHQ 12 score) has also been examined, and there does not appear to be any other study in which estimated GHQ scores at such small areas in Scotland. Alcohol consumption was also modeled using the *SimAlba* framework. The simulation of data of this nature could be considered valuable to policy makers in showing the differing spatial concentrations

of problem drinkers. Furthermore, obesity and various weight categories were simulated using *SimAlba*. The analysis provides an original dataset to explore health outcomes and behaviors in Scotland at either the individual-level or small area-level geography. The estimation of health-related variables; smoking, alcohol, happiness, and obesity at small area level geography is a step forward in understanding what the patterns of health behaviors or health indicators are likely to be. There is still significant potential to use the microdataset created for future research in a variety of fields. The SimAlba model is also able to estimate other variables, which are present in the SHS (e.g., regular exercise), but this would require a modified spatial microsimulation model. The model presented here could also be used as a basis for future modeling work or as the basis of a framework for other survey data sources, for example, to look at spatial and social patterns of tobacco cessation, condom use for disease prevention, seat belt use, or breastfeeding.

AUTHOR CONTRIBUTIONS

MC collected and analyzed data and wrote the first draft; DB made suggestions regarding the analysis and interpretation and also co-authored and edited the manuscript.

FUNDING

This work was funded by a grant from the ESRC and the Scottish Government.

REFERENCES

1. O'Donoghue C, Ballas D, Clarke G, Hynes S, Morrissey K, editors. Spatial microsimulation for rural policy analysis. *Advances in Spatial Science*. Berlin, Heidelberg: Springer (2013).
2. Tanton R, Edwards K, editors. Spatial microsimulation: a reference guide for users, vol 6. *Understanding Population Trends and Processes*. Netherlands: Springer (2013).
3. Ballas D, Clarke G, Dorling D, Rigby J, Wheeler B. Using geographical information systems and spatial microsimulation for the analysis of health inequalities. *Health Informatics J* (2006) 12(1):65–79. doi:10.1177/1460458206061217
4. Tomintz MN, Clarke GP, Rigby JE. The geography of smoking in Leeds: estimating individual smoking rates and the implications for the location of stop smoking services. *Area* (2008) 40(3):341–53. doi:10.1111/j.1475-4762.2008.00837.x
5. Smith DM, Clarke GP, Ransley J, Cade J. Food access and health: a microsimulation framework for analysis. *Stud Region Sci* (2006) 35(4):909–27. doi:10.2457/srs.35.909
6. Smith DM, Pearce JR, Harland K. Can a deterministic spatial microsimulation model provide reliable small-area estimates of health behaviours? An example of smoking prevalence in New Zealand. *Health Place* (2011) 17(2):618–24. doi:10.1016/j.healthplace.2011.01.001
7. Tanton R. Spatial microsimulation as a method for estimating different poverty rates in Australia. *Popul Space Place* (2011) 17(3):222–35. doi:10.1002/psp.601
8. Ballas D, Clarke G, Dorling D, Eyre H, Thomas B, Rossiter D. SimBritain: a spatial microsimulation approach to population dynamics. *Popul Space Place* (2005) 11(1):13–34. doi:10.1002/psp.351
9. Gray L, Merlo J, Mindell J, Hallqvist J, Tafforeau J, O'Reilly D, et al. International differences in self-reported health measures in 33 major metropolitan areas in Europe. *Eur J Public Health* (2012) 22(1):40–7. doi:10.1093/eurpub/ckq170
10. Hanlon P, Lawder RS, Buchanan D, Redpath A, Walsh D, Wood R, et al. Why is mortality higher in Scotland than in England and Wales? Decreasing influence of socioeconomic deprivation between 1981 and 2001 supports the existence of a 'Scottish Effect'. *J Public Health* (2005) 27(2):199–204. doi:10.1093/pubmed/fdi002
11. Walsh D, Bendel N, Jones R, Hanlon P. It's not 'just deprivation': why do equally deprived UK cities experience different health outcomes? *Public Health* (2010) 124(9):487–95. doi:10.1016/j.puhe.2010.02.006
12. Campbell M, Ballas D, Dorling D, Mitchell R. Mortality inequalities: Scotland versus England and Wales. *Health Place* (2013) 23(0):179–86. doi:10.1016/j.healthplace.2013.06.004
13. Scottish Executive. *Improving Health in Scotland*. Edinburgh: Scottish Executive (2003). Available from: http://www.gov.scot/Publications/2003/03/16747/19929
14. Black D, Morris J, Smith C, Townsend P. *Inequalities in Health: Report of a Research Working Group*. London: Department of Health and Social Security (1980).
15. Acheson D. *Independent Inquiry into Inequalities in Health: Report*. London: Stationery Office (1998).
16. Shaw M, Dorling D, Gordon D, Davey-Smith G. *The Widening Gap: Health Inequalities and Policy in Britain*. Bristol: Policy Press (1999).
17. Dorling D. *Death in Britain*. York: Joseph Rowntree Foundation (1997).
18. Leon DA, Morton S, Cannegieter S, McKee M. *Understanding the Health of the Scottish Population in an International Context*. Glasgow: Public Health Institute of Scotland (2003).
19. George S. It's not just deprivation – or is it? *Public Health* (2010) 124(9):496–7. doi:10.1016/j.puhe.2010.05.012
20. Livingston M, Lee D. "The Glasgow effect?" – the result of the geographical patterning of deprived areas? *Health Place* (2014) 29(0):1–9. doi:10.1016/j.healthplace.2014.05.002
21. McCartney G, Collins C, Walsh D, Batty GD. Why the Scots die younger: synthesizing the evidence. *Public Health* (2012) 126(6):459–70. doi:10.1016/j.puhe.2012.03.007

22. Bramley G, Lancaster S, Gordon D. Benefit take-up and the geography of poverty in Scotland. *Reg Stud* (2000) 34(6):507–19. doi:10.1080/00343400050085639

23. Pacione M. Environments of disadvantage: geographies of persistent poverty in Glasgow. *Scott Geogr J* (2004) 120(1–2):117–32. doi:10.1080/00369220418737196

24. Sridharan S, Tunstall H, Lawder R, Mitchell R. An exploratory spatial data analysis approach to understanding the relationship between deprivation and mortality in Scotland. *Soc Sci Med* (2007) 65(9):1942–52. doi:10.1016/j.socscimed.2007.05.052

25. Stead M, MacAskill S, MacKintosh A-M, Reece J, Eadie D. "It's as if you're locked in": qualitative explanations for area effects on smoking in disadvantaged communities. *Health Place* (2001) 7(4):333–43. doi:10.1016/S1353-8292(01)00025-9

26. Sooman A, Macintyre S. Health and perceptions of the local environment in socially contrasting neighbourhoods in Glasgow. *Health Place* (1995) 1(1):15–26. doi:10.1016/1353-8292(95)00003-5

27. Whitley E, Batty GD, Hunt K, Popham F, Benzeval M. The role of health behaviours across the life course in the socioeconomic patterning of all-cause mortality: the West of Scotland Twenty-07 Prospective Cohort Study. *Ann Behav Med* (2014) 47(2):148–57. doi:10.1007/s12160-013-9539-x

28. Katikireddi SV, McLean JA. Introducing a minimum unit price for alcohol in Scotland: considerations under European Law and the implications for European public health. *Eur J Public Health* (2012) 22(4):457–8. doi:10.1093/eurpub/cks091

29. Shipton D, McCartney G, Whyte B, Walsh D, Craig N, Beeston C. Alcohol-related deaths in Scotland: do country-specific factors affecting cohorts born in the 1940s and before help explain the current trends in alcohol-related trends? *Eur J Public Health* (2014) 24(2):177–8. doi:10.1093/eurpub/cku163.055

30. Hyland A, Hassan LM, Higbee C, Boudreau C, Fong GT, Borland R, et al. The impact of smokefree legislation in Scotland: results from the Scottish ITC Scotland/UK longitudinal surveys. *Eur J Public Health* (2009) 19(2):198–205. doi:10.1093/eurpub/ckn141

31. Bennet N. Health on the agenda in Scottish independence referendum. *Lancet* (2014) 383(9915):397–8. doi:10.1016/S0140-6736(14)60120-3

32. Clarke GP, editor. *Microsimulation for Urban and Regional Policy Analysis*. London: Pion (1996).

33. Ballas D, Clarke GP, Dorling D, Rossiter D. Using SimBritain to model the geographical impact of national government policies. *Geogr Anal* (2007) 39(1):44–77. doi:10.1111/j.1538-4632.2006.00695.x

34. Ballas D. Geographical simulation models of happiness and well-being. In: Stillwell J, Norman P, Thomas C, Surridge P, editors. *Understanding Population Trends and Processes, volume 2: Population, Employment, Health and Well-being*. New York: Springer (2010). p. 53–66.

35. Ballas D, Campbell M, Clarke G, Hanaoka K, Nakaya T, Waley P. A spatial microsimulation approach to small area income estimation in Britain and Japan. *Stud Region Sci* (2012) 42(1):163–87. doi:10.2457/srs.42.163

36. Campbell M, Ballas D. A spatial microsimulation approach to economic policy analysis in Scotland. *Region Sci Policy Pract* (2013) 5(3):263–88. doi:10.1111/rsp3.12009

37. Ballas D. Simulating trends in poverty and income inequality on the basis of 1991 and 2001 census data: a tale of two cities. *Area* (2004) 36(2):146–63. doi:10.1111/j.0004-0894.2004.00211.x

38. Edwards KL, Clarke GP. The design and validation of a spatial microsimulation model of obesogenic environments for children in Leeds, UK: SimObesity. *Soc Sci Med* (2009) 69(7):1127–34. doi:10.1016/j.socscimed.2009.07.037

39. Williamson P, Birkin M, Rees PH. The estimation of population microdata by using data from small area statistics and samples of anonymised records. *Environ Plan A* (1998) 30(5):785–816. doi:10.1068/a300785

40. Smith DM, Clarke GP, Harland K. Improving the synthetic data generation process in spatial microsimulation models. *Environ Plan A* (2009) 41(5):1251–68. doi:10.1068/a4147

41. Haw SJ, Gruer L. Changes in exposure of adult non-smokers to second-hand smoke after implementation of smoke-free legislation in Scotland: national cross sectional survey. *BMJ* (2007) 335(7619):549. doi:10.1136/bmj.39315.670208.47

42. Wilkinson RG, Pickett KE. The problems of relative deprivation: why some societies do better than others. *Soc Sci Med* (2007) 65(9):1965–78. doi:10.1016/j.socscimed.2007.05.041

43. Mok PLH, Leyland AH, Kapur N, Windfuhr K, Appleby L, Platt S, et al. Why does Scotland have a higher suicide rate than England? An area-level investigation of health and social factors. *J Epidemiol Community Health* (2013) 67:63–70. doi:10.1136/jech-2011-200855

44. Riva M, Smith D. Generating small-area prevalence of psychological distress and alcohol consumption: validation of a spatial microsimulation method. *Soc Psychiatry Psychiatr Epidemiol* (2012) 47(5):745–55. doi:10.1007/s00127-011-0376-6

45. Meier PS, Purshouse R, Brennan A. Policy options for alcohol price regulation: the importance of modelling population heterogeneity. *Addiction* (2010) 105(3):383–93. doi:10.1111/j.1360-0443.2009.02721.x

46. Withrow D, Alter DA. The economic burden of obesity worldwide: a systematic review of the direct costs of obesity. *Obes Rev* (2011) 12(2):131–41. doi:10.1111/j.1467-789X.2009.00712.x

47. Popkin BM, Gordon-Larsen P. The nutrition transition: worldwide obesity dynamics and their determinants. *Int J Obes Relat Metab Disord* (2004) 28(S3):S2–9. doi:10.1038/sj.ijo.0802804

48. Seidell JC. Obesity, insulin resistance and diabetes – a worldwide epidemic. *Br J Nutr* (2000) 83(SupplS1):S5–8. doi:10.1017/S000711450000088X

49. Wang Y, Lobstein TIM. Worldwide trends in childhood overweight and obesity. *Int J Pediatr Obes* (2006) 1(1):11–25. doi:10.1080/17477160600586747

50. Ellaway A, Kirk A, Macintyre S, Mutrie N. Nowhere to play? The relationship between the location of outdoor play areas and deprivation in Glasgow. *Health Place* (2007) 13(2):557–61. doi:10.1016/j.healthplace.2006.03.005

51. Macintyre S, McKay L, Cummins S, Burns C. Out-of-home food outlets and area deprivation: case study in Glasgow, UK. *Int J Behav Nutr Phys Act* (2005) 2(1):16. doi:10.1186/1479-5868-2-16

52. Cataife G. Small area estimation of obesity prevalence and dietary patterns: a model applied to Rio de Janeiro city, Brazil. *Health Place* (2014) 26(0):47–52. doi:10.1016/j.healthplace.2013.12.004

53. Whitworth A. *Evaluations and Improvements in Small Area Estimation Methodologies*. National Centre for Research Methods Methodological Review Paper. Southampton: National Centre for Research Methods (2013).

14

Prospects for the Use of New Technologies to Combat Multidrug-Resistant Bacteria

Renata Lima¹*, Fernando Sá Del Fiol² and Victor M. Balcão ³,⁴

¹ LABiToN—Laboratory of Bioactivity Assessment and Toxicology of Nanomaterials, University of Sorocaba, Sorocaba, Brazil, ² CRIA—Antibiotic Reference and Information Center, University of Sorocaba, Sorocaba, Brazil, ³ PhageLab—Laboratory of Biofilms and Bacteriophages, i(bs)²—intelligent biosensing and biomolecule stabilization research group, University of Sorocaba, Sorocaba, Brazil, ⁴ Department of Biology and CESAM, University of Aveiro, Campus Universitário de Santiago, Aveiro, Portugal

*Corespondence
Renata de Lima
renata.lima@prof.uniso.br

The increasing use of antibiotics is being driven by factors such as the aging of the population, increased occurrence of infections, and greater prevalence of chronic diseases that require antimicrobial treatment. The excessive and unnecessary use of antibiotics in humans has led to the emergence of bacteria resistant to the antibiotics currently available, as well as to the selective development of other microorganisms, hence contributing to the widespread dissemination of resistance genes at the environmental level. Due to this, attempts are being made to develop new techniques to combat resistant bacteria, among them the use of strictly lytic bacteriophage particles, CRISPR–Cas, and nanotechnology. The use of these technologies, alone or in combination, is promising for solving a problem that humanity faces today and that could lead to human extinction: the domination of pathogenic bacteria resistant to artificial drugs. This prospective paper discusses the potential of bacteriophage particles, CRISPR–Cas, and nanotechnology for use in combating human (bacterial) infections.

Keywords: multidrug-resistant bacteria, bacteriophage particles, phage therapy, CRISPR–Cas, nanotechnology

BACTERIAL RESISTANCE

Since their discovery in 1929, antibiotics have been widely used in human and veterinary medicine, either for treatments or in attempts to prevent bacterial infections. The excessive use of antibiotics, whether for prevention or treatment, has significantly increased the level of bacterial resistance worldwide (Ali et al., 2018). The associated numbers of human deaths are alarming, reaching 50,000 per year in the United States and Europe (Simlai et al., 2016), with an estimated 10 million deaths per year by 2050, surpassing the current deaths resulting from all types of cancer (approximately 8.2 million) (Jansen et al., 2018).

The first list of antibiotic-resistant pathogens was published by the World Health Organization (WHO) in 2017. This list showed that out of the 12 resistant pathogens, seven were noted to be resistant to beta-lactam antibiotics. Consequently, there is renewed focus on the production of new antibiotics, establishing a goal for future research strategies (WHO, 2017).

The overuse and misuse of antibiotics in humans have led to the selective emergence of bacteria resistant to the currently available antibiotics, as well as resistant non-pathogenic microbiota, hence leading to the generalized dissemination of resistance genes at the environmental level (Nitsch-Osuch et al., 2016). There is greatest concern when this phenomenon occurs with *Enterococcus* spp., *Staphylococcus aureus*, *Klebsiella pneumoniae*, *Acinetobacter baumannii*, *Pseudomonas aeruginosa*, and *Enterobacter* spp., together given the acronym ESKAPE, which highlights the ability of these microorganisms to escape the action of antimicrobial agents (Boucher et al., 2009).

Antimicrobial resistance has become globalized, following the first reports of its appearance in India, with its subsequent spread to Pakistan, the United States, Canada, Japan, and the United Kingdom (Rios et al., 2016). This resistance can occur in different ways, depending on the acquired and selective genetic changes or insertion of external genes, which leads to previously non-existent responses. Several mechanisms of resistance have emerged in recent times, including alteration of the target (by a DNA gyrase), increased efflux (export of a drug out of the microorganism), inactivation of fluoroquinolones (by an aminoglycoside N-acetyltransferase), inhibition of the 30S ribosomal subunit (by aminoglycosides), and protection of the target by DNA-binding proteins (the Qnr family) (Redgrave et al., 2014; Munita and Arias, 2016; Kapoor et al., 2017).

Some of these changes are already well known, such as alteration of the chemical structure of antimicrobial agents (Alekshun and Levy, 2007), decrease of the concentration of the antimicrobial at its site of action (Gonzalez-Bello, 2017; Willers et al., 2017), changes in the target of antimicrobial action (Sieradzki and Markiewicz, 2004), and alteration of membrane permeability (Hao et al., 2018). There are mechanisms of permeability reduction that do not involve porin expression, such as changes in the cell envelope of *P. aeruginosa* that are associated with resistance to polymyxin B (Falagas and Kasiakou, 2005). In addition to antibiotics that act on the cell wall, such as penicillins and glycopeptides, the activities of other antimicrobials that act on the bacterial ribosome may also decrease due to changes in their primary target. This phenomenon mainly affects macrolides and tetracyclines (Poehlsgaard and Douthwaite, 2005; Wu et al., 2005).

The presence of these mechanisms of resistance is increasingly common in large numbers of microorganisms, due to the selective pressure exerted by antimicrobials, leading to a natural selection that results in the dominance of certain groups of resistant bacteria, with concomitant death of sensitive microorganisms (Tello et al., 2012).

In a meta-analysis carried out by Bell et al. (2014), in which 243 studies were evaluated, it was concluded that "Increased consumption of antibiotics may not only produce greater resistance at the individual patient level but may also produce greater resistance at the community, country, and regional levels, which can harm individual patients." Another study of the same year evaluated the consumption of antibiotics worldwide between 2000 and 2010. It was found that the consumption of antibiotics increased by around 36%, with the countries of the BRICS group (Brazil, Russia, India, China, and South Africa) accounting for approximately 76% of the increase (Van Boeckel et al., 2014).

Therefore, the data reflect a worrying trend regarding the treatment of infectious diseases, since not only are these drugs being increasingly used (Van Boeckel et al., 2014), but also their use is directly proportional to the increase in resistance indicators (Bell et al., 2014). In the absence of any significant discovery

of new molecules for the control of resistant microorganisms (Hogberg et al., 2010), there is an urgent need for redefining the relationship of humans with infectious diseases.

In summary, the problem faced in relation to bacterial resistance is a concern that must be urgently addressed, since functional meta-genomic studies of soil microorganisms have revealed a wide range of genetic determinants that confer resistance to antibiotics, of which only one fraction has been described in human pathogens (Forsberg et al., 2014).

Hence, there is a pressing need for a new generation of antimicrobials able to mitigate the spread of antibiotic resistance and preserve beneficial microbiota. Among the possibilities for the solution of problems related to bacterial resistance, the use of nanotechnology, CRISPR–Cas9, and therapy with bacteriophage particles can be highlighted as potential future strategies. These techniques could be employed individually to directly combat microorganisms, as well as in combination in integrated strategies.

The scientific community has indicated that there are no perspectives for any significant clinical introduction of new antimicrobials in the short term. The main recommended approach is rational use of the classical antibiotics that have been used for the past 50 years, together with techniques that enhance their activity. This may be achieved using substances that increase antibiotic activity by reducing or blocking the resistance mechanism, such as beta-lactamase, efflux pump, and quorum sensing inhibitors, as well as bacteriophages and new drug delivery systems, among other techniques (Moo et al., 2019; Mulani et al., 2019; Pham et al., 2019; Vikesland et al., 2019).

CRISPRs

CRISPRs (clustered regularly interspaced short palindromic repeats) are adaptive immune systems derived from bacteria and archaea. CRISPR–Cas systems use RNA for target DNA recognition and the Cas enzyme for subsequent destruction of nucleic acids, so they require only one protein for binding and cleavage. Due to this simplicity, researchers have developed a new molecular tool based on natural CRISPRs (**Figure 1**). This tool has different applications, one of them being the possibility of antimicrobial action, since they are cytotoxic systems that can be directed to kill bacteria, immunizing them against resistant plasmids (Sorek et al., 2013; Bikard et al., 2014; Hsu et al., 2014).

For medical purposes, CRISPR–Cas systems can enable the selective and specific removal of microorganisms. Although there are other antimicrobial approaches, they offer only partial solutions, while CRISPR systems are generalized and programmable strategies (Gomaa et al., 2014) that can be employed to selectively and quantitatively remove individual bacterial strains, based purely on sequence information, hence creating opportunities in the treatment of multidrug-resistant infections.

In studies of the use of these systems as antimicrobials, Gomaa et al. (2014) reported that both heterologous and endogenous systems could selectively kill bacterial species and strains. It was shown that all sequences in the target

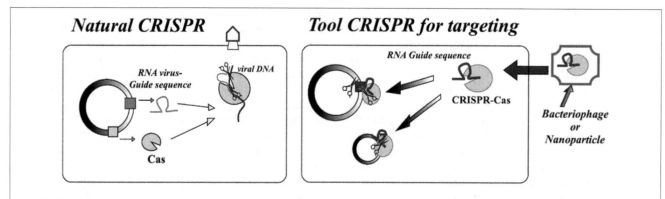

FIGURE 1 | Schematic drawing showing the natural CRISPR–Cas complex found in bacteria, which functions as an "immune system" against viruses, and the CRISPR–Cas tool used as an agent, based on the complex naturally present in bacteria.

genome led to cell death, suggesting that, theoretically, any genomic location could be a distinct target for antimicrobials based on CRISPRs. Another possibility would be the use of this technology for antimicrobial action using RNA-guided nucleases (RGNs), targeting specific resistance genes or undesirable polymorphisms, allowing programmable remodeling of the microbiota (Citorik et al., 2014).

In a study carried out by Fuente-Núñez and Lu (2017) concerning CRISPR–Cas constructs designed to function as precision antimicrobials, these were shown to be capable of eliminating drug-resistant microbes, with CRISPR–Cas selectively targeting genes involved in antibiotic resistance, biofilm formation, and virulence. However, although studies show that CRISPRs are effective, there are still problems to be overcome in relation to an efficient delivery vehicle, which is the next step for the implementation of CRISPR–Cas systems as antimicrobial agents (Beisel et al., 2014). Focusing on the problem of CRISPR transportation and delivery, Pan et al. (2017) were able to identify eight depolymerases in the multi-host bacteriophage K64-1, which, together with K64dep (S2-5), characterized elsewhere, gave a total of nine capsule depolymerases.

Currently, obtaining bacteriophages as carriers of CRISPRs is still a challenge. Shen et al. (2018) succeeded in obtaining positive results in studies aimed at obtaining a *Klebsiella* bacteriophage by genome alteration, which was suggested as a possibility for the use of targeted CRISPRs. One option is to use nanotechnology for the delivery of CRISPRs, which could provide surface modifications that ensure the desired specificity (Yan et al., 2015). As pointed out by Pursey et al., (2018), there is still a great deal to discover concerning the use of CRISPR–Cas in the fight against resistant bacteria, with further research especially needed in relation to its safe use.

Another concern is the possibility that bacteria could present resistance against CRISPR–Cas, since the original mechanisms are present in them. However, in a study by Chen et al. (2019), performed with multidrug-resistant *Shigella*, it was shown that the bacteria that presented resistance genes also presented a decrease in the activity of natural CRISPR–Cas.

If we consider the different possibilities of target genes for CRISPR–Cas, we can conclude that there is a need for

an interdisciplinary study, where there is collaboration of researchers who study sequences, find a safe way of delivery, and evaluate the existence of resistance to technology. Different studies show that bacteria tend to store different genes, and different combinations between virulence and resistance are an alarming threat, as it suggests the feasibility of adaptability. A study carried out by Oliveira Santos et al. (2018), where they showed the possible adaptability of the KPC-2 gene to different mobile elements, is an example of the need to consider different possibilities for the application of CRISPR–Cas. Regarding the onset of carbapenem-resistant *K. pneumoniae*, recent publication showed the introduction of two new DNA editing systems. One is the plasmid pCasKP-pSGKP and the other is the plasmid system pBECKP, where both systems showed efficiency in genome editing, which will facilitate further investigations for treatment of resistance to carbapenems (Wang et al., 2018).

Although the CRISPR–Cas tool offers a new possibility of fighting multidrug bacteria, some studies show that they do not present activity in some strains, as demonstrated by Hullahalli et al. (2017, 2018) in studies with *Enterococcus faecalis* where they present a study that determines the genetic basis of phenotypes associated with CRISPR–Cas tolerance, showing the importance of having a better knowledge of the response of organisms and possible strategies for dealing with conflicts induced by the use of CRISPRS, which may lead to tolerant phenotypes to this tool. Therefore, these studies show that knowledge of the genome and the metabolic pathways of the different resistant multidrug bacteria should be investigated so that resistance problems will not occur in the future in relation to new strategies used to fight resistant bacteria.

NANOTECHNOLOGY IN THE FIGHT AGAINST RESISTANT BACTERIA

Nanotechnology applied to the synthesis of new antibiotics is an important approach, since the use of nanometric size materials can result in greater contact between the compound and the bacteria, with improved bioavailability, increased absorption, faster passage of the drug into the cell, and enhanced mucoadhesion.

There is also the possibility of producing controlled release systems for the targeted delivery of encapsulated or surface adsorbed drugs (Zaidi et al., 2017; Jamil and Imran, 2018). One new approach is to use nanoparticles (NPs) of a metal such as silver, which can affect the bacterial respiration system, inducing the generation of reactive oxygen species (ROS). This approach could be used synergistically with antimicrobials, with effects such as inhibition and alteration of the synthesis of the cell wall, as well as its rupture (Shahverdi et al., 2007; Kumar et al., 2018).

One of the concerns regarding the use of nanoparticles is in relation to the resistance that bacteria can present to them, or the possibility of stimulating the transmission of MultiDrug-Resistant (MDR) genes. An example is provided by the work of Ansari et al. (2014), where Al_2O_3 nanoparticles were observed to promote the horizontal conjugative transfer of MDR genes, hence increasing the resistance to antibiotics.

The use of NPs to eliminate microorganisms can involve microbicidal or microbiostatic effects. In the latter case, the growth of bacteria is interrupted and the metabolic activities are halted, with microbial death then induced by the immune cells of the host. Nanotechnology can also solve problems related to drug solubility, since encapsulation can improve permeation through the membrane, increase circulation times, and enhance efficiency, while there is also the possibility of directing the drug towards the desired site of action in the body (Rodzinski et al., 2016).

The use of nanoparticles appears to have potential for the treatment of infectious diseases, especially considering that NPs may be able to access locations where the pathogens are present. However, there are a number of issues to be resolved, such as the scarcity of toxicity data, few existing preclinical studies, and the need for regulation (Zaidi et al., 2017).

Shaaban et al. (2017) reported that nanoantibiotics produced by incorporating imipenem in PLGA or PCL nanocapsules provided better results, than did classical imipenem. The nanoencapsulated formulations showed antimicrobial and anti-adherent activities in evaluations using clinical isolates of imipenem-resistant bacteria.

Other types of nanoparticles that have received attention are lipid nanoparticles (liposomes) (Derbali et al., 2019) and nanoceramics applied in orthopedic surgeries where systemic drug administration has limitations (Kumar and Madhumathi, 2016).

Gaspar et al. (2017) reported the use of solid lipid nanoparticles containing rifabutin (RFB) for pulmonary administration to treat tuberculosis. The nanoparticles increased the activity of the drug against *M. tuberculosis* infection, suggesting that RFB-solid lipid nanoparticles (SLN) encapsulation could be a promising approach for tuberculosis treatment. A major advantage of encapsulation is that it provides sustained release of the drug, resulting in greater efficiency of treatment, as well as easier absorption, enabling satisfactory results to be achieved with a smaller amount of the active agent.

Although the use of nanoparticles can be advantageous, some studies have shown that the microenvironment where they are released (such as blood and lung fluid) may alter the creation of the nanoparticle–pathogen complex, due to the formation of a corona around the nanoparticle. Siemer et al. (2019) exposed nanoparticles to different bacteria and showed that formation of the pathogen–nanoparticle complex was assisted by its small size and that the presence of a corona significantly inhibited formation of the complex. Therefore, in addition to *in vitro* analyses, new studies are needed that consider the microenvironment in which the nanoparticle will be released and exert its action.

Polymeric Nanoparticles and Nanocrystals

The use of polymeric nanocapsules as carriers for antibiotics, or the use of drug nanocrystals that are stable during delivery, can be successfully applied to a range of commonly used drugs. Polylactide-*co*-glycolide (PLGA) is an especially useful substance that can be employed in nanotechnological drug delivery applications (Kalhapure et al., 2014; Hemeg, 2017; Boya et al., 2017; Shaaban et al., 2017).

Hong et al. (2017) used bacitracin A (BA) modified with PLGA for synthesis of nano-BA, resulting in a core–shell structure with an average diameter of 150 nm. It was found that the nanoparticles strongly increased the antibacterial activity, than does free BA, with effective inhibition of the growth of various types of Gram (+) and Gram (–) bacteria. The formulation provided improved wound healing in rats than did use of a commercial Polysporin® ointment.

Yu et al. (2016) reported the development of a multifunctional release system with encapsulation of gentamicin sulfate/zirconium bis(monohydrogen orthophosphate) (α-ZrP) using chitosan (CHI). The formulation (α-ZrP CHI) extended the release of the drug, than did unencapsulated α-ZrP, which was attributed to the unique lamellar structure and the CHI encapsulation. The methodology provided a model for the future development of new delivery vehicles.

Metallic Nanoparticles

The use of metallic nanoparticles can be a good option in the fight against resistant bacteria. Studies have reported the synthesis and use of different nanoparticulate metals, metal oxides, metal halides, and bimetallic materials showing antimicrobial activity. Nanoparticles have been synthesized consisting of Ag, Au, Zn, Cu, Ti, and Mg, among other metals (Zakharova et al., 2015; Hajipour et al., 2012; Sunitha et al., 2013; Dizaj et al., 2014; He et al., 2016; Senarathna et al., 2017; Eymard-Vernain et al., 2018). However, consideration should be given to their potential toxicity (Lima et al., 2012; Dakal et al., 2016; Durán et al., 2016a).

Eymard-Vernain et al. (2018) showed that MgO nanoparticles presented bactericidal action, mainly affecting the expression of genes related to oxidative stress, together with membrane alteration. Verma et al. (2018) reported excellent antibacterial activity of ZnO nanoparticles, with a size-dependent effect, since the use of smaller nanoparticles resulted in more ROS and increased cell membrane rupture.

Other studies have investigated the bactericidal potential of carbon nanotubes, either plain or functionalized, as well as their use to assist the transport and translocation of antibiotics (Cong et al., 2016; Mocan et al., 2017).

With the development of nanotechnology, many studies have been carried out concerning the application of nanoparticles as antimicrobials. These nanomaterials present different diameters, structures, and modes of action. Some of them have produced good results, showing that nanotechnology can be used as one of the strategies in the fight against multidrug-resistant bacteria in the future (**Supplementary Table 1**).

Silver nanoparticles are the most studied metallic nanoparticles, with their antimicrobial activity having been recognized by the United States Food and Drug Administration (FDA) since the year 1920. The mechanisms of action of silver nanoparticles (AgNP) on bacteria have been exhaustively investigated. There is a consensus that adhesion of the nanoparticles to the cell membrane can lead to electrostatic changes, porosity alteration, rupture, leakage of cytoplasmic content, interference in bacterial respiratory processes, blocking of enzyme activity, and DNA destruction. It has also been observed that there is the production of ROS, with consequent effects on the DNA (Choi and Hu, 2008; Durán et al., 2010; Prabhu and Poulose, 2012; Rai et al., 2012; Kon and Rai, 2013; Yuan et al., 2017).

The adhesion of nanoparticles to bacterial membranes mainly occurs due to the presence of proteoglycans (Kim et al., 2017) and results in rupture or increased porosity of the membrane. This enables access of the nanoparticles into the cell, where they can interact with enzymes and DNA (Grigor'eva et al., 2013; Kasithevar et al., 2017). AgNPs may also interact with membrane proteins, leading to cell stress, or may interact with the lipid part of the membrane, affecting its fluidity (Morones et al., 2005; Chwalibog et al., 2010). Some studies have suggested that the observed effects are actually caused by silver ions released from AgNPs (Jung et al., 2008; Xiu et al., 2011; Xiu et al., 2012; Chernousova and Epple, 2013). Accordingly, the AgNPs only act as vehicles for the delivery of ions that cause adverse effects in the respiratory chain and protein synthesis, as well as DNA alterations (Chen et al., 2011; Li et al., 2014).

The biogenic synthesis of silver nanoparticles (**Figure 2**) has received increasing attention in recent years. These nanoparticles present positive characteristics in terms of their improved stability and dispersion, due to the coating formed during the synthesis. In addition, there may be a positive effect of synergy between the nanoparticles and the compounds originating from the organism used. Biogenic synthesis is considered simple, low cost, and suitable for large-scale nanoparticle production (Lima et al., 2012; Kasithevar et al., 2017).

Biogenic nanoparticles have been found to present lower toxicity, while providing effective bactericidal activity against both Gram (−) and Gram (+) bacteria (Durán et al., 2016b; Kasithevar et al., 2017). These nanoparticles have also shown potential for use in the control of fungi (Balashanmugam and Kalaichelvan, 2015; Ahmad et al., 2016; Guilger et al., 2017).

Nanocages

Nanocages are hollow and porous nanometric structures that may be used for the transport and delivery of antibiotics. They can be synthesized from various substances, including metals, proteins, and polymers, and have been investigated in terms of their potential for combating multidrug-resistant bacteria. Reported advantages of these structures are that they provide greater adhesion, retention at the site of infection, increased systemic circulation, and good biocompatibility (Wang et al., 2016; Mekeer et al., 2018).

Wang et al. (2018) synthesized gold nanocages using membrane coating of macrophages pretreated with *S. aureus*. Clinical treatments performed with local or systemic injection showed that the system provided increased bactericidal effectiveness. Ruozi et al. (2017) synthesized apoferritin-based nanocages, which were used for the encapsulation of streptomycin. The system showed promise for the delivery of antimicrobials, although further characterization, biocompatibility, and efficacy studies were still required. A study by Wu et al. (2019), using silica, silver, and gold nanospheres, showed that the Au–Ag@SiO$_2$ nanocage had broad-spectrum bactericidal properties. The nanocage could be used for antibiotic transport, as well as for infrared-induced hyperthermia therapy against bacterial infection.

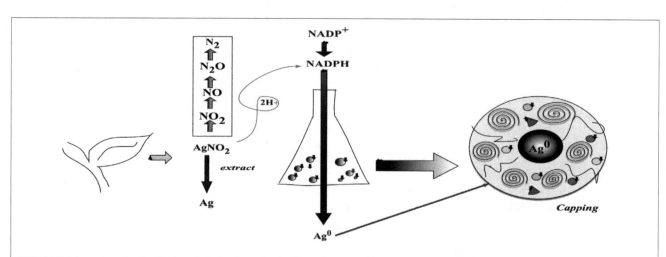

FIGURE 2 | Scheme, based on the literature, illustrating the synthesis of biogenic nanoparticles. The synthesis uses AgNO$_3$ together with extract (or metabolites) and enzymes from the organism. These nanoparticles have a characteristic outer layer (coating) containing metabolites.

BACTERIOPHAGES

Bacteriophages (or phages, for short), which are viruses that only infect bacterial cells, are among the most ubiquitous biological entities, with a total estimated abundance of at least 1,030 types (Chibani-Chennoufi et al., 2004). Despite being known for more than 100 years, only now is renewed interest in phages driving studies of them as potential alternatives or complements to current antibiotics, due to their unique affinities and ability to kill bacteria resistant to antibiotics (Hagens and Loessner, 2010; Hyman and Abedon, 2010; Summers, 2012). The interaction between phage particles and bacteria generally involves specific receptors located in the outer membranes of bacteria. Despite the great potential of phages for treating and/or controlling infections caused by antibiotic-resistant bacteria, only a few clinical trials have been performed in humans and are accepted by public health authorities such as the FDA and the European Medicines Agency (EMA) (Rios et al., 2016).

Phages are ubiquitous in the biosphere and are highly specific to particular bacteria species, acting as natural predators of bacteria. They exhibit high tissue permeability and do not affect the beneficial intestinal microflora (so they do not promote secondary infections). Their exponential growth results in their accumulation in extremely high concentrations where they are needed the most, as long as the bacterial host still exists (Hagens and Loessner, 2010; Wittebole et al., 2013; Rios et al., 2016; Harada et al., 2018). However, phage-based therapy requires that the bacterium responsible for the infection is firstly isolated, before the identification and isolation of a specific and strictly lytic phage can be achieved. In addition, due to their protein nature, plain phage particles may be recognized by the immune system, resulting in a drastic reduction of their therapeutic efficacy (Chan and Abedon, 2012; Wittebole et al., 2013).

Bacterial resistance to phage particles generally occurs due to non-adsorption, membrane coating due to mucilage production by bacteria, and destruction of viral genetic material by restriction endonucleases (Wittebole et al., 2013).

Following oral or intravenous administration, phage particles may affect the major body systems, namely, the cardiovascular, digestive, immune, and nervous systems (Moutinho et al., 2012). Furthermore, due to their protein nature, phage particles are prone to denaturation by conformational changes that may be either reversible or irreversible, or to destruction by the immune system. The solution lies in protecting them, either by encapsulation within nanocarriers (Rios et al., 2018) that are invisible towards the digestive and immune systems, or by binding them to a macroscopic support so that they become insoluble (Balcão et al., 2013; Balcão et al., 2014). The combination of these strategies can provide phages with structural and functional stabilization (Balcão and Vila, 2015), enabling them to be potentially used for the eradication of antibiotic-resistant bacteria.

Several studies have described phage-based CRISPR-driven techniques for the prevention of bacterial drug resistance (Barrangou, 2015; Bikard and Barrangou, 2017; Doss et al., 2017; Hatoum-Aslan, 2018; Pursey et al., 2018). In this approach, bacteriophages are designed to carry and deliver CRISPR–Cas in bacteria, in order to combat multidrug-resistant bacteria. Such systems are being developed by biotechnology companies such as Locus Biosciences (Morrisville, NC, USA) and Eligo Bioscience (Paris, France) (Reardon, 2017).

Recent biotechnological advances therefore open the door to the possibility of tailoring bacteriophage particles to improve their characteristics, including i) enhancing the ability of phages to penetrate bacterial biofilms; ii) increasing phage efficacy; iii) broadening the spectrum of phage lytic activities to infections caused by different bacteria; and iv) making phages more stable and specific (Maura and Debarbieux, 2011; Rios et al., 2016; Harada et al., 2018).

At the present time, due to the increase in bacterial resistance to antibiotics, together with the likely ineffectiveness of antibiotics within a few years, there is an urgent need to develop new antimicrobial strategies. This is a new era, in which the emergence of new solutions and discoveries will be crucial.

FUTURE TRENDS AND POSSIBLE SOLUTIONS

The use of new technologies to combat multidrug-resistant bacteria is ever more necessary, because although there are still effective antibiotics, resistance to them is constantly increasing. The strategies discussed in this paper may provide new ways of fighting multidrug-resistant bacteria. This could include associations between different strategies, as well as their use in combination with antibiotics, in order to combat this critical emerging problem (**Figure 3**).

The use of CRISPRs, a relatively new technology, may be one of the available solutions. Coupled with nanotechnological delivery methods, this technique could be sufficiently specific and provide the activity required to combat multidrug-resistant bacteria. For this, nanocapsules could be synthesized that are able to reach specific targets, which would facilitate the delivery of CRISPRs.

Biogenic metal nanoparticles, such as silver nanoparticles, may be an option in conjugated treatments to combat MDR bacteria. These nanoparticles offer the benefits of synergy between the effects of the metal and the metabolites of the organism used for their production. They present low toxicity and can act to disrupt existing mechanisms of resistance in bacteria.

Bacteriophages can be used successfully to fight multidrug-resistant bacteria, but although it is not difficult to find the correct virus for each specific bacterium host, the task is nevertheless not straightforward. Consequently, the use of bacteriophage particles as carriers for CRISPRs seems to be a faster and more efficient solution, although such delivery may not always be guaranteed. Recent studies show that CRISPR technology can assist in the modification of bacteriophages, making them more specific for the intended purpose.

To conclude, a deeper understanding of these new and innovative therapeutic strategies is of utmost importance. Until such new strategies have been mastered, structured, and made commercially available, it is imperative to control the use of the currently available chemical antibiotics. It is also essential that

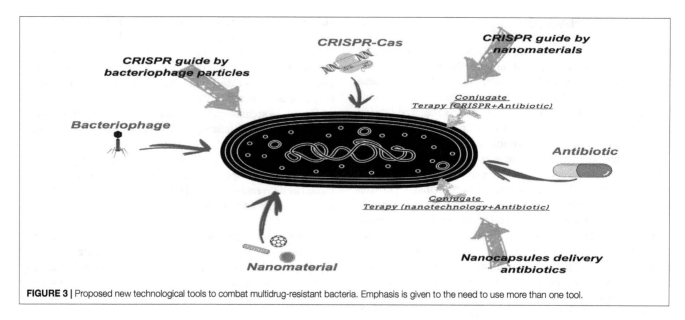

FIGURE 3 | Proposed new technological tools to combat multidrug-resistant bacteria. Emphasis is given to the need to use more than one tool.

health professionals use wisely, and only as a last resort, new antibiotics that may become available in the near future, in order to prevent the emergence and spread of bacterial resistance to them.

AUTHOR CONTRIBUTIONS

All authors participated in writing the manuscript, specifically RL with the themes nanotechnology and CRISPRs, FF with multidrug resistance, and VB with bacteriophage technology.

FUNDING

The funding for this work was provided by the São Paulo State Research Foundation [FAPESP, grants #2016/08884-3 (PneumoPhageColor project), #2016/12234-4 (TransAppIL project), #2018/05522-9 (PsaPhageKill project, BPE fellowship granted to VB), and #2017/13328-5 (Biogenic Metal Nanoparticles project)]. Support was provided by the National Council for Scientific and Technological Development (CNPq), in the form of Research Productivity (PQ) fellowships awarded to VB (grants #306113/2014-7 and #308208/2017-0) and RL (grant #303967/2015-3). Funding support was also provided by CESAM (UID/AMB/50017/2019) and FCT/MCTES.

ACKNOWLEDGMENTS

The authors are grateful to Universidade of Sorocaba/UNISO for supporting the publication charges.

REFERENCES

Ahmad, A., Wei, Y., Syed, F., Tahir, K., Taj, R., Khan, A. U., et al. (2016). Amphotericin B-conjugated biogenic silver nanoparticles as an innovative strategy for fungal infections. *Microb. Pathog.* 99, 271–281. doi: 10.1016/j.micpath.2016.08.031

Alekshun, M. N., and Levy, S. B. (2007). Molecular mechanisms of antibacterial multidrug resistance. *Cell* 128 (6), 1037–1050. doi: 10.1016/j.cell.2007.03.004

Ali, J., Rafiq, Q. A., and Ratcliffe, E. (2018). Antimicrobial resistance mechanisms and potential synthetic treatments. *Future Sci. OA.* 4 (4), Fso290. doi: 10.4155/fsoa-2017-0109

Ansari, M. A., Khan, H. M., Khan, A. A., Cameotra, S. S., Saquib, Q., and Musarrat, J. (2014). Interaction of Al2O3 nanoparticles with Escherichia coli and their cell envelope biomolecules. *J. Appl. Microbiol.* 116 (4), 772–783. doi: 10.1111/jam.12423

Azam, A., Ahmed, A. S., Oves, M., Khan, M. S., Habib, S. S., and Memic, A. (2012). Antimicrobial activity of metal oxide nanoparticles against gram-positive and gram-negative bacteria: a comparative study. *Int. J. Nanomedicine* 7, 6003–6009. doi: 10.2147/IJN.S35347

Balashanmugam, P., and Kalaichelvan, P. T. (2015). Biosynthesis characterization of silver nanoparticles using Cassia roxburghii DC aqueous extract, and coated on cotton cloth for effective antibacterial activity. *Int. J. Nanomedicine* 10 (1), 87–97. doi: 10.2147/IJN.S79984

Balcão, V. M., Barreira, S. V. P., Nunes, T. M., Chaud, M. V., Tubino, M., and Vila, M. M. D. C. (2014). Carbohydrate hydrogels with stabilized phage particles for bacterial biosensing: bacterium diffusion studies. *Appl. Biochem. Biotechnol.* 172, 1194–1214. doi: 10.1007/s12010-013-0579-2

Balcão, V. M., Moreira, A. R., Moutinho, C. G., Chaud, M. V., Tubino, M., and Vila, M. M. (2013). Structural and functional stabilization of phage particles in carbohydrate matrices for bacterial biosensing. *Enzyme Microb. Technol.* 53, 55–69. doi: 10.1016/j.enzmictec.2013.03.001

Balcão, V. M., and Vila, M. M. D. C. (2015). Structural and functional stabilization of protein entities: state-of-the-art. *Adv. Drug Deliv. Rev.* 93, 25–41. doi: 10.1016/j.addr.2014.10.005

Barrangou, R. (2015). The roles of CRISPR–Cas systems in adaptive immunity and beyond. *Curr. Opin. Immunol.* 32, 36–41. doi: 10.1016/j.coi.2014.12.008

Beisel, C. L., Gomaa, A. A., Barrangou, R. (2014). A CRISPR design for next-generation antimicrobials. *Genome Biol.* 15, 516. doi: 10.1186/s13059-014-0516-x

Bell, B. G., Schellevis, F., Stobberingh, E., Goossens, H., and Pringle, M. (2014). A systematic review and meta-analysis of the effects of antibiotic consumption on antibiotic resistance. *Bioorg. Med. Chem. Lett.* 14, 13. doi: 10.1186/1471-2334-14-13

Bikard, D., and Barrangou, R. (2017). Using CRISPR–Cas systems as antimicrobials. *Curr. Opin. Microbiol.* 37, 155–160. doi: 10.1016/j.mib.2017.08.005

Bikard, D., Euler, C. W., Jiang, W., Nussenzweig, P. M., Goldberg, G. W., Duportet, X., et al. (2014). Exploiting CRISPR–Cas nucleases to produce sequence-specific antimicrobials. *Nat. Biotechnol.* 32 (11), 1146–1150. doi: 10.1038/nbt.3043

Boucher, H. W., Talbot, G. H., Bradley, J. S., Edwards, J. E., Gilbert, D., Rice, L. B., et al. (2009). Bad bugs, no drugs: no ESKAPE! an update from the Infectious diseases society of America. Clinical infectious diseases: an official publication of the Infectious. *Dis. Soc. Am.* 48 (1), 1–12. doi: 10.1086/595011

Boya, V. N., Lovett, R., Setua, S., Gandhi, V., Nagesh, P. K. B., Khan, S., et al. (2017). Probin mucin interaction behavior of magnetic nanoparticles. *J. Coll. Inter. Sci.* 488, 258–268.

Brunet, L., Lyon, D. Y., Hotze, E. M., Alvarez, P. J., Wiesner, M. R. (2009). Comparative photoactivity and antibacterial properties of C60 fullerenes and titanium dioxide nanoparticles. *Environ. Sci. Technol.* 43 (12), 4355–4360. doi: 10.1021/es803093t

Chan, B. K., and Abedon, S. T. (2012). "Phage therapy pharmacology phage cocktails," in *Advances in applied microbiology*, vol. 78. Eds. Laskin, A. I., Sariaslani, S., Gadd, G. M. (San Diego: Elsevier Academic Press Inc.), 1–23. doi: 10.1016/B978-0-12-394805-2.00001-4

Chen, M., Yang, Z., Wu, H., Pan, X., Xie, X., Wu, C. (2011). Antimicrobial activity and the mechanism of silver nanoparticle thermosensitive gel. *Int. J. Nanomedicine.* 6, 2873–2877. doi: 10.2147/IJN.S23945

Chen, S., Liu, H., Liang, W., Hong, L., Zhang, B., Huang, L., et al. (2019). Insertion sequences in the CRISPR–Cas system regulate horizontal antimicrobial resistance gene transfer in. shigella strains. *Int. J. Antimicrob. Agents* 53 (2), 109–115. doi: 10.1016/j.ijantimicag.2018.09.020

Chernousova, S., and Epple, M. (2013). Silver as antibacterial agent: ion, nanoparticle, and metal. *Angew. Chem. Int. Ed. Engl.* 52 (6), 1636–1653. doi: 10.1002/anie.201205923

Chibani-Chennoufi, S., Bruttin, A., Dillmann, M.-L., and Brüssow, H. (2004). Phage–host interaction: an ecological perspective. *J. Bacteriol.* 186 (12), 3677–3686. doi: 10.1128/JB.186.12.3677-3686.2004

Choi, O., and Hu, Z. (2008). Size dependent and reactive oxygen species related nanosilver toxicity to nitrifying bacteria. *Environ. Sci. Technol.* 42 (12), 4583–4588. doi: 10.1021/es703238h

Chwalibog, A., Sawosz, E., Hotowy, A., Szeliga, J., Mitura, S., Mitura, K., et al. (2010). Visualization of interaction between inorganic nanoparticles and bacteria or fungi. *Int. J. Nanomedicine.* 5, 1085–1094. doi: 10.2147/IJN.S13532

Citorik, R. J., Mimee, M., and Lu, T. K. (2014). Sequence-specific antimicrobials using efficiently delivered RNA-guided nucleases. *Nat. Biotechnol.* 32 (11), 1141–1145. doi: 10.1038/nbt.3011

Cong, S., Cao, Y., Fang, X., Wang, Y., Liu, Q., Gui, H., et al. (2016). Carbon nanotube macroelectronics for active matrix polymer-dispersed liquid crystal displays. *ACS Nano.* 10 (11), 10068–10074. doi: 10.1021/acsnano.6b04951

Dakal, T. C., Kumar, A., Majumdar, R. S., and Yadav, V. (2016). Mechanistic basis of antimicrobial actions of silver nanoparticles. *Front. Microbiol.* 7, 1831. doi: 10.3389/fmicb.2016.01831

Derbali, R. M., Aoun, V., Moussa, G., Frei, G., Tehrani, S. F., Del'Orto, J. C., et al. (2019). Tailored nanocarriers for the pulmonary delivery of levofloxacin against Pseudomonas aeruginosa: a comparative study. *Mol. Pharm.* 16 (5), 1906–1916. doi: 10.1021/acs.molpharmaceut.8b01256

Dizaj, S. M., Lotfipour, F., Barzegar-Jalali, M., Zarrintan, M. H., and Adibkia, K. (2014). Antimicrobial activity of the metals and metal oxide nanoparticles, mater. *Sci. Eng. C: Mater. Biol. Appl.* 44, 278–284. doi: 10.1016/j.msec.2014.08.031

Doss, J., Culbertson, K., Hahn, D., Camacho, J., and Barekzi, N. (2017). A review of phage therapy against bacterial pathogens of aquatic and terrestrial organisms. *Viruses* 9, 50. doi: 10.3390/v9030050

Durán, N., Durán, M., de Jesus, M. B., Seabra, A. B., Fávaro, W. J., and Nakazato, G. (2016a). Silver nanoparticles: a new view on mechanistic aspects on antimicrobial activity. *Nanomedicine* 12 (3), 789–799. doi: 10.1016/j.nano.2015.11.016

Durán, N., Nakazato, G., and Seabra, A. B. (2016b). Antimicrobial activity of biogenic silver nanoparticles, and silver chloride nanoparticles: an overview and comments. *Appl. Microbiol. Biotechnol.* 100 (15), 6555–6570. doi: 10.1007/s00253-016-7657-7

Durán, N., Marcato, P. D., De Conti, R., Alves, O. L., Costa, F. T. M., and Brocchi, M. (2010). Potential use of silver nanoparticles on pathogenic bacteria, their toxicity and possible mechanisms of action. *J. Braz. Chem. Soc.* 21 (6), 949–959. doi: 10.1590/S0103-50532010000600002

Eymard-Vernain, E., Luche, S., Rabilloud, T., and Lelong, C. (2018). Impact of nanoparticles on the Bacillus subtilis (3610) competence. *Sci. Rep.* 8: 2978, Correction in: *Sci. Rep.* 2018 8, 6486. doi: 10.1038/s41598-018-21402-0

Falagas, M. E., and Kasiakou, S. K. (2005). Colistin: the revival of polymyxins for the management of multidrug-resistant gram-negative bacterial infections. Clinical infectious diseases: an official publication of the. *Infect. Dis. Soc. Am.* 40 (9), 1333–1341. doi: 10.1086/429323

Forsberg, K. J., Patel, S., Gibson, M. K., Lauber, C. L., Knight, R., Fierer, N., et al. (2014). Bacterial phylogeny structures soil resistomes across habitats. *Nature* 509, 612–616. doi: 10.1038/nature13377

Fuente-Núñez, C., and Lu, T. K. (2017). CRISPR–Cas9 technology: applications in genome engineering, development of sequence-specific antimicrobials, and future prospects. *Integr. Biol.* 9, 109–122. doi: 10.1039/c6ib00140h

Gaspar, D. P., Gaspar, M. M., Eleutério, C. V., Grenha, A., Blanco, M., Gonçalves, L. M. D., et al. (2017). Microencapsulated solid lipid nanoparticles as a hybrid platform for pulmonary antibiotic delivery. *Mol. Pharm.* 514 (9), 2977–2990. doi: 10.1021/acs.molpharmaceut.7b00169

Gomaa, A. A., Klumpe, H. E., Luo, M. L., Selle, K., Barrangou, R., and Beisel, C. L. (2014). Programmable removal of bacterial strains by use of genome-targeting CRISPR-Cas systems. *MBio.* 5 (1), e00928–00913. doi: 10.1128/mBio.00928-13

Gonzalez-Bello, C. (2017). Antibiotic adjuvants—a strategy to unlock bacterial resistance to antibiotics. *Bioorg. Med. Chem. Lett.* 27 (18), 4221–4228. doi: 10.1016/j.bmcl.2017.08.027

Grigor'eva, A., Saranina, I., Tikunova, N., Safonov, A., Timoshenko, N., Rebrov, A., et al. (2013). Fine mechanisms of the interaction of silver nanoparticles with the cells of Salmonella typhimurium and staphylococcus aureus. *Biometals* 26 (3), 479–488. doi: 10.1007/s10534-013-9633-3

Guilger, M., Pasquoto-Stigliani, T., Bilesky-José, N., Grillo, R., Abhilash, P. C., Fraceto, L. F., et al. (2017). Biogenic silver nanoparticles based on Trichoderma harzianum: synthesis, characterization, toxicity evaluation and biological activity. *Sci. Rep.* 7, 44421. doi: 10.1038/srep44421

Gurunathan, S., Han, J. W., Dayem, A. A., Eppakayala, V., and Kim, J. H. (2012). Oxidative stress-mediated antibacterial activity of graphene oxide and reduced graphene oxide in Pseudomonas aeruginosa. *Int. J. Nanomedicine* 7, 5901–5914. doi: 10.2147/IJN.S37397

Habash, M. B., Park, A. J., Vis, E. C., Harris, R. J., and Khursigara, C. M. (2014). Synergy of silver nanoparticles and aztreonam against Pseudomonas aeruginosa PAO1 biofilms. *Antimicrob. Agents Chemother.* 58 (10), 5818–5830. doi: 10.1128/AAC.03170-14

Hagens, S., and Loessner, M. J. (2010). Bacteriophage for biocontrol of foodborne pathogens: calculations and considerations. *Curr. Pharm. Biotechnol.* 11 (1), 58–68. doi: 10.2174/138920110790725429

Hajipour, M. J., Fromm, K. M., Ashkarran, A. A., Jimenez de Aberasturi, D., de Larramendi, I. R., Rojo, T., et al. (2012). Antibacterial properties of nanoparticles. *Trends Biotechnol.* 30 (10), 499–511. doi: 10.1016/j.tibtech.2012.06.004

Hao, M., Ye, M., Shen, Z., Hu, F., Yang, Y., Wu, S., et al. (2018). Porin deficiency in carbapenem-resistant enterobacter aerogenes strains. *Microb. Drug Resist.* 24 (9), 1–7. doi: 10.1089/mdr.2017.0379

Harada, L. K., Silva, E. C., Campos, W. F., Del Fiol, F. S., Vila, M., Dąbrowska, K., et al. (2018). Biotechnological applications of bacteriophages: state of the art. *Microbiol. Res.* 212–213, 38–58. doi: 10.1016/j.micres.2018.04.007

Hatoum-Aslan, A. (2018). Phage genetic engineering using CRISPR–Cas systems. *Viruses* 10, 335. doi: 10.3390/v10060335

He, Y., Ingudam, S., Reed, S., Gehring, A., Strobaugh, T. P., Jr., and Irwin, P. (2016). Study on the mechanism of antibacterial action of magnesium oxide nanoparticles against foodborne pathogens. *J. Nanobiotechnology* 14, 54. doi: 10.1186/s12951-016-0202-0

Hemeg, H. A. (2017). Nanomaterials for alternative antibacterial therapy. *Int. J. Nanomedicine* 12, 8211–8225. doi: 10.2147/IJN.S132163

Hogberg, L. D., Heddini, A., and Cars, O. (2010). The global need for effective antibiotics: challenges and recent advances. *Trends Pharmacol. Sci.* 31 (11), 509–515. doi: 10.1016/j.tips.2010.08.002

Hong, W., Gao, X., Qiu, P., Yang, J., Qiao, M., Shi, H., et al. (2017). Synthesis, construction, and evaluation of self-assembled nano-bacitracin A as an efficient antibacterial agent in vitro and in vivo. *Int. J. Nanomedicine* 12, 4691–4708. doi: 10.2147/IJN.S136998

Hsu, P. D., Lander, E. S., and Zhang, F. (2014). Development and applications of CRISPR-Cas9 for genome engineering. *Cell* 157 (6), 1262–1278. doi: 10.1016/j.cell.2014.05.010

Hullahalli, K., Rodrigues, M., and Palmer, K. L. (2017). Exploiting CRISPR–cas to manipulate enterococcus faecalis populations. *Elife* 6, e26664. doi: 10.7554/eLife.26664

Hullahalli, K., Rodrigues, M., Nguyen, U. T., and Palmer, K. (2018). An attenuated CRISPR–Cas system in Enterococcus faecalis permits DNA acquisition. *MBio.* 9 (3), e00414–18. doi: 10.1128/mBio.00414-18

Hyman, P., and Abedon, S. T. (2010). "Bacteriophage host range and bacterial resistance," in *Advances in applied microbiology*, vol. 70. Eds. Laskin, A. I., Sariaslani, S., Gadd, G. M. (San Diego: Elsevier Academic Press Inc.), 217–248. doi: 10.1016/S0065-2164(10)70007-1

Jamil, B., and Imran, M. (2018). Factors pivotal for designing of nanoantimicrobials: an exposition. *Crit. Rev. Microbiol.* 44 (1), 79–94. doi: 10.1080/1040841X.2017.1313813

Jansen, K. U., Knirsch, C., and Anderson, A. S. (2018). The role of vaccines in preventing bacterial antimicrobial resistance. *Nat. Med.* 24 (1), 10–19. doi: 10.1038/nm.4465

Jung, W. K., Koo, H. C., Kim, K. W., Shin, S., Kim, S. H., and Park, Y. H. (2008). Antibacterial activity and mechanism of action of the silver ion in Staphylococcus aureus and. escherichia coli. *Appl. Environm. Microbiol.* 74 (7), 2171–2178. doi: 10.1128/AEM.02001-07

Kalhapure, R. S., Suleman, N., Mocktar, C., Seedat, N., Govender, T. (2014). Nanoengineered drug delivery systems for enhancing antibiotic therapy. *J. Pharm. Sci.* 104 (3), 872–905. doi: 10.1002/jps.24298.

Kapoor, G., Saigal, S., and Elongavan, A. (2017). Action and resistance mechanisms of antibiotics: a guide for clinicians. *J. Anaesthesiol. Clin. Pharmacol.* 33 (3), 300–305. doi: 10.4103/joacp.JOACP_349_15

Kasithevar, M., Periakaruppan, P., Muthupandian, S., and Mohan, M. (2017). Antibacterial efficacy of silver nanoparticles against multi-drug resistant clinical isolates from post-surgical wound infections. *Microb. Pathog.* 107, 327–334. doi: 10.1016/j.micpath.2017.04.013

Khan, S., Alam, F., Azam, A., and Khan, A. U. (2012). Gold nanoparticles enhance methylene blue-induced photodynamic therapy: a novel therapeutic approach to inhibit Candida albicans biofilm. *Int. J. Nanomedicine* 7, 3245–3257. doi: 10.2147/IJN.S31219

Kim, S. Y., Li, B., and Linhardt, R. J. (2017). Pathogenesis and inhibition of flaviviruses from a carbohydrate perspective. *Pharmaceuticals* 10, 44. doi: 10.3390/ph10020044

Kon, K., and Rai, M. (2013). Metallic nanoparticles: mechanism of antibacterial action and influencing factors. *J. Comp. Clin. Pathol. Res.* 2, 160–174.

Kumar, M., Curtis, A., and Hoskins, C. (2018). Application of nanoparticle technologies in the combat against anti-microbial resistance. *Pharmaceutics* 10 (1), 11. doi: 10.3390/pharmaceutics10010011

Kumar, T. S., and Madhumathi, K. (2016). Antibiotic delivery by nanobioceramics. *Ther. Deliv.* 7 (8), 573–588. doi: 10.4155/tde-2016-0025

Li, J., Rong, K., Zhao, H., Li, F., Lu, Z., and Chen, R. (2013). Highly selective antibacterial activities of silver nanoparticles against Bacillus subtilis. *J. Nanosci. Nanotechnol.* 13 (10), 6806–6813. doi: 10.1166/jnn.2013.7781

Li, J., Qiao, Y., Zhu, H., Meng, F., and Liu, X. (2014). Existence, release, and antibacterial actions of silver nanoparticles on Ag–PIII TiO2 films with different nanotopographies. *Int. J. Nanomedicine* 9, 3389–3402. doi: 10.2147/IJN.S63807

Lima, R., Seabra, A. B., and Durán, N. (2012). Silver nanoparticles: a brief review of cytotoxicity and genotoxicity of chemically and biogenically synthesized nanoparticles. *J. Appl. Toxicol.* 32 (11), 867–879. doi: 10.1002/jat.2780

Maura, D., and Debarbieux, L. (2011). Bacteriophages as twenty-first century antibacterial tools for food and medicine. *Appl. Microbiol. Biotechnol.* 90 (3), 851–859. doi: 10.1007/s00253-011-3227-1

Meeker, D. G., Wang, T., Harrington, W. N., Zharov, V. P., Johnson, S. A., Jenkins, S. V., et al. (2018). Versatility of targeted antibiotic-loaded gold nanoconstructs for the treatment of biofilm-associated bacterial infections. *Int. J. Hyperthermia* 34 (2), 209–219. doi: 10.1080/02656736.2017.1392047

Mocan, T., Matea, C. T., Pop, T., Mosteanu, O., Buzoianu, A. D., Suciu, S., et al. (2017). Carbon nanotubes as anti-bacterial agents. *Cell. Mol. Life Sci.* 74 (19), 3467–3479. doi: 10.1007/s00018-017-2532-y

Moo, C. L., Yang, S. K., Yusoff, K., Ajat, M., Thomas, W., Abushelaibi, A., et al. (2019). Mechanisms of antimicrobial resistance (AMR) and alternative approaches to overcome AMR. *Curr. Drug Discov. Technol.* doi: 10.2174/15701 6381666619030412219

Morones, J. R., Elechiguerra, J. L., Camacho, A., Holt, K., Kouri, J. B., Ramírez, J. T., et al. (2005). The bactericidal effect of silver nanoparticles. *Nanotechnology* 16 (10), 2346–2353. doi: 10.1088/0957-4484/16/10/059

Moutinho, C. G., Matos, C. M., Teixeira, J. A., and Balcão, V. M. (2012). Nanocarrier possibilities for functional targeting of bioactive peptides and proteins: state-of-the-art. *J. Drug Target.* 20, 114–141. doi: 10.3109/1061186X.2011.628397

Mulani, M. S., Kamble, E. E., Kumkar, S. N., Tawre, M. S., and Pardesi, K. R. (2019). Emerging strategies to combat ESKAPE pathogens in the era of antimicrobial resistance: a review. *Front. Microbiol.* 10, 539. doi: 10.3389/fmicb.2019.00539

Munita, J. M., and Arias, C. A. (2016). Mechanisms of antibiotic resistance. *Microbiol. Spectr.* 4 (2). doi: 10.1128/microbiolspec.VMBF-0016-2015

Oliveira Santos, I. C., Albano, R. M., Asensi, M. D., and D'Alincourt Carvalho-Assef, A. P. (2018). Draft genome sequence of KPC-2-producing Pseudomonas aeruginosa recovered from a bloodstream infection sample in Brazil. *J. Glob. Antimicrob. Resist.* 15, 99–100. doi: 10.1016/j.jgar.2018.08.021

Nitsch-Osuch, A., Gyrczuk, E., Wardyn, A., Życinska, K., and Brydak, L. (2016). Antibiotic prescription practices among children with influenza. *Adv. Exp. Med. Biol.* 905, 25–31. doi: 10.1007/5584_2015_198

Pan, Y.-J., Lin, T.-L., Chen, C.-C., Tsai, Y.-T., Cheng, Y.-H., Chen, Y.-Y., et al. (2017). Klebsiella phage ΦK64-1 encodes multiple depolymerases for multiple host capsular types. *J. Virol.* 91, e02457–02416. doi: 10.1128/JVI.02457-16

Pham, T. N., Loupias, P., Dassonville-Klimpt, A., and Sonnet, P. (2019). Drug delivery systems designed to overcome antimicrobial resistance. *Med. Res. Rev.* 2019, 1–54. doi: 10.1002/med.21588

Poehlsgaard, J., and Douthwaite, S. (2005). The bacterial ribosome as a target for antibiotics. *Nat. Rev. Microbiol.* 3 (11), 870–881. doi: 10.1038/nrmicro1265

Prabhu, S., and Poulose, E. K. (2012). Silver nanoparticles: mechanism of antimicrobial action, synthesis, medical applications, and toxicity effects. *Int. Nano Lett.* 2, 32. doi: 10.1186/2228-5326-2-32

Pursey, E., Sünderhauf, D., Gaze, W. H., Westra, E. R., and van Houte, S. (2018). CRISPR-Cas antimicrobials: challenges and future prospects. *PLoS Pathog.* 14 (6), e1006990. doi: 10.1371/journal.ppat.1006990

Rai, M. K., Deshmukh, S. D., Ingle, A. P., and Gade, A. K. (2012). Silver nanoparticles: the powerful nanoweapon against multidrug-resistant bacteria. *J. Appl. Microbiol.* 112 (5), 841–852. doi: 10.1111/j.1365-2672.2012.05253.x

Redgrave, L. S., Sutton, S. B., Webber, M. A., and Piddock, L. J. V. (2014). Fluoroquinolone resistance: mechanisms, impact on bacteria, and role in evolutionary success. *Trends Microbiol.* 22 (8), 438–445. doi: 10.1016/j.tim.2014.04.007

Rios, A. C., Vila, M. M. D. C., Lima, R., Del Fiol, F. S., Tubino, M., Teixeira, J. A., et al. (2018). Structural and functional stabilization of bacteriophage particles within the aqueous core of a W/O/W multiple emulsion: a potential biotherapeutic system for the inhalational treatment of bacterial pneumonia. *Process Biochem.* 64, 177–192. doi: 10.1016/j.procbio.2017.09.022

Rios, A. C., Moutinho, C. G., Pinto, F. C., Del Fiol, F. S., Jozala, A., Chaud, M. V., et al. (2016). Alternatives to overcoming bacterial resistances: state-of-the-art. *Microbiol. Res.* 191, 51–80. doi: 10.1016/j.micres.2016.04.008

Rodzinski, A., Guduru, R., Liang, P., Hadjikhani, A., Stewart, T., Stimphil, E., et al. (2016). Targeted and controlled anticancer drug delivery and release with magnetoelectric nanoparticles. *Sci. Rep.* 6, 20867. doi: 10.1038/srep20867

Ruozi, B., Veratti, P., Vandelli, M. A., Tombesi, A., Tonelli, M., Forni, F., et al. (2017). Apoferritin nanocage as streptomycin drug reservoir: technological optimization of a new drug delivery system. *Int. J. Pharm.* 518 (1-2), 281–288. doi: 10.1016/j.ijpharm.2016.12.038

Salem, W., Leitner, D. R., Zingl, F. G., Schratter, G., Prassl, R., Goessler, W., et al. (2015). Antibacterial activity of silver and zinc nanoparticles against Vibrio cholerae and enterotoxic Escherichia coli. *Int. J. Med. Microbiol.* 305 (1), 85–95. doi: 10.1016/j.ijmm.2014.11.005

Senarathna, U. L. N. H., Fernando, S. S. N., Gunasekara, T. D. C. P., Weerasekera, M. M., Hewageegana, H. G. S. P., Arachchi, N. D. H., et al. (2017). Enhanced antibacterial activity of TiO2 nanoparticle surface modified with Garcinia zeylanica extract. *Chem. Cent. J.* 11, 7. doi: 10.1186/s13065-017-0236-x

Shaaban, M. I., Shaker, M. A., and Mady, F. M. (2017). Imipenem/cilastatin encapsulated polymeric nanoparticles for destroying carbapenem-resistant bacterial isolates. *J. Nanobiotechnology* 15 (1), 29. doi: 10.1186/s12951-017-0262-9

Shahverdi, A., Fakhimi, A., Shahverdi, H., and Minaian, S. (2007). Synthesis and effect of silver nanoparticles on the anti-bacterial activity of different antibiotics against staphylococcus aureus and. escherichia coli. *Nanomed. Nanotechnol. Biol. Med.* 3, 168–171. doi: 10.1016/j.nano.2007.02.001

Shen, J., Zhou, J., Chen, G. Q., and Xiu, Z. L. (2018). Efficient genome engineering of a virulent Klebsiella bacteriophage using CRISPR-Cas9. *J. Virol.* 92 (17), e00534–00518. doi: 10.1128/JVI.00534-18

Siemer, S., Westmeier, D., Barz, M., Eckrich, J., Wünsch, D., Seckert, C., et al. (2019). Biomolecule-corona formation confers resistance of bacteria to nanoparticle-induced. *Biomaterials* 192, 551–559. doi: 10.1016/j.biomaterials. 2018.11.028

Sieradzki, K., and Markiewicz, Z. (2004). Mechanism of vancomycin resistance in methicillin resistant Staphylococcus aureus. *J. Microbiol.* 53 (4), 207–14.

Simlai, A., Mukherjee, K., Mandal, A., Bhattacharya, K., Samanta, A., and Roy, A. (2016). Partial purification and characterization of an antimicrobial activity from the wood extract of mangrove plant Ceriops decandra. *EXCLI. J.* 15, 103–112.

Sorek, R., Lawrence, C. M., and Wiedenheft, B. (2013). CRISPR-mediated adaptive immune systems in bacteria and archaea. *Annu. Rev. Biochem.* 82, 237–266. doi: 10.1146/annurev-biochem-072911-172315

Summers, W. C. (2012). The strange history of phage therapy. *Bacteriophage* 2 (2), 130–133. doi: 10.4161/bact.20757

Sunitha, A., Rimal, I. R. S., Sweetly, G., Sornalekshmi, S., Arsula, R., and Praseetha, P. K. (2013). Evaluation of antimicrobial activity of biosynthesized iron and silver nanoparticles using the fungi Fusarium oxysporum and Actinomycetes sp. on human pathogens. *Nano. Biomed. Eng.* 5 (1), 39–45. doi: 10.5101/nbe. v5i1.p39-45

Tello, A., Austin, B., and Telfer, T. C. (2012). Selective pressure of antibiotic pollution on bacteria of importance to public health. *Environ. Health Perspect.* 120 (8), 1100–1106. doi: 10.1289/ehp.1104650

Tran, N., Mir, A., Mallik, D., Sinha, A., Nayar, S., and Webster, T. J. (2010). Bactericidal effect of iron oxide nanoparticles on Staphylococcus aureus. *Int. J. Nanomedicine* 5, 277–283. doi: 10.2147/IJN.S9220

Van Boeckel, T. P., Gandra, S., Ashok, A., Caudron, Q., Grenfell, B. T., Levin, S. A., et al. (2014). Global antibiotic consumption 2000 to 2010: an analysis of national pharmaceutical sales data. *Lancet Infect. Dis.* 14 (8), 742–750. doi: 10.1016/ S1473-3099(14)70780-7

Verma, S. K., Jha, E., Panda, P. K., Das, J. K., Thirumurugan, A., Suar, M., et al. (2018). Molecular aspects of core–shell intrinsic defect induced enhanced antibacterial activity of ZnO nanocrystals. *Nanomedicine (Lond)* 13 (1), 43–68. doi: 10.2217/nnm-2017-0237

Vikesland, P., Garner, E., Gupta, S., Kang, S., Maile-Moskowitz, A., and Zhu, N. (2019). Differential drivers of antimicrobial resistance across the world. *Acc. Chem. Res.* 52 (4), 916–924. doi: 10.1021/acs.accounts.8b00643

Wang, C., Wang, Y., Zhang, L., Miron, R. J., Liang, J., Shi, M., et al. (2018). Pretreated macrophage-membrane-coated gold nanocages for precise drug delivery for treatment of bacterial infections. *Adv. Mater.* 30 (46), e1804023. doi: 10.1002/adma.201804023

Wang, Y., Wan, J., Miron, R. J., Zhao, Y., and Zhang, Y. (2016). Antibacterial properties and mechanisms of gold–silver nanocages. *Nanoscale* 8 (21), 11143–11152. doi: 10.1039/C6NR01114D

Wang, Y., Wang, S., Chen, W., Song, L., Zhang, Y., Shen, Z., et al. (2018). CRISPR–Cas9 and CRISPR-assisted cytidine deaminase enable precise and efficient genome editing in Klebsiella pneumoniae. *Appl. Environ. Microbiol.* 84 (23), e01834–01818. doi: 10.1128/AEM.01834-18

Weitz, I. S., Maoz, M., Panitz, D., Eichler, S., and Segal, E. (2015). Combination

of CuO nanoparticles and fluconazole: preparation, characterization, and antifungal activity against Candida albicans. *J. Nanopart. Res.* 17 (8), 342. doi: 10.1007/s11051-015-3149-4

Willers, C., Wentzel, J. F., du Plessis, L. H., Gouws, C., and Hamman, J. H. (2017). Efflux as a mechanism of antimicrobial drug resistance in clinical relevant microorganisms: the role of efflux inhibitors. *Expert Opin. Ther. Targets* 21 (1), 23–36. doi: 10.1080/14728222.2017.1265105

Wittebole, X., de Roock, S., and Opal, S. M. (2013). A historical overview of bacteriophage therapy as an alternative to antibiotics for the treatment of bacterial pathogens. *Virulence* 4 (8), 1–10. doi: 10.4161/viru.25991

World Health Organization. (2017). Global priority list of antibiotic-resistant bacteria to guide research, discovery, and development of new antibiotics.

Wu, J. Y., Kim, J. J., Reddy, R., Wang, W. M., Graham, D. Y., and Kwon D. H. (2005). Tetracycline-resistant clinical Helicobacter pylori isolates with and without mutations in 16S rRNA-encoding genes. *Antimicrob. Agents Chemother.* 49 (2), 578–583. doi: 10.1128/AAC.49.2.578-583.2005

Wu, S., Li, A., Zhao, X., Zhang, C., Yu, B., Zhao, N., et al. (2019). Silica-coated gold–silver nanocages as photothermal antibacterial agents for combined anti-infective therapy. *ACS. Appl. Mater. Interfaces.* 11 (19), 17177–17183. doi: 10.1021/acsami.9b01149

Xiu, Z. M., Ma, J., and Alvarez, P. J. (2011). Differential effect of common ligands and molecular oxygen on antimicrobial activity of silver nanoparticles versus silver ions. *Environ. Sci. Technol.* 45 (20), 9003–9008. doi: 10.1021/es201918f

Xiu, Z. M., Zhang, Q. B., Puppala, H. L., Colvin, V. L., and Alvarez, P. J. (2012). Negligible particle-specific antibacterial activity of silver nanoparticles. *Nano. Lett.* 12 (8), 4271–4275. doi: 10.1021/nl301934w

Yan, M., Wen, J., Liang, M., Lu, Y., Kamata, M., and Chen, I. S. Y. (2015). Modulation of gene expression by polymer nanocapsule delivery of DNA cassettes encoding small RNAs. *PLoS ONE* 10 (6), e0127986. doi: 10.1371/ journal.pone.0127986

Yu, S., Gao, X., Zhang, R., Li, Z., Tan, Z., and Su, H. (2016). Synthesis and characterization of α-ZrP@CHI drug deliver system. *J. Nanosci. Nanotechnol.* 16 (4), 3628–3631. doi: 10.1166/jnn.2016.11859

Yuan, Y.-G., Peng, Q.-L., and Gurunathan, S. (2017). Effects of silver nanoparticles on multiple drug-resistant strains of Staphylococcus aureus and Pseudomonas aeruginosa from mastitis-infected goats: an alternative approach for antimicrobial therapy. *Int. J. Mol. Sci.* 18, 569. doi: 10.3390/ijms18030569

Zakharova, O. V., Godymchuk, A. Y., Gusev, A. A., Gulchenko, S. I., Vasyukova, I. A., Kuznetsov, D. V. (2015). Considerable variation of antibacterial activity of Cu nanoparticles suspensions depending on the storage time, dispersive medium, and particle sizes. *BioMed Research International* 2015, Article ID 412530, 11. doi: 10.1155/2015/412530

Zaidi, S., Misba, L., and Khan, A. U. (2017). Nano-therapeutics: a revolution in infection control in post antibiotic era. *Nanomedicine* 13 (7), 2281–2301. doi: 10.1016/j.nano.2017.06.015

15

Increasing Incidence of Colorectal Cancer in Adolescents and Young Adults Aged 15–39 Years in Western Australia 1982–2007: Examination of Colonoscopy History

Lakkhina Troeung[1]*, Nita Sodhi-Berry[1,2], Angelita Martini[1], Eva Malacova[1,3], Hooi Ee[4], Peter O'Leary[5,6], Iris Lansdorp-Vogelaar[7] and David B. Preen[1]

[1]Centre for Health Services Research, School of Population Health, The University of Western Australia, Perth, WA, Australia, [2]Occupational Respiratory Epidemiology, School of Population Health, The University of Western Australia, Perth, WA, Australia, [3]Department of Health, Safety and Environment, School of Public Health, Curtin University, Perth, WA, Australia, [4]Department of Gastroenterology, Sir Charles Gairdner Hospital, Queen Elizabeth II Medical Centre, Nedlands, WA, Australia, [5]Health Policy and Management, Faculty of Health Sciences, School of Public Health, Curtin University, Perth, WA, Australia, [6]School of Women's and Infants' Health, The University of Western Australia, Perth, WA, Australia, [7]Department of Public Health, Erasmus MC University Medical Centre, Rotterdam, Netherlands

Correspondence:
Lakkhina Troeung
lakkhina.troeung@uwa.edu.au

Aims: To examine trends in colorectal cancer (CRC) incidence and colonoscopy history in adolescents and young adults (AYAs) aged 15–39 years in Western Australia (WA) from 1982 to 2007.

Design: Descriptive cohort study using population-based linked hospital and cancer registry data.

Method: Five-year age-standardized and age-specific incidence rates of CRC were calculated for all AYAs and by sex. Temporal trends in CRC incidence were investigated using Joinpoint regression analysis. The annual percentage change (APC) in CRC incidence was calculated to identify significant time trends. Colonoscopy history relative to incident CRC diagnosis was examined and age and tumor grade at diagnosis compared for AYAs with and without pre-diagnosis colonoscopy. CRC-related mortality within 5 and 10 years of incident diagnosis were compared for AYAs with and without pre-diagnosis colonoscopy using mortality rate ratios (MRRs) derived from negative binomial regression.

Results: Age-standardized CRC incidence among AYAs significantly increased in WA between 1982 and 2007, APC = 3.0 (95% CI 0.7–5.5). Pre-diagnosis colonoscopy was uncommon among AYAs (6.0%, 33/483) and 71% of AYAs were diagnosed after index (first ever) colonoscopy. AYAs with pre-diagnosis colonoscopy were older at CRC diagnosis (mean 36.7 ± 0.7 years) compared to those with no prior colonoscopy (32.6 ± 0.2 years), $p < 0.001$. At CRC diagnosis, a significantly greater proportion of AYAs with pre-diagnosis colonoscopy had well-differentiated tumors (21.2%) compared to those without (5.6%), $p = 0.001$. CRC-related mortality was significantly lower for AYAs with pre-diagnosis colonoscopy compared to those without, for both 5-year

[MRR = 0.44 (95% CI 0.27–0.75), p = 0.045] and 10-year morality [MRR = 0.43 (95% CI 0.24–0.83), p = 0.043].

Conclusion: CRC incidence among AYAs in WA has significantly increased over the 25-year study period. Pre-diagnosis colonoscopy is associated with lower tumor grade at CRC diagnosis as well as significant reduction in both 5- and 10-year CRC-related mortality rates. These findings warrant further research into the balance in benefits and harms of targeted screening for AYA at highest risk.

Keywords: colorectal cancer screening, young adults, colonoscopy, colorectal cancer, incidence trends

INTRODUCTION

Australia and New Zealand have the highest rates of colorectal cancer (CRC) internationally (1). The average age at incident CRC diagnosis is 70 years with sharp increases in incidence from 50 years of age (2). Accordingly, current Australian guidelines recommend biennial CRC screening through fecal occult blood tests commencing from 50 years of age for all asymptomatic average-risk persons (3). In the United States (US), CRC incidence and mortality in persons over 50 years have declined over the past decade owing in part to screening initiatives (4). In particular, increased uptake of screening colonoscopy is suggested to be the main driver of declining CRC rates in this age group (5), with early detection and removal of premalignant lesions yielding significant reductions in CRC morbidity and mortality (6–10).

In direct contrast to trends in those over 50 years of age, an increasing incidence of CRC among adolescents and young adults (AYAs) has been reported internationally (11–15) as well as in Australia (16, 17) over the past two decades. A recent report showed that from 1990 to 2010, CRC incidence increased by between 85 and 100% in Australians aged 20–29 years and by 35% in those aged 30–39 years (17). The mechanisms underlying the rising incidence of CRC among AYAs are currently not well understood (15, 18); however, this increasing trend is a population health concern (18). Given the observed benefits of screening colonoscopy in the older population (5), questions have been raised in relation to current CRC screening practices in younger populations and whether average-risk CRC screening should be initiated at an earlier age (18–20). However, there is currently a lack of empirical data on the impact of screening in age groups <50 years to inform decision-making.

We examined trends in CRC incidence and colonoscopy history among AYAs aged 15–39 years in Western Australia (WA) from 1982 to 2007, before implementation of the National Bowel Cancer Screening Program (NBCSP), using whole-population linked hospital and Cancer Registry data. While the AYA age group is currently exempt from the NBCSP framework, it is possible that raised awareness of bowel cancer through the NBCSP may have impacted screening behaviors in the younger population. We therefore selected 2007 as our endpoint to examine pre-NBCSP colonoscopy history in AYAs. Specifically, we sought to (1) examine temporal trends in age-standardized and age-specific CRC incidence rates, (2) examine colonoscopy history in AYAs, and (3) compare age at diagnosis, tumor grade,

and 10-year CRC-related mortality for AYAs with and without a record of pre-diagnosis colonoscopy.

MATERIALS AND METHODS

Data Sources

Data were obtained on all persons aged 15–39 years with an incident diagnosis of malignant neoplasm in WA between 1st January 1982 and 31st December 2007, as registered with the WA Cancer Registry (WACR). The age range of 15–39 years for AYA classification is based on that used previously (16, 21). Since 1981, notifications of all malignancies within 6 months of diagnosis have been a statutory requirement in WA, with 86% of cases confirmed histologically (22). Extracted WACR records included information on sociodemographic (age, sex, Indigenous status, and area of residence) and tumor characteristics (diagnosis date, tumor site, morphology, behavior, and grade). Hospital records from 1982 to 2007 for the cohort were obtained through probabilistic matching of WACR records to the WA Hospital Morbidity Data System (HMDS) through the WA Data Linkage System (23). The HMDS is a statutory data collection which captures data for all public and private hospitalizations in WA. All colonoscopies in WA are hospital-based procedures and thus captured in the HMDS. Death records for cohort were also obtained through linkage with the WA Mortality Registry (1982–2007).

Trends in CRC Incidence

Incident primary cases of CRC were ascertained from WACR records using the International Classification of Diseases (ICD) version 9 with Clinical Modifications (ICD-9-CM) codes (153-154) and ICD version 10 with Australian Modification (ICD-10-AM) codes (C18-C21). Incidence rates were calculated by including only the first-ever primary CRC diagnosis for each person (i.e., subsequent CRC diagnoses, even if at different sites, were not counted). Persons registered in the WACR with another type of malignancy prior to CRC diagnosis were included, with date of first-ever CRC used for the analysis.

Five-year age-specific and age-standardized incidence rates of CRC were calculated for all AYAs and by sex using the number of incident CRC cases for each age group in each period as the numerator and the corresponding WA population for each age group in each period as the denominator. Denominators were obtained from population estimates provided by the Australian

Bureau of Statistics (24). Age-standardized rates were adjusted by direct standardization against the 5-year age distribution of the Australian population in the 2001 Census.

Temporal trends in CRC incidence over the study period were investigated using Joinpoint regression analyses (25). Joinpoint analysis uses an algorithm to define segments where statistically significant changes in temporal trends occur. The annual percentage change (APC) in each Joinpoint segment represents the rate of change in cancer incidence per year in a given time period and is calculated using generalized linear models assuming a Poisson distribution (26). Changes in rates include shifts in magnitude or direction where a positive APC indicates an increase in cancer incidence for a given segment while a negative APC indicates decreasing incidence. Joinpoint regression analyses were performed using the Joinpoint Regression Program 4.3.1 from the US National Cancer Institute (25).

Colonoscopy History

Hospital admissions for colonoscopy were ascertained from any of the 11 procedure fields in HMDS records using ICD-9-CM codes (45.21, 45.22, 45.23, 45.24, 45.25, 45.42, 48.24) for admissions between January 1982 and June 1999 and ICD-10-AM codes (32090-00, 56549-01, 32090-02, 32090-01, 90308-00, 90959-00, 90315-00, 32093-00, 32023-00, 32023-03, 32093-00, 32023-02, 32023-01, 32023-05, 32023-04, 32023-01, 92097-02, 32090-00, 32084-00, 32084-02, 32084-01, 90308-00, 90959-00, 90315-00, 32087-00, 30375-23, 56549-01, 32075-00, 32075-01, 32078-00, 32081-00) for hospitalizations from July 1999 onward. We incorporated a 1-year clearance period which excluded 18 AYAs diagnosed with CRC in 1982. A further 16 cases were excluded as they had no hospital records prior to or during the period of cancer diagnosis from which colonoscopy history could be ascertained.

To describe the cohort's colonoscopy history, we divided all colonoscopies into three categories based on the timing of colonoscopy relative to incident CRC diagnosis. "Pre-diagnosis" colonoscopies were defined as any recorded colonoscopy greater than 6 months preceding the date of incident CRC diagnosis as registered with the WACR. "Diagnostic" colonoscopies were defined as any colonoscopies performed which resulted in a diagnosis of CRC within 6 months. "Post-diagnosis" colonoscopies were defined as any colonoscopy admission occurring after date of incident CRC diagnosis. Due to the limitations of administrative data and ICD coding standards, we were unable to determine whether pre-diagnosis colonoscopies were screening/surveillance (i.e., asymptomatic) or diagnostic colonoscopies (i.e., symptomatic colonoscopy).

Age and tumor grade at incident CRC diagnosis was compared between AYAs with and without a record of pre-diagnosis colonoscopy using t-tests and chi-square tests. Tumor grade was examined as data on cancer stage is not documented in the WACR.

CRC Mortality

Deaths within 5 and 10 years of incident CRC diagnosis were identified using WA Death Registry records. CRC-related deaths were ascertained from the underlying cause of death field in death records using the following codes: ICD-9-CM 153-154 and ICD-10-AM C18-C21. CRC-related mortality rate ratios (MRRs) were compared for AYAs with and without pre-diagnosis colonoscopy using negative binomial regression to account for overdispersion of death data in Stata 14.0. Analyses were adjusted for sex and age at incident CRC diagnosis and Charlson comorbidity index. We restricted our analysis to only individuals who had 5 (i.e., diagnosed 1982-2002; $n = 251$) and 10 years (i.e., diagnosed 1982-1997; $n = 234$) of follow-up time, respectively. Differential person-years of risk for each person were accounted for by including time at risk as an offset variable in negative binomial models. Analysis of mortality rates was selected over survival rates to minimize the effect of lead-time bias commonly observed in cancer screening studies.

Ethics Statement

Ethics approval for this study was obtained from the University of Western Australia Research Ethics Committees (reference number: RA/4/1/2228).

RESULTS

A total of 517 incident cases of CRC among AYAs aged 15-39 years were registered with the WACR between 1982 and 2007. There were 256 females (49.6%) and 261 males (50.4%). Mean age at incident CRC diagnosis was 33.7 ± 5.3 years (range 15.2-39.9 years). CRC accounted for 4.2% of all cancers diagnosed in AYAs between 1982 and 2007 in WA.

CRC Incidence and Trends

Five-year age-standardized and age-specific incidence rates for CRC in AYAs are presented in **Table 1** alongside Joinpoint regression results using annual incidence data. An increasing trend in age-standardized incidence rates for CRC in AYAs was observed over the study period (**Figure 1**). The overall age-standardized incidence of CRC significantly increased from 2.1 to 4.8 per 100,000 AYA population between 1982 and 2007, APC = 3.0 (95% CI 0.7-5.5), $p = 0.024$ (**Table 1**). The age-standardized incidence of CRC among female AYAs also significantly increased over the study period, APC = 3.4 (95% CI 1.1-5.7), $p = 0.014$. While an increasing trend in CRC incidence was observed for male AYAs, this was not statistically significant, APC = 2.6 (95% CI −1.0 to 5.2), $p = 0.06$.

An upward trend in CRC incidence was observed in all age groups but the 15-19 years category, for both males and females (**Figure 1**). However, none of the trends were statistically significant for males. For female AYAs, significant increases in CRC incidence were observed across all age groups except in the 15- to 19-year group. The greatest APC was observed for younger female AYAs, particularly those aged 20-24 years, APC = 10.1 (3.3-17.5), $p = 0.014$, and 25-29 years, APC = 4.9 (1.8-14.3), $p = 0.050$.

Colonoscopy History

Colonoscopies were recorded for 77.8% (376/483) of the AYA CRC cohort, with 1,377 total hospital admissions for colonoscopy between 1982 and 2007. Almost a quarter of the cohort had no

TABLE 1 | Five-year age-specific and age-standardized and Joinpoint analysis of annual colorectal cancer incidence rates per 100,000 in adolescents and young adults aged 15–39 years in Western Australia during 1982–2007.

	1982–1984	1985–1989	1990–1994	1995–1999	2000–2004	2005–2007	APC (95% CI) 1982–2007[a]	p
All persons								
Age-specific rates								
15–19 years	0.7	0.1	0.1	0.4	0.1	0.5	2.4 (−10.5 to 17.2)	0.649
20–24 years	0.3	0.9	0.6	0.3	1.6	3.4	8.3 (−2.6 to 20.4)	0.106
25–29 years	1.5	1.5	1.8	1.7	2.1	3.8	3.6 (0.6–6.8)*	0.029
30–34 years	3.1	3.7	3.3	3.3	4.5	6.5	2.7 (0.1–5.4)*	0.050
35–39 years	4.4	6.3	7.3	5.9	8.8	9.1	2.4 (0.1–4.7)*	0.047
Age-standardized rate	2.1	2.6	2.7	2.4	3.5	4.8	3.0 (0.7–5.5)*	0.024
Males								
Age-specific rates								
15–19 years	1.4	0.1	0.1	0.6	0.3	0.5	−4.9 (−14.7 to 6.0)	0.269
20–24 years	0.5	1.2	0.6	0.3	1.2	3.6	6.6 (−2.2 to 16.1)	0.110
25–29 years	1.0	1.2	2.8	3.1	2.4	2.0	2.4 (−4.0 to 9.2)	0.373
30–34 years	3.4	3.8	2.9	2.3	3.5	7.2	2.7 (−2.4 to 8.0)	0.235
35–39 years	4.7	7.1	7.4	5.7	8.5	10.4	2.2 (−0.6 to 5.0)	0.105
Age-standardized rate	2.3	2.8	2.8	2.4	3.3	4.8	2.6 (−0.9 to 5.2)	0.061
Females								
Age-specific rates								
15–19 years	0.2	0.3	0.1	0.3	0.1	0.5	2.0 (−4.3 to 8.7)	0.426
20–24 years	0.3	0.6	0.6	0.3	1.9	3.2	10.1 (3.3–17.5)*	0.014
25–29 years	2.0	1.8	0.9	0.3	1.8	5.6	4.9 (1.8–14.3)*	0.050
30–34 years	2.9	3.7	3.7	4.3	5.4	5.7	2.8 (1.6–4.0)*	0.002
35–39 years	4.2	5.5	7.2	6.1	9.1	7.8	2.6 (0.1–5.3)*	0.050
Age-standardized rate	2.0	2.5	2.7	2.4	3.9	4.7	3.4 (1.1–5.7)*	0.014

APC, annual percentage change.
*APC is statistically significant at a 0.05 level.
[a]The model with 0 Joinpoints (i.e., 1982–2007) was most optimal in all analyses.

recorded colonoscopy over the study period (22.2%, 107/483). For these individuals, CRC was diagnosed during surgical procedure with no follow-up colonoscopies recorded over the study period.

The majority of colonoscopies (70.5%, 971/1,377) were performed post-CRC diagnosis for surveillance purposes to prevent metachronous cancer (**Figure 2**). Colonoscopy was uncommon among AYAs prior to CRC diagnosis, with only 6.8% (33/483) of the cohort with any record of pre-diagnosis colonoscopy. Mean age at index colonoscopy for the cohort was 34.3 ± 5.7 years (range: 16–52 years). For the majority of AYAs, the index colonoscopy was performed during the hospital admission where CRC diagnosis was made (70.5%, 265/376). Only 8.8% of AYAs (33/376) had their index colonoscopy in the pre-diagnosis period, while 20.7% (78/376) had their index colonoscopy during treatment follow-up.

Age and Tumor Grade at Diagnosis

Adolescents and young adults with a recorded pre-diagnosis colonoscopy were significantly younger at index colonoscopy (29.7 ± 6.8 years) compared to those with index colonoscopy at CRC diagnosis (34.8 ± 5.4 years), p < 0.001 (**Table 2**). AYAs with pre-diagnosis colonoscopy were also significantly older at time of incident CRC diagnosis (36.7 ± 0.7 years) compared to those with no pre-diagnosis colonoscopy (32.6 ± 0.2 years), p < 0.001. At CRC diagnosis, a significantly greater proportion of AYAs with pre-diagnosis colonoscopy had low grade (well-differentiated) tumors (21.2%) compared to those with no pre-diagnosis

colonoscopy (5.6%), p = 0.001. A greater proportion of AYAs with no pre-diagnosis colonoscopy had high grade (poorly differentiated) tumors (34.1%) compared to AYAs with pre-diagnosis colonoscopy (24.2%), p = 0.001.

Five- and Ten-Year Mortality

A total of 146 and 117 AYAs died within 5 and 10 years of incident CRC diagnosis, respectively (**Table 3**). There was no significant difference in all-cause 5- or 10-year mortality rates for AYAs with and without a pre-diagnosis colonoscopy. CRC-related 5-year mortality was 56% lower in the group with pre-diagnosis colonoscopy than those without, MRR = 0.44 (95% CI 0.27–0.75), p = 0.045. Similarly, CRC-related 10-year mortality was 57% lower for those with pre-diagnosis colonoscopy compared to those without, MRR = 0.43 (95% CI 0.24–0.83), p = 0.043.

DISCUSSION

While the overall age-standardized incidence of CRC among AYAs in WA remains low (4.8 per 100,000) relative to the overall incidence in all age groups [62 per 100,000 in 2012 (27)], our results show a clear and significant upward trend in CRC incidence in this younger age group. Between 1982 and 2007, a 3.0% annual increase in CRC incidence was observed among AYAs in WA. In particular, CRC incidence in female AYAs rose significantly in all age groups with the exception of those aged 15–19 years.

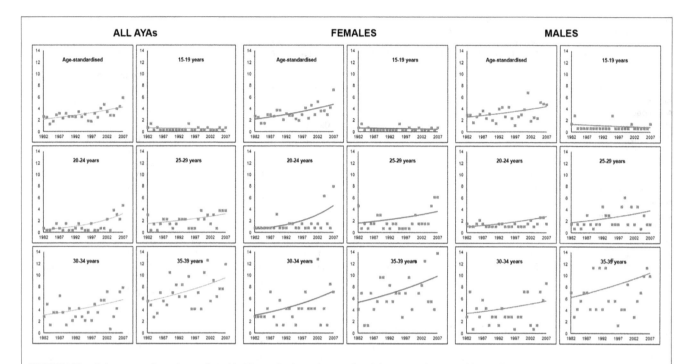

FIGURE 1 | Trends in age-specific and age-adjusted incidence of colorectal cancer for adolescents and young adults aged 15–39 years in Western Australia, 1982–2007. Markers represent observed incidence rates and solid lines represent the Joinpoint regression model trend line.

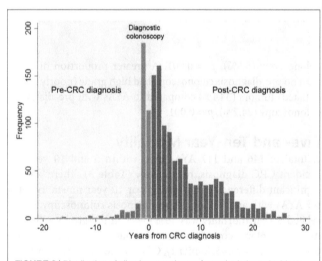

FIGURE 2 | Distribution of all colonoscopies performed relative to incident colorectal cancer (CRC) diagnosis in adolescents and young adults in Western Australia during 1982–2007.

TABLE 2 | Comparison of age and tumor grade at colorectal cancer (CRC) diagnosis between adolescents and young adults (AYAs) with and without pre-diagnosis colonoscopy (n = 483).

	Pre-diagnosis colonoscopy (n = 33)	No pre-diagnosis colonoscopy (n = 450)
Age at index colonoscopy, n (%)		
15–19 years	<5 (3.0)	0 (0)
20–24 years	<5 (9.1)	15 (4.2)
25–29 years	5 (15.2)	34 (9.5)
30–34 years	6 (18.2)	74 (20.7)
35–39 years	18 (54.6)	235 (65.6)
Mean age at index colonoscopy ± SD	33.7 ± 1.5*	37.1 ± 0.4
Age at incident CRC diagnosis, n (%)		
15–19 years	0 (0)	10 (2.1)
20–24 years	0 (0)	36 (7.4)
25–29 years	<5 (12.1)	64 (13.2)
30–34 years	10 (30.3)	133 (27.5)
35–39 years	19 (57.6)*	241 (49.8)
Mean age at incident CRC diagnosis ± SD	36.7 ± 0.7*	32.6 ± 0.2
Tumor grade, n (%)		
1: Low or well-differentiated	24 (16.2)*	62 (6.6)
2: Intermediate or moderately differentiated	9 (27.3)	142 (29.3)
3: High or poorly differentiated	8 (24.2)*	165 (34.1)
9: Not determined	9 (27.3)	149 (30.8)

*$p < 0.05$, significantly different from AYAs with no pre-diagnosis colonoscopy.

Increasing trends in CRC incidence were also observed for male AYAs, although trends were not statistically significant.

Our results are consistent with a growing number of studies demonstrating a significant increase in CRC incidence in those aged under 50 internationally. In the US, Bailey et al. (28) recently showed that at the present rate, the incidence of CRC among young adults will almost double by 2030 while simultaneously declining by more than 30% in adults over 50 years of age. The reasons underlying the rise in CRC in the younger population are currently not well understood (15, 18). However, modern Westernized lifestyle and behaviors have been implicated as potential contributors, including high consumption of takeaway and processed food and red meat in addition to obesity and low

TABLE 3 | Five- and ten-year colorectal cancer (CRC)-related mortality for adolescents and young adults with and without pre-diagnosis colonoscopy.

			Five-year mortality (n = 351)			Ten-year mortality (n = 234)			
	n	Deaths	MRR (95% CI)	*p*	*n*	Deaths	MRR (95% CI)	*p*
All-cause deaths								
Pre-diagnosis colonoscopy	21	11	0.63 (0.27–1.28)	0.061	15	10	0.68 (0.09–1.46)	0.085
No pre-diagnosis colonoscopy	330	135			219	107		
CRC-related deaths								
Pre-diagnosis colonoscopy	21	9	0.44 (0.27–0.75)	0.045*	15	8	0.43 (0.24–0.83)	0.043*
No pre-diagnosis colonoscopy	330	131			219	100		

*$p < 0.05$.
MRR, mortality rate ratio based on negative binomial regression adjusted for sex and age at incident CRC diagnosis and Charlson comorbidity index; CI, confidence interval.

physical activity, which are known risk factors for CRC (29–31) and prevalent in contemporary Australian society (29, 32). Although smoking rates among Australian AYAs have reduced drastically over the past two decades (33), excessive alcohol consumption among AYAs has substantially increased (34) and may also partially account for the rising incidence of CRC in this population (35, 36).

Pre-diagnosis colonoscopy was uncommon among AYAs in our cohort with only 6.8% with a recorded pre-diagnosis colonoscopy and 71% being diagnosed with CRC at index colonoscopy. In Australia, national guidelines recommending routine CRC screening in adults over 50 years were introduced in 1999 with the NBCSP subsequently launched in 2006 (37). An Australian report on adults aged 45 years and above showed that screening colonoscopy was associated with a 50% reduction in risk of subsequent CRC diagnosis compared to no screening (38). In the US, successful implementation of CRC screening programs in the older population have been credited as the main driver of declining CRC rates in those aged above 50 years (5, 39). Austin et al. (5) demonstrated a significant inverse correlation between state-level APC of CRC incidence and colonoscopy rates in the US between 1998 and 2009 in adults aged 50 years and over. Specifically, states with greater reduction in CRC incidence rates over the study period tended to have higher rates of screening colonoscopy. A significant inverse correlation between CRC mortality rates and CRC screening rates between 1990–1994 and 2003–2007 has also been demonstrated in the older US population (39).

Interestingly, a number of studies have found that AYAs with CRC exhibit more advanced disease at diagnosis compared to older adults and receive more aggressive cancer treatment (15, 40–42). While it is currently unclear why this phenomenon occurs, some researchers have suggested that young-onset CRC may represent a different, more aggressive underlying disease process compared to later-onset CRC (43), although robust evidence of a more rapid adenoma-carcinoma sequence in younger adults is yet to be established. Others have implicated the absence of routine screening in this age group. As younger persons are currently omitted from routine CRC screening, CRC is typically detected in younger patients only when it becomes symptomatic or emergent and generally at more advanced stage of disease (15, 18, 20, 42). Thus, more aggressive treatment is required due to delayed diagnosis (42). Consistent with this hypothesis, we found that just under a

quarter of our AYA cohort were likely emergency presentations with no admission for colonoscopy prior to CRC diagnosis and incident diagnosis made during a surgical procedure. Over 60% of our cohort had moderately or poorly differentiated tumors at CRC diagnosis. The opportunity for cancer prevention through detection and removal of premalignant lesions is also not available to young Australians. A recent study forecasted that due to late detection and accelerated progression of disease, CRC patients younger than 50 years will have the worst outcomes of any age group (20).

While colonoscopy prior to CRC diagnosis was uncommon among AYAs in our cohort, our results highlight some potential benefits of pre-diagnosis colonoscopy for younger adults, which may warrant further investigation. On average, AYAs with a pre-diagnosis colonoscopy were diagnosed with CRC at an older age relative to those with no pre-diagnosis colonoscopy history. Over 20% of AYAs with pre-diagnosis colonoscopy had well-differentiated tumors at presentation compared to only 5% of those without. Moreover, both 5- and 10-year CRC-related mortality rates were reduced by over 50% for AYAs with pre-diagnosis colonoscopy compared to AYAs without any colonoscopy history prior to diagnosis. These findings likely highlight the opportunity for early detection and removal of any premalignant adenoma through pre-diagnosis colonoscopy which could both delay CRC onset and enhance survival.

Our current findings add to an emerging body of research calling for action to address the rising incidence of CRC in the younger population (17, 18, 42). While the simplest suggestion may be to initiate average-risk CRC screening at an earlier age given the demonstrated benefits of screening colonoscopy in the older population (44), the costs and risks of widespread application of colonoscopy screening need to be carefully balanced with potential benefits (18, 44). CRC screening in average-risk persons younger than 50 years is unlikely to be cost-effective given that young-onset CRC comprises less than 7% of all CRC cases (19).

Risk-stratified screening for CRC in the average-risk population is a growing area of interest and may offer the most optimal solution (45–47). Current CRC screening models assume equal risk of CRC in the average-risk population with undifferentiated screening approaches for adults aged 50 years and above. However, research suggests that the population presently considered at "average risk" is not homogenous in terms of CRC risk and could be further stratified into distinct risk groups with tailored screening approaches and intervals for each risk level (46, 48, 49).

5

Tailored screening for AYAs with higher than average risk for CRC likely offers a more cost-effective method of CRC screening for this group. A number of risk stratification models for advanced neoplasia and CRC have been developed in recent years; however, most are developed for the older population and their current predictive power is suboptimal (48). To better target population level screening interventions for CRC, future risk models need to simultaneously consider the average-risk population under 50 years given the demonstrated rising incidence of CRC in this age group. The challenge for researchers and policymakers remains how to best identify persons, including AYAs, at-risk of CRC and for whom early screening would be beneficial (42).

Limitations and Directions for Future Research

Our findings show an increasing trend in CRC incidence in WA over 25 years; however, trends over the most recent decade could not be explored due to lack of post-2007 data as our analysis was based on an existing data source with end date of 2008. However, our results are consistent with other Australian and international research (11–17) showing a rising incidence of CRC in the AYA population over recent years. To date, trends in CRC incidence among Australian AYAs have only been explored to 2010 (17), with very limited other research examining colonoscopy use and costs and benefits in the younger population. Future research examining CRC incidence trends and colonoscopy uptake in Australian AYAs over the most recent decade will provide valuable insight into whether extending average risk screening into the younger population is warranted. Other limitations include

we were unable to quantify the number of Lynch syndrome cases and investigate trends in hereditary vs. sporadic CRC cases over time as the WACR does not document this data, and we were unable to examine cancer stage at presentation in our analyses as this data is not collected by the WACR.

CONCLUSION

In summary, our study found a growing increase in CRC incidence in AYAs in WA. Pre-diagnosis colonoscopy was rare in AYAs but where performed it was associated with later age and lower tumor grade at diagnosis and a greater than 50% reduction in CRC-related mortality within 10 years of incident diagnosis. Future research identifying strategies for early CRC detection in the AYA population is warranted.

AUTHOR CONTRIBUTIONS

LT designed the study, designed and performed the statistical analysis, and drafted and revised the manuscript. NS-B, AM, EM, and IL-V revised the draft manuscript. HE and PO obtained funding and revised the draft manuscript. DP obtained funding, revised the draft manuscript, and provided study supervision.

FUNDING

This study was supported by a Cancer Council Western Australia Capacity Building and Collaboration Grant.

REFERENCES

1. Cancer IAfRo. *GLOBOCAN 2012. Colorectal Cancer: Estimated Incidence, Mortality and Prevalence Worldwide in 2012*. Lyon, France: World Health Organization (2016).
2. (AIHW) AIoHaW. *Cancer in Australia: An Overview: AIHW*. (2014). Available from: http://www.aihw.gov.au/WorkArea/DownloadAsset. aspx?id=60129550202
3. Royal Australian College of General Practitioners. *Guidelines for Preventive Activities in General Practice*. 8th ed. East Melbourne: Royal Australian College of General Practitioners (2012).
4. Siegel RL, Ward EM, Jemal A. Trends in colorectal cancer incidence rates in the United States by tumor location and stage, 1992–2008. *Cancer Epidemiol Prev Biomarkers* (2012) 21(3):411–6. doi:10.1158/1055-9965.EPI-11-1020
5. Austin H, Henley SJ, King J, Richardson LC, Eheman C. Changes in colorectal cancer incidence rates in young and older adults in the United States: what does it tell us about screening. *Cancer Causes Control* (2014) 25(2):191–201. doi:10.1007/s10552-013-0321-y
6. Winawer SJ, Zauber AG, Ho MN, O'Brien MJ, Gottlieb LS, Sternberg SS, et al. Prevention of colorectal cancer by colonoscopic polypectomy. *N Engl J Med* (1993) 329(27):1977–81. doi:10.1056/NEJM199312303292701
7. Schoen RE, Pinsky PF, Weissfeld JL, Yokochi LA, Church T, Laiyemo AO, et al. Colorectal-cancer incidence and mortality with screening flexible sigmoidoscopy. *N Engl J Med* (2012) 366(25):2345–57. doi:10.1056/NEJMoa1114635
8. Atkin WS, Edwards R, Kralj-Hans I, Wooldrage K, Hart AR, Northover JMA, et al. Once-only flexible sigmoidoscopy screening in prevention of colorectal cancer: a multicentre randomised controlled trial. *Lancet* (2010) 375(9726):1624–33. doi:10.1016/S0140-6736(10)60551-X
9. Nishihara R, Wu K, Lochhead P, Morikawa T, Liao X, Qian ZR, et al. Long-term colorectal-cancer incidence and mortality after lower endoscopy. *N Engl J Med* (2013) 369(12):1095–105. doi:10.1056/NEJMoa1301969
10. Zauber AG, Winawer SJ, O'Brien MJ, Lansdorp-Vogelaar I, van Ballegooijen M, Hankey BF, et al. Colonoscopic polypectomy and long-term prevention of colorectal-cancer deaths. *N Engl J Med* (2012) 366(8):687–96. doi:10.1056/NEJMoa1100370
11. Aziz H, Pandit V, DiGiovanni RM, Ohlson E, Gruessner AC, Jandova J, et al. Increased incidence of early onset colorectal cancer in Arizona: a comprehensive 15-year analysis of the Arizona Cancer Registry. *J Gastrointest Dig Syst* (2015) 5(5):345–48. doi:10.4172/2161-069X.1000345
12. Wu X, Groves FD, McLaughlin CC, Jemal A, Martin J, Chen VW. Cancer incidence patterns among adolescents and young adults in the United States. *Cancer Causes Control* (2005) 16(3):309–20. doi:10.1007/s10552-004-4026-0
13. Siegel RL, Jemal A, Ward EM. Increase in incidence of colorectal cancer among young men and women in the United States. *Cancer Epidemiol Biomarkers Prev* (2009) 18(6):1695–8. doi:10.1158/1055-9965.epi-09-0186
14. Teng A, Lee DY, Cai J, Patel SS, Bilchik AJ, Goldfarb MR. Patterns and outcomes of colorectal cancer in adolescents and young adults. *J Surg Res* (2016) 205:19–27. doi:10.1016/j.jss.2016.05.036
15. O'Connell JB, Maggard MA, Liu JH, Etzioni DA, Livingston EH, Ko CY. Rates of colon and rectal cancers are increasing in young adults. *Am Surg* (2003) 69(10):866.

16. Haggar FA, Preen DB, Pereira G, Holman CD, Einarsdottir K. Cancer incidence and mortality trends in Australian adolescents and young adults, 1982-2007. *BMC Cancer* (2012) 12(1):151. doi:10.1186/1471-2407-12-151

17. Young JP, Win AK, Rosty C, Flight I, Roder D, Young GP, et al. Rising incidence of early-onset colorectal cancer in Australia over two decades: report and review. *J Gastroenterol Hepatol* (2015) 30(1):6–13. doi:10.1111/jgh.12792

18. Ahnen DJ, Wade SW, Jones WF, Sifri R, Silveiras JM, Greenamyer J, et al., editors. The increasing incidence of young-onset colorectal cancer: a call to action. *Mayo Clinic Proceedings*. Denver: Elsevier (2014).

19. Inra JA, Syngal S. Colorectal cancer in young adults. *Dig Dis Sci* (2015) 60(3):722–33. doi:10.1007/s10620-014-3464-0

20. Amri R, Bordeianou LG, Berger DL. The conundrum of the young colon cancer patient. *Surgery* (2015) 158(6):1696–703. doi:10.1016/j.surg.2015.07.018

21. Weir HK, Marrett LD, Cokkinides V, Barnholtz-Sloan J, Patel P, Tai E, et al. Melanoma in adolescents and young adults (ages 15-39 years): United States, 1999-2006. *J Am Acad Dermatol* (2011) 65(5):S38. e1–S. e13. doi:10.1016/j.jaad.2011.04.038

22. Health WADo. *Cancer Incidence and Mortality in Western Australia, 2014.* Perth, WA: WA Department of Health (2015).

23. Department of Health Government of Western Australia. *Data Linkage Western Australia 2015.* (2015). Available from: http://www.datalinkage-wa.org

24. Statistics ABo. *2001 Census Data.* (2001). Available from: http://www.abs.gov.au/websitedbs/censushome.nsf/home/historicaldata2001?opendocument

25. National Cancer Institute. *Joinpoint Regression Program, Version 4.5.0.1; Statistical Methodology and Applications Branch, Surveillance Research Program.* Bethesda, MD: National Cancer Institute (2017).

26. Kim H-J, Fay MP, Feuer EJ, Midthune DN. Permutation tests for Joinpoint regression with applications to cancer rates. *Stat Med* (2000) 19(3):335–51. doi:10.1002/(SICI)1097-0258(20000215)19:3<335::AID-SIM336>3.3.CO;2-Q

27. Australia C. *Bowel Cancer (Colorectal Cancer) in Australia.* (2016). Available from: https://bowel-cancer.canceraustralia.gov.au/statistics

28. Bailey CE, Hu C-Y, You YN, Bednarski BK, Rodriguez-Bigas MA, Skibber JM, et al. Increasing disparities in age-related incidence of colon and rectal cancer in the United States, 1975-2010. *JAMA Surg* (2015) 150(1):17. doi:10.1001/jamasurg.2014.1756

29. Crino M, Sacks G, Vandevijvere S, Swinburn B, Neal B. The influence on population weight gain and obesity of the macronutrient composition and energy density of the food supply. *Curr Obes Rep* (2015) 4(1):1–10. doi:10.1007/s13679-014-0134-7

30. Ananthakrishnan AN, Du M, Berndt SI, Brenner H, Caan BJ, Casey G, et al. Red meat intake, NAT2, and risk of colorectal cancer: a pooled analysis of 11 studies. *Cancer Epidemiol Biomarkers Prev* (2015) 24(1):198–205. doi:10.1158/1055-9965.EPI-14-0897

31. Campbell PT, Patel AV, Newton CC, Jacobs EJ, Gapstur SM. Associations of recreational physical activity and leisure time spent sitting with colorectal cancer survival. *J Clin Oncol* (2013) 31:876–85. doi:10.1200/JCO.2012.45.9735

32. Rahman A, Harding A. Prevalence of overweight and obesity epidemic in Australia: some causes and consequences. *J P J Biostat* (2013) 10(1):31.

33. Scollo M, Winstanley M. *Tobacco in Australia: Facts and Issues Melbourne, Australia: Cancer Council Victoria.* (2016). Available from: www.TobaccoInAustralia.org.au

34. Kelly AB, Chan GC, Toumbourou JW, O'Flaherty M, Homel R, Patton GC, et al. Very young adolescents and alcohol: evidence of a unique suscepti bility to peer alcohol use. *Addict Behav* (2012) 37(4):414–9. doi:10.1016/j.addbeh.2011.11.038

35. Phipps AI, Robinson J, Campbell PT, Win AK, Figueiredo J, Lindor NM, et al. Prediagnostic alcohol consumption and colorectal cancer survival: the Colon Cancer Family Registry. *Cancer Res* (2016) 76(14 Suppl):3425. doi:10.1158/1538-7445.AM2016-3425

36. Cho E, Lee JE, Rimm EB, Fuchs CS, Giovannucci EL. Alcohol consumption and the risk of colon cancer by family history of colorectal cancer. *Am J Clin Nutr* (2012) 95(2):413–9. doi:10.3945/ajcn.111.022145

37. Health AGDo. *National Bowel Cancer Screening Program: Australian Government.* (2016). Available from: http://www.cancerscreening.gov.au/internet/screening/publishing.nsf/content/bowel-screening-1

38. Steffen A, Weber MF, Roder DM, Banks E. Colorectal cancer screening and subsequent incidence of colorectal cancer: results from the 45 and up study. *Med J Aust* (2014) 201(9):523–7. doi:10.5694/mja14.00197

39. Naishadham D, Lansdorp-Vogelaar I, Siegel R, Cokkinides V, Jemal A. State disparities in colorectal cancer mortality patterns in the United States. *Cancer Epidemiol Biomarkers Prev* (2011) 20(7):1296–302. doi:10.1158/1055-9965.EPI-11-0250

40. You Y, Xing Y, Feig BW, Chang GJ, Cormier JN. Young-onset colorectal cancer: Is it time to pay attention? *Arch Intern Med* (2012) 172(3):287–9. doi:10.1001/archinternmed.2011.602

41. Edwards BK, Ward E, Kohler BA, Eheman C, Zauber AG, Anderson RN, et al. Annual report to the nation on the status of cancer, 1975-2006, featuring colorectal cancer trends and impact of interventions (risk factors, screening, and treatment) to reduce future rates. *Cancer* (2010) 116(3):544–73. doi:10.1002/cncr.24760

42. Abdelsattar ZM, Wong SL, Regenbogen SE, Jomaa DM, Hardiman KM, Hendren S. Colorectal cancer outcomes and treatment patterns in patients too young for average-risk screening. *Cancer* (2016) 122(6):929–34. doi:10.1002/cncr.29716

43. Minardi AJ Jr, Sittig KM, Zibari GB, McDonald JC. Colorectal cancer in the young patient. *Am Surg* (1998) 64(9):849.

44. Turaga KK. Screening young adults for nonhereditary colorectal cancer. *JAMA Surg* (2015) 150(1):22–3. doi:10.1001/jamasurg.2014.1765

45. Wong MCS, Ching JYL, Wong SH, Ng SC, Shum JP, Chan VCW, et al. The cost-effectiveness of adopting risk-scoring systems for population-based colorectal cancer screening. *Clin Gastroenterol Hepatol* (2015) 13(7):e86. doi:10.1016/j.cgh.2015.04.070

46. Wong MC, Wong SH, Ng SC, Wu JC, Chan FK, Sung JJ. Targeted screening for colorectal cancer in high-risk individuals. *Best Pract Res Clin Gastroenterol* (2015) 29:941–51. doi:10.1016/j.bpg.2015.09.006

47. Schroy PC, Duhovic E, Chen CA, Heeren TC, Lopez W, Apodaca DL, et al. Risk stratification and shared decision making for colorectal cancer screening: a randomized controlled trial. *Med Decis Making* (2016) 36:526–35. doi:10.1177/0272989x15625622

48. Ma G, Ladabaum U. Personalizing colorectal cancer screening: a systematic review of models to predict risk of colorectal neoplasia. *Clin Gastroenterol Hepatol* (2014) 12:1624–34. doi:10.1016/j.cgh.2014.01.042

49. Win AK, MacInnis RJ, Hopper JL, Jenkins MA. Risk prediction models for colorectal cancer: a review. *Cancer Epidemiol Biomarkers Prev* (2012) 21(3):398–410. doi:10.1158/1055-9965.EPI-11-0771

16

Kawasaki Disease and the Use of the Rotavirus Vaccine in Children

Natália Gibim Mellone[1], Marcus Tolentino Silva[1], Mariana Del Grossi Paglia[1], Luciane Cruz Lopes[1], Sílvio Barberato-Filho [1], Fernando de Sá Del Fiol[1] and Cristiane de Cássia Bergamaschi[1]*

[1] *Pharmaceutical Science Graduate Course, University of Sorocaba, Sorocaba, Brazil,*

[2] *Federal University of Amazonas, Faculty of Medicine, Manaus, Brazil*

Correspondence:
Cristiane de Cássia Bergamaschi
cristiane.motta@prof.uniso.br

Background: The vaccine against the rotavirus is an effective measure in reducing hospitalizations and mortality caused by the virus. However, its use can result in serious adverse effects. The available evidence on Kawasaki disease has not yet been reported in the literature. This study investigated the risk of developing Kawasaki disease with the use of rotavirus vaccines in children.

Methods: This is a systematic review of data collected from studies retrieved on the following databases: Cochrane, MEDLINE, Embase, CINAHL, Scopus, Web of Science, HealthSTAR, Lilacs, Clinical trial.gov, and International Clinical Trials Registry Platform, up to the 15th of August 2018, with no restrictions on language or date of publication. The outcomes measured were incidence of Kawasaki disease, risk of developing the disease, and rate of discontinuation of the vaccination schedule. Four reviewers independently selected the studies, performed data extraction, and assessed the quality of evidence. A meta-analysis of random effects was performed.

Results: A total of 13 publications were included, with a population of 164,434 children included in the meta-analysis. The incidence of Kawasaki disease (24 cases per 100,000, 95% CI = 11.98–48.26) in the vaccinated children was low. No difference between the vaccines was found in the prevalence rate of adverse effects (RR = 1.55, 95% CI = 0.41–5.93). Use of the vaccines was not associated with risk of developing Kawasaki disease (low-quality evidence). None of the studies reported the rate of discontinuation of the vaccination schedule.

Conclusions: The vaccines were associated with a low incidence of developing Kawasaki disease, showing no association with this serious adverse effect.

Keywords: Kawasaki disease, rotavirus vaccine, safety, systematic review, adverse effect

INTRODUCTION

The rotavirus is the leading cause of severe diarrhea in infants and children worldwide, particularly in developing countries representing one of the main causes of morbidity in young children globally (Uhlig et al., 2014; Yin et al., 2015). The deaths caused by gastroenteritis due to infection by the rotavirus have been high in low-to-medium income Latin American countries (Bryce et al., 2005) and the Caribbean (Linhares et al., 2011).

Two vaccines are recommended by the World Health Organization (WHO) for use against the rotavirus, referred to as the pentavalent vaccine and the monovalent vaccine, introduced into immunization programs of some countries from 2006 onwards (Uhlig et al., 2014; World Health Organization, 2014). Other vaccines are commercially available, such as the oral monovalent Lanzhou lamb rotavirus in China (Yin et al., 2015), the monovalent Rotavin-M vaccine in Vietnam, and the monovalent Rotavac vaccine in India (Kollaritsch et al., 2015).

In 2009, and again in 2013, the WHO recommended the introduction of one of these vaccines into all national immunization programs (Soares-Weiser et al., 2012). The vaccines are administered *via* the oral route in babies, in two doses for the monovalent vaccine and three for the pentavalent vaccine. The monovalent vaccine is administered at between the 6th and 15th week of life while the pentavalent vaccine is given as a three-dose series between the 6th and 32nd week (Shatsky and Vaccine, 2006).

The most common adverse reactions associated with the use of the vaccine are cough, nasal discharge, diarrhea, irritability, loss of appetite, fever, and vomiting (Bravo et al., 2014). However, its use can also cause serious adverse effects, such as intussusception (Maglione et al., 2014) and Kawasaki disease (Soares-Weiser et al., 2012).

Kawasaki disease was included as a serious adverse effect in the package insert of the pentavalent vaccine after being reviewed by the manufacturer and approved by the Food and Drug Administration (FDA) in 2007, when a pre-licensure clinical trial revealed the presence of this effect in children after use of the vaccine (Hua et al., 2009).

Kawasaki disease has features compatible with common viral infections and mainly affects children, where almost 100% of cases occur in children younger than 5 years and genetically predisposed individuals (Makino et al., 2018). Children of Japanese and Asian-Pacific Island descent have the highest rates, and males have higher rates than females (Fuller, 2019).

In Asian countries, the incidence rates of Kawasaki disease are high (Singh et al., 2015). Recent Japanese data revealed the highest global annual incidence of disease in children under 5 years of age (Makino et al., 2018), with second and third highest rates reported for South Korea (Kim et al., 2014) and Taiwan (Lin et al., 2015), respectively. However, other Asian countries have a steadily increasing incidence of this disease (Saundankar et al., 2014; Wu et al., 2017). In Canada (Lin et al., 2010), the United States (Uehara and Belay, 2012), and Europe (Salo et al., 2012; Jakob et al., 2016), Kawasaki disease rates are significantly lower. The marked differences in incidence rates among different ethnicities strongly support the idea of a strong genetic basis of susceptibility (Holman et al., 2010).

Abbreviations: CINAHL, Cumulative Index to Nursing and Allied Health Literature; GRADE, Grading of Recommendations Assessment Development, and Evaluation; FDA, Food and Drug Administration; WHO, World Health Organization; PRISMA, Preferred Reporting Items for Systematic Reviews and Meta-Analyses; RCT, randomized clinical trials; CENTRAL, Cochrane Central Register of Controlled Trials; PROSPERO, International Prospective Register of Systematic Reviews; VHL, Virtual Health Library; ICTRP, International Clinical Trials Registry Platform.

The disease presents a variety of signs and symptoms, such as persistent fever for longer than 5 days, non-exudative bilateral conjunctivitis, erythema of the lips and oral mucosa, swelling of the extremities, cutaneous eruption, gastrointestinal symptoms, and lymphadenopathy. Aneurysm of the coronary artery or ectasia can develop in 20–25% of cases, along with other complications in untreated children, where the condition may evolve to myocardial infarction, ischemic heart disease, and death (Abrams et al., 2015).

Although most epidemiologic and immunologic evidence suggests that an infectious agent causes Kawasaki disease (Geier et al., 2008), this is not conclusive. Besides, the infectious agent and the genetic characteristics of susceptible children have yet to be elucidated (Principi et al., 2013); it is possible that vaccination play some role in the pathogenesis of Kawasaki disease (Burgner and Harnden, 2005; Rowley and Shulman, 2007). The distinctive immune system characteristics of children with Kawasaki disease could suggest that they respond to all antigenic stimulations, including those due to vaccines (Esposito et al., 2016) in a way that differs from that observed in healthy children. However, the motive, based on biochemical and immunological mechanisms, by which the rotavirus vaccines leads to Kawasaki disease, were not found in the literature.

The available evidence on risk of Kawasaki disease with the use of rotavirus vaccines has not yet been reported in the literature. This knowledge can help guide health professionals in clinical decision-making. This systematic review sought to answer the following PICO question: "what is the risk of Kawasaki disease in children who made use of rotavirus vaccines compared to those who did not?" Therefore, the objective of this study was to investigate the risk of developing Kawasaki disease with the use of rotavirus vaccines in children.

METHODS

Protocol and Registration

The systematic review was performed according to the recommendations specified in the Cochrane Manual of Interventionist Reviews and reported according to the Preferred Reporting Items for Systematic Reviews and Meta-Analyses (PRISMA) checklist (Liberati et al., 2009; Moher et al., 2010; Higgins JPT, 2011)

This protocol was registered on the International Prospective Register of Systematic Reviews (PROSPERO: CRD4201604633, https://www.crd.york.ac.uk/prospero/display_record.php?RecordID=46334).

Eligibility Criteria
Inclusion Criteria

This study included randomized clinical trials (RCT) and quasi-randomized and observational studies (case report, ecological, case series, adverse event report, cross-sectional, case-control, and cohort studies) involving children up to 32 weeks of age in use of vaccines (monovalent or pentavalent) against rotavirus.

Exclusion Criteria
Abstracts published in congresses not providing data on the incidence of the adverse effect were excluded.

Search for Primary Studies
Electronic Searches
The following electronic databases were searched: Cochrane Central Register of Controlled Trials (CENTRAL), MEDLINE (*via* Ovid), Embase, Cumulative Index to Nursing and Allied Health Literature (CINAHL), Web of Science, HealthSTAR (*via* Ovid), Scopus, LILACS, Clinical trial.gov, and International Clinical Trials Registry Platform, up to the 15th of August 2018, with no restrictions on language or date of publication.

Other Search Resources
The references from the eligible studies, the systematic reviews on the rotavirus vaccine, and FDA data were reviewed to identify other eligible studies. The National Health Surveillance Agency in Brazil and the National Brazilian Immunization Program were contacted by email *via* the individuals in charge to check for the existence of reports of Kawasaki disease associated with the vaccines. Information was requested for notifications of the disease as well as related signs and symptoms. Google Scholar (to find unindexed journals), ProQuest Dissertation and Theses Database, the Brazilian Digital Library of Thesis and Dissertations, and the Thesis and Dissertation Catalog of Coordenação de Aperfeiçoamento de Pessoal de Nível Superior (CAPES) were also consulted.

Search Strategies
The following Mesh descriptors and their combinations (entry terms) were used: rotavirus vaccines (or vaccines, rotavirus) and mucocutaneous lymph node syndrome (or Kawasaki syndrome or lymph node syndrome or mucocutaneous, or Kawasaki disease) for the article search. Search strategies for each database used are available in **Supplementary Data Sheet 1**.

Outcomes Assessed
The primary outcome was the incidence of Kawasaki disease associated with the vaccines (number of cases of the disease/total number of children vaccinated for rotavirus). The secondary outcomes were risk of Kawasaki disease comparing each rotavirus vaccine with a control group, and the rate of discontinuation of the vaccination schedule. Given the lack of a standard case definition for the disease, the diagnostic criteria adopted by the studies was used.

The rate of adverse effects was expressed according to the following categories: very common ≥1/10 (≥10%), common ≥1/100 and <1/10 (≥1% and <10%), uncommon ≥1/1,000 and <1/100 (≥0.1% and <1%), rare ≥1/10,000 and <1/1,000 (≥0.01% and <0.1%), and very rare <1/10,000 (<0.01%) (Meyboom and Egberts, 1999).

Study Selection
The reviewers (NM and CB), working independently, selected the potentially relevant studies and applied the eligibility criteria. The full texts of all the potentially eligible articles were obtained and then the reviewers (NGB and MP, FSD-F, and SB-F) assessed the eligibility of each full article. Disagreements were resolved by consensus and, when necessary, submitted to a third reviewer (LL). The Endnote X7 software package was employed for study selection.

Data Extraction
The data were extracted by all reviewers, working independently, using a data extraction form. In the case of articles published only as abstracts or those with key information missing, their respective authors were contacted to obtain the necessary information. Disagreements were again resolved by consensus and, when necessary, submitted to a third reviewer.

Information was collected on: i) the characteristics of the studies (objectives, study design, country where the study was conducted, type of vaccine, data collection period, and conclusions) and ii) the study population (age, gender, race, sample size [number of children vaccinated]), vaccination status (doses of rotavirus vaccine given to child prior to onset of Kawasaki disease), diagnostic method for Kawasaki's disease, time to disease onset after vaccination (days of rotavirus vaccination until the cases developed the disease), and other concomitant vaccinations, when available.

Subgroup analyses were proposed for age, gender, race, and country, where applicable. The heterogeneity of the studies was determined using the χ^2 test and I^2 statistic. The following heterogeneity was considered: 0–25% (low heterogeneity), 50% (moderate heterogeneity), and 75% (high heterogeneity) (Higgins et al., 2003).

Assessment of Risk of Bias
The quality of the observational studies was determined using the tool described by Munn et al. (2014). This step was performed by all reviewers, working in pairs and independently. This tool includes 10 items for critical assessment of the methodological quality of prevalence studies. For each criterion, the study was attributed "yes" or "no" or "not applicable." The total number of "yes" answers per study was tallied. A higher number of "yes" answers indicates a lower risk of bias of the study. The risk of bias of clinical trials was that reported by the systematic review (Soares-Weiser et al., 2012), which used the Cochrane risk of bias tool to assess the following criteria: sequence; allocation concealment; blinding of the patient, healthcare professionals, outcome assessors, data collectors, and data analysts; incomplete outcome data; selective outcome reporting; and major baseline imbalance.

Data Synthesis
The random-effect meta-analysis was performed using the STATA software package (version 14.2) (Montori et al., 2008). Given that this was a systematic review of adverse effect, RCTs and cohort studies were included in the meta-analysis, where both study designs allow information on adverse effects to be collected. Data were summarized according to incidence of the disease per 100,000 vaccinated children and relative risk (RR) with a 95% confidence interval (95% CI). When the meta-analysis was not suitable, a narrative summary of the studies was provided.

Quality of Evidence

The quality of evidence of the studies was assessed using the Grading of Recommendations Assessment, Development, and Evaluation (GRADE) approach (Guyatt et al., 2011). In this approach, RCTs start with high-quality evidence but can be assessed by one or more of the five categories of limitation of the studies: risk of bias, inconsistency, indirect measurement, imprecision, and publication bias. Observational studies start with low-quality evidence, which can increase according to the assessment of the categories.

RESULTS

Literature Search Results

A total of 1,051 publications were revised (after duplicates removed) and 52 potential eligible publications selected. Of these articles, 13 publications (total 14 studies) were included.

One of the publications, a package inserts by the FDA, contained information on two studies: a phase III trial and a phase IV study (**Figure 1**). There were no Brazilian studies or notifications reported in Brazil on Kawasaki disease due to use of the rotavirus vaccines. A search for articles in the references of the systematic review (Soares-Weiser et al., 2012) led to the identification of a further three clinical trials (Phua et al., 2005; Phua et al., 2009; Salinas et al., 2005), which were subsequently included in the study.

Description of Studies Included in Narrative Syntheses

The characteristics and outcomes of the studies included are given in **Table 1** (descending order of year of publication). This review found information in: two case reports (Uhlig et al., 2014; Chang and Islam, 2018), four cohort studies (Belongia et al., 2010; Loughlin et al., 2012; Layton et al., 2018; RotaTeq, 2017),

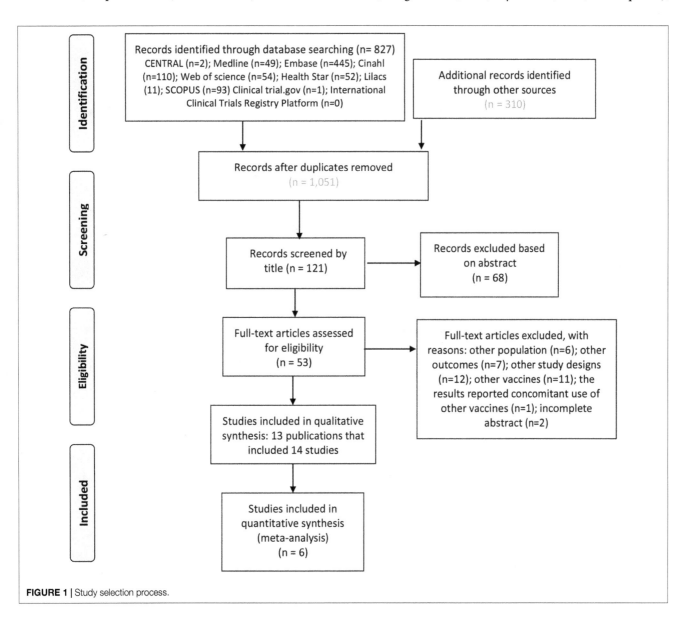

FIGURE 1 | Study selection process.

TABLE 1 | Characteristics of the studies and outcomes found in children vaccinated against the rotavirus.

Author (year)	Study design	Data collection period	Country	Vaccines	Diagnostic methods of KD	N of KD cases	Total (N of children vaccinated)	Total of children with AE	OR or RR (95% CI)
Chang and Islam (2018)	Case report	NR	USA	RV1	Standard (AHA)	1	1	1	Not applicable
Layton et al. (2018)	Cohort	2006–2014	USA	RV1 and RV5	ICD	23	2,468,002	NR	RR = 0.54 (0.20–1.48)
Yin et al. (2015) (Park et al., 2011)	Case report	2015	China	LLR	NR	1	1	1	Not applicable
Paulke-Korinek et al. (2013)	Adverse event reports	2010–2011	Austria	RV1 and RV5	NR	0	NR	823	Not applicable
Loughlin et al. (2012)	Cohort	2006–2007	USA	RV5	ICD	3	85,150	NR	RR = 0.4 (0.01–8.47)
Belongia et al. (2010)	Cohort	2006–2008	USA	RV5	Medical record	16	207,621	NR	OR = 0.28 (0.07–1.09)
Oberle et al. (2010)	Cross-sectional	2001–2009	Germany	RV5	Medical record	4	NR	1.088	OR = 3.1 (1.1–9.1)
Information from package insert (phase III trial) (M. U.S. Food and Drug Administration)	RCT	NR	NR	RV5	NR	5	36,150	NR	RR = 4.9 (0.6–239.1)
Information from package insert (phase IV study) (M. U.S. Food and Drug Administration)	Cohort	NR	NR	RV5	NR	1	17,433	NR	RR = 0.7 (0.01–55.56)
Hua et al. (2009)	Adverse event reports	1990–2007	USA	RV5	Medical records	16	NR	239,535	NR
Phua et al. (2009)	RCT	2003–2005	Hong Kong, Singapore, and Taiwan	RV1	NR	1	4,272	NR	RR = 2.9 (0.12–72.83)
Geier et al. (2008)	Adverse event reports	2006–2007	USA	RV5	NR	16	NR	1,526	NR
Phua et al. (2005)	RCT	2001–2003	Singapore	RV1	NR	2	1,811	NR	RR = 1.8 (0.09–37.53)
Salinas et al. (2005)	RCT	2001–2003	Brazil, Mexico, and Venezuela	RV1	NR	1	1,618	NR	RR = 1.0 (0.04–24.44)

USA, United States of America; AHA, American Heart Association; KD, Kawasaki disease; AE, adverse effect; OR, odds ratio; RR, relative risk; 95% CI, 95% confidence interval; NR, not reported; RV1, monovalent vaccine; RV5, pentavalent vaccine; ICD, International Classification of Disease; LLR, Lanzhou lamb rotavirus; RCT, randomized clinical trial.

one cross-sectional study (Oberle et al., 2010), three adverse event reports (Geier et al., 2008; Hua et al., 2009; Paulke-Korinek et al., 2013), and four RCTs (Phua et al., 2005; Salinas et al., 2005; Phua et al., 2009; RotaTeq, 2017).

One case report described a 4-month-old Caucasian child, presenting classic Kawasaki disease shortly after receiving vaccines (pneumococcal 13, diphtheria–tetanus–pertussis, polio, Hepatitis B, and rotavirus vaccine). The case supports that vaccines may be associated with vasculitis and Kawasaki disease and that ongoing, systematic surveillance of such events is warranted (Chang and Islam, 2018).

Only one study reported the use of the Lanzhou lamb rotavirus vaccine. It consisted of a clinical case report of a 20-month-old Chinese child with Kawasaki disease after use of the rotavirus vaccine concomitantly with the hepatitis A vaccine. According to the authors, the rotavirus vaccine may have played a key role in the development of the disease, but no causal relationship between the effect and the vaccine could be established based on a single case (Yin et al., 2015).

A cohort study of commercial insurance data investigated the risk of adverse events associated with rotavirus vaccines. Most children received a concomitant diphtheria–tetanus–pertussis vaccine. Of a total of 2,468,002 vaccines, 23 cases of Kawasaki disease were found (Layton et al., 2018).

An adverse event report study determined the prevalence of adverse events associated with the monovalent and pentavalent vaccines using the sentinel surveillance system. A total of 833 adverse events were associated with the vaccines, but no cases of Kawasaki disease were reported (Paulke-Korinek et al., 2013).

The cohort study identified post-marketing adverse effects after routine use of the pentavalent vaccine from records held on an electronic database. Of the 85,150 children that received the rotavirus vaccine, there were 3 cases of Kawasaki disease in the intervention group (only 1 case was confirmed to have occurred within 30 days of vaccination) and 1 in the control group (recipients of diphtheria–tetanus–acellular pertussis vaccine). No increased risk of developing the disease due to the vaccine was observed (Loughlin et al., 2012).

Another cohort study assessed the risk of intussusception and other adverse events using the Vaccine Adverse Event Reporting System (VAERS) database among children aged 4–48 weeks who received the pentavalent vaccine (intervention group) compared to a non-exposed group. Similarly, no association of developing Kawasaki disease with use of the pentavalent vaccine was found (Geier et al., 2008).

A cross-sectional study used the database of the Paul Ehrlich Institute to assess the cases of Kawasaki disease associated with the use of monovalent and pentavalent vaccines (between 2001 and 2010). Four cases of the disease were reported from a total of 1,088 adverse events associated with the use of the pentavalent vaccine in children aged 2–5 months. The study reported the day on which the effect occurred (average of 6.3 days after vaccination). Three children were in use of another vaccine concomitantly (Oberle et al., 2010).

An adverse event report study assessed the data on adverse events associated with the pentavalent vaccine using the VAERS database. A total of 1,526 adverse events were associated with the pentavalent vaccine. Of 16 children found to have Kawasaki disease, 5 used this vaccine (Belongia et al., 2010).

Another study also searched the VAERS information to identify Kawasaki disease in children following use of vaccines with licensure in the United States. The authors identified a total of 239,535 events, including 107 cases of Kawasaki disease, 16 of which were following the use of the pentavalent vaccine. The study did not specify the number of pentavalent vaccines administered (Hua et al., 2009).

The package inserts by the FDA for the pentavalent vaccine described the results of two studies (a post-marketing study—phase IV and phase III clinical trials—the Rotavirus Efficacy Safety Trial/REST). The cohort study compared the data on the disease in 17,433 children who received the pentavalent vaccine *versus* a control group of 12,339 that received a diphtheria, tetanus, and pertussis vaccine, revealing only one case of Kawasaki disease within 30 days of vaccination (RotaTeq, 2017).

The clinical trial found five cases of Kawasaki disease in 36,160 vaccinated children and one case in 35,536 children who received a placebo (42 days after the use of the pentavalent vaccine). The other three clinical trials also found no association of the adverse effect with the use of the monovalent vaccine (Phua et al., 2005; Phua et al., 2009; Salinas et al., 2005).

Risk of Bias of the Studies

The cohort studies had risk of bias, having failed to account for possible confounding factors and/or to perform subgroup analyses. The cross-sectional and adverse event report studies had shortcomings for a larger number of assessed criteria that included the problems observed in the cohort studies plus those of data analysis with problems of underestimation of prevalence data for Kawasaki disease (**Table 2**).

It was not possible to assess risk of bias of the studies described in the package insert of the pentavalent vaccine because some information pertaining to these studies could not be accessed (RotaTeq, 2017). According to a systematic review (Soares-Weiser et al., 2012), one of the clinical studies (Phua et al., 2009) fulfilled all the assessment criteria for risk of bias and, therefore, had minimum bias risk. Another clinical trial (Salinas et al., 2005) had risk of bias for allocation and reporting of selective outcomes, whereas one study (Phua et al., 2005) had risk of bias for most of the criteria assessed.

Results of Outcome Evaluated and Quality of Evidence

None of the studies reported the rate of discontinuation of the vaccination schedule. Some studies were not included in the meta-analysis because they failed to report data on the incidence of Kawasaki disease.

The meta-analysis revealed a rare incidence of cases of Kawasaki disease, with 24 cases per 100,000 vaccinated children for both vaccines (95% CI = 11.98–48.26). No differences between vaccines were found for incidence of the adverse effect (relative risk = 1.55 95% CI = 0.41–5.93) (**Figure 2**).

TABLE 2 | Risk of bias of observational studies according to criteria adopted by Munn et al. (2014).

Study author and year	Was the sample representative of the target population?	Were study participants recruited in an appropriate way?	Was the sample size adequate?	Were the study subjects and setting described in detail?	Was the data analysis conducted with sufficient coverage of the identified sample?	Were objective, standard criteria used for measurement of the condition?	Was the condition measured reliably?	Was there appropriate statistical analysis?	Are all important confounding factors/subgroups/differences identified and accounted for?	Were subpopulation identified using objective criteria?	Total number of "yes"
Layton et al. (2018)	Yes	Yes	Yes	Yes	Yes	Not applicable	Not applicable	Yes	No	Not applicable	6
Paulke-Korinek et al. (2013)	Yes	Yes	Yes	Yes	No	No	Not applicable	Yes	No	Not applicable	5
Loughlin et al. (2012)	Yes	Yes	Yes	Yes	Yes	Yes	Not applicable	Yes	No	No	7
Belongia et al. (2010)	Yes	Yes	Yes	Yes	No	Yes	Not applicable	Yes	No	No	6
Oberle et al. (2010)	Yes	Yes	Yes	Yes	No	Yes	Not applicable	Yes	No	No	6
Hua et al. (2009)	Yes	Yes	Yes	Yes	No	Yes	Not applicable	Not applicable	No	No	5
Geier et al. (2008)	Yes	Yes	Yes	Yes	No	No	Not applicable	No	No	No	4

The risk of developing Kawasaki disease in the group of children receiving the vaccines did not differ to the comparator group, where no statistical difference was found between them. No heterogeneity was observed among the studies (**Figure 3**). However, the quality of the evidence according to the GRADE criteria for this outcome was considered low for both the vaccines, due to the high risk of bias, and imprecision in the results obtained.

Subgroup analyses were performed between studies conducted in the West (Salinas et al., 2005; Loughlin et al., 2012) and Asian-Pacific (Phua et al., 2005; Phua et al., 2009) countries. There was a higher incidence of disease in Asian-Pacific (57 per 100,000, $I^2 = 49.4\%$) compared to Western (23 per 100,000, $I^2 = 60.5\%$) countries. Subgroup analyses were not carried out for age, gender, and race due to the absence of information in the eligible studies.

DISCUSSION

Summary of Findings and Their Interpretation With the Available Literature

The findings of this review showed that the occurrence of Kawasaki disease is rare in children that received the monovalent or pentavalent vaccines. In addition, the risk of having the disease in the children receiving the vaccines against the rotavirus did not differ to comparator group.

A total of 13 publications reporting the frequency of the Kawasaki disease were included, the majority of which were conducted in the United States of America and Asian countries. The studies reported information on both the monovalent and pentavalent vaccines, where only one case report was found on the Lanzhou lamb rotavirus, marketed solely in China.

In general, the studies concluded that there was no increased risk or causal relationship of the adverse effect with use of the vaccines. However, some publications (Geier et al., 2008; Hua et al., 2009; Belongia et al., 2010) reported the need for monitoring the use of these vaccines in order to gather further information on their safety.

The rate of discontinuation of the vaccination schedule was not reported in included studies. This occurred either because the cross-sectional studies described the adverse effects reported in the databases or because the longitudinal studies did not bother to collect this outcome, important for endemic control programs.

The studies that involved the collection of information in databases were not included in the meta-analysis owing to the absence of data enabling the incidence of the adverse effect to be determined. The authors of these studies highlighted some shortcomings in the collection of the information in the databases used. The difficulty establishing a causal relationship between Kawasaki disease and the use of the vaccine stems, in part, from uncertainties regarding the information reported in the databases (Paulke-Korinek et al., 2013), and from the concomitant use of the rotavirus vaccine with vaccines against diphtheria, tetanus, and pertussis and/or pneumococcus, among others (Hua et al., 2009; Oberle et al., 2010; Layton et al., 2018), demonstrating that other vaccines could also cause the disease.

In the researched literature, we found studies that evaluated the use of vaccines in children, such as measles, mumps, rubella,

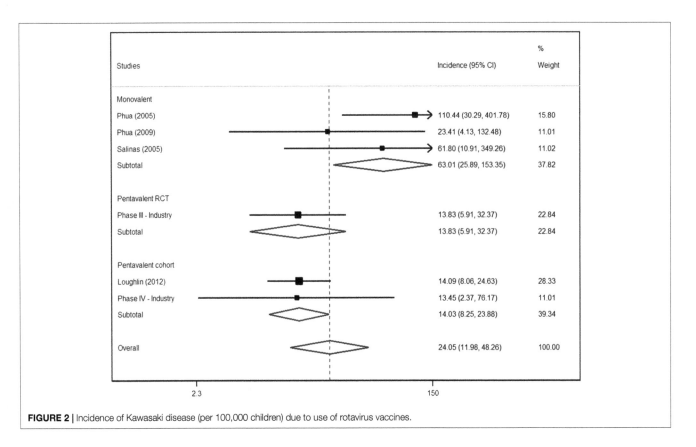

FIGURE 2 | Incidence of Kawasaki disease (per 100,000 children) due to use of rotavirus vaccines.

and varicella (MMRV) vaccine; measles, mumps, and rubella (MMR) vaccine (Holman et al., 2010); and pneumococcal vaccine (Park et al., 2011) and observed no association between vaccination and Kawasaki disease. We found no studies that evaluated the risk of Kawasaki disease due to combination of the rotavirus vaccine with any other vaccine (diphtheria, tetanus, and pertussis and/or pneumococcus).

In the present study, higher incidence of disease in Asian-Pacific countries compared to Western countries was observed. These results agree with the literature that have reported higher incidence of the disease in children of Asian and Japanese ethnicities (Holman et al., 2010; Park et al., 2011). However, the genetic characteristics of those children susceptible remain only partially elucidated (Principi et al., 2013). Subgroups analysis for age, gender, and race were not performed due to the absence of information in the eligible studies.

In addition, some studies failed to report how Kawasaki disease was diagnosed or reported, such as the studies based on data from the VAERS (Geier et al., 2008; Hua et al., 2009). The authors noted that the rates of notifications obtained by the system could not be interpreted as real, given possible under-reporting of the adverse effects, which in turn may have been largely due to difficulties confirming the disease diagnosis and to the way this is recorded on the systems.

The revision of the package insert of pentavalent vaccine carried out in 2007, which included Kawasaki as a serious adverse effect, which led to an increase in the number of notifications of this disease (Hua et al., 2009; Hua et al., 2010; Oberle et al., 2010).

The study of Hua et al. (2009) noted a rise in the number of annual cases from 0.65 to 2.78 per 100,000 children less than 5 years of age followed for up to 30 days post-vaccination, after amendment of the insert.

Assessment of Study Validity: Limitations and Strengths

The difficulty in the description of the information registered on the systems/databases reported by the studies is a limitation of the present investigation. Measurement bias was also observed, owing to problems concerning the description of method of disease diagnosis (or absence of standard for diagnosis), which was not reported by some of the studies. This might be explained, in part, by difficulties studying Kawasaki disease, given the lack of a standard case definition coupled with insufficient knowledge of etiology.

The lack of a standard for diagnosing the disease can lead to the inherent underreporting of data on these databases. However, this occurred mainly in cross-sectional and adverse event report studies, which were not included in the meta-analysis.

In cases where the information on some RCTs proved inaccessible, the diagnostic criteria for the disease were described as "not reported." However, the design of this type of study ensures, with some confidence, that the adverse effect was measured rigorously. With regard to the observational studies, it is important to emphasize that the results found in the meta-analysis do not imply causation, since there is always the possibility of residual confounding in these studies.

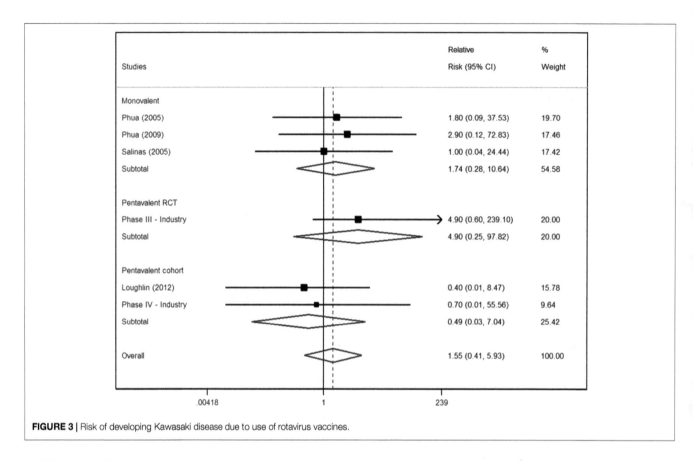

FIGURE 3 | Risk of developing Kawasaki disease due to use of rotavirus vaccines.

Despite the broad search of scientific articles in several different databases and exhaustive attempts to obtain the missing information for some of the selected studies, few studies contained all the information required, as exemplified by some information from clinical trials provided by the systematic review and the absence of details in some studies described (such as number of doses of the rotavirus vaccine given prior to onset of Kawasaki disease, time to onset of Kawasaki disease after rotavirus vaccination, use of concomitant vaccinations, among others), hampering the analysis of bias risk. This study did not search specific databases for Asian and Japanese children, in whom the literature indicates a possible higher prevalence of the disease.

Notwithstanding, this systematic review and meta-analysis pooled the incidence of Kawasaki disease due to use of the rotavirus vaccine. The results exhibited no heterogeneity across studies, partly due to the high number of participants. Moreover, the method employed in this study was rigorous with explicit eligibility criteria and a broad search. The assessment of the quality of evidence was based on an independent assessment of bias risk, imprecision, consistency, indirect measures, and publication bias.

Clinical Implications and Future Perspectives

The results of the present study suggest no association of Kawasaki disease with the use of monovalent and pentavalent vaccines. However, these results should be interpreted with

caution due to low quality of the evidence from the studies included in the meta-analysis. The difficulty in conducting studies that did not associate rotavirus vaccine with other vaccines is due to the age of children who are receiving many of them. This difficulty finds robust epidemiological evidence to associate this adverse effect with the rotavirus vaccine. Then, future studies should be concerned with minimizing these biases.

The study also showed that observational studies assessing the incidence and causality of this adverse effect in the literature are scarce. This information underscores the importance of the use of vaccines, in view of the risks of contamination by the rotavirus in children under 5 years and the efficacy of these in preventing the infection (Tate and Parashar, 2014; Kollaritsch et al., 2015; Santos et al., 2016). However, the literature studied highlights the need for notification of adverse effects related to the vaccines in order to ensure continuous monitoring of these and other possible effects associated with the vaccines.

Although the results indicate low incidence of Kawasaki disease in children that used the rotavirus vaccines, it is important that health professionals and society at large report these and other adverse effects associated with the vaccines, rendering notification common practice, thereby contributing to the monitoring of safety data on the use of vaccines. This study reports the evidence on risk of Kawasaki disease with the use of rotavirus vaccines, and this finding can help guide health professionals in clinical decision-making.

CONCLUSION

The results of the present study indicate that the monovalent and pentavalent vaccines were associated with a low incidence of developing Kawasaki disease, showing no association with this serious adverse effect. However, further studies involving larger samples are needed to confirm these findings.

AUTHOR CONTRIBUTIONS

NM is the principal investigator, participated in all stages of the study, and oversaw the writing of the manuscript. CB and MS are the project managers and co-investigators, were involved in study selection and extraction and statistical analysis, and contributed to the writing and revision of the manuscript. LL, MM, FDF, and SB-F are co-investigators, took part in study selection and extraction and contributed to the writing and revision of the manuscript. All authors read and approved the final manuscript.

FUNDING

This project is funded by the governmental Program Graduate Education Institutions-PROSUP-CAPES/UNISO.

REFERENCES

Abrams, J. Y., Weintraub, E. S., Baggs, J. M., McCarthy, N. L., Schonberger, L. B., Lee, G. M., et al. (2015). Childhood vaccines and Kawasaki disease, Vaccine Safety Datalink, 1996-2006. *Vaccine* 33, 382–387. doi: 10.1016/j.vaccine.2014.10.044

Belongia, E. A., Irving, S. A., Shui, I. M., Kulldorff, M., Lewis, E., Yin, R., et al. (2010). Real-time surveillance to assess risk of intussusception and other adverse events after pentavalent, bovine-derived rotavirus vaccine. *Pediatr. Infect. Dis. J.* 29, 1–5. doi: 10.1097/INF.0b013e3181af8605

Bravo, L., Chitraka, A., Liu, A., Choudhury, J., Kumar, K., Berezo, L., et al. (2014). Reactogenicity and safety of the human rotavirus vaccine, Rotarix in The Philippines, Sri Lanka, and India: a post-marketing surveillance study. *Hum. Vaccin. Immunother.* 10, 2276–2283. doi: 10.4161/hv.29280

Bryce, J., Boschi-Pinto, C., Shibuya, K., and Black, R. E. (2005). WHO estimates of the causes of death in children. *Lancet* 365, 1147–1152. doi: 10.1016/S0140-6736(05)71877-8

Burgner, D., and Harnden, A. (2005). Kawasaki disease: what is the epidemiology telling us about the etiology? *Int. J. Infect. Dis.* 9, 185–194. doi: 10.1016/j.ijid.2005.03.002

Chang, A., and Islam, S. (2018). Kawasaki disease and vasculitis associated with immunizations. *Pediatr. Int.* 60 (7), 613–617. doi: 10.1111/ped.13590

Esposito, S., Bianchini, S., Dellepiane, R. M., and Principi, N. (2016). Vaccines and Kawasaki disease. *Expert Rev. Vaccines* 15, 417–424. doi: 10.1586/14760584.2016.1128329

Fuller, M. G. (2019). Kawasaki disease in infancy. *Adv. Emergency Nurs. J.* 41, 222–228. doi: 10.1097/TME.0000000000000253

Geier, D. A., King, P. G., Sykes, L. K., and Geier, M. R. (2008). RotaTeq vaccine adverse events and policy considerations. *Med. Sci. Monit.* 14, Ph9–P16. doi: 10.2188/jea.je20110131

Guyatt, G. H., Oxman, A. D., Kunz, R., Woodcock, J., Brozek, J., Helfand, M., et al. (2011). GRADE guidelines: 7. Rating the quality of evidence—inconsistency. *J. Clin. Epidemiol.* 64, 1294–1302. doi: 10.1016/j.jclinepi.2011.03.017

Higgins JPT, Green S (Eds) (2011). *Cochrane Handbook for Systematic Reviews of Interventions Version 5.1.0.* The Cochrane Collaboration. Available from: http://handbook.cochrane.org.

Higgins, J. P., Thompson, S. G., Deeks, J. J., and Altman, D. G. (2003). Measuring inconsistency in meta-analyses. *Bmj* 327, 557–560. doi: 10.1136/bmj.327.7414.557

Holman, R. C., Belay, E. D., Christensen, K. Y., Folkema, A. M., Steiner, C. A., and Schonberger, L. B. (2010). Hospitalizations for Kawasaki syndrome among children in the United States, 1997-2007. *Pediatr. Infect. Dis. J.* 29, 483–488. doi: 10.1097/INF.0b013e3181cf8705

Holman, R. C., Christensen, K. Y., Belay, E. D., Steiner, C. A., Effler, P. V., Miyamura, J., et al. (2010). Racial/ethnic differences in the incidence of Kawasaki syndrome among children in Hawaii. *Hawaii Med. J.* 69, 194.

Hua, W., Izurieta, H. S., Slade, B., Belay, E. D., Haber, P., Tiernan, R., et al. (2009). Kawasaki disease after vaccination: reports to the vaccine adverse event reporting system 1990-2007. *Pediatr. Infect. Dis. J.* 28, 943–947. doi: 10.1097/INF.0b013e3181a66471

Hua, W., Tiernan, R., and Steffey, A. (2010). Postmarketing safety review for rotarix1: data from the vaccine adverse event reporting system (VAERS), April 2008-October 2009. *Pharmacoepidemiol. Drug Saf.* 19, 326–327.

Jakob, A., Whelan, J., Kordecki, M., Berner, R., Stiller, B., Arnold, R., et al. (2016). Kawasaki disease in Germany: a prospective, population-based study adjusted for underreporting. *Pediatr. Infect. Dis. J.* 35, 129–134. doi: 10.1097/INF.0000000000000953

Kim, G. B., Han, J. W., Park, Y. W., Song, M. S., Hong, Y. M., Cha, S. H., et al. (2014). Epidemiologic features of Kawasaki disease in South Korea: data from nationwide survey, 2009-2011. *Pediatr. Infect. Dis. J.* 33, 24–27. doi: 10.1097/INF.0000000000000010

Kollaritsch, H., Kundi, M., Giaquinto, C., and Paulke-Korinek, M. (2015). Rotavirus vaccines: a story of success. *Clin. Microbiol. Infect.* 21, 735–743. doi: 10.1016/j.cmi.2015.01.027

Layton, J. B., Butler, A. M., Panozzo, C. A., and Brookhart, M. A. (2018). Rotavirus vaccination and short-term risk of adverse events in US infants. *Pediatr. Perinat. Epidemiol.* 32 (5), 448–457. doi: 10.1111/ppe.12496

Liberati, A., Altman, D. G., Tetzlaff, J., Mulrow, C., Gøtzsche, P. C., Ioannidis, J. P., et al. (2009). The PRISMA statement for reporting systematic reviews and meta-analyses of studies that evaluate health care interventions: explanation and elaboration. *PLoS Med.* 6, e1000100. doi: 10.1371/journal.pmed.1000100

Lin, Y. T., Manlhiot, C., Ching, J. C., Han, R. K., Nield, L. E., Dillenburg, R., et al. (2010). Repeated systematic surveillance of Kawasaki disease in Ontario from 1995 to 2006. *Pediatr. Int.* 52, 699–706. doi: 10.1111/j.1442-200X.2010.03092.x

Lin, M. C., Lai, M. S., Jan, S. L., and Fu, Y. C. (2015). Epidemiologic features of Kawasaki disease in acute stages in Taiwan, 1997–2010: effect of different case definitions in claims data analysis. *J. Chin. Med. Assoc.: JCMA* 78, 121–126. doi: 10.1016/j.jcma.2014.03.009

Linhares, A. C., Stupka, J. A., Ciapponi, A., Bardach, A. E., Glujovsky, D., Aruj, P. K., et al. (2011). Burden and typing of rotavirus group A in Latin America and the Caribbean: systematic review and meta-analysis. *Rev. Med. Virol.* 21, 89–109. doi: 10.1002/rmv.682

Loughlin, J., Mast, T. C., Doherty, M. C., Wang, F. T., Wong, J., and Seeger, J. D. (2012). Postmarketing evaluation of the short-term safety of the pentavalent rotavirus vaccine. *Pediatr. Infect. Dis. J.* 31, 292–296. doi: 10.1097/INF.0b013e3182421390

Maglione, M. A., Das, L., Raaen, L., Smith, A., Chari, R., Newberry, S., et al. (2014). Safety of vaccines used for routine immunization of U.S. children: a systematic review. *Pediatrics* 134, 325–337. doi: 10.1542/peds.2014-1079

Makino, N., Nakamura, Y., Yashiro, M., Sano, T., Ae, R., Kosami, K. et al. (2018). Epidemiological observations of Kawasaki disease in Japan, 2013–2014. *Pediatr. Int.* 60 (6), 581–587. doi: 10.1111/ped.13544

Meyboom, R. H., and Egberts, A. C. (1999). Comparing therapeutic benefit and risk. *Therapie* 54, 29–34.

Moher, D., Liberati, A., Tetzlaff, J., and Altman, D. G. (2010). Preferred reporting items for systematic reviews and meta-analyses: the PRISMA statement. *Int. J. Surg.* 8, 336–341. doi: 10.1016/j.ijsu.2010.02.007

Montori, V., Guyatt, G., Oxman, A., Cook, D., and Drummond, R. (2008). Fixed-effects and random-effects models. *JAMA's Users' Guides to the Medical Literature: A Manual for Evidence-Based Clinical Practice.* 555–562.

Munn, Z., Moola, S., Riitano, D., and Lisy, K. (2014). The development of a critical appraisal tool for use in systematic reviews addressing questions of prevalence. *Int. J. Health Policy Manage.* 3, 123–128. doi: 10.15171/ijhpm.2014.71

Oberle, D., Pönisch, C., Weißer, K., Keller-Stanislawski., B., and Mentzer, D. (2010). Schutzimpfung gegen Rotavirusgastroenteritis. Assoziation mit dem Kawasaki-Syndrom? *Monatsschrift Kinderheilkunde* 158, 1253–1260. doi: 10.1007/s00112-010-2309-y

Park, Y. W., Han, J. W., Hong, Y. M., Ma, J. S., Cha, S. H., Kwon, T. C., et al. (2011). Epidemiological features of Kawasaki disease in Korea, 2006-2008. *Pediatr. Int.: Off. J. Jpn. Pediatr. Soc.* 53, 36–39. doi: 10.1111/j.1442-200X.2010.03178.x

Paulke-Korinek, M., Kollaritsch, H., Aberle, S. W., Zwazl, I., Schmidle-Loss, B., Vecsei, A., et al. (2013). Sustained low hospitalization rates after four years of rotavirus mass vaccination in Austria. *Vaccine* 31, 2686–2691. doi: 10.1016/j.vaccine.2013.04.001

Phua, K. B., Quak, S. H., Lee, B. W., Emmanuel, S. C., Goh, P., Han, H. H., et al. (2005). Evaluation of RIX4414, a live, attenuated rotavirus vaccine, in a randomized, double-blind, placebo-controlled phase 2 trial involving 2464 Singaporean infants. *J. Infect. Dis.* 192 Suppl (1), S6–s16. doi: 10.1086/431511

Phua, K. B., Lim, F. S., Lau, Y. L., Nelson, E. A., Huang, L. M., Quak, S. H., et al. (2009). Safety and efficacy of human rotavirus vaccine during the first 2 years of life in Asian infants: randomised, double-blind, controlled study. *Vaccine* 27, 5936–5941. doi: 10.1016/j.vaccine.2009.07.098

Principi, N., Rigante, D., and Esposito, S. (2013). The role of infection in Kawasaki syndrome. *J. Infect.* 67, 1–10. doi: 10.1016/j.jinf.2013.04.004

RotaTeq (Rotavirus vaccine, live, oral, pentavalent) (2017). United States Prescribing Information. Revised February 2017, US Food & Drug Administration. Available online at: https://www.fda.gov/vaccines-blood-biologics/approved-vaccine-products/rotavirus-vaccine-live-oral-pentavalent (Accessed on March 07, 2017).

Rowley, A. H., and Shulman, S. T. (2007). New developments in the search for the etiologic agent of Kawasaki disease. *Curr. Opin. Pediatr.* 19, 71–74. doi: 10.1097/MOP.0b013e328012720f

Salinas, B., Perez Schael, I., Linhares, A. C., Ruiz Palacios, G. M., Guerrero, M. L., Yarzabal, J. P., et al. (2005). Evaluation of safety, immunogenicity and efficacy of an attenuated rotavirus vaccine, RIX4414: a randomized, placebo-controlled trial in Latin American infants. *Pediatr. Infect. Dis. J.* 24, 807–816. doi: 10.1097/01.inf.0000178294.13954.a1

Salo, E., Griffiths, E. P., Farstad, T., Schiller, B., Nakamura, Y., Yashiro, M., et al. (2012). Incidence of Kawasaki disease in Northern European countries. *Pediatr. Int. Off. J. Jpn. Pediatr. Soc.* 54, 770–772. doi: 10.1111/j.1442-200X.2012.03692.x

Santos, V. S., Marques, D. P., Martins-Filho, P. R., Cuevas, L. E., and Gurgel, R. Q. (2016). Effectiveness of rotavirus vaccines against rotavirus infection and hospitalization in Latin America: systematic review and meta-analysis. *Infect. Dis. Poverty* 5, 83. doi: 10.1186/s40249-016-0173-2

Saundankar, J., Yim, D., Itotoh, B., Payne, R., Maslin, K., Jape, G., et al. (2014). The epidemiology and clinical features of Kawasaki disease in Australia. *Pediatrics* 133, e1009–e1014. doi: 10.1542/peds.2013-2936

Shatsky, M., and Vaccine, Rotavirus (2006). Live, Oral, Pentavalent (RotaTeq) for prevention of rotavirus gastroenteritis. *Am. Family Physician* 74, 1014–1015.

Singh, S., Vignesh, P., and Burgner, D. (2015). The epidemiology of Kawasaki disease: a global update. *Arch. Dis. Childhood* 100, 1084–1088. doi: 10.1136/archdischild-2014-307536

Soares-Weiser, K., Maclehose, H., Bergman, H., Ben-Aharon, I., Nagpal, S., Goldberg, E., et al. (2012). Vaccines for preventing rotavirus diarrhoea: vaccines in use. *Cochrane Database Syst. Rev.* 14 (11), CD008521. doi: 10.1002/14651858.CD008521.pub2

Tate, J. E., and Parashar, U. D. (2014). Rotavirus vaccines in routine use. *Clin. Infect. Dis.* 59, 1291–1301. doi: 10.1093/cid/ciu564

Uehara, R., and Belay, E. D. (2012). Epidemiology of kawasaki disease in Asia, Europe, and the United States. *J. Epidemiol.* 1201310285–1201310285. 22 (2), 79–85. doi: 10.2188/jea.JE20110131

Uhlig, U., Kostev, K., Schuster, V., Koletzko, S., and Uhlig, H. H. (2014). Impact of rotavirus vaccination in Germany: rotavirus surveillance, hospitalization, side effects and comparison of vaccines. *Pediatr. Infect. Dis. J.* 33, e299–e304. doi: 10.1097/INF.0000000000000441

World Health Organization. (2014). Safety profile of a novel live attenuated rotavirus vaccine. *WER.* 89, 326–327.

Wu, M.-H., Lin, M.-T., Chen, H.-C., Kao, F.-Y., and Huang, S.-K. (2017). Postnatal risk of acquiring Kawasaki disease: a nationwide birth cohort database study. *J. Pediatr.* 180, 80–86. e2. doi: 10.1016/j.jpeds.2016.09.052

Yin, S., Liubao, P., Chongqing, T., and Xiaomin, W. (2015). The first case of Kawasaki disease in a 20-month old baby following immunization with rotavirus vaccine and hepatitis A vaccine in China: a case report. *Hum. Vaccin. Immunother.* 11, 2740–2743 doi: 10.1080/21645515.2015.1050571

Efficacy and Safety of Brinzolamide as Add-On to Prostaglandin Analogues or β-Blocker for Glaucoma and Ocular Hypertension

Yuanzhi Liu[1], Junyi Zhao[1,2], Xiaoyan Zhong[1], Qiming Wei[1] and Yilan Huang[1]*

[1] Department of Pharmacy, The Affiliated Hospital of Southwest Medical University, Luzhou, China,

[2] College of Pharmacy, Southwest Medical University, Luzhou, China

*Corresponding author:
Yilan Huang
hyl3160131@163.com

Background: Brinzolamide as a carbonic anhydrase inhibitor could be combined with other intraocular pressure (IOP) lowering drugs for glaucoma and ocular hypertension (OHT), but the efficacy was controversial. So, this study was used to assess the efficacy and safety of brinzolamide as add-on to prostaglandin analogues (PGAs) or β-blocker in treating patients with glaucoma or OHT who fail to adequately control IOP.

Methods: We searched PubMed, Embase, MEDLINE, Cochrane Library, and clinicaltrials.gov from inception to October 4, 2018. Randomized controlled trials of brinzolamide as add-on to PGAs or β-blocker for glaucoma and OHT were included. Meta-analysis was conducted by RevMan 5.3 software.

Results: A total of 26 trials including 5,583 patients were analyzed. Brinzolamide produced absolute reductions of IOP as an adjunctive therapy for patients with glaucoma or OHT. Brinzolamide and timolol were not significantly different in lowering IOP as add-on to PGAs (9 am: $P = 0.07$; 12 am: $P = 0.66$; 4 pm: $P = 0.66$). Likewise, brinzolamide was as effective as dorzolamide in depressing IOP (9 am: $P = 0.59$; 12 am: $P = 0.94$; 4 pm: $P = 0.95$). For the mean diurnal IOP at the end of treatment duration, there were no statistical differences in above comparisons ($P > 0.05$). Compared with brimonidine (b.i.d.), there was a significant reduction of IOP in brinzolamide (b.i.d.) at 9 am ($P < 0.0001$); however, the difference was cloudy in thrice daily subgroup ($P = 0.44$); at 12 am, brinzolamide (b.i.d.) was similar to brimonidine (b.i.d.) in IOP-lowering effect ($P = 0.23$), whereas brimonidine (t.i.d.) led to a greater effect than brinzolamide (t.i.d.) ($P = 0.02$). At 4 pm, brinzolamide (b.i.d.) was superior IOP-lowering effect compared with brimonidine (b.i.d.) ($P = 0.0003$); conversely, the effect in brinzolamide (t.i.d.) was lower than brimonidine (t.i.d.) ($P < 0.0001$). For the mean diurnal IOP, brinzolamide was lower in twice daily subgroup ($P < 0.00001$); brimonidine was lower in thrice daily subgroup ($P < 0.00001$). With regard to the safety, brinzolamide and dorzolamide had a higher incidence of taste abnormality; moreover, brinzolamide resulted in more frequent blurred vision;

dorzolamide resulted in more frequent ocular discomfort and eye pain. Timolol resulted in more frequent blurred vision and less conjunctival hyperemia. Brimonidine resulted in more frequent ocular hyperemia. As to other adverse events (AEs) (conjunctivitis, eye pruritus, foreign body sensation in eyes, and treatment-related AEs), brinzolamide was similar to other three active comparators.

Conclusions: Brinzolamide, as add-on to PGAs or β-blocker, significantly decreased IOP of patients with refractory glaucoma or OHT and the AEs were tolerable.

Keywords: brinzolamide, prostaglandin analogues, β-blocker, glaucoma, ocular hypertension, systematic review

INTRODUCTION

Glaucoma is an acquired disease of irreversible blindness and the second leading cause of blindness worldwide, characterized by optic neuropathies and intraocular pressure (IOP) elevation (Peters et al., 2014). Primary open-angle glaucoma (POAG), one of the most prevalent types, will have threatened 76.0 million people by 2020 and 111.8 million people by 2040 (Tham et al., 2014). There are no significant symptoms in the early stage of glaucoma, but once showing impaired vision, the patients have lost nearly 1 million of their retinal ganglion cell (RGCS) (Weinreb et al., 2014; Sharif, 2018). Therefore, the early diagnosis and treatment are particularly important for glaucoma.

Currently, pharmacotherapy is still a common and effective way to treat glaucoma and ocular hypertension (OHT). There are a variety of IOP-lowering agents containing carbonic anhydrase inhibitors (CAIs), beta-blockers, α2-adrenergic agonists, and prostaglandin analogues (PGAs). PGAs are the first-line treatment option, while their monotherapies may offer insufficient IOP control, so they need to be combined with other therapies, such as latanoprost and travoprost, which are combined with brinzolamide or dorzolamide or brimonidine or timolol for patients failing to control IOP (Cheng et al., 2009; Dzhumataeva, 2016; Lusthaus and Goldberg, 2017). Timolol, one of the β-blockers, has an obvious effect on diurnal IOP, but it is also insufficient to hold a stable IOP over the long term (Konstas et al., 2016). Brimonidine, an α2-adrenergic agonist, is popularized due to the positive effect of AQH and neuroprotective actions (Lusthaus and Goldberg, 2017). Brinzolamide and dorzolamide could inhibit carbonic anhydrase in ciliary epithelium to reduce IOP, increase retinal blood flow, and the efficacy of brinzolamide would be enhanced after improving the drug-delivery system (Iester, 2008; Konstas et al., 2013; Dong et al., 2018; Wang et al., 2018). However, brinzolamide and dorzolamide are restricted by lacking efficacy and brimonidine has a higher AE. It is, therefore, essential to combine multiple agents.

According to the differences of mechanisms, brinzolamide could be used in combination with other IOP-lowering drugs for glaucoma and OHT. However, there were no relevant systematic reviews to compare the efficacy and safety between brinzolamide and other active drugs as add-on treatment. Thus, basing on published and unpublished randomized controlled trials (RCTs) of patients with glaucoma or OHT, we did a systematic review to assess the efficacy and safety of brinzolamide compared with other anti-glaucoma agents as add-on treatment.

METHODS

This systematic review was conducted in accordance with the Preferred Reporting Items for Systematic Reviews and Meta-Analyses (PRISMA) statement (Knobloch et al., 2011).

Data Sources and Search Strategy

We systematically searched using databases including PubMed, Embase, MEDLINE, and Cochrane Library from inception to September 4, 2018, with a language restriction (English). The unpublished data were also searched from clinicaltrials.gov. We used the following terms: "brinzolamide," "CAS No. 138890-62-7," "carbonic anhydrase inhibitors (CAI)," "glaucoma," and "ocular hypertension." These terms were adjusted to adhere to the relevant rules in each database.

Two independent reviewers screened titles and abstracts of all retrieved citations, and subsequently examined potentially eligible studies in full text. All discrepancies were resolved through discussion and added to the third reviewer when necessary.

Study Selection and Data Extraction

We included RCTs if they met the following criteria: 1) patients aged > 18 years; 2) a clinical diagnosis of glaucoma (POAG, exfoliation glaucoma, pigmentary glaucoma) or OHT in at least one eye (study eye); 3) the patients without lowering IOP adequately by the monotherapies of antiglaucomatous drugs (PGA: IOP ≥ 18 mmHg; β-blocker: IOP ≥ 20 mmHg) or the patients with IOP ≥ 20 mmHg without medication (including washout schedule); 4) the patients using brinzolamide as a monotherapy or a combination therapy for safety analysis; 5) no history of glaucoma surgery before the study; 6) Snellen visual acuity ≥ 0.1 or Snellen score ≥ 20/100 in the study eye(s); 7) duration: follow-up time ≥ 4 weeks; and 8) outcome variables: a) IOP changes from baseline; b) the mean diurnal IOP at the end of treatment duration; c) AEs.

Exclusion criteria were as follows: 1) a history of chronic or recurrent severe ocular inflammatory disease; 2) ocular trauma or intraocular surgery within 6 months or laser eye surgery within 3 months of screening; 3) ocular infection, endophthalmitis, or retinal disease; 4) hypersensitivity to any of the excipients in the study medications; 5) maximum corrected visual acuity ≤ 0.2 (decimal acuity) or an anterior chamber angle grade < 2 in either eye; 6) quantify visual acuity < 0.6 logarithm of the minimal angle resolution; 7) optic nerve with a cup-disc ratio > 0.8; 8) previous or current evidence of a severe illness or any other condition that could make the patient unsuitable for the study; 9) treatment with stable doses of any medication within 30 days of the start of the study that could affect IOP; and 10) pregnant or lactating, or intending to become pregnant during the study period.

Data Extraction and Risk of Bias Assessment

The data extraction was implemented by two independent reviewers (YL and QW) according to the inclusion criteria. The information extracted from the trials includes study characteristics, interventions, types of glaucoma, duration of treatment, background therapy, and efficacy outcomes and AEs.

The methodological quality of eligible studies was assessed using the Cochrane risk-of-bias tool (Higgins et al., 2011). The predefined key domains included: randomization, allocation concealment, blinding, intent-to-treat (ITT) analysis, and a description of losses to follow-up.

We chose doses of the study drugs including brinzolamide 1% b.i.d. or t.i.d., which were the most commonly used doses in clinical treatments. In addition, our studies included 23 articles published and 3 articles unpublished. All studies are assessed under the same criteria.

Statistical Analysis

The statistical analysis was performed by 5.3 software and Stata 12 software. For the efficacy (IOP changes from baseline, the mean diurnal IOP at the end of treatment duration), we assessed them by the weighted mean difference (WMD) with 95% confidence intervals (CIs). For the safety, we assessed the incidences of AEs by risk ratios (RRs) with 95% CIs. Heterogeneity was evaluated with the chi-square test and the I^2 statistic. We planned to explore heterogeneity with a sensitivity analysis when I^2 was higher than 50% (Higgins et al., 2003). We also conducted egger analysis to assess the potential publication bias when three or more studies offered relevant data, and defined significant publication bias with the P value < 0.1.

RESULTS

Search Results and Study Characteristics

We identified 831 articles from four databases search through the search strategy, and 472 with duplicate were removed. After excluding reviews, meta-analysis, non-human studies, and non-clinical human studies, 109 were left. By further reviewing the full text, we included 26 articles with a total of 5,683 patients (**Figure 1**). The basic characteristics of the included studies were shown in **Supplementary Table 1**. All trials were randomized and active-controlled involving the study drugs added on PAG

in 11 articles (Hollo et al., 2006; Reis et al., 2006; Feldman et al., 2007; Day and Hollander, 2008; Miura et al., 2008; Bournias and Lai, 2009; Nakamura et al., 2009; Pfeiffer, 2011; Konstas et al., 2013; Alcon, 2016; Aihara et al., 2017), added on timolol 0.5% in two articles (Michaud and Friren, 2001; Martinez and Sanchez-Salorio, 2009), and added on the combination therapy of latanoprost and a beta-blocker in one article (Tsukamoto et al., 2005). Main clinical diagnosis of patients were POAG and OHT; a few were other glaucoma (exfoliation glaucoma, pigmentary glaucoma). Duration of intervention ≥ 4 weeks.

Bias Risk Analysis

Supplementary Table 2 presented the bias risk analysis of the included RCTs. All studies were randomized, multicenter clinical trials; six trials (Silver, 1998; Miura et al., 2008; Bournias and Lai, 2009; Manni et al., 2009; Katz et al., 2013; Aung et al., 2014) described the sequence generation. Twelve studies (Silver, 1998; Sall, 2000; March and Ochsner, 2000; Hollo et al., 2006; Feldman et al., 2007; Day and Hollander, 2008; Kaback et al., 2008; Miura et al., 2008; Bournias and Lai, 2009; Pfeiffer, 2011; Katz et al., 2013; Aung et al., 2014) offer the details of concealment procedures (Martinez and Sanchez-Salorio, 2009; Research, 2013a; Research, 2013b; Alcon, 2016). Sixteen trials performed ITT analyses (Sall, 2000; March and Ochsner, 2000; Michaud and Friren, 2001; Hollo et al., 2006; Feldman et al., 2007; Kaback et al., 2008; Bournias and Lai, 2009; Martinez and Sanchez-Salorio, 2009; Manni et al., 2009; Pfeiffer, 2011; Research, 2013a; Research, 2013b; Katz et al., 2013; Nguyen et al., 2013; Whitson et al., 2013; Aung et al., 2014) and all studies described withdraws or dropouts. All studies were funded by the company.

Efficacy Analysis
Brinzolamide vs Timolol

The changes of IOP from baseline between brinzolamide and timolol were shown in **Figure 2**. Both drugs significantly decreased IOP as adjunctive therapies to PGAs. There were no statistically significant differences (9 am: WMD 0.50 mmHg, 95%CI [−0.04 to 1.04], $P = 0.07$, $I = 37\%$; 12 am: WMD 0.25 mmHg, 95%CI [−0.70 to 1.19], $P = 0.61$, $I = 60\%$; 4 pm: WMD 0.41 mmHg, 95%CI [−1.16 to 1.97], $P = 0.66$, $I = 87\%$). For the high level of heterogeneity at 12 am, we removed one trial (Hollo et al., 2006) whose designs slightly differ from others, and the heterogeneity was eliminated without affecting the overall estimate (WMD 0.77 mmHg, 95%CI [−0.02 to 1.57], $P = 0.06$, $I = 0\%$). At 4 pm, we did not use a sensitivity analysis due to only including two trials. Likewise, the mean diurnal IOPs at the end of treatment duration did not differ between brinzolamide and timolol (WMD 0.38 mmHg, 95%CI [−0.18 to 0.94], $P = 0.18$, $I = 21\%$) (**Figure 3**). There was no publication bias on egger test ($P ≥ 0.1$; **Supplementary Table 3**).

Brinzolamide vs Dorzolamide

The changes of IOP from baseline between brinzolamide and dorzolamide were shown in **Figure 4**. Both drugs significantly decreased IOP as adjunctive therapies to PGAs and/or beta-blocker, and the brinzolamide was as effective as dorzolamide

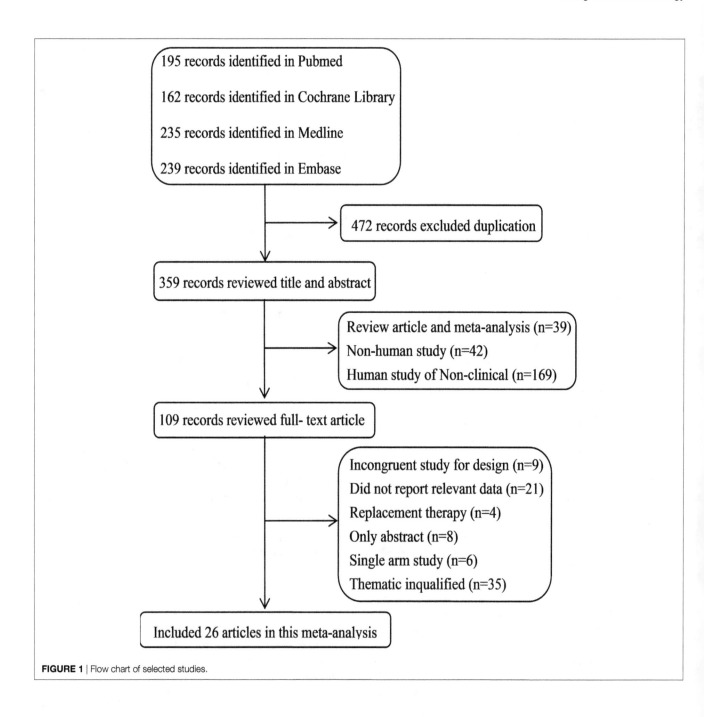

FIGURE 1 | Flow chart of selected studies.

in depressing IOP (9 am: WMD −0.04 mmHg, 95%CI [−0.20 to 0.11], $P = 0.59$, $I = 0\%$; 12 am: WMD −0.01 mmHg, 95%CI [−0.16 to 0.14], $P = 0.94$, $I = 0\%$; 4 pm: WD 0 mmHg, 95%CI [−0.16 to 0.17], $P = 0.95$, $I = 0\%$). The mean diurnal IOPs at the end were also similar (WMD 0.07 mmHg, 95%CI [−0.20 to 0.34], $P = 0.63$, $I = 0\%$) (**Figure 3**). No publication bias on egger test was found ($P \geq 0.1$; **Supplementary Table 3**).

Brinzolamide vs Brimonidine

The changes of IOP from baseline between brinzolamide and brimonidine were shown in **Figure 5**. Both drugs significantly

decreased IOP as adjunctive therapies to PGAs. At 9 am, a significant reduction of IOP was found in the brinzolamide (b.i.d.) compared to brimonidine (b.i.d.) (WMD −1.11 mmHg, 95%CI [−1.60 to −0.61], $P < 0.0001$, $I = 0\%$); however, the difference was not significant in thrice daily subgroup (WMD −0.60 mmHg, 95%CI [−2.13 to −0.96], $P = 0.44$). At 12 am, brinzolamide (b.i.d.) was similar to brimonidine (b.i.d.) in IOP-lowering effect, with a statistically significant heterogeneity (WMD −0.53 mmHg, 95%CI [−1.40 to −0.34], $P = 0.23$, $I = 53\%$). When thrice daily, brimonidine led to a greater IOP-lowering effect than brinzolamide, with statistically significant

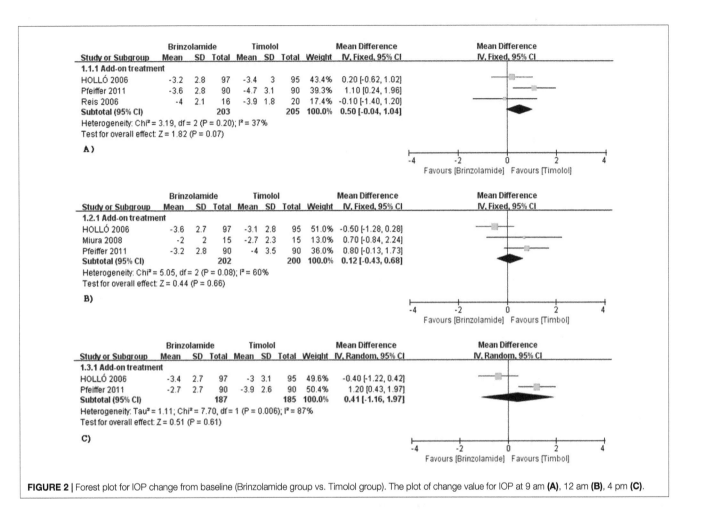

FIGURE 2 | Forest plot for IOP change from baseline (Brinzolamide group vs. Timolol group). The plot of change value for IOP at 9 am **(A)**, 12 am **(B)**, 4 pm **(C)**.

heterogeneity (WMD 2.07 mmHg, 95%CI [0.37 to 3.78], P = 0.02, I = 70%). In this analysis, we did not perform a sensitivity analysis due to only including two trials in each dose group. At 4 pm, brinzolamide (b.i.d.) had a superior IOP-lowering effect compared with brimonidine (b.i.d.) (WMD −0.97 mmHg, 95%CI [−1.51 to −0.44], P = 0.0003, I = 0%); conversely, the effect in brinzolamide (t.i.d.) was lower than brimonidine (t.i.d.) (WMD 1.19 mmHg, 95%CI [0.74 to 1.64], P < 0.0001, I = 0%). With regard to the mean diurnal IOPs at the end, brinzolamide was lower in twice daily subgroup (WMD −1.20 mmHg, 95%CI [−1.31 to 1.08], P < 0.00001, I = 0%), brimonidine was lower in thrice daily subgroup (WMD 1.41 mmHg, 95%CI [1.02 to 1.80], P < 0.00001, I = 0%), and the results were also consistent with their IOP changes. There were no publication biases on egger test (P ≥ 0.1 for each group; **Supplementary Table 3**). The changes of IOP between brinzolamide and brimonidine could be related to their plasma concentrations and pharmacokinetics (detailed descriptions in the Discussion section).

Safety Analysis

To obtain a more comprehensive safety profile, we compared the common AEs between brinzolamide and other anti-glaucoma agents, including monotherapies and add-on therapies.

Blurred Vision and Conjunctival Hyperemia

Blurred vision was one of the most common AEs of brinzolamide. Compared with active comparators (dorzolamide, brimonidine), a greater proportion of patients suffered from blurred vision in brinzolamide (**Table 1**). However, the difference between brinzolamide and timolol was not significant (**Table 1**). For conjunctival hyperemia, the incidence was significantly increased in brinzolamide compared to timolol (**Table 1**); there were no significant differences when comparing brinzolamide with other active comparators (dorzolamide, brimonidine) (**Table 1**).

Occurrence of Taste Abnormality

Occurrence of taste abnormality was analyzed to have a similar incidence between brinzolamide and dorzolamide (**Table 1**). However, compared with other active comparators (timolol, brimonidine), the reports of occurrence of taste abnormality were significantly higher in brinzolamide (**Table 1**).

Ocular Discomfort, Eye Pain, and Ocular Hyperemia

Ocular discomfort and eye pain were analyzed to have significantly lower incidences in brinzolamide compared to dorzolamide (**Table 1**); but the differences between

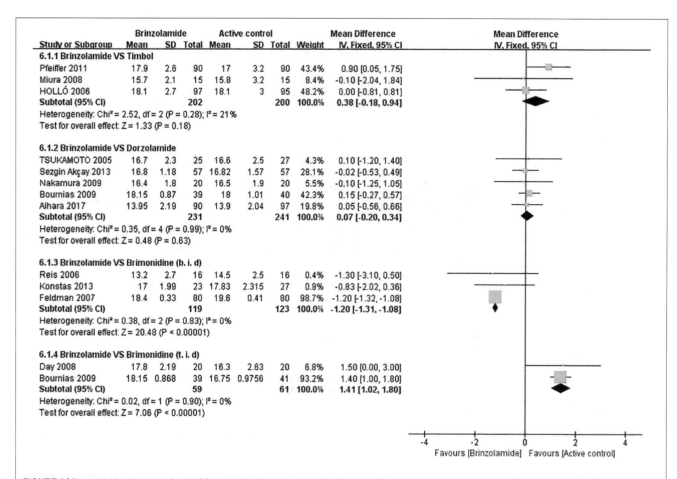

FIGURE 3 | Forest plot for the mean diurnal IOP at the end of treatment duration (Brinzolamide group vs. active control group).The mean diurnal IOP between Brinzolamide group and Timolol group (6.1.1); between Brinzolamide group and Dozorlamide group (6.1.2); between Brinzolamide group and Brimonidine group (b.i.d) (6.1.3), (t.i.d) (6.1.4).

brinzolamide and other active (timolol, brimonidine) were not significant (**Table 1**). For ocular hyperemia, the incidence was significantly lower in brinzolamide than brimonidine (**Table 1**); nevertheless, the differences between brinzolamide and other active comparators (timolol, dorzolamide) were not significant (**Table 1**).

Other Adverse Events

There were no significant differences in the incidence of occurrence of conjunctivitis, eye pruritus, foreign body sensation in eyes, and treatment-related AEs when we compared brinzolamide with active comparators (timolol, dorzolamide, and brimonidine) (all $P > 0.05$; **Table 1**). Besides, no severe AEs were reported in most studies.

DISCUSSION

In the present systematic review, we assessed 26 RCTs, containing a comparison between brinzolamide and timolol in 7 studies

(Silver, 1998; March and Ochsner, 2000; Hollo et al., 2006; Reis et al., 2006; Kaback et al., 2008; Miura et al., 2008; Pfeiffer, 2011), brinzolamide and dorzolamide in 10 studies (Sall, 2000; Michaud and Friren, 2001; Tsukamoto et al., 2005; Bournias and Lai, 2009; Martinez and Sanchez-Salorio, 2009; Manni et al., 2009; Nakamura et al., 2009; Sezgin Akcay et al., 2013; Alcon, 2016; Aihara et al., 2017), and brinzolamide and brimonidine in 9 studies (Feldman et al., 2007; Day and Hollander, 2008; Katz et al., 2013; Konstas et al., 2013; Nguyen et al., 2013; Research, 2013a; Research, 2013b; Whitson et al., 2013; Aung et al., 2014). Patients with POAG or OHT have a common characteristic as elevated IOP, which is closely associated with progression of visual field deterioration. Currently, IOP level control is a primary goal for the treatment of POAG and OHT.

Our analyses found that brinzolamide had similar efficacies to timolol in lowering IOP at three time points (9 am, 12 am, 4 pm) and holding the mean diurnal IOP at the end of treatment duration, as add-on therapies to a PGA, which were not inconsistent with the effects as monotherapies. In a previous meta-analysis, monotherapies were adopted to treat patients with POAG or OHT, and the relative

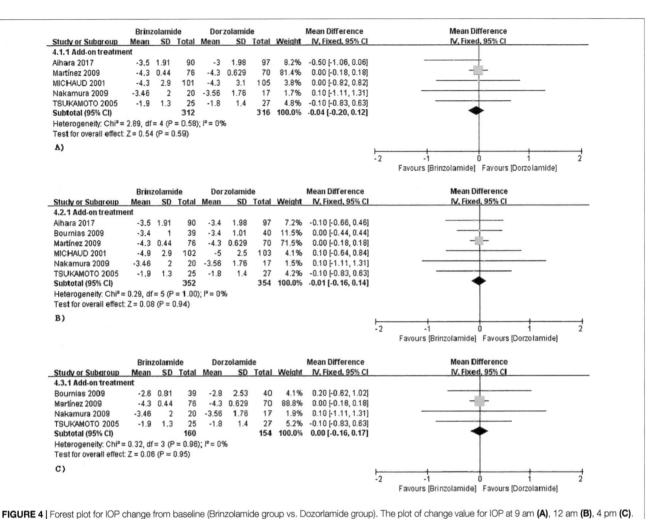

FIGURE 4 | Forest plot for IOP change from baseline (Brinzolamide group vs. Dozorlamide group). The plot of change value for IOP at 9 am **(A)**, 12 am **(B)**, 4 pm **(C)**.

peaks of reduction in IOP were 17% and 27% for brinzolamide and timolol, respectively (van der Valk et al., 2005). Timolol and brinzolamide could reduce formation of AQH; the former decreases blood flow to the iris root–ciliary body while the latter inhibits CAI, and timolol has a stronger effect on the process than brinzolamide (Costagliola et al., 2002; Shoji et al., 2005). PGAs, besides exporting the first-line effect, could enhance the activity of CAI, so brinzolamide is added on PGAs benefiting patients with glaucoma or OHT to achieve further reductions in IOP (Puscas and Coltau, 1995; Miura et al., 2008). However, there is not an interaction between timolol and PGAs. Thus, the efficacy of brinzolamide was similar to timolol as added on PGAs in daytime. Moreover, brinzolamide also lowered the nighttime IOP, although the effect was smaller than during daytime (Liu et al., 2004; Liu et al., 2009). The performance may be explained by the fact that brinzolamide is weaker in reducing the formation of AQH during the nocturnal period than during the diurnal period (Ingram and Brubaker, 1999). In contrast, timolol has no similar effect, because there are normally reductions of endogenous circulating catecholamines in night-time (Topper and Brubaker, 1985; Liu et al., 2004; Liu et al., 2009; Konstas et al., 2016).

As for brinzolamide and dorzolamide, they had same mechanisms that lowered IOP by inhibiting the activity of carbonic anhydrase and enhanced ocular hemodynamic function by retarding the release of intracellular Ca^{2+} (Chandra et al., 2016; Dong et al., 2018). Accumulating evidences showed that visual field defect was highly related to the reduction in ocular blood flow (Deokule et al., 2010; Calvo et al., 2012). Therefore, it was reasonable to our results that brinzolamide and dorzolamide had a similar effect in lowering IOP at three time points (9 am, 12 am, 4 pm) and same mean diurnal IOPs at the end of treatment duration, as add-on therapy to a PGA or beta-blocker.

In terms of the comparisons between brinzolamide and brimonidine where some changes had been generated, we implemented subgroup analysis on medication times. At 9 am, brinzolamide was more effective than brimonidine when added to PGAs, and a similar tendency occurred in the brinzolamide group (b.i.d.) at 4 pm. Interestingly, this tendency had reversed in brimonidine (t.i.d.) at 12 am and 4 pm, respectively. However, the difference was not statistically significant comparing brimonidine (b.i.d.) with brimonidine (b.i.d.) at 12 am. In addition, brinzolamide

TABLE 1 | Meta-analysis for the efficacy and safety outcomes.

Outcome	Interventions	Studies, (n)	Participants analyzed, n		RR	P value	I^2/%
			Brinzolamide	Comparator	(95% CI)		
Blurred vision	Brinzolamide VS timolol	3	489	323	2.43 [0.95, 5.76]	0.07	0
	Brinzolamide VS dorzolamide	9	988	993	3.24 [1.89, 3.60]	<0.00001	0
	Brinzolamide VS brimonidine	9	1,287	1,260	4.38 [1.36, 14.17]	0.01	63
Ocular discomfort (burning and stinging)	Brinzolamide VS timolol	4	586	418	0.74 [0.27, 1.98]	0.55	52
	Brinzolamide VS dorzolamide	7	711	719	0.21 [0.14, 0.31]	<0.00001	0
	Brinzolamide VS brimonidine	3	90	90	0.85 [0.29, 2.48]	0.76	0
Occurrence of taste abnormality	Brinzolamide VS timolol	3	489	323	6.41 [1.51, 27.16]	0.01	0
	Brinzolamide VS dorzolamide	6	808	806	1.04 [0.69, 1.56]	0.85	0
	Brinzolamide VS brimonidine	9	1,243	1,219	9.61 [5.23, 17.67]	<0.00001	5
Ocular hyperemia	Brinzolamide VS timolol	2	324	250	3.02 [0.48, 19.10]	0.24	0
	Brinzolamide VS dorzolamide	4	545	540	0.45 [0.18, 1.10]	0.08	13
	Brinzolamide VS brimonidine	8	1,053	1,025	0.41 [0.23, 0.73]	0.002	45
Occurrence of conjunctivitis	Brinzolamide VS timolol	2	315	148	0.48 [0.09, 2.70]	0.41	0
	Brinzolamide VS dorzolamide	3	339	336	0.45 [0.15, 1.40]	0.17	13
	Brinzolamide VS brimonidine	4	316	310	0.53 [0.15, 1.93]	0.34	0
Eye pruritus	Brinzolamide VS timolol	3	367	363	1.23 [0.33, 4.52]	0.76	14
	Brinzolamide VS dorzolamide	4	347	350	0.50 [0.17, 1.46]	0.2	59
	Brinzolamide VS brimonidine	4	885	865	0.97 [0.41, 2.26]	0.94	0
Treatment-related adverse events	Brinzolamide VS timolol	3	361	342	1.33 [0.93, 1.91]	0.11	50
	Brinzolamide VS dorzolamide	4	532	543	0.83 [0.49, 1.42]	0.49	79
	Brinzolamide VS brimonidine	5	402	395	1.05 [0.80, 1.39]	0.72	0
Eye pain	Brinzolamide VS timolol	2	324	232	0.88 [0.24, 3.20]	0.85	0
	Brinzolamide VS dorzolamide	2	277	274	0.25 [0.07, 0.88]	0.03	56
	Brinzolamide VS brimonidine	9	1,103	1,075	1.05 [0.61, 1.81]	0.86	0
Foreign body sensation in eyes	Brinzolamide VS timolol	3	421	345	1.56 [0.50, 4.84]	0.44	21
	Brinzolamide VS dorzolamide	4	486	475	0.70 [0.23, 2.16]	0.53	58
	Brinzolamide VS brimonidine	5	507	485	1.29 [0.46, 3.67]	0.63	0
Conjunctival hyperemia	Brinzolamide VS timolol	3	367	363	2.20 [1.14, 4.23]	0.02	0
	Brinzolamide VS dorzolamide	1	98	101	1.03 [0.07, 16.25]	0.98	—
	Brinzolamide VS brimonidine	4	885	865	0.72 [0.31, 1.71]	0.46	0

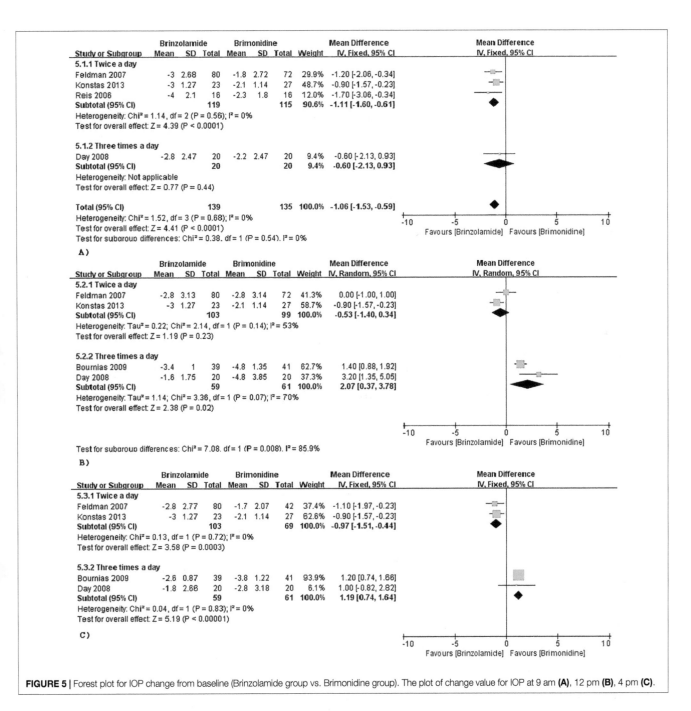

FIGURE 5 | Forest plot for IOP change from baseline (Brinzolamide group vs. Brimonidine group). The plot of change value for IOP at 9 am **(A)**, 12 pm **(B)**, 4 pm **(C)**.

had a lower mean diurnal IOP in twice daily subgroup, but brimonidine had a lower mean diurnal IOP in thrice daily subgroup. The reasons leading to variabilities for therapeutic effect were listed as follows. On the one hand, brinzolamide worked within 30 min and reached a peak after 1–2 h after administration (Silver, 1998). But for brimonidine, the effect was only observed within 1 h, and the peak effect occurred by 2–3 h (Walters, 1996). Nevertheless, the IOP lowering effect of two drugs dropped back to a trough over 10 h after doses (Anderson, 2003; Lusthaus and Goldberg, 2017). On the other hand, the plasma concentrations of two drugs (t.i.d.) were greater than the drugs (b.i.d.), which were more beneficial to the effect of brimonidine than brinzolamide (Fudemberg et al., 2008).

Safety profile of brinzolamide was similar to the other three active comparators when they were used as either monotherapies or adjunctive therapies, but there were some AEs with diverse frequencies. The incidences of blurred vision and taste abnormality were outstanding in brinzolamide. Differing from brinzolamide, ocular discomfort and eye pain were common in dorzolamide; ocular hyperemia was common in brimonidine; timolol led to a low risk of conjunctival hyperemia. All AEs of the four drugs were usually mild and superficial depending on their unique structures; furthermore, brinzolamide with a physiological pH could also ameliorate tolerability and adherence (Silver, 1998).

The present study still had some limitations. First, all articles in our study were published in English; there was a potential risk that we failed to involve some papers that were published in other languages. Second, people with glaucoma and OHT eventually ended up with visual field loss. The patient's visual field directly reflected the disease progression. However, there was not a precise and accepted visual field detection method at present. Therefore, we evaluated the treatment effect of study drugs by IOP changes from baseline as well as the mean diurnal IOP at the end of treatment duration to restrict the potential bias. Third, due to the lack of data, we did not compare the nocturnal IOP, which also played a dominant role responding to the control level of the disease. It was necessary that more researches were still needed for the available guidance. Finally, there was a lack of cost-effectiveness studies of brinzolamide as an adjunctive therapy.

CONCLUSION

This meta-analysis indicated that brinzolamide, as add-on to PGAs or β-blocker, could significantly decrease IOP of people with refractory glaucoma or OHT, and the AEs of brinzolamide were tolerable. Therefore, it could be used as a replacement therapy for patients whose IOP became uncontrollable with a PGA or timolol alone; or as an alternative treatment to patients with contraindications of timolol and brimonidine.

AUTHOR CONTRIBUTIONS

YH contributed to devising the topic and writing the manuscript. YL and JZ contributed equally to this work (contributed by writing the manuscript and analyzing the data). XZ and QW contributed to checking the data.

REFERENCES

Aihara, M., Adachi, M., Matsuo, H., Togano, T., Fukuchi, T., and Sasaki, N. (2017). Additive effects and safety of fixed combination therapy with 1% brinzolamide and 0.5% timolol versus 1% dorzolamide and 0.5% timolol in prostaglandin-treated glaucoma patients. *Acta Ophthalmol.* 95, e720–e726. doi: 10.1111/aos.13401

Alcon, a.N.C. (2016). Comparison of Intraocular Pressure (IOP)-Lowering Efficacy and Safety of AZORGA® Ophthalmic Suspension and COSOPT® Ophthalmic Solution. (NCT02325518). Available online at: https://www.clinicaltrials.gov/

Anderson, D. R. (2003). Collaborative normal tension glaucoma study. *Curr. Opin. Ophthalmol.* 14, 86–90. doi: 10.1097/00055735-200304000-00006

Aung, T., Laganovska, G., Hernandez Paredes, T. J., Branch, J. D., Tsorbatzoglou, A., and Goldberg, I. (2014). Twice-daily brinzolamide/brimonidine fixed combination versus brinzolamide or brimonidine in open-angle glaucoma or ocular hypertension. *Ophthalmology* 121, 2348–2355. doi: 10.1016/j.ophtha.2014.06.022

Bournias, T. E., and Lai, J. (2009). Brimonidine tartrate 0.15%, dorzolamide hydrochloride 2%, and brinzolamide 1% compared as adjunctive therapy to prostaglandin analogs. *Ophthalmology* 116, 1719–1724. doi: 10.1016/j.ophtha.2009.03.050

Calvo, P., Ferreras, A., Polo, V., Guerri, N., Seral, P., Fuertes-Lazaro, I., et al. (2012). Predictive value of retrobulbar blood flow velocities in glaucoma suspects. *Invest. Ophthalmol. Vis. Sci.* 53, 3875–3884. doi: 10.1167/iovs.11-8817

Chandra, S., Muir, E. R., Deo, K., Kiel, J. W., and Duong, T. Q. (2016). Effects of dorzolamide on retinal and choroidal blood flow in the DBA/2J mouse model of glaucoma. *Invest. Ophthalmol. Vis. Sci.* 57, 826–831. doi: 10.1167/iovs.15-18291

Cheng, J. W., Li, Y., and Wei, R. L. (2009). Systematic review of intraocular pressure-lowering effects of adjunctive medications added to latanoprost. *Ophthalmic Res.* 42, 99–105. doi: 10.1159/000225963

Costagliola, C., Del Prete, A., Verolino, M., Antinozzi, P., Fusco, R., Parmeggiani, F., et al. (2002). Effect of 0.005% latanoprost once daily on intraocular pressure in glaucomatous patients not adequately controlled by beta-blockers twice daily: a 3-year follow-up. *Graefes Arch. Clin. Exp. Ophthalmol.* 240, 379–386. doi: 10.1007/s00417-002-0469-8

Day, D. G., and Hollander, D. A. (2008). Brimonidine purite 0.1% versus brinzolamide 1% as adjunctive therapy to latanoprost in patients with glaucoma or ocular hypertension. *Curr. Med. Res. Opin.* 24, 1435–1442. doi: 10.1185/030079908X301848

Deokule, S., Vizzeri, G., Boehm, A., Bowd, C., and Weinreb, R. N. (2010). Association of visual field severity and parapapillary retinal blood flow in open-angle glaucoma. *J. Glaucoma* 19, 293–298. doi: 10.1097/IJG.0b013e3181b6e5b9

Dong, Y. R., Huang, S. W., Cui, J. Z., and Yoshitomi, T. (2018). Effects of brinzolamide on rabbit ocular blood flow in vivo and ex vivo. *Int. J. Ophthalmol.* 11, 719–725. doi: 10.18240/ijo.2018.05.03

Dzhumataeva, Z. A. (2016). Prostaglandin analogues in glaucoma treatment. *Vestn. Oftalmol.* 132, 62–67. doi: 10.17116/oftalma2016132462-67

Feldman, R. M., Tanna, A. P., Gross, R. L., Chuang, A. Z., Baker, L., Reynolds, A., et al. (2007). Comparison of the ocular hypotensive efficacy of adjunctive brimonidine 0.15% or brinzolamide 1% in combination with travoprost 0.004%. *Ophthalmology* 114, 1248–1254. doi: 10.1016/j.ophtha.2007.03.012

Fudemberg, S. J., Batiste, C., and Katz, L. J. (2008). Efficacy, safety, and current applications of brimonidine. *Expert Opin. Drug Saf.* 7, 795–799. doi: 10.1517/17425250802457609

Higgins, J. P., Altman, D. G., Gotzsche, P. C., Juni, P., Moher, D., Oxman, A. D., et al. (2011). The Cochrane Collaboration's tool for assessing risk of bias in randomised trials. *BMJ* 343, d5928. doi: 10.1136/bmj.d5928

Higgins, J. P., Thompson, S. G., Deeks, J. J., and Altman, D. G. (2003). Measuring inconsistency in meta-analyses. *BMJ* 327, 557–560. doi: 10.1136/bmj.327.7414.557

Hollo, G., Chiselita, D., Petkova, N., Cvenkel, B., Liehneova, I., Izgi, B., et al. (2006). The efficacy and safety of timolol maleate versus brinzolamide each given twice daily added to travoprost in patients with ocular hypertension or primary open-angle glaucoma. *Eur. J. Ophthalmol.* 16, 816–823. doi: 10.1177/112067210601600606

Iester, M. (2008). Brinzolamide. *Expert Opin. Pharmacother.* 9, 653–662. doi: 10.1517/14656566.9.4.653

Ingram, C. J., and Brubaker, R. F. (1999). Effect of brinzolamide and dorzolamide on aqueous humor flow in human eyes. *Am. J. Ophthalmol* 128, 292–296. doi: 10.1016/S0002-9394(99)00179-8

Kaback, M., Scoper, S. V., Arzeno, G., James, J. E., Hua, S. Y., Salem, C., et al. (2008). Intraocular pressure-lowering efficacy of brinzolamide 1%/timolol 0.5% fixed combination compared with brinzolamide 1% and timolol 0.5%. *Ophthalmology* 115, 1728–1734, 1734.e1721-1722. doi: 10.1016/j.ophtha.2008.04.011

Katz, G., Dubiner, H., Samples, J., Vold, S., and Sall, K. (2013). Three-month randomized trial of fixed-combination brinzolamide, 1%, and brimonidine, 0.2%. *JAMA Ophthalmol.* 131, 724–730. doi: 10.1001/jamaophthalmol.2013.188

Knobloch, K., Yoon, U., and Vogt, P. M. (2011). Preferred reporting items for systematic reviews and meta-analyses (PRISMA) statement and publication bias. *J. Craniomaxillofac. Surg.* 39, 91–92. doi: 10.1016/j.jcms.2010.11.001

Konstas, A. G., Hollo, G., Haidich, A. B., Mikropoulos, D. G., Giannopoulos, T., Voudouragkaki, I. C., et al. (2013). Comparison of 24-hour intraocular pressure reduction obtained with brinzolamide/timolol or brimonidine/timolol fixed-combination adjunctive to travoprost therapy. *J. Ocul. Pharmacol. Ther.* 29, 652–657. doi: 10.1089/jop.2012.0195

Konstas, A. G., Quaranta, L., Bozkurt, B., Katsanos, A., Garcia-Feijoo, J., Rossetti L., et al. (2016). 24-h Efficacy of glaucoma treatment options. *Adv. Ther.* 33, 481–517. doi: 10.1007/s12325-016-0316-7

Liu, J. H., Kripke, D. F., and Weinreb, R. N. (2004). Comparison of the nocturnal effects of once-daily timolol and latanoprost on intraocular pressure. *Am. J. Ophthalmol* 138, 389–395. doi: 10.1016/j.ajo.2004.04.022

Liu, J. H., Medeiros, F. A., Slight, J. R., and Weinreb, R. N. (2009). Comparing diurnal and nocturnal effects of brinzolamide and timolol on intraocular pressure in patients receiving latanoprost monotherapy. *Ophthalmology* 116, 449–454. doi: 10.1016/j.ophtha.2008.09.054

Lusthaus, J. A., and Goldberg, I. (2017). Brimonidine and brinzolamide for treating glaucoma and ocular hypertension: a safety evaluation. *Expert Opin. Drug Saf.* 16, 1071–1078. doi: 10.1080/14740338.2017.1346083

Manni, G., Denis, P., Chew, P., Sharpe, E. D., Orengo-Nania, S., Coote, M. A., et al. (2009). The safety and efficacy of brinzolamide 1%/timolol 0.5% fixed combination versus dorzolamide 2%/timolol 0.5% in patients with open-angle glaucoma or ocular hypertension. *J. Glaucoma* 18, 293–300. doi: 10.1097/IJG.0b013e31818fb434

March, W. F., and Ochsner, K. I. (2000). The long-term safety and efficacy of brinzolamide 1.0% (azopt) in patients with primary open-angle glaucoma or ocular hypertension. The Brinzolamide Long-Term Therapy Study Group. *Am. J. Ophthalmol* 129, 136–143. doi: 10.1016/S0002-9394(99)00343-8

Martinez, A., and Sanchez-Salorio, M. (2009). A comparison of the long-term effects of dorzolamide 2% and brinzolamide 1%, each added to timolol 0.5%, on retrobulbar hemodynamics and intraocular pressure in open-angle glaucoma patients. *J. Ocul. Pharmacol. Ther.* 25, 239–248. doi: 10.1089/jop.2008.0114

Michaud, J. E., and Friren, B. (2001). Comparison of topical brinzolamide 1% and dorzolamide 2% eye drops given twice daily in addition to timolol 0.5% in patients with primary open-angle glaucoma or ocular hypertension. *Am. J. Ophthalmol.* 132, 235–243. doi: 10.1016/S0002-9394(01)00974-6

Miura, K., Ito, K., Okawa, C., Sugimoto, K., Matsunaga, K., and Uji, Y. (2008). Comparison of ocular hypotensive effect and safety of brinzolamide and timolol added to latanoprost. *J. Glaucoma* 17, 233–237. doi: 10.1097/IJG.0b013e31815072fe

Nakamura, Y., Ishikawa, S., Nakamura, Y., Sakai, H., Henzan, I., and Sawaguchi, S. (2009). 24-hour intraocular pressure in glaucoma patients randomized to receive dorzolamide or brinzolamide in combination with latanoprost. *Clin. Ophthalmol.* 3, 395–400. doi: 10.2147/OPTH.S5726

Nguyen, Q. H., McMenemy, M. G., Realini, T., Whitson, J. T., and Goode, S. M. (2013). Phase 3 randomized 3-month trial with an ongoing 3-month safety extension of fixed-combination brinzolamide 1%/brimonidine 0.2%. *J. Ocul. Pharmacol. Ther.* 29, 290–297. doi: 10.1089/jop.2012.0235

Peters, D., Bengtsson, B., and Heijl, A. (2014). Factors associated with lifetime risk of open-angle glaucoma blindness. *Acta Ophthalmol.* 92, 421–425. doi: 10.1111/aos.12203

Pfeiffer, N. (2011). Timolol versus brinzolamide added to travoprost in glaucoma or ocular hypertension. *Graefes Arch. Clin. Exp. Ophthalmol.* 249, 1065–1071. doi: 10.1007/s00417-011-1650-8

Puscas, I., and Coltau, M. (1995). Prostaglandins with vasodilating effects inhibit carbonic anhydrase while vasoconstrictive prostaglandins and leukotriens B4 and C4 increase CA activity. *Int. J. Clin. Pharmacol. Ther.* 33, 176–181. doi: 10.1097/00004580-199503000-00007

Reis, R., Queiroz, C. F., Santos, L. C., Avila, M. P., and Magacho, L. (2006). A randomized, investigator-masked, 4-week study comparing timolol maleate 0.5%, brinzolamide 1%, and brimonidine tartrate 0.2% as adjunctive therapies to travoprost 0.004% in adults with primary open-angle glaucoma or ocular hypertension. *Clin. Ther.* 28, 552–559. doi: 10.1016/j.clinthera.2006.04.007

Research, A. (2013a). Safety and efficacy of brinzolamide/brimonidine fixed combination. (NCT00961649). Available online at: https://www.clinicaltrials.gov/

Research, A. (2013b). Three month efficacy/safety study with a 3-month safety extension of brinzolamide 1%/brimonidine 0.2% vs. brinzolamide 1% or brimonidine 0.2%. (NCT01297920). Available online at: https://www.clinicaltrials.gov/

Sall, K. (2000). The efficacy and safety of brinzolamide 1% ophthalmic suspension (Azopt) as a primary therapy in patients with open-angle glaucoma or ocular hypertension. Brinzolamide Primary Therapy Study Group. *Surv. Ophthalmol.* 44 Suppl 2, S155–162. doi: 10.1016/S0039-6257(99)00107-1

Sezgin Akcay, B. I., Guney, E., Bozkurt, K. T., Unlu, C., and Akcali, G. (2013). The safety and efficacy of brinzolamide 1%/timolol 0.5% fixed combination versus dorzolamide 2%/timolol 0.5% in patients with open-angle glaucoma or ocular hypertension. *J. Ocul. Pharmacol. Ther.* 29, 882–886. doi: 10.1089/jop.2013.0102

Sharif, N. A. (2018). Glaucomatous optic neuropathy treatment options: the promise of novel therapeutics, techniques and tools to help preserve vision. *Neural Regen. Res.* 13, 1145–1150. doi: 10.4103/1673-5374.235017

Shoji, N., Ogata, H., Suyama, H., Ishikawa, H., Suzuki, H., Morita, T., et al. (2005). Intraocular pressure lowering effect of brinzolamide 1.0% as adjunctive therapy to latanoprost 0.005% in patients with open angle glaucoma or ocular hypertension: an uncontrolled, open-label study. *Curr. Med. Res. Opin.* 21, 503–508. doi: 10.1185/030079905X38222

Silver, L. H. (1998). Clinical efficacy and safety of brinzolamide (Azopt), a new topical carbonic anhydrase inhibitor for primary open-angle glaucoma and ocular hypertension. Brinzolamide Primary Therapy Study Group. *Am. J. Ophthalmol* 126, 400–408. doi: 10.1016/S0039-6257(99)00107-1

Tham, Y. C., Li, X., Wong, T. Y., Quigley, H. A., Aung, T., and Cheng, C. Y. (2014). Global prevalence of glaucoma and projections of glaucoma burden through 2040: a systematic review and meta-analysis. *Ophthalmology* 121, 2081–2090. doi: 10.1016/j.ophtha.2014.05.013

Topper, J. E., and Brubaker, R. F. (1985). Effects of timolol, epinephrine, and acetazolamide on aqueous flow during sleep. *Invest. Ophthalmol. Vis. Sci.* 26, 1315–1319. doi: 10.1097/00004397-198502520-00019

Tsukamoto, H., Noma, H., Matsuyama, S., Ikeda, H., and Mishima, H. K. (2005). The efficacy and safety of topical brinzolamide and dorzolamide when added to the combination therapy of latanoprost and a beta-blocker in patients with glaucoma. *J. Ocul. Pharmacol. Ther.* 21, 170–173. doi: 10.1089/jop.2005.21.170

van der Valk, R., Webers, C. A., Schouten, J. S., Zeegers, M. P., Hendrikse, F., and Prins, M. H. (2005). Intraocular pressure-lowering effects of all commonly used glaucoma drugs: a meta-analysis of randomized clinical trials. *Ophthalmology* 112, 1177–1185. doi: 10.1016/j.ophtha.2005.01.042

Walters, T. R. (1996). Development and use of brimonidine in treating acute and chronic elevations of intraocular pressure: a review of safety, efficacy, dose response, and dosing studies. *Surv. Ophthalmol.* 41 Suppl 1, S19–S26. doi: 10.1016/S0039-6257(96)82028-5

Wang, F., Bao, X., Fang, A., Li, H., Zhou, Y., Liu, Y., et al. (2018). Nanoliposome-encapsulated brinzolamide-hydropropyl-beta-cyclodextrin inclusion complex: a potential therapeutic ocular drug-delivery system. *Front. Pharmacol.* 9, 91. doi: 10.3389/fphar.2018.00091

Weinreb, R. N., Aung, T., and Medeiros, F. A. (2014). The pathophysiology and treatment of glaucoma: a review. *JAMA* 311, 1901–1911. doi: 10.1001/jama.2014.3192

Whitson, J. T., Realini, T., Nguyen, Q. H., McMenemy, M. G., and Goode, S. M. (2013). Six-month results from a Phase III randomized trial of fixed-combination brinzolamide 1% + brimonidine 0.2% versus brinzolamide or brimonidine monotherapy in glaucoma or ocular hypertension. *Clin. Ophthalmol.* 7, 1053–1060. doi: 10.2147/OPTH.S46881

18

Knowledge Translation for Improving the Care of Deinstitutionalized People with Severe Mental Illness in Health Policy

Izabela Fulone[1], Jorge Otavio Maia Barreto[2], Silvio Barberato-Filho[1], Marcel Henrique de Carvalho[3] and Luciane Cruz Lopes[1]*

[1] Pharmaceutical Sciences Graduate Course, University of Sorocaba, UNISO, Sorocaba, Brazil, [2] Fiocruz School of Government, Fiocruz Brasília, Oswaldo Cruz Foundation, Brasília, Brazil, [3] Veredas Institute, Brasília, Brazil

*Correspondence:
Luciane Cruz Lopes
luciane.lopes@prof.uniso.br;
luslopesbr@gmail.com

Background: Knowledge translation (KT) is an effective strategy that uses the best available research evidence to bring stakeholders together to develop solutions and improve public health policy-making. Despite progress, the process of deinstitutionalization in Brazil is still undergoing consolidation, and the changes and challenges that are involved in this process are complex and necessitate evidence-informed decision-making. Accordingly, this study used KT tools to support efforts that aim to improve the care that is available to deinstitutionalized people with severe mental disorders in Brazil.

Methods: We used the Supporting Policy Relevant Reviews and Trials tools for evidence-informed health policymaking and followed eight steps: 1) capacity building; 2) identification of a priority policy issue within a Brazilian public health system; 3) meetings with policy-makers, researchers and stakeholders; 4) development of an evidence brief (EB) that addresses the problem of deinstitutionalization; 5) facilitating policy dialogue (PD); 6) the evaluation of the EB and PD; 7) post-dialogue mini-interviews; and 8) dissemination of the findings.

Results: Capacity building and meetings with key informants promoted awareness about the gap between research and practice. Local findings were used to define the problem and develop the EB. Twenty-four individuals (policy-makers, stakeholders, researchers, representatives of the civil society, and public defense) participated in the PD. They received the EB to subsidise their deliberations during the PD, which in turn were used to validate and improve the EB. The PD achieved the objective of promoting an exhaustive discussion about the problem and proposed options and improved communication and interaction among those who are involved in mental health care. The features of both the EB and PD were considered to be favorable and helpful.

Conclusions: The KT strategy helped participants understand different perspectives and values, the interpersonal tensions that exist among those who are involved in the field of mental health, and the strategies that can bridge the gap between research and policy-making. The present findings suggest that PDs can influence practice by promoting greater engagement among stakeholders who formulate or revise mental health policies.

Keywords: evidence-informed policy, knowledge translation, health policy, policy-making, deinstitutionalization, mental health

BACKGROUND

Knowledge translation (KT) is a dynamic and interactive process that uses evidence to make decisions and take actions that can improve health outcomes and reduce health inequities, particularly in low- and middle-income countries (LMICs) (Boyko et al., 2012).

Overall, there are different complexities and barriers that impede the application of KT for public health action in LMICs: deficits in knowledge production, the application of the available knowledge, and the use of strategies that are based on the best available evidence (Malla et al., 2018). When resources are scarce and there are strong sociocultural interferences, the translation and dissemination of knowledge can be adversely affected by contextual and local limiting factors (Newlin and Webber, 2015).

In order to promote the appropriate use of scientific evidence in the development and implementation of public health policies, KT platforms such as the Evidence-informed Policy Network (EVIPNet), which is supported by the World Health Organization (WHO), have been established to support health policy-making in Africa, Asia, and the Americas (Moat et al., 2014). The main objective of the EVIPNet is to facilitate the use of scientific knowledge in the formulation and implementation of health policies. Specifically, it focuses on the preparation of evidence briefs and policy dialogues, and adopts an approach that is similar to the Supporting Policy Relevant Reviews and Trials (SUPPORT) method (Moat and Lavis, 2014).

KT platforms are change agents that have a positive impact on policy decisions, interest group interactions, and health systems (Ongolo-Zogo et al., 2018). The use of KT platforms in Uganda, Cameroon, and Lebanon demonstrate the positive impact of such platforms: the promotion of awareness, acceptance, and adoption of research-based knowledge, achievement of the health goals, reallocation of resources, and identification of the sources of conflicts (Yehia and El Jardali, 2015; Ongolo-Zogo et al., 2018).

Evidence briefs should rely on the best available systematic reviews to delineate the important aspects of the issue in question. It must integrate global evidences and local knowledge to inform deliberations about health policies among policy-makers and stakeholders (Lavis et al., 2009a). Policy dialogues use the evidence brief as primary input to subsidise the deliberations followed by the views, experiences and tacit knowledge of different actors, who will be affect or involved by future decisions (Lavis et al., 2009b; El-Jardali et al., 2014; Yehia and El Jardali, 2015).

Since its inception in Brazil in 2007, EVIPINet has been focusing on promoting the use of scientific knowledge in the decision-making processes of the Brazilian Health System, the development of innovative strategies in health management, and the facilitation of technical cooperation regarding KT among the participant countries (Evipnet-Brazil, 2019). The Brazilian network consists of the representatives of different institutions and subject-matter experts (Dias et al., 2014).

Accordingly, in response to the need for and challenges in the promotion of evidence-informed health policy-making in the largest city in the state of São Paulo (Sorocaba), a working group was constituted at the University of Sorocaba in 2016. This team, which consisted of researchers, doctoral students, and health professionals, was denominated as *Seriema* (Evidence Services for Monitoring & Evaluation in Health Policy).

The Seriema group aims to suggest and contribute to health initiatives and formulate evidence-based public policies. This group works collaboratively with the Health Department of Sorocaba, which oversees 48 additional cities in São Paulo that are together inhabited by more than three million individuals (Brazil, 2018).

This group seeks to design research studies in accordance with the needs of Brazilian policy-makers specially supporting deinstitutionalization in Brazil (mainly in region of Sorocaba).

Mental Health in the Region of Sorocaba

In the 1980s, the history of Brazilian mental health was marked by serious denunciations of mistreatment, lack of hygiene and care for patients with mental disorders who lived in psychiatric hospitals, mainly in the region of Sorocaba (São Paulo), Rio de Janeiro (Rio de Janeiro), and Barbacena (Minas Gerais) (Vidal et al., 2008; Emerich and Yasui, 2016). Social and political mobilizations that advocated for psychiatric reform and the approval of Federal law no. 10216 in 2001 accelerated the process of deinstitutionalization. It also led to the understanding that hospitalization must be the last treatment option for patients with mental disorders. Consequently, the right to receive community care services was promulgated (Brazil, 2001; Silva and Rosa, 2014).

Sorocaba has a population of approximately 671,186 inhabitants and a high human development index (0.8), and its economy is based on industries and commerce (Brazil, 2019). The city has an adequate health-care infrastructure, and its hospitals provide services to the (almost three million) inhabitants of the tertiary care level of 48 municipalities in southwest São Paulo (Brazil, 2018). These municipalities are smaller than Sorocaba, their economies are diversified, and their high human development index ranges from 0.6 to 0.8 (Brazil, 2019). Mental health care services are not available in all 48 municipalities. Therefore, these municipalities belong to a network of mental health care institutions that are connected at the primary, secondary, and tertiary level (Brazil, 2019).

The Sorocaba region housed the largest mental asylum in the country (i.e. high number of psychiatric beds) (Cayres, 2015). The seven asylums in this region were among the ten largest Brazilian asylums that had the highest mortality rate between 2004 and 2011. Most of these deaths were due to an unknown cause, and they were especially common during the colder months of the year; the age of the youngest patient who died under these circumstances was approximately 53 years (Garcia, 2012; Cayres, 2015). In addition, there was a high number of resident patients who did not have the requisite civil documentation, and the number of mental health professionals was less than half of the number that was specified by the federal legislation (Garcia, 2012; Emerich and Yasui, 2016).

During the second half of the 1990s, there were 72,514 psychiatric beds in the Brazilian public health sector. In Brazil, the number of beds had reduced to 52,962 in 2001; in 2014, there were 25,988 psychiatric beds across the 167 psychiatric hospitals that were located in the 116 municipalities of the 23 states (Brazil, 2005; Brazil, 2015). In 2014, the Psychosocial Census of the State of São Paulo identified 53 psychiatric hospitals across 39 municipalities, seven of which were located within the Sorocaba region and together housed 2,273 patients (Cayres, 2015).

On the basis of the aforementioned census data, the federal, state, and municipal bodies signed an agreement that they would ensure the gradual deinstitutionalization of patients with mental disorders and the closure of the seven asylums in the region (Brazil, 2012). However, the deinstitutionalization process did not proceed in the same manner across the different regions of Brazil. Specifically, in regions where the number of patients that were admitted to the hospitals was very high, the institutions were underequipped to provide ambulatories and community services. This demonstrated the insufficiency and fragility of the services that were available to meet the demands of the patients (Vidal et al., 2008). However, a few community mental health care services (e.g. Psychosocial Care Center, Therapeutic Residential Service, and the Back Home Federal Program) have been found to be effective (Brazil, 2015). Nevertheless, some of the key principles that have been recommended by the WHO are not

adhered to, primarily due to the following reasons: insufficient funding, qualitative and quantitative human resource deficiency, poor infrastructure, a lack of political resources and intensive follow-up care, the absence of an integration between services and fragile social mobilization (WHO, 2014; Brazil, 2015).

In October 2016, the Seriema organised the first workshop on evidence-based health policy during which the deinstitutionalization of patients with mental disorders was ascribed the highest priority among all other health policy-related issues. Subsequently, the State Health Department of the Sorocaba region contacted the Seriema group with the objective of signing a partnership and helping them formulate public policies that are related to deinstitutionalization. This represented an important opportunity to subsidise the policy and collaborate with the State Health Department. This allowed them to adapt their actions and strategies to improve the care of deinstitutionalized individuals with mental disorders in Sorocaba and the neighboring regions.

Since the use of KT is one of the challenges that is currently faced by the health systems in LMICs, the present study investigated the means by which the care of deinstitutionalized individuals with severe mental disorders can be enhanced using KT tools.

METHODS

We used the SUPPORT Tools (Lavis et al., 2009a; Lavis et al., 2009b) for evidence-informed health Policymaking, which includes the following eight steps (**Figure 1**) for KT:

1) Capacity building

There was a need to conduct capacity building workshops that addressed evidence-informed policy-making and provided technical training on the use of SUPPORT tools for relevant stakeholders. Therefore, in 2016 and 2017, three workshops were conducted to provide training and raise awareness. In addition, there was the possibility of addressing topics of interest.

2) Prioritizing and supporting evidence-informed policy-making

The first step was to prioritise policy-related issues. The Seriema group provided a set of criteria that were to be used to

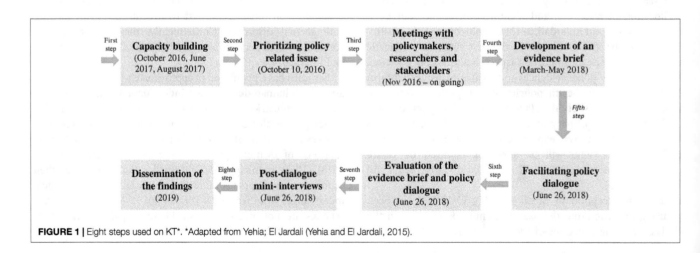

FIGURE 1 | Eight steps used on KT*. *Adapted from Yehia; El Jardali (Yehia and El Jardali, 2015).

select important topics, and it included questions about public perceptions and the impact of the problem (see **Supplementary Materials—Table S1**).

In the first workshop, 40 participants fulfilled the criteria and they discussed their most pressing issues. Deinstitutionalization was identified as the most important health policy-related issue by the workshop participants. With regard to the means by which the care of deinstitutionalized people with severe mental disorders can be improved, the participants underscored the need for further evidence and to address policy-related challenges at both the national and regional levels. The chronology of events that have led to the current state of the mental health care systems in Brazil can be summarised as follows: (i) asylums provided inadequate services to their patients with mental disorders; (ii) there was immense pressure to shut down the seven psychiatric hospitals in the region; and (iii) important changes have been made to Brazilian mental health policies.

3) Meetings with policy-makers researchers and stakeholders

A number of meetings were organised with policy-makers and stakeholders to clarify and define the problem, gather information about the status quo that could promote dialogue, and identify other key informants who could provide further insights.

4) The development of a policy brief that addresses the problem of deinstitutionalization

Once the issue of deinstitutionalization was prioritised, the focus was geared towards gathering a wide range of evidence on the various aspects of the issue. Therefore, a systematic review of literature was undertaken. First, a well-defined search strategy was used to retrieve relevant research articles from research databases. The search focused elements for policies that were related to the care of deinstitutionalized patients with mental disorders (see **Supplementary Materials Data Sheet 1**).

Between March and May 2018, we prepared a policy brief, which defined the problem and five evidence-based options to address the issue of deinstitutionalization. The evidence was contextualized to the Brazilian scenario, based on the recommendations of the policy-makers, subject-matter experts, and experts in the field of mental health.

5) Facilitating policy dialogue

The policy brief was circulated to the participants 30 days prior to the dialogue to inform them of the deliberations of the meeting. A group of 24 individuals, which entailed an equal representation of policy-makers, health-care providers, researchers, and representatives of the community and public defense sectors, participated in the policy dialogue (see **Table 1**).

The dialogue was conducted in accordance with the method that has been described by the SUPPORT tools and Chatham House rules. It was intended to achieve the following: participant commitment and transparency, an appropriate duration of dialogue, adequate group size and representation of the participants, skilful facilitation of problem-focused discussions (i.e. five options to address the policy issue), equity, key implementation considerations, and role distribution.

TABLE 1 | A profile of the stakeholders who participated in the policy dialogue.

Stakeholder category	N = 24 (100%)
Policy-makers[a]	5 (20.8%)
Health-care providers[b]	11 (45.8%)
Researchers in the field of public and mental health[c]	6 (25%)
Civil society organization[d]	1 (4.2%)
Public defense representative[e]	1 (4.2%)

[a]Policy-makers at the federal, state, and municipal level; [b]Health care providers included mental health specialists, public health specialists, psychologists, psychiatrists, occupational therapists, nurses, and social workers; [c]Researchers from Brazilian public and private universities, EVIPNet-Brazil members, and Seriema members; [d]The Brazilian anti-asylum movement; [e]Public defense representative from the state of São Paulo who was involved in mental health-related legislations.

6) The evaluation of the evidence brief and policy dialogue

The evaluation of the evidence brief and the policy dialogue was based on an adapted version of Lavis (2009) (Lavis et al., 2009a; Lavis et al., 2009b). Specifically, two surveys were administered to the participants (i.e. prior to dialogue and during the dialogue for those who did not complete it the first time). It consisted of items that required the respondent to assess the evidence brief and indicate the extent to which the policy dialogue was helpful on a rating scale that ranged from 1 (very unhelpful) to 7 (very helpful).

7) Post-dialogue mini-interviews

During the policy dialogue, the stakeholders were invited to participate in a video-recorded interview. In this interview, they were required to describe the insights that they gained from the dialogue. For this purpose, we posed the following two questions: a) How did the policy dialogue change your perspective about the problem in question? and b) What actions should be taken to address the problem in question?

8) Dissemination of the findings

The evidence brief was uploaded to the EVIPNet-Brazil secretariat webpage (http://brasil.evipnet.org/), where it is currently available for free download by all who are interested. A summary of the evidence brief and the policy dialogue will also be made available. Further, the federal government will order 100 prints of the evidence brief.

RESULTS

The results that are presented in the following sections summarise the main findings that pertain to the evidence brief; this section is followed by a discussion of the results that belong to the policy dialogue.

Defining the Problem

What are the most important challenges that impede the improvement of mental health care that is available to deinstitutionalized people with severe mental disorders in Brazil?

The participants reviewed the findings that were presented in the evidence brief, highlighted what is already known about the problem, and provided an enriching analysis of the brief; this process consumed the most time. They individually and collectively focused on the prominent challenges: (i) insufficient and fragile community care services to meet patient needs; (ii) unequal access to community care across the different regions of Brazil; (iii) insufficient funding and a lack of political resources; (iv) qualitative and quantitative human resource deficiencies; (v) a lack of intensive follow-up care; and (vi) the absence of integration and communication between services.

All the participants agreed that it is necessary to expand and strengthen community care services for all Brazilians. Indeed, the process of deinstitutionalization did not progress in the same manner across different Brazilian regions. In some of them, such as region of Sorocaba (main manicomial pole), where the number of patients admitted to hospital beds was very high, the deinstitutionalization process exceeded the capacity of assimilation of services offered in community.

Some participants observed that, despite progress, community care services are still precarious with regard to a wide range of issues (i.e. from physical infrastructure to human resources). They noted that many professionals still retain an "asylum mentality," and that there is insufficient communication among mental health professionals and services, and between the municipal, state, and federal governmental bodies. The participants contended that the lack of communication and continued education adversely affects the follow-up care and rehabilitation of patients with mental disorders.

The participants expressed their concerns about the process of deinstitutionalization (i.e. the withdrawal of patients from psychiatric hospitals) and trans-institutionalization (i.e. the transfer of patients from asylums to other inappropriate institutions). Indeed, these can lead to social neglect and have profound repercussions for the community, such as increased rates of homelessness, incarceration, drug addiction (primarily, cocaine), depression, suicide, and an overloading of emergency services. All participants agreed that deinstitutionalization requires efforts that extend beyond deinstitutionalization and trans-institutionalization. They also agreed that the "Ministry of Health must have a serious commitment to those patients who leave the psychiatric hospitals."

The participants contended that the issue of deinstitutionalization is also complicated by financial conflicts of interests that pertain to psychiatric hospitalizations. This suggests that there is a "mercantilization of life of an especially vulnerable population." Finally, the participants also recognised that the health care that is available to deinstitutionalized individuals has significantly advanced across the years; however, the socio-cultural treatment of these individuals remains problematic.

Options to Address the Problem of Deinstitutionalization

The five mutually non-exclusive options to address the problem of deinstitutionalization that was articulated in the evidence brief are presented in **Table 2**.

TABLE 2 | The definitions of the options to address deinstitutionalization that were presented in the evidence brief.

Option	Definition
Option 1: Expand and Improve the Implementation of a Psychiatric Day Hospital	It is a hospital unit that offers intensive care to patients with acute mental disorders based on a multidisciplinary approach and early discharge policy (Marshall et al., 2011).
Option 2: Provide Psychoeducational programs	Psychoeducation provides patients and their families or caregivers with information about the disease, its treatment, and its prognosis (Xia et al., 2011; Zhao et al., 2015).
Option 3: Develop Community Mental Health Teams	Multidisciplinary teams provide specialized mental health care to patients with mental disorders in the community, facilitate early intervention, and lower the rates of hospital admissions and suicides (Malone et al., 2007).
Option 4: Implement and Monitor the Practice of Intensive Case Management	It is a flexible model of mental health services that is characterised by intensive case management and patient care that is provided to individuals with mental disorders in the community. It is available throughout the day, and the follow-up care is provided by a multidisciplinary team to a small group of patients. They aim to improve social reintegration, psychosocial functioning, and autonomy development, and decrease the rate of hospitalization and treatment abandonment (Dieterich et al., 2010).
Option 5: Promote assisted living	Structuring housing intended to accommodate patients with mental disorders who have been hospitalized in psychiatric institutions for many years, and are currently homeless and unable to return to their families (Leff et al., 2009).

The deliberations that pertained to the options are summarised in the following sections.

Option 1: Expand and Improve the Implementation of a Psychiatric Hospital Day

This option caused much polemic and controversy among the participants of the policy dialogue, possibly because of a misunderstanding of the option. A majority of the participants opposed this option because they considered traditional psychiatric hospitals to be regressive: "*something that did not work in the past, which isolates and excludes.*" At the same time that the policy dialogue was conducted, the national policy on mental health was being reformulated with a strong aim to reopen the psychiatric hospitals; evidently, many of the participants were aware of this. However, other participants understood this option more accurately and were in favor of such an approach because it entails the early discharge policy of psychiatric day hospitals. However, they suggested that the name of the option be changed to "Strengthening interventions for acute psychiatric episodes" in order to convey that this option endorses institutions that provide humane treatment to individuals who present with acute psychiatric episodes, and hospitalize briefly such individuals only when necessary.

Option 2: Provide Psychoeducational Programs

This option was wholeheartedly supported and endorsed by the participants. Further, a majority of the studies that were reviewed supported the effectiveness of this option. The Brazilian Health System does not offer psychoeducational programs. According to some of the participants, this may have been attributable to the preconceived notions that managers hold about mental health professionals. They also recommended the implementation of a few psychoeducational techniques.

Option 3: Develop Community Mental Health Teams

Only one of the systematic reviews (Malone et al., 2007) addressed this option. Nevertheless, the conclusions of the review suggested that this option promotes greater acceptance of the treatment and greater patient satisfaction, when compared to standard treatment paradigms. In addition, the hospitalization rate was significantly lower; this suggests that the number of suicides and deaths under suspicious circumstances was also lower. The participants considered this option to be interesting and promising. However, the Brazilian mental health policy does not have provisions for such community mental health teams. Although Brazil does have other community teams, they comply with only a few of the principles of the proposed team.

Option 4: Implement and Monitor the Practice of Intensive Case Management

Model that is similar to those of intensive case management are practiced in some communities in Brazil. Every participant considered this model to be extremely important to all Brazilian cities. However, several small towns do not comply with this model. Therefore, the participants highlighted the importance of expanding and strengthening this model.

Option 5: Promote Assisted Living

The participants underscored the importance of and challenges that are involved in implementing assisted living in such a manner that it does not result in trans-institutionalization.

Two participants observed issues that pertained to the inadequacy of housing, infrastructure, and food, and the absence of leisure-time activities.

Many participants agreed that cohabitating a space with individuals who differ in age, diagnosis, and the severity of the diagnosis facilitates social reintegration: "caring and helping each other are positive factors observed in their daily lives."

The Evidence Brief and Policy Dialogue: Evaluation Results

Eight and nine individuals out of the 24 participants completed the evaluation surveys for the evidence brief and policy dialogue, respectively. The response rate was low despite repeated attempts to administer the survey, and it can be attributed to time limitations and the busy lives that the participants led.

Despite the low response rate, the average item scores were positive, and they ranged from 5.0 to 7.0 for the evidence brief evaluation survey. The features that received the highest ranking (i.e. very helpful) were as follows: employ a graded-entry format

and use systematic and transparent methods to identify, select, and assess synthesized research evidence (see **Supplementary Materials—Table S2**).

The results of the policy dialogue evaluation were also positive, and the scores ranged from 4.6 to 6.6. The following features were considered to be very useful: rely on a facilitator to assist with the deliberation, address high-priority policy issues, do not aim for consensus, provide an exhaustive discussion, and ensure a fair representation of those who will be involved in or affected by future decisions that are related to the respective issue (see **Supplementary Materials—Table S3**).

Post-Dialogue Mini-Interviews

Approximately 10 individuals agreed to participate in the post-dialogue mini-interviews, which were video-recorded. The findings of the study suggest that many participants demonstrated the positive insights that they gained during the policy dialogue (see **Table 3**).

DISCUSSION

Main Findings

The application of KT tools to support efforts to improve the care of deinstitutionalized patients with mental disorders and to contribute to the promulgation of evidence-informed mental health policies was a promising and innovative experience in Sorocaba. This experience entailed eight steps, and it demonstrated to policy-makers that the process of KT can bridge the gap between research and practice.

TABLE 3 | Participant opinions (insights) about the policy dialogue.

- "Very important space to discuss and align the thoughts so that the actions are more articulated"
- "Moment of interaction between different visions and access to information that goes well beyond global evidence ... greatly influenced by different views and experiences"
- "It is extremely important that managers, members of civil society and academia come together to discuss mental health issues. Articulation between Ministry of Health, universities and various actors involved in mental health policy will contribute to the advancement of public health policies in mental health"
- "The opportunity to listen to people who work in different areas of mental health was very important to understand better the problem and to contextualize the policy brief developed"
- "Policy dialogue is very interesting because it is not a debate; people dialogue and reflect to evolve in a particular concept or a specific implementation policy ... it allows the communication between the services of several levels"
- "Opportunity to bring together research and management ... the research shows the theoretical component that management does not have"
- "An important approach between research and practice ... does not seek a consensus, seeks a listening..."
- "It provides an expanded view of how deep the needs are around psychiatric reform in Brazil, and how divergent the opinions are from collecting local evidence from different actors in society (local, federal, professional, and civil society managers)...representing an environment of democratic discussion"
- "Listening to the most diverse opinions on the same subject, same problem ... there are several actors involved and each one with a participation, experience and a point of view ... very important this exchange, because it is very difficult to see from another prism"

The application of evidence in mental health practice and the exchange of knowledge between health-care providers, researchers, and community representatives were positively appraised. The entire process also helped those who are likely to be involved in or be affected by future policy-related decisions gain valuable insights. The features of the evidence brief and policy dialogue were considered to be very helpful, and they believed that it promoted an exhaustive discussion about the issue of deinstitutionalization.

A Comparison of the Present and Past Findings

Capacity building, which was the first step of the process, made the participants aware of the importance of the following: using KT tools to make evidence-informed policy decisions, align research at the University of Sorocaba with policy priorities, and build partnerships between policy-makers, stakeholders, and researchers. Training workshops have been found to improve knowledge and comprehension about the use of evidence in policy decision making in other countries as well (Uneke et al., 2012; Waqa et al., 2013; El-Jardali et al., 2014). The workshops also strengthened partnerships and enhanced the interaction between the Seriema group and the Health Departments of Sorocaba and the neighboring regions.

The evidence brief was prepared based on the best evidence available on the issue at hand. However, a majority of the systematic reviews focused on high-income countries (e.g. the United States of America, the United Kingdom, Canada, Australia), and none of them were conducted in Brazil. This demonstrated a knowledge gap regarding mental health care in Brazil (Amaral et al., 2018; Votruba et al., 2018). This led to many difficulties because the relationship between evidence and policy-making depends on country-specific features (e.g. social, organizational, and public factors), the specific policy issue, resources allocation, and contextual factors, which are very different (and in some cases, deficient) in LMICs (Tricco et al., 2013; Votruba et al., 2018). This difference can be attributed to the following features that characterise LMICs: low research capacity, an obscure policy-making process, a high risk of political instability, limited financial resources, a lack of interaction between researchers and policy-makers, and lack of empowerment of civil society (Young, 2005).

Furthermore, our findings corroborate the gap between research and practice that has been observed in LMICs, as well as the difficulties and complexities that mental health care entails. Despite the global burden of mental disorders (e.g. disability and lower disability-adjusted life years), mental health is not a policy priority in LMICs (Patel, 2007; Votruba et al., 2018). Mental health policy issues differ from other policy issues because they pertain to a highly heterogeneous set of conditions (i.e. mental, behavioral, or neurodevelopmental disorders), the presence of comorbidities, a lack of consensus on the best possible approach to treatment and care, a high rate of untreated patients, and the incumbent stigma (Votruba et al., 2018).

The definition of the problem and the options were discussed exhaustively, without the aim of reaching a consensus. The problem was perceived to be critical, and many of the participants (policy-makers, health-care providers, researchers, and representative of civil society, and public defense) conceptualized the problem based on their rich practical experience, and they echoed a majority of the challenges that were already presented in the evidence brief. In other words, the policy dialogue deliberations validate the evidence brief (Yehia and El Jardali, 2015). Thus, it is noteworthy that option 2 (*Provide psychoeducational programs*) was strongly supported by findings as well as the participants. On the other hand, option 1 (*Expand and improve the implementation of a Psychiatric Day Hospital*) was strongly opposed by a majority of the participants due to local findings; further, there were differences of opinion between international and local researches. Many of the participants were aware of the grave and inhumane treatment that patients with mental disorders had been subjected to in psychiatric hospitals in this region; they were also cognisant of the struggles that were required to shut down all the hospitals. The regulation of care with regard to crisis management and the treatment of acute episodes appear to be the most unclear albeit critical aspects of mental health care in Brazil (Amaral et al., 2018).

There is no KT strategy that is singularly effective across all contexts. Therefore, it is important to report about the context-specific utility of each strategy, so that they can be modified and utilised by other interested decision makers (Larocca et al., 2012). In this study, the participants provided positive evaluations of the evidence brief and of policy dialogue; they considered it to be favorable and useful, and these results corroborate past findings (Yehia and El Jardali, 2015; Boyko et al., 2016; Mc Sween-Cadieux et al., 2018). Similar findings emerged from the mini-interviews that were conducted at the end of the policy dialogue; specifically, all participant opinions were positive in tone. The use of a facilitator be to assist with the deliberation was considerate the most helpful feature of the policy dialogue. Past findings corroborate these results and emphasize the role of the facilitator as an unbiased agent which support KT platform (El-Jardali et al., 2014; Yehia and El Jardali, 2015).

Evidence briefs and summaries of policy dialogues (i.e. products of KT) can be used in public health policy-making only if the local and federal authorities are receptive to such efforts; unfortunately, often not the case (Cabieses and Espinoza, 2011).

Although the application of KT in public health policy-making is relatively new in LMCIs, the situation is changing. There is an increased use of evidence-informed policy frameworks (Cabieses and Espinoza, 2011; Votruba et al., 2018) and an increased demand for KT products from policy-makers. This has been proven by the EVIPNet-Brazil, which has expanded and consolidated its network (Dias et al., 2014). This practice needs to become a priority for Brazilian policy-makers because evidence-based public health models are powerful frameworks that can be used to identify the most effective health strategies and ensure that the resources are spent appropriately (Milat and Li, 2017).

Limitations and Strengths

The present study was the first attempt to use KT tools to improve some aspects of mental health care in Brazil (e.g. deinstitutionalization), which is a priority topic of regional and national importance. The policy dialogue brought together stakeholders who are involved in the process of deinstitutionalization (e.g. researchers, policy-makers, health-care providers, and representatives from public defense and civil society), which enriched the deliberations and provided the participants with an opportunity to acquire new knowledge and learn from each other.

The present study has a few limitations. A large part of the KT framework and the best evidence available were developed in high-income countries (e.g. the United Kingdom, Canada, Australia) that's can bring indirectness evidence. Further, we could not examine budgetary impact because the studies did not present cost analyses. Additionally, some of the options that were identified were difficult to understand because they were articulated using obscure terminologies. The variability in the quality of the reviewed studies and the lack of information about the options that can be implemented are a few other limitations. The low response rate that was evidenced for the evidence brief and policy dialogue evaluation surveys was attributed to time limitations and the busy lives that our participants led; therefore, some of our results may be underestimated. Although we have conducted an exhaustive and in-depth discussion, some topics that pertained to implementation were not discussed due to the paucity of time. However, since some aspects of implementation vary across communities, they should be discussed in accordance with the conditions of each municipality.

CONCLUSIONS

The KT process that was adopted was considered to be a useful means to discuss important policy issues, bring together policy-makers, health care providers, researchers, and representatives of civil society and public defense, enhance interaction and partnerships between evidence-producers and evidence-users, and promote the dissemination and application of global and local evidence in practice.

The present study did not seek to examine causal relationships. Nevertheless, a longer study period will allow future researchers to capture the positive changes in mental health care that result from KT. Future investigations are required to understand whether and how evidence briefs and policy dialogue can be used to improve the care of deinstitutionalized people with severe mental disorders and their contributions to Brazilian mental health policy.

Researchers and other stakeholders who are interested in using KT tools should consider the lessons that were learnt during the course of our study.

AUTHOR CONTRIBUTIONS

LL conceptualized the study. IF, JB, LL designed the study. IF, SB, MC and LL led data collection, carried out the analysis and drafted the initial manuscript. All authors read (IF, LL, JB, SB and MC) provided critical revision and approved the final manuscript.

FUNDING

This article was funded by FAPESP grants 2017/20668-7 and EVIPNet Brazil/Ministry of Health SCON2017-02502.

ACKNOWLEDGMENTS

The authors thank the Health Departments of the Sorocaba region.

REFERENCES

Amaral, C. E., Onocko-Campos, R., De Oliveira, P. R. S., Pereira, M. B., Ricci, E. C., Pequeno, M. L., et al. (2018). Systematic review of pathways to mental health care in Brazil: narrative synthesis of quantitative and qualitative studies. *Int. J. Ment Health Syst.* 12, 65. doi: 10.1186/s13033-018-0237-8

Boyko, J. A., Lavis, J. N., Abelson, J., Dobbins, M., and Carter, N. (2012). Deliberative dialogues as a mechanism for knowledge translation and exchange in health systems decision-making. *Soc. Sci. Med.* 75, 1938–1945. doi: 10.1016/j.socscimed.2012.06.016

Boyko, J. A., Kothari, A., and Wathen, C. N. (2016). Moving knowledge about family violence into public health policy and practice: a mixed method study of a deliberative dialogue. *Health Res. Policy Syst.* 14, 31. doi: 10.1186/s12961-016-0100-9

Brazil. (2001). Lei nº 10.216, de 6 de abril de 2001, que dispõe sobre a proteção e os direitos das pessoas portadoras de transtornos mentais e redireciona o modelo assistencial em saúde mental. 2001. Available at: https://hpm.org.br/wp-content/uploads/2014/09/lei-no-10.216-de-6-de-abril-de-2001.pdf (Accessed May 10 2017).

Brazil. (2005). Ministério da Saúde. Secretaria de Atenção à Saúde. Departamento de Ações Programáticas Estratégicas. Coordenação Geral de Saúde Mental.

Reforma psiquiátrica e política de saúde mental no Brasil. Documento apresentado à Conferência Regional de Reforma dos Serviços de Saúde Mental: 15 anos depois de Caracas. OPAS. Brasília: DF, 2005.

Brazil. (2012). SÃO PAULO (Estado). Ministério Público. Procuradoria Geral da Justiça. Termo de Ajuste e Conduta (TAC). São Paulo, 18 de dezembro de 2012. Available at: http://pfdc.pgr.mpf.mp.br/temas-de-atuacao/saude-mental/atuacao-do-mpf/tac-desinstitucionalizacao-de-hospitais-psiquiatricos-2012 (Accessed Jul 20 2017).

Brazil. (2015). Ministério da Saúde. Secretaria de Atenção à Saúde. Departamento de Ações Programáticas Estratégicas. Coordenação Geral de Saúde Mental, Álcool e Outras Drogas. Saúde Mental em Dados – 12, Ano 10, nº 12. Brasília: Informativo eletrônico de dados sobre a Política Nacional de Saúde Mental, 2015, 48p. Available at: http://www.mhinnovation.net/sites/default/files/downloads/innovation/reports/Report_12-edicao-do-Saude-Mental-em-Dados.pdf (Accessed Jan 10 2017).

Brazil. (2018). São Paulo. SP Notícias. Novo Hospital Regional de Sorocaba será referência em alta complexidade. Available at: http://www.saopaulo.sp.gov.br/spnoticias/ultimas-noticias/em-sorocaba-alckmin-entrega-hospital-de-alta-complexidade-com-260-leitos/ (Accessed Jul 13 2019).

Brazil. (2019). The Brazilian Institute of Geography and Statistics – IBGE. Cidades e Estados. Available at: https://ww2.ibge.gov.br/english/disseminacao/eventos/missao/instituicao.shtm (Accessed Apr 25 2019).

Cabieses, B., and Espinoza, M. A. (2011). La investigación traslacional y su aporte para la toma de decisiones en políticas de salud. *Rev. Peruana Med. Exp. y Salud. Publica* 28, 288–297. doi: 10.1590/S1726-46342011000200017

Cayres, A. Z. F. E. A. (2015). Secretaria da Saúde. Caminhos para a desinstitucionalização no Estado de São Paulo: censo psicossocial 2014. São Paulo: FUNDAP, 2015. Available at: http://www.saude.sp.gov.br/resources/ses/perfil/profissional-da-saude/grupo-tecnicodeacoesestrategicasgtae/saudemental/censopsicossocial/censo_psicossocial_2014.pdf (Accessed Jun 10 2019).

Dias, R. I. D. B., Barreto, J. O. M., and Souza, N. M. (2014). Desenvolvimento atual da Rede de Políticas Informadas por Evidências (EVIPNet Brasil): relato de caso. *Rev. Panam Salud. Publica* 36, 50–56.

Dieterich, M., Irving, C. B., Park, B., and Marshall, M. (2010). Intensive case management for severe mental illness. *Cochrane Database Syst. Rev.* (10) doi: 10.1002/14651858.CD007906.pub2

El-Jardali, F., Lavis, J., Moat, K., Pantoja, T., and Ataya, N. (2014). Capturing lessons learned from evidence-to-policy initiatives through structured reflection. *Health Res. Policy Syst.* 12, 2. doi: 10.1186/1478-4505-12-2

Emerich, B. F., and Yasui, S. (2016). O hospital psiquiátrico em diálogos atemporais. *Interface* 20, 207–216. doi: 10.1590/1807-57622015.0264

Evipnet-Brazil. (2019). Rede para Políticas Informadas por Evidências. Ministério da Saúde - Departamento de Ciência e Tecnologia (Decit). Available at: http://brasil.evipnet.org/sobre/ (Accessed Marc 20 2019).

Garcia, M. R. V. (2012). A mortalidade nos manicômios da região de Sorocaba e a possibilidade da investigação de violações de direitos humanos no campo da saúde mental por meio do acesso aos bancos de dados públicos. *J. Rev. Psicologia Política* 12, 105–120.

Larocca, R., Yost, J., Dobbins, M., Ciliska, D., and Butt, M. (2012). The effectiveness of knowledge translation strategies used in public health: a systematic review. *BMC Public Health* 12, 751. doi: 10.1186/1471-2458-12-751

Lavis, J. N., Permanand, G., Oxman, A. D., Lewin, S., and Fretheim, A. (2009a). Support Tools for evidence-informed health Policymaking (STP) 13: Preparing and using policy briefs to support evidence-informed policymaking. *Health Res. Policy Syst.* 7 Suppl 1, S13. doi: 10.1186/1478-4505-7-S1-S13

Lavis, J. N., Boyko, J. A., Oxman, A. D., Lewin, S., and Fretheim, A. (2009b). Support tools for evidence-informed health Policymaking (STP) 14: organising and using policy dialogues to support evidence-informed policymaking. *Health Res. Policy Syst.* 7 Suppl 1, S14. doi: 10.1186/1478-4505-7-S1-S14

Leff, H. S., Chow, C. M., Pepin, R., Conley, J., Allen, I. E., and Seaman, C. A. (2009). Does one size fit all? What we can and can't learn from a meta-analysis of housing models for persons with mental illness. *Psychiatr. Serv.* 60, 473–482. doi: 10.1176/ps.2009.60.4.473

Malla, C., Aylward, P., and Ward, P. (2018). Knowledge translation for public health in low- and middle- income countries: a critical interpretive synthesis. *Glob Health Res. Policy* 3, 29. doi: 10.1186/s41256-018-0084-9

Malone, D., Newron-Howes, G., Simmonds, S., Marriot, S., and Tyrer, P. (2007). Community mental health teams (CMHTs) for people with severe mental illnesses and disordered personality. *Cochrane Database Syst. Rev.* (3). doi: 10.1002/14651858.CD000270.pub2

Marshall, M., Crowther, R., Sledge, W. H., Rathbone, J., and Soares-Weiser, K. (2011). Day hospital versus admission for acute psychiatric disorders. *Cochrane Database Syst. Rev.* (2). doi: 10.1002/14651858.CD004026.pub2

Mc Sween-Cadieux, E., Dagenais, C., and Ridde, V. (2018). A deliberative dialogue as a knowledge translation strategy on road traffic injuries in Burkina Faso: a mixed-method evaluation. *Health Res. Policy Syst.* 16, 113. doi: 10.1186/s12961-018-0388-8

Milat, A. J., and Li, B. (2017). Narrative review of frameworks for translating research evidence into policy and practice. *Public Health Res. Pract.* 27 (1), e2711704. doi: 10.17061/phrp2711704

Moat, K. A., and Lavis, J. N. (2014). Suporte para uso de evidências de pesquisa nas Américas através do "one-stop shop" eletrônico: EVIPNet. *Cadernos Saúde Pública* 30, 2697–2701. doi: 10.1590/0102-311x00110214

Moat, K. A., Lavis, J. N., Clancy, S. J., El-Jardali, F., and Pantoja, T. (2014). Evidence briefs and deliberative dialogues: perceptions and intentions to act on what was learnt. *Bull. World Health Organ* 92, 20–28. doi: 10.2471/BLT.12.116806

Newlin, M., and Webber, M. (2015). Effectiveness of knowledge translation of social interventions across economic boundaries: a systematic review. *Eur. J. Soc. Work* 18, 543–568. doi: 10.1080/13691457.2015.1025710

Ongolo-Zogo, P., Lavis, J. N., Tomson, G., and Sewankambo, N. K. (2018). Assessing the influence of knowledge translation platforms on health system policy processes to achieve the health millennium development goals in Cameroon and Uganda: a comparative case study. *Health Policy Plan* 33, 539–554. doi: 10.1093/heapol/czx194

Patel, V. (2007). Mental health in low- and middle-income countries. *Br. Med. Bull.* 81–82, 81–96. doi: 10.1093/bmb/ldm010

Silva, E. K. B. D., and Rosa, L. C. D. S. (2014). Desinstitucionalização Psiquiátrica no Brasil: riscos de desresponsabilização do Estado. *Rev. Katálysis* 17, 252–260. doi: 10.1590/S1414-49802014000200011

Tricco, A. C., Cogo, E., Ashoor, H., Perrier, L., Mckibbon, K. A., Grimshaw, J. M., et al. (2013). Sustainability of knowledge translation interventions in healthcare decision-making: protocol for a scoping review. *BMJ Open* 3, e002970. doi: 10.1136/ bmjopen-2013-002970

Uneke, C. J., Ezeoha, A. E., Ndukwe, C. D., Oyibo, P. G., and Onwe, F. (2012). Promotion of evidence-informed health policymaking in Nigeria: bridging the gap between researchers and policymakers. *Glob Public Health* 7, 750–765. doi: 10.1080/17441692.2012.666255

Vidal, C. E. L., Bandeira, M., and Gontijo, E. D. (2008). Reforma psiquiátrica e serviços residenciais terapêuticos. *J. Brasileiro Psiquiatria* 57, 70–79. doi: 10.1590/S0047-20852008000100013

Votruba, N., Ziemann, A., Grant, J., and Thornicroft, G. (2018). A systematic review of frameworks for the interrelationships of mental health evidence and policy in low- and middle-income countries. *Health Res. Policy Syst.* 16, 85. doi: 10.1186/s12961-018-0357-2

Waqa, G., Mavoa, H., Snowdon, W., Moodie, M., Nadakuitavuki, R., Mc Cabe, M., et al. (2013). Participants' perceptions of a knowledge-brokering strategy to facilitate evidence-informed policy-making in Fiji. *BMC Public Health* 13, 725. doi: 10.1186/1471-2458-13-725

WHO. (2014). World Health Organization and the Gulbenkian Global Mental Health Plataform. Innovation in deinstitutionalization: a WHO expert survey. Geneva: World Health Organization, 2014.

Xia, J., Merinder, L. B., and Belgamwar, M. R. (2011). Psychoeducation for schizophrenia. *Cochrane Database Syst. Rev.* (6) doi: 10.1002/14651858. CD002831.pub2

Yehia, F., and El Jardali, F. (2015). Applying knowledge translation tools to inform policy: the case of mental health in Lebanon. *Health Res. Policy Syst.* 13, 29. doi: 10.1186/s12961-015-0018-7

Young, J. (2005). Research, policy and practice: why developing countries are different. *J. Int. Dev.* 17, 727–734. doi: 10.1002/jid.1235

Zhao, S., Sampson, S., Xia, J., and Jayaram, M. B. (2015). Psychoeducation (brief) for people with serious mental illness. *Cochrane Database Syst. Rev.* (4). doi: 10.1002/14651858.CD010823.pub2

19

Efficacy and Safety in the Continued Treatment with a Biosimilar Drug in Patients Receiving Infliximab: A Systematic Review in the Context of Decision-Making from a Latin-American Country

Edward Mezones-Holguin[1]*, Rocio Violeta Gamboa-Cardenas[2], Gadwyn Sanchez-Felix[3], José Chávez-Corrales[4], Luis Miguel Helguero-Santin[5], Luis Max Laban Seminario[5], Paula Alejandra Burela-Prado[6], Maribel Marilu Castro-Reyes[6] and Fabian Fiestas[6]

[1] Universidad San Ignacio de Loyola (USIL), Centro de Excelencia en Estudios Económicos y Sociales en Salud, Lima, Peru, [2] Seguro Social en Salud (EsSalud), Hospital Nacional Guillermo Almenara Irigoyen, Servicio de Reumatologia, Lima, Peru, [3] Seguro Social en Salud (EsSalud), Hospital Nacional Edgardo Rebagliati Martins, Servicio de Dermatología, Lima, Peru, [4] Seguro Social en Salud (EsSalud), Hospital Nacional Edgardo Rebagliati Martins, Servicio de Reumatologia, Lima, Peru, [5] Universidad Nacional de Piura (UNP), Facultad de Ciencias de la Salud, Sociedad Científica de Estudiantes de Medicina (SOCIEMUNP), Piura, Peru, [6] Seguro Social en Salud (EsSalud), Instituto de Evaluación de Tecnologías Sanitarias e Investigación (IETSI), Lima, Peru

*Correspondence:
Edward Mezones-Holguin
emezones@gmail.com;
emezones@usil.edu.pe

Introduction: Biological products, including infliximab (INF), are a therapeutic option for various medical conditions. In the Peruvian Social Security (EsSalud), infliximab is approved for the treatment of rheumatoid arthritis, psoriasis, psoriatic arthropathy, ankylosing spondylitis, ulcerative colitis and Crohn's disease (in cases refractory to conventional treatment). Biosimilars are a safe and effective alternative approved for these diseases in patients who start treatment with infliximab. Nevertheless, there are people in treatment with the biological reference product (BRP), in whom the continuing therapy with a biosimilar biological product (BBP) must be evaluated.

Objectives: To synthesize the best available evidence, calculate a preliminary financial impact and conduct technical discussions about the interchangeability into biosimilar in patients receiving treatment with original infliximab for medical conditions approved in EsSalud.

Methodology: We carried out a systematic review of controlled clinical trials. Primary search was performed in Pubmed- MEDLINE, SCOPUS, WOS, EMBASE, TRIPDATABASE, DARE, Cochrane Library, NICE, AHRQ, SMC, McMaster-PLUS, CADTH, and HSE until June-2018. We used the Cochrane Collaboration tool to assess the risk of bias. Also, we implemented a preliminary financial analysis about the impact of biosimilar introduction on institutional purchasing budget. Moreover, technical meetings with medical doctors specialized in rheumatology, gastroenterology and dermatology were held for discussing findings.

Results: In primary search, 1136 records were identified, and 357 duplicates were removed. From 799 records, we excluded 765 after title and abstract evaluation. From 14 full-text appraised documents, we included five clinical trials in the risk of bias assessment: four studies evaluated CTP-13 and one tested SB2. Two double-blind clinical trials reported no differences in efficacy and safety profiles between maintenance group (INF/INF) and interchangeability group in all diseases included (INF/CTP-13) and rheumatoid arthritis (CTP13 and SB2). In the other three studies, open-label extension of primary clinical trials, no differences were founded in efficacy and safety profiles between CTP-13/CTP-13 and INF/CTP-13 groups. In financial analysis, the inclusion of biosimilars implied savings around S/7'642,780.00 (1USD=S/3.30) on purchasing budget of EsSalud. In technical meetings, beyond certain concerns, specialists agreed with the findings.

Conclusions: Evidence from clinical trials support that there are no differences in efficacy or safety of continuing the treatment with Infliximab BRP or exchanging into its biosimilar in patients with medical conditions approved in EsSalud. Financial analysis shows that the biosimilar introduction produce savings in purchasing institutional budget. Therefore, based on cost-opportunity principle, exchanging into biosimilar in patients receiving the original Infliximab, is a valid therapeutic alternative in the Peruvian Social Security.

Keywords: Infliximab, biosimilar, interchangeability, decision making, Latin-American

INTRODUCTION

Biological products are therapeutic options for different diseases. These drugs are molecules with a complex structure, large and often highly specific and are derived from living organisms (Pombo et al., 2009; Wang and Singh, 2013; Auclair, 2019). Biologic drugs are used to treat various diseases, including conditions that involve the immune system, randomized studies have shown their efficacy for reducing symptoms and improving the quality of life in people undergoing treatment (Wang and Singh, 2013; Zelikin et al., 2016). However, a significant number of patients do not respond, have an inadequate response to initial treatment (primary failure), lose response over time (secondary failure), or may develop adverse effects potentially limiting the therapy (Auclair, 2019). One of these drugs is infliximab (REMICADE®), a tumor necrosis factor alpha inhibitor (TNFa) (Ecker et al., 2015). Infliximab has been approved for the treatment of rheumatoid arthritis (RA), severe psoriasis, ankylosing spondylitis, Crohn's disease, and ulcerative colitis, among other diseases.(Acevedo and Gaitan, 2012; European Medicines Agency (EMA), 2018; Food and Drug Administration, 2018). Efficacy, effectiveness, and safety of this biological drug has been tested in different studies (Li et al., 2017). Hence, infliximab is currently included in the pharmacological petition of the Peruvian Social Security (EsSalud). (Seguro Social en Salud (EsSalud), 2017).

On the other hand, the biosimilar biological products (BBP) are an efficient treatment alternative to the biological reference products (BRP). They usually offering similar effects and lower cost (Declerck et al., 2017; Gutka et al., 2018). BBP contains the active component of BRP with similar characteristics in its pharmacological activity, efficacy and safety (Gamez-Belmonte et al., 2018; Gutka et al., 2018). The equivalence of BBP has been reported from comparison – in equal terms - with BRP in various randomized clinical trials (Portela et al., 2017; Uhlig and Goll, 2017), where infliximab is one the most studied drugs (Gutka et al., 2018). Based on this information, international guidelines for its regulation have been spread and adopted in several countries (Garcia and Araujo, 2016; Sheets, 2017; Tsai, 2017; Zahl, 2017). The Peruvian health system is fragmented, segmented and inequitable (Sánchez-Moreno, 2014), where around 25% of population are affiliated to EsSalud (Mezones-Holguin et al., 2019). The General Directorate of Medicines, Supplies and Drugs (DIGEMID, from Spanish Acronym) as the national health authority, approved the commercialization of some infliximab biosimilars in Peru (Ministerio de Salud, Dirección General de Medicamentos, Insumos y Drogas (DIGEMID), 2016). Therefore, certain public institutions, supported by the Peruvian Government contracting laws, including the Social Security, have purchased BBP. Currently, in EsSalud there are two kinds of patients: those who will start treatment with Infliximab and those who continue their therapy with Infliximab. In the first group, the use of biosimilar is accepted as valid; however, in the other group, there are certain concerns with respect to the continuation with BBP.

Based on the context described, a decision should be made regarding the continuation with a biosimilar in patients undergoing treatment with original infliximab in EsSalud. Although, there are several definitions on interchangeability, in our manuscript it means a transition from using BRP to BBP (Gutka et al., 2018; Trifirò et al., 2018). At the moment, there is an interesting debate about interchangeability with active participation of distinct actors from different health care systems;

thus, international regulations have been proposed to the use of BBP and the transition from its BRP (Portela et al., 2017; Tsai, 2017; Cohen et al., 2018; Niazi, 2018). Nevertheless, in Peru, and specifically in EsSalud, there is no explicit decree for it. Therefore, the Institute for Health Technology Assessment and Research (IETSI, from Spanish acronym) - as technical entity in EsSalud - must evaluate the best available scientific evidence to inform decision-making in the Peruvian Social Security.

In light of the above mentioned, the aim of our study was to synthesize the best available evidence, calculate a preliminary financial impact, and conduct a technical discussion concerning the interchangeability into biosimilar in patients undergoing treatment with original infliximab for medical conditions approved in EsSalud. Although there are systematic reviews published (Chingcuanco et al., 2016; Cohen et al., 2018; McKinnon et al., 2018; Feagan et al., 2019), our study incorporates two key elements used in the decision-making process for health systems with limited resources: institutional budget and clinical experience. Consequently, our article is a description of this complexity in Peru and shows the use of the best scientific evidence in the real world.

METHODS

In our manuscript, we describe the three main activities performed in order to inform the decision-making process in EsSalud regarding infliximab interchangeability:

a) Systematic review based on PRISMA guidelines (Moher et al., 2009),
b) Preliminary financial analysis about the direct impact on institutional purchasing budget of EsSalud, and
c) Technical meeting with rheumatologists, dermatologists and gastroenterologists for discussing the results from clinical practice perspective.

SYSTEMATIC REVIEW

Clinical Question (PICOS)

The population(P) was circumscribed to adults with rheumatoid arthritis, psoriasis, ulcerative colitis, Crohn's disease and ankylosing spondylitis undergoing treatment with the original Infliximab. Intervention(I) was to exchange into a biosimilar, and comparison(C) was the continuation with original Infliximab. The outcomes(O) were efficacy and safety. In accordance with current legal regulations in EsSalud, we included only controlled clinical studies(S) in biosimilar drugs approved by DIGEMID for their commercialization in Peru (CTP-13 and SB2).

Search Strategy and Selection of Study

We conducted a search without language restrictions until June 2018. Primary strategy formulation included controlled and free terms according to PICOS question. Studies were restricted to clinical trials in humans of any age, gender or nationality. We searched in: PubMed-MEDLINE, SCOPUS, Web of Science

(WOS), Excerpta Medica (EMBASE), Translating Research into Practice (TRIPDATABASE), Database of Abstracts of Reviews of Effects (DARE), Cochrane Central Register of Controlled Trials (CENTRAL), National Institute for Health and Care Excellence (NICE), The Agency for Healthcare Research and Quality (AHRQ), The Scottish Medicines Consortium (SMC), McMaster PLUS, The Canadian Agency for Drugs and Technologies in Health (CADTH), and The Health Systems Evidence (HSE). Primary search strategies for each database are explicitly presented as annexes (A-N) (**Supplementary Table 1**). Additionally, we reviewed the list of references. Poster and oral presentations in scientific meetings were not considered.

Article Selection

Records found were collected in an electronic folder using Mendeley® (Elsevier Inc, NY, USA) and we generated a Research Information Systems (RIS) file. Duplicates were removed by automatic and manual methods; then, we exported a new file to Rayyan® (Qatar Computer Research Institute, Doha, Qatar). Two authors (LHS and LLS) completed a blind and independent selection based on abstract and title, third author (EMH) had diriment decision. Then, two authors (LH-S and LL-S) selected articles in full-text evaluation with third author as diriment (EM-H). Afterward, two evaluators (LHS and LLS) codified the articles and uploaded them in Google Drive® folder (Google Inc, CA, USA).

Risk of Bias Assessment

Two authors (LHS and LLS) acted upon blind and independent appraisal of clinical trials using the Cochrane Collaboration tool(Higgins et al., 2011). Disagreements were resolved by consensus and diriment participation (EMH).

Statistical Synthesis

Although a meta-analysis was initially proposed, it was not performed due to clinical and methodological heterogeneity.

Preliminary Financial Analysis

We implemented an analysis about the impact of biosimilar introduction in the institutional purchasing budget based on the official reports of EsSalud and Electronic Government Procurement System of Peru (SEACE, from Spanish Acronym).

Technical Meeting

We held several face-to-face meetings to present and discuss the results of the systematic review and financial analysis. A group of rheumatologists, dermatologists and gastroenterologists working in hospitals of EsSalud in Lima, participated in these reunions.

RESULTS

Selection and Characteristics of Studies

We identified a total of 1136 records in the primary search, from which we removed 357 duplicates. From 799 screened records, we excluded 765 in title and abstract evaluation. Then, we appraised 14 full-text documents, and included five clinical trials for risk of bias assessment and data extraction (**Figure 1**).

We found five controlled studies, that corresponded to five publications, which evaluated the interchangeability between Infliximab and its PBB. Only one assessed SB2 biosimilar (Smolen et al., 2018), and the four remaining studies evaluated biosimilar CTP-13. Two publications were double-blind Randomized controlled studies (RCT), while the remaining three were open-label continuation of clinical trials that initially compared the PBR with PBB. Three studies focused specifically on patients with rheumatoid arthritis, one in ankylosing spondylitis and another, in addition to these two diseases, included Crohn's

disease, ulcerative colitis, psoriatic arthritis and chronic plaque psoriasis. In **Table 1** we present the general characteristics of trials included.

Only two articles respond directly to the PICO question, since they evaluated the exchange of the original Infliximab to the biosimilar compared to the maintenance of the original biotherapy: Smolen et al. (2018) and Jørgensen et al. (2017), who tested SB2 and CTP-13, respectively. In both cases, they did not find statistical differences in efficacy or safety between maintenance and exchanging groups.

The other three publications did not respond directly to PICOS question. These studies did not contain primary safety or efficacy data in a blind setting. Instead, they provided complementary

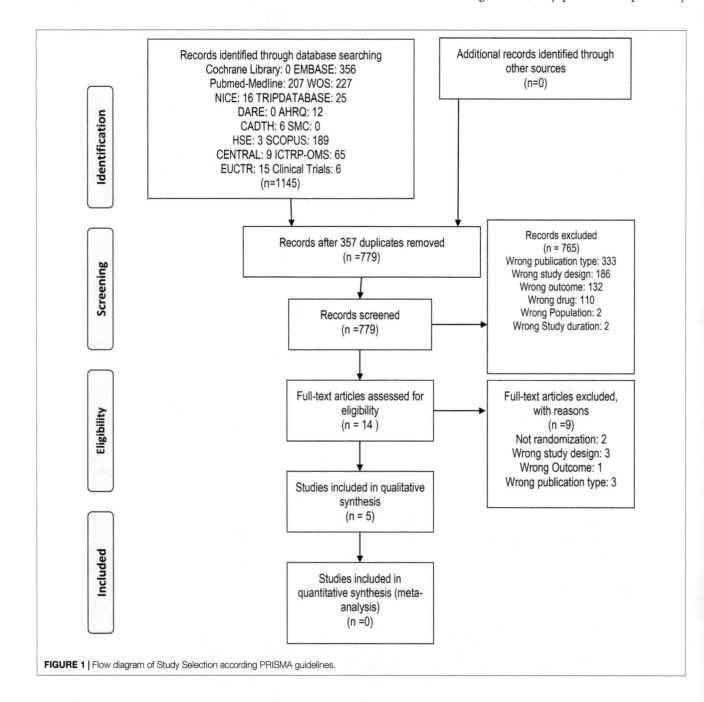

FIGURE 1 | Flow diagram of Study Selection according PRISMA guidelines.

TABLE 1 | Characteristics of primary studies included in the analysis.

Author (Year)	Design (Founding)	Population	Countries	Comparison (Pre/ post exchange)*	Average time (Pre/post exchange)	Conclusion
Biosimilar: SB2						
Smolen et al. (2018)	Randomized double-blind phase 3 trial(Samsung Bioepis Co Ltd.)	Rheumatoid arthritis	Bulgaria Colombia Czech Republic Hungary Republic of Korea Lithuania Mexico Poland Ukraine UK	INF/INF (n=101) SB2/SB2 (n=201) INF/SB2 (n=92)	(54/46 weeks)	The efficacy, safety and immunogenicity profiles were similar between the groups: INF/SB2,INF/INF and SB2/ SB2.No emergent treatment or clinically relevant problems were observed after the change from INF to SB2
Biosimilar: CT-P13						
Jørgensen et al. (2017)	Randomized double-blind non-inferiority phase 4 trial(Government of Norway)	Crohn's disease, ulcerative colitis, rheumatoid arthritis, spondylarthritis, psoriatic arthritis, chronic plaque psoriasis	Norway	CT-P13/ CT-P13 (n=241) INF/CT-P13 (n=241)	(26/52 weeks)**	The change from INF to CT-P13 showed no inferiority to the continuous treatment with INF in terms of safety and immunogenicity for all the diseases studied.However, there was not enough statistical power to demonstrate non-inferiority for each disease.
Tanaka (2017)	Open label extension of phase 2 trial(Celltrion Inc)	Rheumatoid arthritis	Japan	CT-P13/ CT-P13 (n=38) INF/CT-P13 (n=33)	(52/72 weeks)***	CT-P13 was well tolerated with persistent efficacy for both groups. Likewise, stable clinical efficacy was shown in patients with RA.
Yoo et al. (2017)	Open label extension of the phase 3-PLANETRA trial(Celltrion Inc)	Rheumatoid arthritis	Bosnia Bulgaria Chile Colombia Italy Latvia Lithuania Mexico Peru Poland Philippines Romania Slovakia Spain UK Ukraine	CT-P13/ CT-P13 (n=158) INF/CT-P13 (n=144)	(54/48 weeks)	The efficacy and tolerability observed was similar between patients who were switched from INF to CTP-13 and those who had a long-term treatment with CT-P13 for two years.
Park et al. (2017)	Open-label extension of a phase 3-PLANETAS trial(Celltrion Inc)	Ankylosing spondylitis	Bulgaria Chile Colombia Republic of Korea Latvia Mexico Poland Portugal Spain Ukraine	CT-P13/ CT-P13 (n=388) INF/CT-P13 (n=86)	(54/48 weeks)	The exchange from the original biological reference product into biosimilar is possible without negative effects on safety and efficacy in patients with ankylosing spondylitis.

* The number of patients corresponds to exchanging started time.
** Randomization was applied in patients who already had treatment with the original infliximab drug for a minimum of 6 months.
*** The initial phase of treatment ended at 54 weeks. The first dose of the second stage started eight weeks later in week 62.

information with the purpose of expanding the perspective of clinical use in potential EsSalud scenarios. Those publications reported the evaluation of open-label continuation of primary clinical trials: Tanaka et al. (2017), Yoo et al. (2017), and Park et al. (2017). In these publications no differences were found in efficacy or safety between patients who switched from original infliximab to biosimilar (INF/CTP-13), and maintained biosimilar treatment (CTP-13/CTP-13).

Risk of Bias

In **Table 2**, we show the appraisal for each study included. Trials with direct response to PICOS question had lower risk of bias, mainly due to randomization and blinding.

Description of Evidence

We briefly described efficacy and safety outcomes for each study: one for SB2 and four for CTP-13. We describe efficacy and safety outcomes.

Biosimilar SB2

Smolen et al. (2018) "**Safety, Immunogenicity And Efficacy After Switching From Reference Infliximab To Biosimilar SB2 Compared With Continuing Reference Infliximab And SB2 In Patients With Rheumatoid Arthritis: Results Of A Randomized, Double-Blind, Phase III Transition Study.**" **Annals Of The Rheumatic Diseases; 7:234-40.**

A randomized, double-blind, phase 3 clinical study was carried out in people with rheumatoid arthritis. This study had two initial groups. Patients were randomized into two groups for 52 weeks: 293 were treated with Infliximab (INF) and 292 received biosimilar (SB2). Then, a new randomization was performed, INF group was divided into a maintenance group (INF/INF n=101) or exchanging group (INF/SB2 n=94). Meanwhile, the group initially assigned to SB2 continued with biosimilar (SB2/SB2 n=201). Efficacy, safety and immunogenicity profiles were not different among the groups up to week 78.

Efficacy

The major findings of this study are presented in **Table 3A**. We describe the findings according the clinical scale used.

American College Of Rheumatology (ACR20, ACR50 And ACR70)

Authors found that the percentage of patients who showed a 20% improvement (ACR20) at week 78 of follow-up was not statistically different between the three groups: INF/INF (68.8%), SB2/SB2 (65.7%) and INF/SB2 (63.5%) (p-value:0.7316). Also, there was no statistically significant difference between groups in the proportion of patients with 50% improvement (ACR50)

(p-value:0.3249). Moreover, in 70% improvement (ACR70), no significant differences were found in (p-value: 0.3071): INF/INF group (31.2%), SB2/SB2 (25.6%) and INF/SB2 (22.4%).

European League Against Rheumatology Score (EULAR)

EULAR response criteria scores were measured at week 78, no statistically significant differences were observed. Good or moderate responses were 84.9% in INF/INF group, 87.3% in SB2/SB2 group and 84.7% in INF/SB2 group (p-value: 0.8074). Regarding the proportion of patients with good response, there was no significant difference between groups: INF/INF (34.4%), SB2/SB2 (35.6%) and INF/SB2 (32.9%) (p= 0.8740).

Diseases Activity Score 28 (DAS28), Simple Disease Activity Index (SDAI) And Clinical Diseases Activity Index (CDAI)

These three instruments were used to measure the activity of the disease and there were no significant statistical differences between randomized groups. DAS28 values were (mean±sd): INF/INF (4,1±1,5), SB2/SB2 (4,0±1,4), y INF/SB2 (3,9±1,3). SDAI score in each group were: INF/INF (15,2±12,0), SB2/SB2 (initial 14,6±12,2), and INF/SB2 (13,2±10,0). Regarding CDAI, patients obtained similar scores: INF/INF (15,2±12,0), SB2/SB2 (initial 14,6±12,2), and INF/SB2 (13,2±10,0). No point values were reported at the end of the follow-up at week 78; authors showed graphically the evolution of the scores during the post interchange period, there is no difference between the three groups evaluated (**Table 3A**).

Safety
Adverse Events

No differences were observed in the frequency of adverse events (AE) among the three post-exchange groups: Specifically, for any AE were: INF/INF (35,6%), SB2/SB2 (40,3%), and INF/SB2 (36,2%) of patients presenting any AE (p=0.546). Regarding serious AE post-exchange, frequencies were: 6.4% in INF/SB2, 3% in INF/INF and 3.5% in SB2/SB2 (p=0.456). Similarly, no differences were found in the frequency of discontinuation due to AE (p=0.625) (**Table 3E**).

TABLE 2 | Risk of bias assessment in each study according Cochrane Collaboration Tool.

Author (Year)	Selection Bias		Performance bias	Detection bias	Attrition bias	Reporting bias	Others
	Randomization	Allocation concealment	Blinding of participants and staff	Blinding of outcome assessors and results	Monitoring, exclusion and abandonment	Selective reporting of results	Other biases
Smolen et al. (2018)*	Low	Low	Low	Low	Low	Low	Low
Jorgensen et al. (2017)*	Low	Low	Low	Low	Low	Low	Low
Tanaka (2017)	High	High	High	High	Low	Low	Low
Yoo et al. (2017)	High	High	High	High	Low	Low	Low
Park et al. (2017)	High	High	High	High	Low	Low	Low

These articles respond directly PICOs question.

Efficacy and Safety in the Continued Treatment with a Biosimilar Drug in Patients Receiving...

167

TABLE 3A | Efficacy outcomes in patients with rheumatoid arthritis.

Author (Year)	Time	Groups (patients allocated)	ACR20* n(%)	ACR50 n(%)	ACR70 n(%)	DAS28 (media±ds)	EULAR n (%)
Smolen et al. (2018)	Exchange: Week 54 End: Week 78	INF/INF (n=101)	End: 68.8%	End: 47.3%	End: 31.2%	Baseline: 4.1±1.5 End:**	End (93 patients): No response: 14 (15.1%) Moderate: 47 (50.5%) Good: 32 (34.4%)
		INF/SB2 (n=94)	End: 63.5%	End: 37.6%	End: 22.4%	Baseline: 3.9±1.3 End:**:	End (85 patients): No response: 13 (15.3%) Moderate: 44 (51.8%) Good: 28 (32.9%)
		SB2/SB2 (n=94)	End: 68.3%	End: 40.6%	End: 25.6%	Baseline: 4.0±1.4 End:**:	End (180 patients): No response: 23 (12.8%) Moderate: 93 (51.7%) Good: 64 (35.6%)
		Estimated p-value	p=0.7316	p=0.3249	p=0.3071	NA	P=0.8074***
Tanaka et al. (2017)	Exchange: Week 62 End: Week 167	CT-P13/CTP-13 n=38	End: 29(78.4%)	End: 26 (70.3%)	End: 20(54.1%)	Baseline: -2.66 ± 1.57 End: -2.78 ± 1.59	End: Moderate or Good: 31(83.8%)
		INF/CTP-13 n=33	End: 62.5%)	End: 17(53.1%)	End: 13 (40.6%)	Baseline: -2,01 ± 1.33 End -2,03 ± 1.73	End: Moderate or Good: 22 (68.8%)
		Estimated p-value	P=0.1535	P=0.14	P=0.26	P=0.612	P=0.1498***
Yoo et al. (2017)	Exchange: Week 54 End: Week 102	CT-P13/CTP-13 n=168	End: 117 (74.1%)	End: 78 (49.4%)	End: 39(24.7%)	Baseline: -2,40±1.27 End: -2.40 ± 1.42	End: No response: 15 (9.9%) Moderate: 80 (52.6%) Good: 43 (28.3%)
		INF/CTP-13 n=144	End: 111(77.1%)	End: 78 (54.2%)	End: 38 (26.4%)	Baseline: -2.37±1.22 End: -2,48±1.43	End: No response: 12 (8.5%) Moderate: 69 (48.6%) Good: 46 (32.4%)
		Estimated p-value	p=0.54	p=0.40	p=0.7341	p=0.99	p=0.669***

ACR20, ACR50 y ACR70: Improvement in 20%, 50% and 70% according to the American College of Rheumatology criteria.

DAS28, Score of activity of the disease in 28 joints with reactive protein C (PCR).

EULAR, European League against Rheumatism.

*Jorgensen et al. study included patients with rheumatoid arthritis, however, the random assignment and the sample calculation were for all pathologies. Because it was a subgroup analysis, no results were reported for RA in this table. Baseline corresponds to time of exchanging.

**No differences were founded between the DAS28 indices for each group, no point values were reported at the end of follow-up. The article did not report any differences using graphic methods.

***Comparison for moderate or good classification.

Immunogenicity

Post-exchange immunogenicity levels were very similar among groups: INF/INF (14.9%), SB2/SB2 (14.1%) and INF/SB2 (14.6%) (p=0.98) (p=0.98) (**Table 3E**).

Biosimilar CTP-13

Jørgensen et al., 2017. **"Switching from Originator Infliximab to Biosimilar CT-P13 Compared with Maintained Treatment with Originator Infliximab (NOR-SWITCH): A 52-Week, Randomized, Double-Blind, Non-Inferiority Trial."** Lancet 389 (10086): 2304–16 (Jørgensen et al., 2017).

The authors conducted a phase 4, randomized double-blind non-inferiority trial. Patients with Crohn's disease, ulcerative colitis, rheumatoid arthritis, spondylarthrosis, psoriatic arthritis and chronic plaque psoriasis receiving original infliximab were enrolled and randomized in two arms:: maintenance group with the original biological component (INF/INF), and exchanging group from the original biological into its biosimilar (INF/CT-P13). The exchange group showed non-inferiority to the ongoing treatment with INF on efficacy and safety for all diseases investigated. However, there was not enough statistical power to demonstrate the non-inferiority for each disease studied. This research was financed by the Norwegian Government.

Efficacy

Different measurements were used according to clinical population studied. Authors define two main types of variables: a) *categorical (state):* percentage of patients with a specified condition (deterioration or remission) based on clinical scales, and b) *numerical (change):* any variation in the score of clinical scales at the end of the follow-up with respect to the baseline (exchange time).

TABLE 3B | Efficacy findings in clinical trials in patients with ankylosing spondylitis.

Author (Year)	Start / end time	Groups (Patients allocated)	ASAS20 n(%)	ASAS40 n(%)	ASAS PR n(%)	BASDAI (mean)	BASFI (mean)	ASDAS Global Score (mean)	BASMI (mean)
Park et al. (2017)	*Exchange:* Week 54	CT-P13/CT-P13 (n=88)	*End:* 67/83 (80.7)	*End:* 53/83 (63.9)	*End:* 16/83 (19.3)	*End:* 3.19	*End:* 3.24	*End:* 1.86	*End:* 2.4
	End: Week 102	INF/CT-P13 (n=86)	*End:* 60/78 (76.9)	*End:* 48/78 (61.5)	*End:* 18/78 (23.1)	*End:* 3.23	*End:* 3.25	*End:* 1.97	*End:* 2.6
		Estimated p value	*0.506*	*0.672*	*0.275*	*NS**	*NS**	*NS**	*NS**

ASAS, *The Assessment of Spondylarthritis International Society;* PR, *Partial Remission;* BASDAI, *The Bath Ankylosing Spondylitis Disease Activity Index;*
BASFI, *Bath Ankylosing Spondylitis Functional Index;* ASDAS, *Ankylosing Spondylitis Disease Activity Score;* BASMI, *Bath Ankylosing Spondylitis Metrology Index;*
ASDAS, *Ankylosing Spondylitis Disease Activity Score.*
* Standard deviation was not reported. Authors only compared graphically.

Deterioriation During Follow-Up

This was the primary outcome for all patients based on specific clinical scales for each of the six diseases studied. In the ITT analysis, frequency of deterioration in all diseases were 22.4% in the INF/INF group, and a 26.3% in the INF/CTP-13 group (p=0.3259). Although the frequency of decline of the six diseases was defined, there was not enough statistical power to test non-inferiority of each disease; thus, we only report the frequencies for exploratory purposes (**Table 3C**).

Remission During Follow-Up

Approximately 60% of patients in each group achieved remission (p=0.8810) (**Table 3C**). There was not enough statistical power to evaluate the non-inferiority for each disease.

Quality of Life: SF36 and EQ5D

Health-related quality of life (QoL) for all diseases were assessed using SF36 and EQ5D; two validated and widely used instruments. In the first group, statistically significant differences during the follow-up period regarding physical limitations (p=0.0069) and emotional limitations were found (p=0.026); with a greater average of deterioration (decrease in score) in the maintenance group (-0.4) and exchange group (-1.1). There were not statistical differences in the others components. Meanwhile, there were different changes on the clinical global impressions scale of EQ5D in both groups (p=0.999) (**Table 3D**).

Safety

There were no statistically significant differences between patients of two groups in safety variables.

Adverse Events

Frequencies of serious AE were 10% in maintenance patients and 9% in exchanging group. Discontinuation due to AE was 4% and 3%, respectively.

Immunogenecity

Frequency of patients with post transition ADA were: 7% (INF/INF) and 8% (INF/CTP-13) (**Table 3E**).

Tanaka et al., 2017. **"Safety and Efficacy of CT-P13 in Japanese Patients with Rheumatoid Arthritis in an Extension Phase or after Switching from Infliximab." Modern Rheumatology 27 (2): 237–45** (Tanaka et al. 2017).

This open label study, RA patients were randomized in two arms: INF/CTP-13 and CTP-13/CTP-13. There were no statistical differences in efficacy and safety assessed by clinical scales.

Efficacy
ACR20, ACR50 and ACR70

No differences were found in frequency of patients who improved in the three categories proposed by the American College of Rheumatology: ACR20%, ACR50% and ACR70%. In CTP-13/CTP-13 (78.4%, 70.3% and 54.1%) and INF/CTP-13 (62.5%, 53.1% and 40.6%), respectively (**Table 3A**).

TABLE 3C | Frequency of deterioration and remission during follow-up in patients with Crohn's disease, ulcerative colitis, spondylarthritis, rheumatoid arthritis, psoriatic arthritis, and chronic plaque psoriasis.

				Worsening during follow-up							Remission during follow-up
Author (Year)	Time	Groups	Patients allocated	All diseases	Rheumatoid arthritis	Psoriatic arthritis	Psoriasis	Spondylarthritis	Crohn's Disease	Ulcerative colitis	All Diseases
Jorgensen et al. (2017)	*Start:* Week 0	INF/INF	241	54 (22.4%)	11(28.2%)	7 (50%)	2 (11.1%)	17 (37.8%)	14 (17.9%)	3 (6.4%)	145 (60.2%)
	End: Week 52	INF/CT-P13 *Estimated p-value*	240	63 (26.3%) p=0.3259	*10 (26.3%)* NE	*8 (50.0%)* NE	2 (11.8%) NE	*14 (30.4%)* NE	*24 (31.2%)* NE	5 (10.9%) NE	*146 (60.8%)* p=0.8810

NE, Not estimated due to the low statistical power.

TABLE 3D | Quality of life in patients with Crohn's disease, ulcerative colitis, spondylarthritis, rheumatoid arthritis, psoriatic arthritis, and chronic plaque psoriasis (SF36 and EQ5D).

Author (Year)	Time	Groups (patients allocated)	SF-36 FF	SF-36 LRF	SF-36 Pain	SF-36 SG	SF-36 BE	SF-36 LRE	SF-36 FS	SF-36 EF	SF-36 RCF	SF-36 RCM	EQ 5D
Jørgensen et al. (2017)	*Exchange:* Week 0	INF/INF (n=241)	*Baseline:* 50.6 (11.3)	*Baseline:* 45.6 (11.6)	*Baseline:* 47.2 (8.5)	*Baseline:* 43.5 (10.2)	*Baseline:* 50.0 (9.8)	*Baseline:* 48.8 (10.8)	*Baseline:* 48.0 (10.5)	*Baseline:* 47.1 (10.4)	*Baseline:* 46.4 (10.1)	*Baseline:* 49.1 (10.7)	*Baseline:* 0.8 (0.2)
			End: −1.2 (7.0)	*End:* −1.1 (11.2)	*End:* −0.7 (7.3)	*End:* −1.1 (7.3)	*End:* −1.3 (7.8)	*End:* −0.5 (12.2)	*End:* −0.2 (9.4)	*End:* −1.9 (8.5)	*End:* −1.2 (6.9)	*End:* −0.7 (8.9)	*End:* 0.0 (0.2)
	End: Week 52	INF/CT-P13 (n=240)	*Baseline:* 50.5 (10.9)	*Baseline:* 46.9 (11.3)	*Baseline:* 47.8 (9.5)	*Baseline:* 44.5 (10.2)	*Baseline:* 50.9 (8.9)	*Baseline:* 50.0 (10.4)	*Baseline:* 48.6 (9.5)	*Baseline:* 46.9 (10.2)	*Baseline:* 46.8 (10.3)	*Baseline:* 50.3 (9.3)	*Baseline:* 0.8 (0.2)
			End: 0 (6.3)	*End:* −0.4 (9.4)	*End:* −0.5 (7.7)	*End:* −1.1 (7.1)	*End:* −0.7 (7.8)	*End:* −2.4 (10.5)	*End:* −0.6 (10.4)	*End:* 0.5 (8.3)	*End:* 0.2 (6.6)	*End:* −1.3 (8.9)	*End:* 0.0 (0.2)
		Estimated p-value	0.103	0.0069	0.4096	0.6677	0.999	0.026	0.1183	0.7129	0.4921	*0.999*	*0.999*

SF-36, 36-Item Short Form Health Survey; FF, Physical functioning; LRF, Limitation of physical roles; SG, General Health; BE, Emotional wellbeing; LRE, Limitation of emotional roles; FS, Social Functioning; EF, Energy or Fatigue; RCF, Physical component summary; RCM, Mental component summary; Baseline, exchanging time; End, Conclusion of follow-up.

DAS28

There were also no differences in the average scores at the end of the follow-up between maintenance group (2.78) and exchange group (2.03) (p=0.612) (**Table 3A**).

EULAR

Frequency of good or moderate response after the follow-up period did not show significant statistical difference between the two groups: 83% in maintenance patients and 68.8% in exchanging people (**Table 3A**).

Safety
Adverse Events

In maintenance group, 5.3% of patients had serious AE and 10.5% discontinuing the prescription due to AE. Meanwhile, in CTP-13 exchanging group participants had 12.1% of serious AE and 24.2% discontinued the treatment due to AE. These differences were not statistically significant (**Table 3E**).

Immunogenicity

In post-transition stage, frequency of patients with ADA were 10.6% in maintenance group and 12.1% in exchanging group. (p=0.901) (**Table 3E**).

"**Efficacy and Safety of CT-P13 (Biosimilar Infliximab) in Patients with Rheumatoid Arthritis: Comparison between Switching from Reference Infliximab to CT-P13 and Continuing CT-P13 in the PLANETRA Extension Study**." **Annals of the Rheumatic Diseases 76 (2): 355–63** (Yoo et al., 2017).

Authors compared two groups of Rheumatoid arthritis patients: maintenance (CTP-13/CTP-13) and exchanging (INF/CTP13). Efficacy, tolerability and safety observed were non different between groups.

ACR20, ACR50 and ACR70

Frequencies of 20%, 50% and 70% responses according to the ACR criteria were: 74.1%, 49.4% and 24.7% in CTP-13/CTP-13,

and 77.1%, 54.2% and 26.4% in INF/CTP-13 group. There was no evidence of statistically significant differences between groups (**Table 3A**).

DAS28

The average final scores were not statistically different between maintenance (2.40) and exchanging (2.48) groups (**Table 3A**).

EULAR

Frequency of patients with a good or moderate criterion according to EULAR were 80.9% and 81% in maintenance and exchanging arms, respectively. There were no statistical differences between groups (p=0.669) (**Table 3A**).

Safety
Adverse Events

In maintenance group, 7.5% of patients had serious AE, and 10% discontinued their treatment due to AE. These frequencies did not differ than exchanging group (9% and 5.6%, respectively) (**Table 3E**).

Park et al., 2017. "**Efficacy and Safety of Switching from Reference Infliximab to CT-P13 Compared with Maintenance of CT-P13 in Ankylosing Spondylitis: 102-Week Data from the PLANETAS Extension Study**" **Annals of the Rheumatic Diseases 76 (2): 346–54** (Park et al., 2017).

This trial was carried out in patients with ankylosing spondylitis. Participants were randomized in two groups: maintenance (CTP-13/CTP-13) and exchanging (INF/CTP-13). No statistically significant differences were observed between group in terms of efficacy or safety.

Efficacy
Assessment of Spondylarthritis international Society (ASAS20, ASAS40 and ASAS PR)

Non statistical differences were found between groups according ASAS measurements for 20%, 40% and partial remission

TABLE 3E | Safety outcomes in all primary studies included.

Author (Year)	Conditions	Exchanging Time	Intervention Groups	Patients allocated	Immunogenicity (ADA)	Patients with adverse events (post exchange)
Smolen et al. (2018)	Rheumatoid arthritis	Exchange: Week 54	INF/INF	101	Post-transition: 14.9%	Any AE: 36(35.6%)Serious AE: 3 (3%) Discontinuation due to AE: 1 (1%)
		End: Week 78	SB2/SB2	201	Post-transition: 14.1%	Any AE:81(40.3%)Serious AE: 7(3.5%) Discontinuation due to AE: 3 (1.5%)
			INF/SB2	94	Post-transition: 14.6%	Any AE: 34(36. 2%)Serious AE: 6 (6.4%) Discontinuation due to AE: 3 (3.2%)
		Estimated p-value			p=0.98	
Jorgensen et al. (2017)*	Crohn's disease. Ulcerative colitis. Rheumatoid arthritis. Spondylarthritis. Psoriatic arthritis. Chronic plaque psoriasis	Exchange: Week 0 End: Week 52	INF/INF	241	Post-transition: 17 (7.1%)	Any AE: 168 (70%)Serious AE: 24 (10%) Discontinuation due to AE: 9(4%)
			INF/CT-P13	240	Post-transition: 19 (7.9%)	Any AE: 164 (68%)Serious AE: 21(9%) Discontinuation due to AE: 8(3%)
		Estimated p-value			0.911	
Tanaka et al. (2017)*	Rheumatoid arthritis	Exchange: Week 54 End: Week 167	CT-P13/CT-P13	38	Post-transition: 4 (10.6%)	Any AE: 34(89. 5%)Serious AE: 2(5.3%) Discontinuation due to AE: 4(10.5%)
			INF/CT-P13	33	Post-transition: 4 (12.1%)	Any AE: 29 (87.9%)Serious AE: 4 (12.1%) Discontinuation due to AE: 8 (24.2%)
		Estimated p-value			0.901	
Yoo et al. (2017)	Rheumatoid arthritis	Exchange: Week 54 End: Week 102	CT-P13/CT-P13	158	Post-transition: 64(40.5%)	Any AE: 85 (53.8%) Serious AE: 12(7.5%) Discontinuation due to AE: 16 (10.1%)
			INF/CT-P13	144	Post-transition: 64 (44.4%)	Any AE: 77 (53.5%) Serious AE: 13(9.0%) Discontinuation due to AE: 8 (5.6%)
		Estimated p-value			0.48	
Park et al. (2017)	Ankylosing spondylitis	Exchange: Week 54 End: Week 102	CT-P13/CT-P13	88	Post-transition: 21 (23.3%)	Any AE: 44 (50%) Serious AE: 4 (4.5%) Discontinuation due to AE: 3 (3.3%)
			INF/CT-P13	86	Post-transition: 23 (27.4%)	Any AE: 60 (69.7%)Serious AE: 4 (4.6%) Discontinuation due to AE: 4 (4.6%)
		Estimated p-value			0.60	

ADA, Anti-drug antibody; NR, Not reported; EA, Adverse Events. Primary outcome was cumulative incidence of AE.

of disease: in maintenance (80.7%, 63.9% and 19.3%) and exchanging (76.9%, 61.5% and 23.1%) patients (**Table 3B**).

Bath Ankylosing Spondylitis Disease Activity Index (BASDAI), Bath Ankylosing Spondylitis Functional Index (BASFI), Ankylosing Spondylitis Disease Activity Score (ASDAS) and Bath Ankylosing Spondylitis Metrology Index (BASMI)

Authors reported - using graphical methods - non differences in average at the end of follow-up between maintenance and exchanging groups: BASDAI (3.19 vs. 3.23), BASFI (3.1 vs. 3.25), ASDAS (1.86 vs. 1.97), and BASMI (2.4 vs. 2.6) (**Table 3B**).

Safety
Adverse Events
In maintenance group, 4.5% and 3.3% of allocated patients had serious AE and discontinued treatment due to AE, respectively. Meanwhile, in exchanging group frequencies were 4.6% in both

measures. There are no evidence of statistical differences between arms (**Table 3E**).

Immunogenicity
In post-exchange period, there were non statistical differences in proportion of patients with ADAs between groups. Authors reported 23.3% in CTP-13/CTP-13 and 27.4% in INF/CTP-13 groups (**Table 3E**).

Preliminary Financial Analysis
First, we present the estimate of annual costs per patient based on price for each vial offered by each provider, S/2040.00 (S/: Peruvian soles) for BRP and S/857 for BBP; and number of vials required per patient (annual average). This implies annual savings around S/24843 per-patient with biosimilar. Secondly, we estimated the cost differences based on annual requirement of Infliximab from EsSalud (6460 vials); thus, the biosimilar introduction could produce savings around S/7´642,780.00 (1 USD: S/3.30) (**Table 4**).

TABLE 4 | Preliminary financial analysis about the cost related to treatment with infliximab an its biosimilar in EsSalud (1USD = S/3.30).

Biological Product	Supplier	Estimation of annual costs per patient				EsSalud Annual Purchase	
		Unit cost per vial*	Average requirement per application per patient **	Frequency of annual application***	Average annual cost per patient	Annual requirement****	Total annual cost
Infliximab Original	Johnson& Johnson	S/2,040.00	3 vials	7 times	S/42,840.00	6460 vials	S/13,178,400.00
Biosimilar	AC Farma	S/857.00			S/17,997.00		S/5,536,220.00
Difference		-S/1,183.00			-S/24,843.00		-S/7,642,780.00

*Based on what was sold by the suppliers in the last purchase of the biological product registered in the SEACE platform for a vial of infliximab of 100 mg.
**Estimated for 60 kg person on average at a dose of 5mg / kg.
***The application is every 8 weeks on average; the annual estimate has been rounded.
****The total requirement corresponds to what was requested by EsSalud for the year 2018.

Technical Discussion With Medical Doctors

In first meeting, we received questions and feedback from rheumatologists, dermatologists and gastroenterologists. In second meeting, we discussed those questions an related legal aspects, and we also defined scope and limitations of analysis performed. At the last meeting, we presented and received the approbation of final technical document. The main concerns expressed by doctors were not being able to conclude for each disease separately, nocebo effect and using of generic questionnaires to assess the quality of life. We address them in the discussion.

DISCUSSION

Our findings reflect the best primary evidence available related to continuation with a biological biosimilar drug in patients that receive Infliximab -as biological reference drug - in conditions approved by the Peruvian Social Security. While only two of the studies respond directly to PICOS question using Infliximab as original maintenance drug, we included all controlled trials that evaluated interchangeability from the original Infliximab into its biosimilar. All primary studies did not find statistical and clinical differences between maintenance and exchanging groups in efficacy and safety profiles. Moreover, in comparison with infliximab, the use of its biosimilar produce a substantial savings in EsSalud purchasing budget. In addition, both analyzes were discussed and accepted by rheumatologists, dermatologists and gastroenterologists working in EsSalud. In this sense, our manuscript is an integrated technical piece, which embraces scientific evidence, institutional budget and clinical experience about infliximab interchangeability in the complexity of Peruvian Health System, where EsSalud is one of the foremost public institutions with assurance, provision and health care functions (Sánchez-Moreno, 2014; Mezones-Holguin et al., 2019). Consequently, we described a mixed methodological approach to inform making-decisions with the best available evidence in low and middle-income countries context.

In the academic realm, other systematic reviews have addressed the interchangeability from original into biosimilar drugs. First, *Chingcuanco* et al., performed a SR in Pubmed, EMBASE, CENTRAL and LILACS until April-2016; they concluded that there is primary evidence that supports interchangeability from Biological reference products to biosimilar drugs in TNF-α family (Chingcuanco et al., 2016). Second, *Cohen et al.*, carried out a SR including interventional and observational clinical studies in MEDLINE and EMBASE until June-2017; in this review the risk of events related to immunogenicity and declination of efficacy did not change after exchanging from original to biosimilar (Cohen et al., 2018). Third, *McKinnon et al.*, published an SR performed in Pubmed, EMBASE and Cochrane Library until June-2017 to evaluate the efficacy and safety of biosimilar interchangeability. There were still gaps to determining safety and efficacy of interchangeability of biosimilar was their conclusion, although they did not provide any specific conclusion about infliximab (McKinnon et al., 2018). Fourth, *Feagan et. al*, recently published a SR, they searched until January-2018 in Medline for articles and EMBASE for abstract congress. Six RCT and 64 observational studies were included. The authors described that "the evidence revealed no clinically important efficacy or safety signals associated with switching" (Feagan et al., 2019). Consequently, none of those synthesis studies reported differences in efficacy or safety between maintenance or exchanging into biosimilar, however there are different opinions in recommending the continuation with biosimilar drug.

In technical meetings with specialists, some concerns were exposed. The first was the inability to make specific comparisons for each disease separately- due to low statistical power- specifically in the clinical trial financed by the Government of Norway conducted in patients with rheumatoid arthritis, severe psoriasis, ulcerative colitis, Crohn's disease and spondylarthrosis. (Jørgensen et al., 2017). Although the authors performed subgroup analyses for each disease and reported findings with no statistically significant differences for several specific outcomes, their results were exploratory and could be affected by selection bias (Assmann et al., 2000; Brookes et al., 2004). However, valid conclusions were obtained for all diseases studied. In this regard, the authors report three main outcomes of efficacy (worsening of the disease, remission of the disease, and quality of life) and two safety outcomes (adverse effects and immunogenicity) for all diseases included. They observed non statistical differences between groups with adequate statistical power. (Jørgensen et al., 2017). Therefore, the first two outcomes of efficacy were the total percentage of patients who had worsening or remission of the disease in each group. Definition of state was based on medical evaluation supported by validated and accepted specific clinical scales for each disease (Jørgensen et al., 2017).

On the other hand, the use of generic questionnaires to assess quality of life (QoL) across the diseases was the second concern. *Jorgensen* et al. did not find differences in the SF-36 and EQ5D between the maintenance and switched groups (Jørgensen et al., 2017). QoL is widely recognized as a valid outcome in clinical studies and as basis for calculating utility measurements (Drummond et al., 2005; Bottomley et al., 2018). SF-36 and EQ5D can be used in any health conditions; both scales has been used by National Institute of Clinical Excellence (NICE) to assess efficacy of interventions in several diseases, including: rheumatological, dermatological and gastroenterological (Longworth et al., 2014). It is noteworthy that these two generic indices allow us to estimate utilities measures - as Quality of life adjusted life years (QALY) - for comparing across different health conditions (Rabarison et al., 2015). In the following two paragraphs we provide a succinct description of those tools in relation to diseases evaluated.

The SF-36 is widely used worldwide and it has evidence of validity and reliability in Peru (Salazar and Bernabé, 2015). A series of SR show that this tool has adequate psychometric properties in patients with RA (Matcham et al., 2014), it allows to quantify worsening psoriasis in clinical trials (Ali et al., 2017) and it is a valid outcome in patients with psoriatic arthritis that receive biological drugs (Druyts et al., 2017). In addition, for inflammatory bowel disease, SR described that SF-36 is useful to assess the quality of life and it provides evidence of variations in stages of activity and inactivity of the disease (Knowles et al., 2018) and a Cochrane systematic review describe that SF-36 is a valid and reliable instrument to evaluate the effect of biological therapy. (LeBlanc et al., 2015). Moreover, other SRs argue that this questionnaire has psychometric validity (Yarlas et al., 2018a) and serves to estimate the burden of disease in patients with ulcerative colitis (Yarlas et al., 2018b). Also, SF-36 is useful to assess QoL in patients with ankylosing spondylitis (Yang et al., 2016).

The EQ5D is a tool developed by EUROQOL that, with appropriate contextualization, serves as the basis for the calculation of QALYs (Brazier et al., 2017; Dakin et al., 2018). There is a Peruvian version of EQ5D (Szende et al., 2007; Brooks et al., 2013). In patients with rheumatoid arthritis its use has been described in the estimation of utility measures (Boyadzieva et al., 2018), clinical practice (Hiligsmann et al., 2018), also it has a good correlation with disease activity (Skacelova et al., 2017). EQ-5D is a valid and reliable instrument in the assessment of worsening in clinical trials conducted in patients with psoriasis. (Ali et al., 2017). Also, it is used in patients with plaque psoriasis, psoriatic arthritis (Longworth et al., 2014; Yang et al., 2016) and multicenter studies of skin diseases (Balieva et al., 2017). A Cochrane SR described that EQ-5D was adequate in the evaluation of the effectiveness of treatment with biological drugs in patients with inflammatory bowel disease (LeBlanc et al., 2015). Likewise, EQ-5D is an adequate tool to measure quality of life in ankylosing spondylitis patients (Boonen et al., 2007) and high correlation with specific scales of the disease has been observed (Mlcoch et al., 2017).

Similarly, safety is a highly important outcome studied. We defined immunogenicity and adverse events as main safety results. Immunogenicity is a relevant marker in the biotherapeutics research, since the production of anti-drug antibodies is clearly associated with therapeutic failure and side effects of protein drugs (Ingrasciotta et al., 2018). Also, immunogenicity of Infliximab biosimilar can be extrapolated to the different diseases treated (Ben-Horin et al., 2015). Moreover, the adverse events, especially the serious ones, are valid safety outcomes for a biological drug in the context of clinical trials (Tridente, 2013). Subsequently, we incorporated two main safety measures in the biosimilars arena.

Our study has potential limitations. First, we did not include unpublished studies from the gray literature (reports, conference proceedings, doctoral theses/dissertations, etc.), which may imply a selection bias. But, critical appraisal of the evidence is essential for developing a SR, since, although the findings can be made known, we cannot evaluate their quality, which has repercussions on the validity and reliability of a synthesis study (Bolaños-Díaz et al., 2011). Second, non-inclusion of observational studies could be a selection bias source, even more when the academy recognizes them as a valid source of clinical evidence (Greenfield, 2017; Corrao and Cantarutti, 2018). Nevertheless, our manuscript is circumscribed in a specific decision-making environment, where there is an institutional regulatory framework. In EsSalud, IETSI has defined that– based on internal validity criterion- randomized clinical trials are the main source of evidence to inform making-decisions; in addition, the overall results of SRs - that included observational studies - did not differ from RCT findings and provide consistency to our results. Third, we did not carry out a quantitative synthesis of the studies, due to the enormous clinical and methodological heterogeneity, but in this situation performing meta-analysis is not advisable (Melsen et al., 2014). Fourth, we have not considered drop-out rates and nocebo effect, which could potentially exist in switched patients (from original into biosimilar) (Kristensen et al., 2018; Odinet et al., 2018); education provided prior to switch -among other interventions - is a valuable tool that can greatly help overcome this effect (Pouillon et al., 2019). Fifth, in the financial analysis, we do not have the official information of short-term patients and long-term chronic patients in each disease approved; however, our estimation is valid since it was based on absolute institutional annual requirement of infliximab. Sixth, we did not have a national representative sample of physicians; however, participants were working in the main healthcare networks of EsSalud.

Beyond the limitations and based on cost-opportunity as a legitimate principle of collective health, our findings support the use of a biosimilar to continue the treatment in patients receiving infliximab in EsSalud. Therefore, biosimilar constitute a valid therapeutic alternative for the management of medical conditions approved in EsSalud. Access to biological drugs is a struggle for health care systems, especially in low and middle-income economies, where a key aspect is the price of these innovative medicines, which leads to a significant economic exertion from Governments and their public budgets. In this sense, infliximab biosimilars are an alternative that could be efficient in the Peruvian Social Security context.

AUTHOR CONTRIBUTIONS

EM-H, FF, MC-R, PB-P, GS-F, RG-C, and JC-C participated in the conception of the study and the research question. EM-H, LL-S, and LH-S designed the systematic review, developed the search strategy, and selected the articles. EM-H, FF, PB-P, GS-F, MC-R, JC-C, and RG-C defined and discussed the outcomes of interest. EM-H, LL-S, and LH-S performed the extraction and preliminary drafting of the results. EM-H, FF, PB-P, and MC-R carried out the cost estimates. EM-H, FF, PB-P, GS-F, MC-R, JC-C, and RG-C reviewed the results and delineated the discussion. EM-H, LL-S, and LH-S made the first version of the article. EM-H, FF, MC-R, PB-P, LH-S, LL-S, JC-C, GS-F, and RG-C made substantial contributions to the manuscript. All authors agreed with the published version of the article and assume responsibility for its content.

REFERENCES

Acevedo, A. D. M., and Gaitan, M. F., (2012). *Infliximab: Pharmacology, Uses and Limitations*. Hauppauge, New York, USA: Nova Science Publishers, Incorporated.

Ali, F. M., Cueva, A. C., Vyas, J., Atwan, A. A., Salek, M. S., Finlay, A. Y., et al. (2017). A systematic review of the use of quality-of-life instruments in randomized controlled trials for psoriasis. *Br. J. Dermatol.* 176, 577–593. doi: 10.1111/bjd.14788

Assmann, S. F., Pocock, S. J., Enos, L. E., and Kasten, L. E. (2000). Subgroup analysis and other (mis)uses of baseline data in clinical trials. *The Lancet* 355, 1064–1069. doi: 10.1016/S0140-6736(00)02039-0

Auclair, J. R. (2019). Regulatory Convergence for biologics through capacity building and training. *Trends Biotechnol.* 37, 5–9. doi: 10.1016/j.tibtech.2018.06.001

Balieva, F., Kupfer, J., Lien, L., Gieler, U., Finlay, A. Y., Tomás-Aragonés, L., et al. (2017). The burden of common skin diseases assessed with the EQ5D™: a European multicentre study in 13 countries. *Br. J. Dermatol.* 176, 1170–1178. doi: 10.1111/bjd.15280

Ben-Horin, S., Heap, G. A., Ahmad, T., Kim, H., Kwon, T., and Chowers, Y. (2015). The immunogenicity of biosimilar infliximab: can we extrapolate the data across indications? *Expert Rev. Gastroenterol. Hepatol.* 9 (Suppl 1), 27–34. doi: 10.1586/17474124.2015.1091307

Bolaños-Díaz, R., Mezones-Holguín, E., Gutiérrez-Aguado, A., and Málaga, G. (2011). Synthesis studies as the basis for economic evaluations in health: the need for their quality appraisal. *Rev. Peru. Med. Exp. Salud Pública* 28, 528–534. doi: 10.1590/S1726-46342011000300019

Boonen, A., van der Heijde, D., Landewé, R., van Tubergen, A., Mielants, H., Dougados, M., et al. (2007). How do the EQ-5D, SF-6D and the well-being rating scale compare in patients with ankylosing spondylitis? *Ann. Rheum. Dis.* 66, 771–777. doi: 10.1136/ard.2006.060384

Bottomley, A., Pe, M., Sloan, J., Basch, E., Bonnetain, F., Calvert, M., et al. (2018). Moving forward toward standardizing analysis of quality of life data in randomized cancer clinical trials. *Clin. Trials* 15, 624–630. doi: 10.1177/1740774518795637

Boyadzieva, V. V., Stoilov, N., Stoilov, R. M., Tachkov, K., Kamusheva, M., Mitov, K., et al. (2018). Quality of life and cost study of rheumatoid arthritis therapy With biological medicines. *Front. Pharmacol.* 9, 794. doi: 10.3389/fphar.2018.00794

Brazier, J., Ratcliffe, J., Saloman, J., and Tsuchiya, A. (2017). *Measuring and valuing health benefits for economic evaluation*. New York, USA: Oxford University Press.

Brookes, S. T., Whitely, E., Egger, M., Smith, G. D., Mulheran, P. A., and Peters, T. J. (2004). Subgroup analyses in randomized trials: risks of subgroup-specific analyses. *J. Clin. Epidemiol.* 57, 229–236. doi: 10.1016/j.jclinepi.2003.08.009

Brooks, R., Rabin, R., and de Charro, F. (2013). *The measurement and valuation of health status using EQ-5D: A European Perspective: Evidence from the EuroQol BIOMED Research Programme*. Dordrecht, Netherlands: Springer Science & Business Media.

Chingcuanco, F., Segal, J. B., Kim, S. C., and Alexander, G. (2016). Bioequivalence of biosimilar tumor necrosis factor-α inhibitors compared with their reference biologics: a systematic review. *Ann. Intern. Med.* 165, 565–574. doi: 10.7326/M16-0428

Cohen, H. P., Blauvelt, A., Rifkin, R. M., Danese, S., Gokhale, S. B., and Woollett, G. (2018). Switching reference medicines to biosimilars: a systematic literature review of clinical outcomes. *Drugs* 78, 463–478. doi: 10.1007/s40265-018-0881-y

Corrao, G., and Cantarutti, A. (2018). Building reliable evidence from real-world data: needs, methods, cautiousness and recommendations. *Pulm. Pharmacol. Ther.* 53, 61–67. doi: 10.1016/j.pupt.2018.09.009

Dakin, H., Abel, L., Burns, R., and Yang, Y. (2018). Review and critical appraisal of studies mapping from quality of life or clinical measures to EQ-5D: an online database and application of the MAPS statement. *Health Qual. Life Outcomes* 16, 31. doi: 10.1186/s12955-018-0857-3

Declerck, P., Danesi, R., Petersel, D., and Jacobs, I. (2017). The language of biosimilars: clarification, definitions, and regulatory aspects. *Drugs* 77, 671–677. doi: 10.1007/s40265-017-0717-1

Drummond, M. F., Sculpher, M. J., Torrance, G. W., O'Brien, B. J., and Stoddart, G. L. (2005). *Methods for the Economic Evaluation of Health Care Programmes*. New York, USA: Oxford University Press.

Druyts, E., Palmer, J. B., Balijepalli, C., Chan, K., Fazeli, M. S., Herrera, V., et al. (2017). Treatment modifying factors of biologics for psoriatic arthritis: a systematic review and Bayesian meta-regression. *Clin. Exp. Rheumatol.* 35, 681–688.

Ecker, D. M., Jones, S. D., and Levine, H. L. (2015). The therapeutic monoclonal antibody market. *mAbs* 7, 9–14. doi: 10.4161/19420862.2015.989042

European Medicines Agency (EMA). (2018).Remicade (Infliximab). *Eur. Med. Agency*. Accessed.

Feagan, B. G., Lam, G., Ma, C., and Lichtenstein, G. R. (2019). Systematic review: efficacy and safety of switching patients between reference and biosimilar infliximab. *Aliment. Pharmacol. Ther.* 49, 31–40. doi: 10.1111/apt.14997

Food and Drug Administration (2018). Remicade (infliximab). Accessed.

Gamez-Belmonte, R., Hernandez-Chirlaque, C., Arredondo-Amador, M., Aranda, C. J., Gonzalez, R., Martinez-Augustin, O., et al. (2018). Biosimilars: Concepts and controversies. *Pharmacol. Res.* 133, 251–264. doi: 10.1016/j.phrs.2018.01.024

Garcia, R., and Araujo, D. V. (2016). The regulation of biosimilars in Latin America. *Curr. Rheumatol. Rep.* 18, 16. doi: 10.1007/s11926-016-0564-1

Greenfield, S. (2017). Making real-world evidence more useful for decision making. *Value Health J. Int. Soc. Pharmacoeconomics Outcomes Res.* 20, 1023–1024. doi: 10.1016/j.jval.2017.08.3012

Gutka, H. J., Yang, H., and Kakar, S. (2018). *Biosimilars: Regulatory, Clinical, and Biopharmaceutical Development*. Cham, Switzerland: Springer.

Higgins, J. P. T., Altman, D. G., Gøtzsche, P. C., Jüni, P., Moher, D., Oxman, A. D., et al. (2011). The Cochrane Collaboration's tool for assessing risk of bias in randomised trials. *BMJ* 343, d5928. doi: 10.1136/bmj.d5928

Hiligsmann, M., Rademacher, S., Kaal, K. J., Bansback, N., and Harrison, M. (2018). The use of routinely collected patient-reported outcome measures in rheumatoid arthritis. *Semin. Arthritis Rheum.* 48, 357–366. doi: 10.1016/j.semarthrit.2018.03.006

Ingrasciotta, Y., Cutroneo, P. M., Marcianò, I., Giezen, T., Atzeni, F., and Trifirò, G. (2018). Safety of Biologics, Including Biosimilars: Perspectives on Current Status and Future Direction. *Drug Saf.* 41, 1013–1022. doi: 10.1007/s40264-018-0684-9

Jørgensen, K. K., Olsen, I. C., Goll, G. L., Lorentzen, M., Bolstad, N., Haavardsholm, E. A., et al. (2017). Switching from originator infliximab to biosimilar CT-P13 compared with maintained treatment with originator infliximab (NOR-SWITCH): a 52-week, randomised, double-blind, non-inferiority trial. *The Lancet* 389, 2304–2316. doi: 10.1016/S0140-6736(17)30068-5

Knowles, S. R., Graff, L. A., Wilding, H., Hewitt, C., Keefer, L., and Mikocka-

Walus, A. (2018). Quality of life in inflammatory bowel disease: a systematic review and meta-analyses-part I. *Inflamm. Bowel Dis.* 24, 742–751. doi: 10.1093/ibd/izx100

Kristensen, L. E., Alten, R., Puig, L., Philipp, S., Kvien, T. K., Mangues, M. A., et al. (2018). Non-pharmacological effects in switching medication: the nocebo effect in switching from originator to biosimilar agent. *BioDrugs Clin. Immunother. Biopharm. Gene Ther.* 32, 397–404. doi: 10.1007/s40259-018-0306-1

LeBlanc, K., Mosli, M. H., Parker, C. E., and MacDonald, J. K. (2015). The impact of biological interventions for ulcerative colitis on health-related quality of life. *Cochrane Database Syst. Rev.*, CD008655. doi: 10.1002/14651858.CD008655.pub3

Li, P., Zheng, Y., and Chen, X. (2017). Drugs for autoimmune inflammatory diseases: from small molecule compounds to anti-TNF biologics. *Front. Pharmacol.* 8, 460. doi: 10.3389/fphar.2017.00460

Longworth, L., Yang, Y., Young, T., Mulhern, B., Hernández Alava, M., Mukuria, C., et al. (2014). Use of generic and condition-specific measures of health-related quality of life in NICE decision-making: a systematic review, statistical modelling and survey. *Health Technol. Assess. Winch. Engl.* 18, 1–224. doi: 10.3310/hta18090

Matcham, F., Scott, I. C., Rayner, L., Hotopf, M., Kingsley, G. H., Norton, S., et al. (2014). The impact of rheumatoid arthritis on quality-of-life assessed using the SF-36: a systematic review and meta-analysis. *Semin. Arthritis Rheum.* 44, 123–130. doi: 10.1016/j.semarthrit.2014.05.001

McKinnon, R. A., Cook, M., Liauw, W., Marabani, M., Marschner, I. C., Packer, N. H., et al. (2018). Biosimilarity and interchangeability: principles and evidence: a systematic review. *BioDrugs Clin. Immunother. Biopharm. Gene Ther.* 32, 27–52. doi: 10.1007/s40259-017-0256-z

Melsen, W. G., Bootsma, M. C. J., Rovers, M. M., and Bonten, M. J. M. (2014). The effects of clinical and statistical heterogeneity on the predictive values of results from meta-analyses. *Clin. Microbiol. Infect. Off. Publ. Eur. Soc. Clin. Microbiol. Infect. Dis.* 20, 123–129. doi: 10.1111/1469-0691.12494

Mezones-Holguin, E., Amaya, E., Bellido-Boza, L., Mougenot, B., Murillo, J. P., Villegas-Ortega, J., et al. (2019). [Health insurance coverage: the peruvian case since the universal insurance act]. *Rev. Peru. Med. Exp. Salud Publica* 36, 196–206. doi: 10.17843/rpmesp.2019.362.3998

Ministerio de Salud, Dirección General de Medicamentos, Insumos y Drogas (DIGEMID) (2016). Reglamento que regula la presentación y contenido de los documentos requeridos en la inscripción y reinscripción de productos biológicos que opten por la vía de la similaridad.

Mlcoch, T., Sedova, L., Stolfa, J., Urbanova, M., Suchy, D., Smrzova, A., et al. (2017). Mapping the relationship between clinical and quality-of-life outcomes in patients with ankylosing spondylitis. *Expert Rev. Pharmacoecon. Outcomes Res.* 17, 203–211. doi: 10.1080/14737167.2016.1200468

Moher, D., Liberati, A., Tetzlaff, J., and Altman, D. G. (2009). Preferred reporting items for systematic reviews and meta-analyses: the PRISMA statement. *Ann. Intern. Med.* 151, 264–269. doi: 10.7326/0003-4819-151-4-200908180-00135

Niazi, S. K. (2018). *Biosimilars and Interchangeable Biologics: Strategic Elements.* Boca Raton, FL, USA: CRC Press.

Odinet, J. S., Day, C. E., Cruz, J. L., and Heindel, G. A. (2018). The biosimilar nocebo effect? a systematic review of double-blinded versus open-label studies. *J. Manag. Care Spec. Pharm.* 24, 952–959. doi: 10.18553/jmcp.2018.24.10.952

Park, W., Yoo, D. H., Miranda, P., Brzosko, M., Wiland, P., Gutierrez-Ureña, S., et al. (2017). Efficacy and safety of switching from reference infliximab to CT-P13 compared with maintenance of CT-P13 in ankylosing spondylitis: 102-week data from the PLANETAS extension study. *Ann. Rheum. Dis.* 76, 346. doi: 10.1136/annrheumdis-2015-208783

Pombo, M. L., Di Fabio, J. L., and Cortés, M. de L. (2009). Review of regulation of biological and biotechnological products in Latin American and Caribbean countries. *Biol. J. Int. Assoc. Biol. Stand.* 37, 271–276. doi: 10.1016/j.biologicals.2009.07.003

Portela, M., da, C. C., Sinogas, C., Albuquerque de Almeida, F., Baptista-Leite, R., and Castro-Caldas, A. (2017). Biologicals and biosimilars: safety issues in Europe. *Expert Opin. Biol. Ther.* 17, 871–877. doi: 10.1080/14712598.2017.1330409

Pouillon, L., Danese, S., Hart, A., Fiorino, G., Argollo, M., Selmi, C., et al. (2019). Consensus report: clinical recommendations for the prevention and management of the nocebo effect in biosimilar-treated IBD patients. *Aliment. Pharmacol. Ther.* 49, 1181–1187. doi: 10.1111/apt.15223

Rabarison, K. M., Bish, C. L., Massoudi, M. S., and Giles, W. H. (2015). Economic evaluation enhances public health decision making. *Front. Public Health* 3, 164. doi: 10.3389/fpubh.2015.00164

Salazar, F. R., and Bernabé, E. (2015). The Spanish SF-36 in Peru: factor structure, construct validity, and internal consistency. *Asia. Pac. J. Public Health* 27, NP2372–NP2380. doi: 10.1177/1010539511432879

Sánchez-Moreno, F. (2014). El sistema nacional de salud en el Perú. *Rev. Peru. Med. Exp. Salud Publica* 31, 747–753. doi: 10.17843/rpmesp.2014.314.129

Seguro Social en Salud (EsSalud), *Petitorio Farmacológico EsSalud*, 2017, Available at: http://www.essalud.gob.pe/ietsi/pdfs/normas/compilacion_petitorio_farmacologico_ESSALUD_2017.xlsx [Accessed].

Sheets, R. (2017). *Fundamentals of Biologicals Regulation: Vaccines and Biotechnology Medicines.* London, UK: Academic Press.

Skacelova, M., Pavel, H., Hermanova, Z., and Langova, K. (2017). Relationship between rheumatoid arthritis disease activity assessed with the US7 score and quality of Life measured with questionnaires (HAQ, EQ-5D, WPAI). *Curr. Rheumatol. Rev.* 13, 224–230. doi: 10.2174/1573397113666170517160726

Smolen, J. S., Choe, J.-Y., Prodanovic, N., Niebrzydowski, J., Staykov, I., Dokoupilova, E., et al. (2018). Safety, immunogenicity and efficacy after switching from reference infliximab to biosimilar SB2 compared with continuing reference infliximab and SB2 in patients with rheumatoid arthritis: results of a randomised, double-blind, phase III transition study. *Ann. Rheum. Dis.* 77, 234–240. doi: 10.1136/annrheumdis-2017-211741

Szende, A., Oppe, M., and Devlin, N. (2007). *EQ-5D Value Sets: Inventory, Comparative Review and User Guide.* Dordrecht, Netherlands: Springer Science & Business Media.

Tanaka, Y., Yamanaka, H., Takeuchi, T., Inoue, M., Saito, K., Saeki, Y., et al. (2017). Safety and efficacy of CT-P13 in Japanese patients with rheumatoid arthritis in an extension phase or after switching from infliximab. *Mod. Rheumatol.* 27, 237–245. doi: 10.1080/14397595.2016.1206244

Tridente, G. (2013). *Adverse Events with Biomedicines: Prevention Through Understanding.* Dordrecht, Netherlands: Springer Science & Business Media.

Trifirò, G., Marcianò, I., and Ingrasciotta, Y. (2018). Interchangeability of biosimilar and biological reference product: updated regulatory positions and pre- and post-marketing evidence. *Expert Opin. Biol. Ther.* 18, 309–315. doi: 10.1080/14712598.2018.1410134

Tsai, W.-C. (2017). Update on biosimilars in asia. *Curr. Rheumatol. Rep.* 19, 47. doi: 10.1007/s11926-017-0677-1

Uhlig, T., and Goll, G. L. (2017). Reviewing the evidence for biosimilars: key insights, lessons learned and future horizons. *Rheumatol. Oxf. Engl.* 56, iv49–iv62. doi: 10.1093/rheumatology/kex276

Wang, W., and Singh, M. (2013). *Biological Drug Products: Development and Strategies.* Weinheim, Germany: Wiley.

Yang, X., Fan, D., Xia, Q., Wang, M., Zhang, X., Li, X., et al. (2016). The health-related quality of life of ankylosing spondylitis patients assessed by SF-36: a systematic review and meta-analysis. *Qual. Life Res. Int. J. Qual. Life Asp. Treat. Care Rehabil.* 25, 2711–2723. doi: 10.1007/s11136-016-1345-z

Yarlas, A., Bayliss, M., Cappelleri, J. C., Maher, S., Bushmakin, A. G., Chen, L. A., et al. (2018a). Psychometric validation of the SF-36® health survey in ulcerative colitis: results from a systematic literature review. *Qual. Life Res. Int. J. Qual. Life Asp. Treat. Care Rehabil.* 27, 273–290. doi: 10.1007/s11136-017-1690-6

Yarlas, A., Rubin, D. T., Panés, J., Lindsay, J. O., Vermeire, S., Bayliss, M., et al. (2018b). Burden of ulcerative colitis on functioning and well-being: a systematic literature review of the SF-36® health survey. *J. Crohns Colitis* 12, 600–609. doi: 10.1093/ecco-jcc/jjy024

Yoo, D. H., Prodanovic, N., Jaworski, J., Miranda, P., Ramiterre, E., Lanzon, A., et al. (2017). Efficacy and safety of CT-P13 (biosimilar infliximab) in patients with rheumatoid arthritis: comparison between switching from reference infliximab to CT-P13 and continuing CT-P13 in the PLANETRA extension study. *Ann. Rheum. Dis.* 76, 355–363. doi: 10.1136/annrheumdis-2015-208786

Zahl, A. (2017). *International Pharmaceutical Law and Practice.* Bolingbrook, IL, USA: LexisNexis.

Zelikin, A. N., Ehrhardt, C., and Healy, A. M. (2016). Materials and methods for delivery of biological drugs. *Nat. Chem.* 8, 997. doi: 10.1038/nchem.2629

20

Propensity Score Methods in Health Technology Assessment: Principles, Extended Applications and Recent Advances

M Sanni Ali[1,2,3]*, Daniel Prieto-Alhambra[2,4], Luciane Cruz Lopes[5], Dandara Ramos[3], Nivea Bispo[3], Maria Y. Ichihara[3,6], Julia M. Pescarini[3], Elizabeth Williamson[1], Rosemeire L. Fiaccone[3,6,7], Mauricio L. Barreto[3,6] and Liam Smeeth[1,3]

[1] Faculty of Epidemiology and Population Health, London School of Hygiene and Tropical Medicine, London, United Kingdom, [2] Nuffield Department of Orthopaedics, Rheumatology and Musculoskeletal Sciences (NDORMS), Center for Statistics in Medicine (CSM), University of Oxford, Oxford, United Kingdom, [3] Centre for Data and Knowledge Integration for Health (CIDACS), Instituto Gonçalo Muniz, Fundação Osvaldo Cruz, Salvador, Brazil, [4] GREMPAL Research Group (Idiap Jordi Gol) and Musculoskeletal Research Unit (Fundació IMIM-Parc Salut Mar), Universitat Autònoma de Barcelona, Barcelona, Spain, [5] University of Sorocaba–UNISO, Sorocaba, São Paulo, Brazil, [6] Institute of Public Health, Federal University of Bahia (UFBA), Salvador, Brazil, [7] Department of Statistics, Federal University of Bahia (UFBA), Salvador, Brazil

*Correspondence:
M Sanni Ali
Sanni.ali@lshtm.ac.uk;
sanni.ali@ndorms.ox.ac.uk

Randomized clinical trials (RCT) are accepted as the gold-standard approaches to measure effects of intervention or treatment on outcomes. They are also the designs of choice for health technology assessment (HTA). Randomization ensures comparability, in both measured and unmeasured pretreatment characteristics, of individuals assigned to treatment and control or comparator. However, even adequately powered RCTs are not always feasible for several reasons such as cost, time, practical and ethical constraints, and limited generalizability. RCTs rely on data collected on selected, homogeneous population under highly controlled conditions; hence, they provide evidence on efficacy of interventions rather than on effectiveness. Alternatively, observational studies can provide evidence on the relative effectiveness or safety of a health technology compared to one or more alternatives when provided under the setting of routine health care practice. In observational studies, however, treatment assignment is a non-random process based on an individual's baseline characteristics; hence, treatment groups may not be comparable in their pretreatment characteristics. As a result, direct comparison of outcomes between treatment groups might lead to biased estimate of the treatment effect. Propensity score approaches have been used to achieve balance or comparability of treatment groups in terms of their measured pretreatment covariates thereby controlling for confounding bias in estimating treatment effects. Despite the popularity of propensity scores methods and recent important methodological advances, misunderstandings on their applications and limitations are all too common. In this article, we present a review of the propensity scores methods, extended applications, recent advances, and their strengths and limitations.

Keywords: bias, confounding, effectiveness, health technology assessment, propensity score, safety, secondary data, observational study

INTRODUCTION

Randomized clinical trials (RCTs) are generally accepted as the gold-standard approaches for measuring the "causal" effects of treatments on outcomes (Sibbald and Roland, 1998; Concato et al., 2000) and the design of choice for health technology assessment (HTA). In causal inference terminology using Rubin's potential outcomes framework (Rubin, 2005), the effect of a certain treatment (Z = 1) versus a control or comparator (Z = 0) on an outcome (Y) involves comparison of potential outcomes under treatment (Y_1)) and an alternative treatment (Y_0)). In RCT, with sufficient numbers of participants and adequate concealment of allocation, randomization ensures that individuals assigned to treatment and control or comparator groups are comparable in all pretreatment characteristics, both measured and unmeasured (Sibbald and Roland, 1998). The only difference is that one group received the treatment (Z = 1) and the other received no treatment or the alternative treatment (Z = 0); hence, any difference in outcomes between the two groups can be attributable to the effect of the treatment. In other words, the "causal" effect of treatment in the study population (the average treatment effect, ATE) on outcomes can be estimated by a direct comparison of the outcomes between the treatment and the comparator groups (Equation 1) (Concato et al., 2000). However, even adequately powered RCT may not always be feasible for reasons such as cost, time, ethical, and practical constraints (Sibbald and Roland, 1998). RCTs also rely on data collected on selected, homogeneous population under highly controlled conditions; hence, they provide evidence on efficacy rather than on effectiveness of interventions or treatments (Eichler et al., 2011).

$$ATE = E[Y_1 - Y_0] = E[Y_1] - E[Y_0] \qquad (1)$$

With steadily increasing costs of health care and the introduction of novel, yet very expensive, pharmaceutical products and diagnostics, HTA agencies such as the UK National Institute for Health and Care Excellence (NCIE) are inquiring robust methods for evaluation of relative effectiveness and safety of medications, devices, and diagnostics in daily clinical practice. In contrast to efficacy, relative effectiveness of an intervention or treatment is "the extent to which an intervention does more good than harm, when compared to one or more alternative intervention(s)" when used under the routine setting of health care practice" (Eichler et al., 2011; Schneeweiss et al., 2011). In addition, for medical devices and diagnostics, waiting for evidence from RCTs when the health technology is diffusing in the clinical practice could be costly for the payers, inefficient from policy perspective, and methodologically questionable (Tarricone et al., 2016). On the other hand, regulators' and HTA agencies' perception of the importance of real-world data in complementing evidence on the relative effectiveness of health technologies has been steadily increasing (Makady et al., 2017; Yuan et al., 2018).

The effect of a particular health technology, e.g., a medication, on a certain outcome event could also be investigated using non-randomized studies (i.e., observational or quasi-experimental)

using routinely collected data (Schneeweiss et al., 2011, Ali et al., 2016, Bärnighausen et al., 2017). In observational studies, however, treatment selection is mainly influenced by the patient, the physician, and, to a certain extent, the health system characteristics. Hence, treated and untreated groups differ not only in receiving the treatment but also in other pretreatment characteristics, leading to non-comparability or non-exchangeability, a phenomenon leading to confounding bias (Greenland and Morgenstern, 2001). This means that differences in outcomes between the two groups, treated versus untreated, could be explained by either the treatment, or other pretreatment variables, or both. In other words, direct comparison of outcome events between the two groups leads to biased estimate of the treatment effect. Hence, any systematic difference in pretreatment characteristics between treatment should be accounted for by design, or analysis, or both (Rubin, 1997). Over the years, several methodologies have been developed to control for confounding bias in observational studies (**Figure 1**); the propensity score methods (Rosenbaum and Rubin, 1983) are among the popular approaches in pharmacoepidemiology and health technology evaluations (Ali et al., 2015).

Propensity score approaches were first introduced by Rosenbaum and Rubin in 1983 (Rosenbaum and Rubin, 1983), and their use to control for confounding has been increasing in the previous decade. Propensity score (PS) is a scalar summary of all measured pretreatment characteristics (often called potential confounders); stated formally, the propensity score e(X) is the conditional probability of receiving a certain treatment, versus a comparator or no treatment, given the measured pretreatment characteristics (Rosenbaum and Rubin, 1983), X, denoted as

$$e(X) = pr(Z = 1|X), \qquad (2)$$

where Z = 1 for individuals in the treatment group and Z = 0 for individuals in the comparison group (Rosenbaum and Rubin, 1983; Rosenbaum and Rubin, 1984). Treated and untreated individuals with similar propensity scores have, on average, similar or comparable pretreatment characteristics, a situation similar to an RCT. However, this comparability, conditional on the propensity score, of the treatment groups is limited only to measured pretreatment characteristics included in the propensity score model and may not hold for unmeasured ones (Rosenbaum and Rubin, 1983). Hence, balancing these pretreatment potential confounders through propensity scores enables researchers to obtain a "quasi-randomization" of treatment groups to reduce confounding and hence to get a better estimate of the treatment effect. Implicitly, researchers assume "Strongly Ignorable Treatment Assignment" (SITA) given the measured covariates; this comprises "unconfoundedness" and "positivity" (Rosenbaum and Rubin, 1983). Unconfoundedness implies that all relevant pretreatment characteristics are measured and included in the propensity score model; hence, given these measured covariates are included in the propensity score, there is no unmeasured confounding. Positivity, on the other hand, implies that every individual has a non-zero (positive) probability of receiving all values of the treatment variable: $0 < P(Z = 1|X) < 1$ for all values of Z (Rosenbaum and Rubin, 1983).

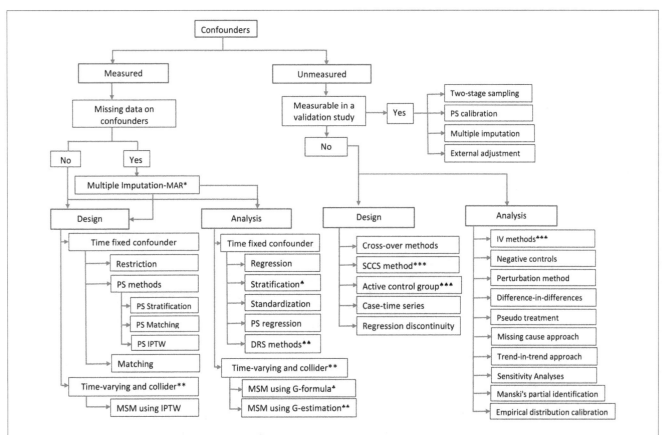

FIGURE 1 | Methods to control for confounding in observational studies.*Multiple imputation is valid when the assumption of Missing at Random (MAR) holds;**if time-varying confounder is affected by previous treatment, all PS-based methods except marginal structural model (MSM) using inverse probability of treatment weight (IPTW) will give biased estimate;***self-controlled case-series design; ♠)stratification using effect modifier and adjustment within the strata to account for other covariates; ♠♠)Disease risk score (prognostic score) method; ♠♠♠)restriction or choosing an active comparison group vs non-user group; ♣)G-formula and ♣♣)G-estimation of structural nested models, which rely on specification of the outcome model; ♣♣♣)instrumental variable methods. (Adapted in part from Schneeweiss (2006), Uddin et al. (2016), and Zhang et al. (2018)).

In the last decade, the propensity score methods have been popular among clinical researchers, their use in pharmacoepidemiology and HTAs has been ubiquitous, and they have undergone substantial methodological advances. On the other hand, confusions and misunderstandings on what a propensity score method can and cannot do as well as errors in the design, analysis, interpretation, and reporting of propensity score-based analyses are unfortunately all too common (Ali et al., 2015). With increasing availability of routinely collected electronic medical records for evaluation of effects (both comparative effectiveness and safety) of health technologies, and relatively rapid development of the methods, an up-to-date review of the methods and their characteristics is necessary. In this article, we aim to introduce propensity score methods with an emphasis on important aspects of the methods; describe their extended applications and recent developments; and discuss their strengths and limitations.

The manuscript, including the introduction, is organized into eight sections: the section *Introduction* has introduced RCT, observational studies, and propensity score in relation to HTA; the section *Variable Selection and Propensity Score Estimation* discusses variable selection and propensity score estimation

approaches; the section *Covariate Balance Assessment* describes methods for assessment of covariate balance in propensity score methods; the section *Propensity Score Methods* summarizes the different types of propensity score methods; the section *Extended Applications* describes extended applications of propensity scores; the section *Advantages and Limitations of Propensity Score Methods* summarizes strengths and limitations of the propensity score methodology; the section *Reporting* highlights on reporting of propensity score based analysis; and the section *Conclusion* concludes the discussion.

VARIABLE SELECTION AND PROPENSITY SCORE ESTIMATION

Observational studies using administrative or clinical databases often involve high dimensionality with respect to the number of pretreatment covariates available for analysis including socioeconomic characteristics, demographics, comorbidities, comedications, and health system characteristics, among others. The inclusion of a large number of covariates in conventional regression models, particularly in nonlinear models such as logistic regression and Cox regression models, requires sufficient number of outcome events (approximately 10 outcome events per covariate) (Peduzzi et al., 1995; Peduzzi et al., 1996; Cepeda et al., 2003). For example, to adjust for 5 confounders using logistic regression model, one would need to have 5*10 = 50 outcome events. However, many practical settings in pharmacoepidemiology and other HTAs involve relatively few or rare outcome events; hence, confounding adjustment using regression methods requires selection of a limited number of covariates to avoid problems such as over-fitting (Peduzzi et al., 1995). Alternatively, the use of propensity score methods to summarize a large pool of covariates into a single score, the propensity score, avoids over-fitting and collinearity issues in estimating treatment effects (Cepeda et al., 2003). When the number of covariates available in the study dataset is relatively small, it is common practice to include all the pretreatment covariates in the propensity score model; however, covariate selection might be required when researchers are presented with very large number (several hundreds) of covariates and limited number of outcome events (Schneeweiss et al., 2009).

Covariates selection in propensity score is often based on prior subject-matter knowledge on the relationships underlying the covariates in the study data, statistical tests on the association between the covariates and the outcome event (using p-values or change in effect estimates) (Brookhart et al., 2006; Patrick et al., 2011; Ali et al., 2015; Adelson et al., 2017), strength of associations with the treatment and/or the outcome event (Patrick et al., 2011; Ali et al., 2015; Adelson et al., 2017), and machine learning methods such as generalized boosted models (McCaffrey et al., 2004). Each approach has its own strengths and limitations; however, emphasis should be given to achieve balance on important prognostic pretreatment characteristics (Rosenbaum and Rubin, 1983) and not to improve model fit or to predict treatment as well as possible. Hence, the use of p-values, goodness-of-fit tests, and model discrimination tests such as c-statistics should be avoided (Weitzen et al., 2005; Patrick et al., 2011; Westreich et al., 2011). The iterative approach of model fitting, by including interactions and square terms of the covariates, and subsequent balance assessment, which was recommended in the seminal paper by Rosenbaum and Rubin (1983), is still a more robust approach. This application helps to achieve the goal of propensity score modelling, "improving balance" of potential confounders between treatment groups so that the groups are comparable or exchangeable conditional on the propensity score.

One of the greatest strengths of propensity score approaches is the separation of design from analysis, i.e., propensity score methods purposefully disregard outcome information at this stage of the design (Rubin, 2004b; Leacy and Stuart, 2014). That would also mean, as in the classical implementation of the methods, association between the covariates and the outcome event in the study data is not assessed for selection of covariates while constructing the propensity score model. However, this approach is not without disadvantages: failure to exclude colliders (variables that are common effects of the treatment and the outcome) and strong instruments (variables that are strongly related to treatment but independent of both the

confounders and the outcome) can lead to increased bias in the estimated treatment effect (Pearl, 2011; Myers et al., 2011a, Myers et al., 2011b; Pearl, 2012; Ali et al., 2016).

It is important to emphasize that, similar to conventional regression modelling, intermediates (variables on the causal pathway between the treatment and the outcome) and colliders should not be included in the propensity score model (Greenland and Morgenstern, 2001) since including these variables will tend to increase (rather than reduce) bias. In addition, strong instruments should also be excluded, particularly when strong unmeasured confounding is a concern thereby avoiding any amplification of the residual bias (Pearl, 2011; Myers et al., 2011a; Myers et al., 2011b; Pearl, 2012; Ali et al., 2016). However, it is not common to come across with such a scenario; the use of propensity score method is meaningful when the assumption of "Strongly Ignorable Treatment Assignment", SITA, is met (i.e., there is no unmeasured confounding given the measured covariates and also there is positivity) (Rosenbaum and Rubin, 1983). Compared to residual confounding by unmeasured characteristics, bias amplification should be considered a secondary concern; hence, researchers should be cautious and are advised to err on the side of including rather than excluding any potential confounder (Myers et al., 2011b; Ali et al., 2017c). Alternatively, when a strong instrument—essentially a proxy measure of difference in treatment—is identified that is independent of confounders and outcome, instrumental variable analysis can be a powerful tool to account for any unmeasured confounding (Angrist et al., 1996).

A common question asked by clinical researchers who have not used propensity score methods is "why do we need to estimate the probability that an individual receives a certain treatment versus a comparator while we certainly know from the data whether that particular individual has received the treatment?" A brief answer to this important question is as follows: propensity score exists both in RCT and in observational studies (Joffe and Rosenbaum, 1999; Rubin, 2004b; Ali et al., 2016). In RCT, the true propensity score is known by design or the treatment allocation mechanism, i.e., randomization. For example, consider a simple two-arm RCT in which individuals are assigned to a treatment versus a comparison group by flipping of a fair coin (also assume that the sample sizes are equal in both treatment groups). The propensity score for every individual, the probability of being assigned to the treatment group versus the comparator group, is equal to 0.5, apart from chance variations. In contrast, in observational studies, the true propensity score for individuals is unknown and is dependent on several pretreatment characteristics, both clinical and nonclinical, under consideration by the physician. As a result, the propensity score should be—and can often be—estimated using the study data (Joffe and Rosenbaum, 1999; Rubin, 2004b; D'Agostino, 2007; Ali et al., 2016). Estimation of the propensity score is needed to create a "quasi-randomized experiment" by using the individual's probability of receiving the treatment as a summary score of all measured pretreatment covariates. It enables appropriate adjustment for measured potential confounders to estimate the effect of the treatment. This explains one of the key properties of the propensity score method: if we find two individuals with the same propensity score, one in the treated group and one in the untreated group, we can assume that these two individuals are more or less "randomly assigned" to one of the treatment groups in the sense of being equally likely to be treated or not, with respect to measured pretreatment characteristics (Ali et al., 2015; Ali et al., 2016).

In practice, the propensity score is often estimated using ordinary logistic regression model, in which treatment status is regressed on measured pretreatment characteristics (Austin, 2008a; Ali et al., 2015). The estimated propensity score is the predicted probability of receiving the treatment derived from the fitted logistic regression model. Logistic regression has several advantages: it is a familiar and well-understood statistical tool for researchers as well as easy to implement using standard statistical software packages (Setoguchi et al., 2008; Westreich et al., 2010; Ali et al., 2016). However, logistic regression is not the only approach; other methods have also been used including recursive partitioning (D'Agostino, 2007) and several machine learning methods, for example, classification and regression trees (CARTs), neural networks, and random forests (Setoguchi et al., 2008; Lee et al., 2010; Westreich et al., 2010; Lee et al., 2011). Comparative simulation studies favor the use of machine learning methods over logistic regression when there is moderate or high nonlinearity (square or cubic terms of covariates) and non-additivity (interactions between pretreatment covariates) in the propensity score models. This could be explained by the fact that machine learning methods include interactions and square terms by default (Setoguchi et al., 2008), compared to logistic regression where the researcher should "manually" include interactions and square terms. When important interaction and square terms are included, the performance of logistic regression is as good as other machine learning methods (Ali et al., 2017b).

COVARIATE BALANCE ASSESSMENT

The aim of propensity score methods is to balance covariates between treatment groups and hence control for measured confounding (Rosenbaum and Rubin, 1983). Therefore, the quality of propensity score model should be assessed primarily on the covariate balance achieved. It should not be evaluated based on how well the propensity score model discriminates between treated and untreated individuals, i.e., whether the treatment assignment is correctly modeled (Rubin, 2004b; Westreich et al., 2011; Ali et al., 2015, Ali et al., 2016) or whether the subsequent estimates of treatment effect are smaller or larger than expected (Rosenbaum and Rubin, 1984; Hansen, 2004). Hence, propensity score modelling can be considered as an iterative step where the propensity score model is updated by adding different covariates, interactions between covariates, or higher-order terms of continuous covariates until an acceptable level of balance on important confounding variables is achieved (Rosenbaum and Rubin, 1984). It is also important to underline that variable selection and covariate balance are inseparably linked; however, covariate balance is often checked on a preselected list of pretreatment covariates (Ali et al., 2015). On the other hand, there are propensity score modelling techniques that optimize covariate balance while estimating the propensity score (Imai and Ratkovic, 2014; Austin, 2019).

It is helpful to start propensity score analysis by examining the distribution of propensity scores using histograms or density plots. This facilitates subjective judgment on whether there is sufficient overlap, also called "the common support," between propensity score distributions of treated and untreated groups (Dehejia and Wahba, 2002). However, such plots should not be considered as proper measures of covariate balance; they can guide the choice of matching algorithms in propensity score matching and the number of strata in propensity score stratification (Ali et al., 2015; Ali et al., 2016). For example, when there is very little overlap in the propensity score distributions, matching treated and untreated individuals with replacement, with or without caliper, can be a better option because it will be challenging to find sufficient number of untreated individuals for the treated individuals (Ali et al., 2016). Inadequate overlap in the propensity score distributions, which can be quantified using overlapping coefficient (Ali et al., 2014), should also warn researchers that the dataset, no matter how large, could not support any causal conclusion about the effect of the treatment on the outcome of interest without relyng o untrustworthy model assumptions (Rubin, 1997; Ali et al., 2016).

To assess covariate-specific balance, several metrics have been proposed in the literature (Austin, 2009; Belitser et al., 2011; Ali et al., 2014). Each balance metric has its own advantages and limitations; the absolute standardized difference in means or proportions (ASMD) (Austin, 2009) is more robust in terms of sample size and covariate distribution requirements in comparison to other balance diagnostics, such as overlapping coefficients (Ali et al., 2014; Ali et al., 2015; Ali et al., 2016). The ASMD is also a familiar, easy-to-calculate and present, and well-understood statistical tool (Austin, 2009; Ali et al., 2015; Ali et al., 2016). Hence, it is recommended for checking and reporting covariate balances in propensity score methods (Austin, 2009; Belitser et al., 2011; Ali et al., 2014; Ali et al., 2015; Ali et al., 2016). The ASMD is calculated for each covariate and can be averaged to compute an overall covariate balance and to compare propensity score models (Belitser et al., 2011; Ali et al., 2014). The covariate-specific ASMD is useful to identify the variable that is still imbalanced and to modify the propensity score model with squares and interaction terms of the variable to improve its balance. Although there is no universal threshold below which the level of covariate imbalance is always acceptable (Imai and Van Dyk, 2004; Ali et al., 2016), the use of arbitrary cutoffs for balance diagnostics (e.g., < 10% for the ASMD) is common in the medical literature (Ali et al., 2015; Ali et al., 2016). Covariate balance is not only a property of the sample means but also of the overall distribution of the covariate; hence, higher-order sample moments of the covariate distribution such as variance should also be evaluated (Rosenbaum and Rubin, 1985; Rubin, 2001; Ho et al., 2007; Austin, 2009; Linden and Samuels, 2013). Rubin (2001) proposed the ratio of variances of treated and untreated groups as an additional check on balance; a variance ratio of 1.0 in the propensity score matched sample indicates a good matching and acceptable balance, and a variance ratio below 2 is generally considered acceptable balance (Rubin, 2001; Linden and Samuels, 2013).

In addition to numerical quantification of the covariate balance achieved by the specified propensity score model, graphical methods such as (weighted) side-by-side box plots, quintile-quintile (Q-Q) plots, plots of ASMD, and empirical density plots of continuous pretreatment covariates provide a simplified overview on whether balance on individual pretreatment covariates has improved, compared to pre-matching, pre-stratification, or pre-weighting (Rosenbaum and Rubin, 1983; Ali et al., 2016).

PROPENSITY SCORE METHODS

Once the propensity score has been estimated, researchers have several options of using the propensity score in the design or analyses, including matching, stratification (also called subclassification), covariate adjustment using the propensity score, inverse probability of treatment weighting, and combinations of these methods (Rosenbaum and Rubin, 1983; Rosenbaum and Rubin, 1984; Rubin and Thomas, 2000; Hirano and Imbens, 2001; Johnson et al., 2018). Each method has its own advantages and disadvantages; the choice of a specific propensity score method is in part determined by the inferential goal of the research (i.e., the type of treatment effect estimand: the average treatment effect in the entire population, ATE, versus the average treatment effect in the treated population, ATT) (Imbens, 2000; Stuart, 2008; Ali et al., 2016). Although it is possible to estimate both ATT and ATE using all of the four propensity score methods, for example, by assigning different weights for the treated and untreated individuals, the default approach in each method might give slightly different estimand. For example, propensity score matching primarily estimates the treatment effect in the treated group, ATT (Imbens, 2004; Stuart, 2008). Therefore, to get an estimate of the average treatment effect in the entire population, ATE, one has to use either full matching (Hansen, 2004) or different weighting (Stuart, 2008, Stuart, 2010; Ali et al., 2015; Ali et al., 2016). The use of a specific propensity score method has also direct implication on the covariate balance assessment (Rosenbaum and Rubin, 1983; Rosenbaum and Rubin, 1984; Ali et al., 2016) and interpretation of the estimated treatment effect (Stuart, 2008; Ali et al., 2015; Ali et al., 2016).

Propensity Score Matching

Propensity score matching, the most common application of propensity score (Ali et al., 2015), entails forming matched groups of treated and untreated individuals having a similar value of the propensity score (Rosenbaum and Rubin, 1983; Rubin and Thomas, 1996). The matching could be done in many ways: one-to-one or one-to-many (1:n, where n is the number of untreated individuals often up to five), exact or caliper matching, matching with or without replacement, stratified matching, and full matching (Hansen, 2004). However, one-to-one caliper matching without replacement is the most common implementation of propensity score matching (Ali et al., 2015; Ali et al., 2016). For detailed discussion on different matching approaches, we refer to the literature (Rosenbaum and Rubin, 1985; Hansen, 2004; Stuart, 2010).

Once a matched sample has been formed, covariate balance can be easily checked between the matched groups using one of the balance diagnostics, preferably ASMD, and then treatment effect can be estimated by directly comparing outcomes between treated and untreated individuals in the matched sample (Rosenbaum and Rubin, 1983; Rubin and Thomas, 1996). With dichotomous or binary outcomes such as the presence or absence of a disease ("Yes" or "No"), the effect of the treatment can be estimated as the difference or the ratio between the proportion of individuals experiencing the outcome event in each of the two treatment groups (treated vs. untreated) in the matched sample. If the outcome is continuous, for example blood pressure measurement or HBA1c level, the effect of the treatment is estimated as the difference between the mean outcome for treated and the mean outcome for untreated individuals in the matched sample (Rosenbaum and Rubin, 1983).

If matching is done with replacement or in one-to-many matching, weights should be incorporated to account for the multiple use of the same untreated individual to match with several treated individuals or the multiple use of the same treated individual to match with several untreated individuals, respectively (Stuart, 2010). Whether or not to account for the matched nature of the data in estimating the variance of the treatment effect, for example, using paired t-test for continuous outcome or McNemar's test for binary outcome, is an ongoing discussion (Schafer and Kang, 2008; Stuart, 2008; Austin, 2008a; Austin, 2011).

The most appealing feature of propensity score matching is that the analysis can partly mimic that of an RCT, meaning that the distribution of measured pretreatment covariates will be, on average, similar between treatment groups. Hence, direct comparison of outcomes between treated and untreated groups within the propensity score matched sample has the potential to give unbiased estimate of the treatment effect, depending on the extent to which the measured variables have captured the potential confounding factors (Rosenbaum and Rubin, 1983). However, RCT, on average, guarantees balance on both measured an unmeasured confounders, whereas propensity score improves balance on measured confounders but those of unmeasured confounders only to the extent that they are related to the measured confounders included in the propensity score model (Rubin, 2004b; Austin, 2011). Other useful features include: separation of the design from analysis *via* preprocessing of the data to improve covariate balance without using outcome data, thereby a minimal reliance on model specification; relatively easy assessment, visualization, and communication of covariate balance using simple statistics or plots; and qualitative indication of whether the dataset at hand is good enough to address the causal question without relying on untrustworthy "model-dependent" extrapolations (Rubin, 2004b; Ho et al., 2007; Ali et al., 2016).

Recently, the use of propensity score for matching has been criticized on the basis of an argument that propensity score matching approximates complete randomization and not completely blocked randomization; hence, it engages in random pruning or exclusion of individuals during matching. "Unlike completely blocked randomization, random exclusion of individuals in propensity score matching, as in complete randomization, means a decrease in sample size leading to covariate imbalance and more model dependence, so called the 'propensity score paradox'" (King and Nielsen, 2016). At first this might seem a valid argument; however, the practical implication of this paradox is very limited, if any (Ali et al., 2017a). This is partly due to the fact that propensity score matching could do better than complete randomization with respect to the balance of measured covariates if variables related to treatment are included in the propensity score model (Joffe and Rosenbaum, 1999). In addition, the use of matching algorithms such as caliper matching or matching with replacement retains the best matches thereby avoiding random pruning or exclusion, and hence the paradox is not a big concern. Furthermore, it is currently a standard practice to check covariate balance in the propensity score matched sample before estimating the treatment effect, further minimizing any risk of exacerbating covariate imbalance (Ali et al., 2015).

Similar to RCT, when there are residual differences in pretreatment characteristics between treatment groups in propensity score matched sample, regression adjustment can be used on the matched sample to reduce bias due to residual differences in important prognostic factors (Rubin and Thomas, 2000; Imai and Van Dyk, 2004; Schafer and Kang, 2008). This method has been described as a doubly robust (DR) approach, i.e., correct specification of either the matching or the regression adjustment, but not necessarily both, is required to obtain unbiased estimate of the treatment effect (Schafer and Kang, 2008; Funk et al., 2011; Nguyen et al., 2017). Propensity score matching primarily estimates the effect of treatment in the treated individuals (ATT), not the effect of treatment in the population (treated and untreated individuals, ATE) (Imbens, 2004; Stuart, 2008). This is because the closest untreated and treated individuals are matched and the remaining untreated individuals that were not matched are often excluded from the analysis (Stuart, 2008; Ali et al., 2016). It is important to emphasize that exclusion of unmatched individuals from the analysis not only affects the precision of the treatment effect estimate but also could have consequences for the generalizability of the findings, even for the ATT (Lunt, 2013; Ali et al., 2016). For example, exclusion of treated individuals due to a lack of closer untreated matches could change the estimand from the effect of treatment in the treated (ATT) to the effect of treatment in those treated individuals for whom we can find untreated matches (ATT) (Lunt, 2013; Ali et al., 2016). However, it is possible to estimate the ATE in the matched sample with slight modifications of the matching algorithms. For example, using full matching that retains all the treated and untreated individuals in the study data, one can estimate either the ATE or ATT (Hansen, 2004; Stuart, 2010). Generally, matching discards some data (often unmatched untreated individuals); however, it may increase the efficiency, reducing the estimated standard error, of the treatment effect estimate by reducing heterogeneity of observations (Ho et al., 2007; Ali et al., 2016).

Propensity Score Stratification

Propensity score stratification, also called propensity score subclassification, involves grouping individuals into strata based on their propensity scores (often 5 groups using quintiles or 10 groups using percentiles). Within these strata, treated and untreated individuals will have a similar distribution of measured covariates; hence, the effect of the treatment can be estimated by direct comparison of outcomes between treated and untreated groups within each strata (Rosenbaum and Rubin, 1984; D'Agostino, 2007; Ali et al., 2017a). The stratum-specific treatment effects can then be aggregated across subclasses to obtain an overall measure of the treatment effect (Rosenbaum and Rubin, 1984).

Rosenbaum and Rubin (1983, 1984) proposed quintile stratification on the propensity score based on their finding that five equal-size propensity score strata removed over 90% of the bias due to each of the pretreatment covariates used to construct the propensity score. However, it is recommended that researchers examine the sensitivity of their results to the number of subclasses by repeating the analysis using different quantiles of the propensity score (Imai and Van Dyk, 2004; Adelson et al., 2017). Similar to matching, residual imbalances after stratification can be accounted for using regression adjustment within each stratum (Rosenbaum and Rubin, 1984; Rubin, 2001). Alternatively, the propensity score, defined as quintiles and deciles, can be used as a categorical variable in a model-based adjustment to estimate treatment effects (Rosenbaum and Rubin, 1984; Ali et al., 2016).

Propensity score stratification can estimate the stratum-specific ATT, or the overall ATT across strata, or the ATE, depending on how the subclass treatment effect estimates are weighted. Weighting stratum-specific estimates by the total number of individuals (treated and untreated) in each stratum yields the ATE. On the other hand, weighting stratum-specific estimates by the proportion of treated individuals in each stratum provides ATT (Stuart, 2010; Ali et al., 2016). Similarly, pooling stratum-specific variances provides pooled estimates of the variance for the pooled ATT or ATE estimate (Imbens, 2004; Ali et al., 2016). Pooling the stratum-specific treatment effect is straightforward when treatment effect is homogeneous among the propensity score strata (Ali et al., 2016). When there is heterogeneity of treatment effect among the strata even after automated iterations of the number and boundaries of propensity score strata (Imbens, 2004; Imbens and Rubin, 2015; Ali et al., 2016), pooling the stratum-specific treatment effect might complicate interpretation of the treatment effect estimate (Ali et al., 2014; Ali et al., 2016). In the presence of treatment effect modification regardless of the presence of confounding, Mantel-Haenszel methods do not estimate a population parameter (ATE); hence, estimating the effect of treatment in the treated (ATT) rather than the whole population (ATE), for example, using propensity score matching is preferable (Stürmer et al., 2006b). Alternatively, one could standardize the stratum-specific estimates to a specified distribution of propensity scores, for example, to calculate a standardized mortality ratio (AMR) from the stratum-specific estimates (Stürmer et al., 2006b; Lunt et al., 2009)

Stratification has several advantages: it is an easy and well-understood method to implement; it is straightforward to evaluate and communicate covariate balance, and to interpret particularly to non-technical audiences; it separates the design of the study from the analysis, like propensity score matching, hence less dependent on parametric models (Rosenbaum and Rubin, 1984); it is less sensitive to nonlinearities in the relationship between propensity scores and outcomes; and it can accommodate additional model-based adjustments (Rosenbaum and Rubin, 1983; Rosenbaum and

Rubin, 1984). However, this propensity score approach is prone to residual confounding, which might be an issue due to propensity score heterogeneity within the strata.

Regression Adjustment Using Propensity Score

The propensity score, as a single summary of all covariates included in the propensity score model, can be included as a covariate in a regression model of the treatment, i.e., the outcome variable is regressed on the treatment variable and the estimated propensity score (Rosenbaum and Rubin, 1983; Ali et al., 2016). Although this approach is very easy to implement, it is generally considered to be a sub-optimal application of the propensity score for several reasons: 1) The treatment effect estimation is highly model-dependent because it mixes the study design and data analysis steps; hence, it requires correct specification of the propensity score model (Rubin, 2004b; Johnson et al., 2018). 2) It also makes additional assumptions unique to regression adjustment; the relationship between the estimated propensity score and the outcome must be linear and there should be no interaction between treatment status and the propensity score (Rosenbaum and Rubin, 1983; Austin, 2011; Ali et al., 2016). However, both assumptions can be checked with the data, and can be relaxed if necessary, for example, by combining with propensity score stratification. 3) It enables estimation of the ATE; however, its interpretation is complicated particularly in nonlinear models such as logistic regression or Cox regression where the estimand of interest is non-collapsible. Non-collapsibility refers to a phenomenon in which, in the presence of a non-null treatment effect, the marginal (overall) treatment effect estimate is different from the conditional (stratum-specific) treatment effect estimate, even in the absence of confounding (Greenland et al., 1999; Austin, 2008b). In addition, assessment and communication of covariate balance are not straightforward (Ali et al., 2016).

Inverse Probability Treatment Weighting

Inverse probability weights (IPW) calculated from propensity score can also be used to create a weighted "artificial" population, also called a "pseudo-population" in which treatment and measured pretreatment characteristics included in the propensity score are independent (Hernán et al., 2000; Robins et al., 2000; Cole and Hernán, 2008; Ali et al., 2016). Hence, treated individuals will be assigned weights equal to the inverse of their propensity scores (1/PS, as they have received the treatment) and untreated individuals will be assigned weights equal to the inverse of one minus their propensity scores [1/(1 − PS)] (D'Agostino, 2007). A particular diagnostic concern in using propensity score weighting is that individuals with extremely large weights may disproportionately influence results and yield estimates with high variance (Lee et al., 2011). When some individuals have probabilities of receiving the treatment close to 0 or 1, the weights for such individuals become extremely high or extremely low, respectively (Ali et al., 2016). Weight stabilization to "normalize" the range of the inverse probabilities is often considered: the "1" in the numerator of the inverse probability weights can be replaced with the proportion of treated individuals and the proportion of untreated individuals for

treated and untreated individuals, respectively (Hernán et al., 2000; Ali et al., 2016).

Alternative approaches such as weight trimming and weight truncation have been suggested (Cole and Hernán, 2008; Lee et al., 2011). Weight trimming involves removing individuals in the tails of the propensity score distributions using percentile cut-points (Cole and Hernán, 2008; Lee et al., 2011), i.e., individuals who have extreme values of the propensity score—both very high and very low are excluded. On the other hand, weight truncation involves setting a maximum allowable weight, W_{ma}), such that individuals with a weight greater than W_{ma}) will be assigned W_{ma}) instead of their actual weights. Both approaches may help stabilize weights, reduce the impact of extreme observations, and can improve the accuracy and precision of parameter estimates; however, both involve bias-variance trade-offs (Lee et al., 2011). For example, trimming the tails excludes some individuals with extreme values and hence changes the population, which might introduce bias depending on the cut-off (Cole and Hernán, 2008). Recently, Li et al. (2018) suggested a different set of weights called "overlapping weights" which weight each individual proportional to its probability of receiving the alternative treatment, i.e., the overlap weight is defined as 1-PS for a treated individual and PS for an untreated individual. Unlike standard IPW, the overlap weights are bounded between 0 and 1; hence, they are less sensitive to extreme weights. It also means that there is no need for arbitrary choice of a cut-off for inclusion in the analysis as well as exclusion of individuals, unlike weight trimming (Li et al., 2018).

In the weighted population, weighted standardized difference can be used to compare means, proportions, higher-order moments, and interactions between treated and untreated individuals. In addition, graphical methods can be employed to compare the distribution of continuous covariates between treated and untreated individuals (Austin and Stuart, 2015). Once sufficient covariate balance is achieved, the effect of the treatment can be estimated by direct comparison of outcomes between treated and untreated groups. The weights can also be used in weighted regression models to estimate the effect of the treatment; and adjustment can be made for covariates that are not sufficiently balanced in the weighted sample. This method focuses on estimating the average treatment effect in the entire population (ATE); modification of the weights allows to estimate the average treatment effect in the treated population (ATT) (Stuart, 2010; Ali et al., 2016). Most importantly, the variance estimation should take into account the weighted nature of the "pseudo-population" since some observations can have weights that are unequal to one another (hence, potentially inducing a within-individual correlation in outcomes), for example, by using the sample weights in robust variance estimation (Hernán et al., 2000; Cole and Hernán, 2008; Austin and Stuart, 2015). Alternatively, bootstrapping could be used to construct 95% confidence intervals, which also takes into account the estimation of the propensity score, in addition to the lack of independence between duplicate observations in the weighted sample (Hernán et al., 2000; Austin and Stuart, 2015; Ali et al., 2016; Ali et al., 2017b).

Inverse probability of treatment weights (IPTW) can be also be used to estimate parameters of marginal structural models (MSMs) to deal with time-varying confounding (Hernán et al., 2000), time-modified confounding (Platt et al., 2009), and competing risks (Hernán et al., 2000; Ali et al., 2017b). Hence, the implementation of propensity scores as inverse probability weights is often referred to as MSM using IPTW. All other propensity score approaches can only be extended to time-varying confounding and treatment settings under certain conditions as described in **Figure 2**. Comparison of the four propensity score approaches is summarized in **Table 1**.

EXTENDED APPLICATIONS

Time-Varying Treatments

In clinical practice, it is common for patients to start on a certain medication, stop or switch to another one (for example, due to intolerance or lack of adequate response); in such cases, treatment might be treated as a time-varying exposure. Consider a cohort study to estimate the effect of antiretroviral zidovudine treatment (AZT) in HIV (human immunodeficiency virus) positive individuals, on progression to AIDS (acquired immune deficiency syndrome), where CD4 count is a confounder. Assuming individuals show up for clinical visits at baseline/pretreatment (t = 0) and then every 6 months (t = 1, 2, 3,...), and CD4 counts are recorded at these visits ($CD4_t$, represented as $CD4_0$, $CD4_1$, $CD4_2$,...). If AZT is a time-varying dichotomous treatment variable indicating whether the individual is on antiretroviral treatment at each of the visits (AZT_t, represented as AZT_0, AZT_1, AZT_2,...), this means, an individual's treatment

plan, at each subsequent visit (t = 1,2,...), is time-varying: the clinician in consultation with the individual decides treatment AZT_t based on the changing values of the individual's clinical and demographic history recorded during the previous and current visits. These include prior treatment history, current CD4 count, and other confounders, which are not included in this discussion and ignored for now for the sake of simplicity. The relationships between treatment, confounder, and outcome are presented using directed acyclic graphs (DAGs) for clarity.

In **Figure 2**, we considered two time points or visits t = 0 (baseline/pretreatment) and t = 1; hence, $CD4_0$ refers to baseline CD4 count and AZT_0 refers to treatment at the first visit. Treatment decision at the first visit AZT_0 is influenced by pretreatment CD4 count ($CD4_0$), represented in **Figure 2A** by the arrow from $CD4_0$ to AZT_0. In the second visit (t = 1), treatment decision AZT_1 is based on previous treatment (AZT_0) and CD4 count at the current visit ($CD4_1$), represented in **Figure 2A** by the arrows from AZT_0 and $CD4_1$ to AZT_1.

In settings such as DAG of **Figure 2A**, where there is no arrow from AZT_0 to $CD4_1$ implying previous treatment does not affect current CD4 count, all the standard propensity score approaches can deal with the time-varying confounder CD4 count by matching, conditioning, stratification, or weighting, for example, by combining with time-varying Cox models to estimate the treatment effect. However, this is not biologically plausible; RCTs have proved that antiretroviral treatment indeed affects CD4 count. It is important

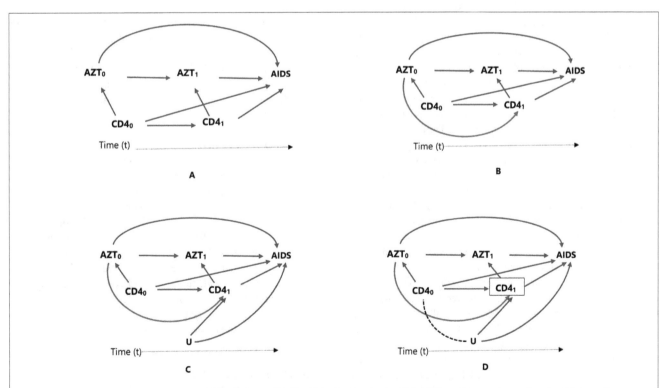

FIGURE 2 | Causal diagrams representing time-varying treatment (AZT), outcome (progression to AIDS, AIDS), and time-varying confounding (CD4 count). Time-varying confounding is not affected by prior treatment **(A)**, time-varying confounding is affected by prior treatment **(B)**, time-varying confounding affected by unmeasured factor U, which is also associated with the outcome **(C)**, and conditioning or stratifying on time-varying confounder, indicated by box around CD41), creates association between time-varying confounder $CD4_0$ and unmeasured factor U **(D)**.

TABLE 1 | Comparison of the different propensity score methods.

Characteristics	Matching[a]	Stratification[b]	Regression[c]	IPTW[d]
Model dependence	Minimum	Minimum	High	Minimum
Application[1]	Easy	Easy	Easy	Complex
Overall transparency	High	High	Low	Medium
Easy to communicate	Yes	Yes	Not always	Not always
Design and analysis	Separated	Separated	Mixed	Separated
Easy to check balance	Yes	Yes	No	Yes
Requires unique assumption[2]	No	No	Yes	No
Excluded individuals from analysis[3]	Yes	No	No	Yes-No
Variance estimation	Not clear	Easy	Easy	Complex
Easy to interpret[4]	Not always	Yes	No	Often
"Propensity score paradox"	Sensitive	No	No	No
Estimand[5]	Often ATT	ATE, ATT	ATE	ATE, ATT
Time-varying confounding[6]	No	No	No	Yes
Multiple treatments	Possible	Complex	Complex	Easier
Multi-level treatment applications	Exist	Exist	None	Exist
Treatment effect modification	Easier	Complex	Easier	Complex

[a]Constructs treated and untreated matched groups with similar propensity scores. [b]Constructs subgroups of treated and untreated individuals, often quintiles or deciles of PS. [c]PS is used, as a single summary of all covariates included in PS model, in regression model. [d]PSs are used as weights to create a pseudo-population in which exposure and measured covariates included in the treatment (PS) model are independent (Ali et al., 2016). [1]Estimation of stabilized weights as well as extension to time-varying treatment and confounding setting in MSMs framework can be complex (Ali et al., 2016). [2]Requires correct specification of PS and outcome model, apart from the basic assumptions that there is positivity and no unmeasured confounding (Ali et al., 2016). [3]Weight trimming excludes some individuals in the tails of the propensity score distribution. [4]In PSM, when treated individuals are excluded, interpretation of the treatment effect may change, not just ATT and in Stratification, when there is treatment effect modification by the PS, in regression adjustment using PS, when non-collapsible effect measures such as odds ratios are used. [5]Modification of the matching or weighting method enable to estimate either ATT or ATE. [6]When time-varying confounder is affected by previous treatment, all the propensity score based methods fail to correctly control for the confounding bias including standard IPWs; however, MSMs using IPWs.

to mention that there are many practical examples where both treatment and confounders are time-varying or dynamic, but previous treatment does not affect time-varying confounder; hence, the DAG in **Figure 2A** may still be valid in other situations.

When a time-varying confounder (such as CD4 count in our example, $CD4_1$) is affected by previous treatment (AZT_0) as in the DAG of **Figure 2B**, the time-varying confounder ($CD4_1$) is also an "intermediate" for the effect of previous treatment (AZT_0) on the outcome (progression to AIDS), represented by the path $AZT_0 \rightarrow CD4_1 \rightarrow AIDS$. Furthermore, if there is an unmeasured common cause (U) of both the time-varying confounder ($CD4_1$) and the outcome (progression to AIDS) as in DAG of **Figure 2C**, the time-varying confounder ($CD4_1$) is also a "collider" on the path $AZT_0 \rightarrow CD4_1 \leftarrow U \rightarrow AIDS$ (the arrows from U and $CD4_0$ collide on $CD4_1$). Hence, the path $AZT_0 \rightarrow CD4_1 \leftarrow U \rightarrow AIDS$ is a closed or non-causal path because it is blocked at $CD4_1$ (using DAG terminologies). It also means that there is no association between AZT_0 and U unless one conditions, matches, or stratifies on this collider, $CD4_1$ (Hernán et al., 2000; Robins et al., 2000). Such a time-dependent variable is a confounder, an intermediate, and also a collider all at the same time; hence, adjustment requires careful consideration.

Conventional statistical approaches including propensity score methods (matching, stratification, and regression adjustment) that condition or stratify on such a covariate will result in a biased estimate of the treatment effect (Hernán et al., 2000; Robins et al., 2000). This happens because conditioning or stratifying on an intermediate will adjust away the indirect effect of the treatment mediated by the cofounder, in this case $CD4_1$; and conditioning or stratifying on a collider creates a spurious association between the treatment and the unmeasured common cause that did not exist before conditioning (creating an open backdoor path $AZT_0 \rightarrow CD4_1,... U \rightarrow AIDS$), which is indicated by using dotted lines in the DAG of **Figure 2D**, leading to collider-stratification bias (Hernán et al., 2000; Cole et al., 2009; Ali et al., 2013).

In such settings, MSM using inverse probability weighting is the method of choice; unlike conditioning or stratification, weighting creates a "pseudo-population" in which the association between the time-varying confounder and treatment is removed (Hernán et al., 2000; Robins et al., 2000). Additional methods are also available to deal with time-varying treatment and confounding including other classes of marginal structural models (g-formula and g-estimation of structural nested models) (Hernán et al., 2000; Robins et al., 2000).

It is straightforward to hypothesize that such a time-varying confounding can also be time-modified, which means not only the confounder (CD4 count) change over time but also its association with the treatment and its impact on the outcome (progression to AIDS) varies during these times. The effects of the confounder change over time mean that the strength of association between $CD4_0$ and AIDS ($CD4_0 \rightarrow AIDS$) is different from that of $CD4_1$ and AIDS ($CD4_1 \rightarrow AIDS$) (Platt et al., 2009). However, time-modified confounding might still exist in longitudinal treatment settings where the confounder is time-invariant or fixed. Standard methods are sufficient to deal with time-modified confounding unless the confounder is both time-varying and affected by previous treatment, which requires the implementation of marginal structural models, such as using inverse probability weighting.

Multiple Treatments

Propensity score methods are often used to estimate the effect of a binary treatment (whether treatment is received: Yes = 1 or No = 0) in observational data. However, with more than two levels of treatment, which is common in pharmacoepidemiology such as comparison of three or more statins (e.g., simvastatin, atorvastatin, fluvastatin, lovastatin, pravastatin, and rosuvastatin) or of multiple doses of a certain medication (e.g., low, medium and high doses), estimation of treatment effects requires additional assumptions and modelling techniques (Imbens, 2000; McCaffrey et al., 2004). These include the use of multinomial logistic and multinomial probit models for nominal treatments and ordinal logistic regression or the proportional odds model for ordinal treatments (Imbens, 2000). Alternatively, generalized boosted model, a machine learning approach involving an iterative process using multiple regression trees to capture complex, nonlinear, and non-additive relationships between treatment assignment and pretreatment covariates without the risk of over-fitting the data, can be used to fit inverse probability weighting for multiple treatments (McCaffrey et al., 2004). However, applications in pharmacoepidemiology using observational data are infrequent partly due to methodological complexities in fitting the models and understanding their assumptions as well as limited availability of guidance documents on these methods.

Multilevel Treatments

Propensity score methods have been extensively studied and widely applied in a single-level treatment (no clustering among participants); however, most healthcare data have a multilevel structure such that individuals are grouped into clusters such as geographical areas, treatment centers (hospital or physician), or insurance plans (Goldstein et al., 2002). The unknown mechanisms that assign individuals to clusters may be associated with individual-level measured confounders (such as race, age, and clinical characteristics) and unmeasured confounders (such as unmeasured severity of disease, aggressiveness in seeking treatment) (Li et al., 2013). These measured and unmeasured confounders might also create a cluster-level variation in treatment and/or outcome. If this variation is correlated with group assignment at the group or cluster level, it might lead to confounding (Greenland, 2000; Li et al., 2013). Hence, the use of standard regression or propensity score methods ignoring the cluster structure should be avoided. This is because ignoring the cluster structure often leads to invalid inferences: not only the standard errors are inaccurate but also the cluster-level effects could be confounded with individual-level effects.

Propensity score matching and weighting are often used in such settings (Arpino and Mealli, 2011; Li et al., 2013). One might consider the use of within-cluster PSM (of treated and untreated individuals), which automatically achieves perfect balance on all the measured cluster characteristics. However, it is very unlikely, particularly in small clusters, to find a sufficient number of untreated matches to treated individuals in the same cluster. Alternatively, PSM could be performed across clusters taking into account the cluster structure in the propensity score estimation model. Preferably, cluster structure should be taken into account in estimation of both the propensity score and the treatment effect (Li et al., 2013).

Multilevel regression models that include fixed effects and/or random effects have been developed (Greenland, 2000; Goldstein et al., 2002), and extended to propensity scores approaches (Arpino and Mealli, 2011). Empirical applications of such methods in medication and device effectiveness and safety are rare. However, simulations studies have shown that multilevel propensity score matching (Arpino and Mealli, 2011) and weighting approaches (Li et al., 2013), without imposing a within-cluster matching or weighting requirement, reduce bias due to unmeasured cluster-level confounders.

Missing Data

Missing data is a common problem in the estimation of treatment effects using routinely collected data. The impact of such missing data on the results of the treatment effect estimation depends on the mechanism that caused the data to be missing and the way missing data are handled. Missing data can be categorized into three distinct classes based on the relationship between the missing data mechanism and the missing and observed values: i) Missing Completely at Random (MCAR), when the missing data mechanism is unrelated to the values of any variable, whether missing or observed. Hence, the observed values are representative of the entire sample without missing values. ii) Missing at Random (MAR), when the missing data mechanism is unrelated to the missing values but may be related to the observed values of other variables. iii) Missing Not at Random (MNAR), when the missing data mechanism is related not only to the observed values of other variables but also to the missing values (Rubin, 1996). For each of the missing data patterns, different statistical techniques are used to correct for its impact on the quality of the inference. It is important to emphasize that MCAR, MAR, and MNAR could exist for different variables in a specific data. However, if one variable is MAR or MNAR, generally, the dataset is considered MAR or MNAR, respectively.

Complete case analysis, including only those individuals who have no missing data in any of the variables that are required for the analysis, performs well when data are MCAR and may be valid under some MAR and MNAR conditions. However, it often results in biased estimate of the treatment effect if missing is at random (MAR) (Rubin, 1996; Sterne et al., 2009). In MAR, as stated before, any systematic difference between the missing values of a variable and the observed values of the variable can be explained by differences in observed data (Sterne et al., 2009). Furthermore, missing data in several variables often lead to exclusion of a substantial proportion of the original sample, which leads to a substantial loss of precision (i.e., power) and hence estimates with wider confidence intervals (Cummings, 2013). Other approaches to deal with missing data include: 1) replacing missing values with values imputed from the observed data (for example, using the mean of the observed values); 2) using a missing category indicator; and 3) using the last observed value to replace missing values particularly in longitudinal studies [often called "last observation carried forward" (LOCF)]. These three approaches are generally statistically invalid, except under certain conditions, and they might lead to serious bias (Rubin, 1996; Sterne et al., 2009). Missing category indicator and LOCF approaches require specific assumptions for validity that are distinct from the MCAR, MAR, and MNAR categorization. On the other hand, single imputation of missing values (mean imputation) usually results in too small standard errors, because it fails to account for the uncertainty about the missing values (Sterne et al., 2009).

A relatively flexible approach to allow for the uncertainty in the missing data is multiple imputation. Multiple imputation involves creating multiple different copies of the dataset with the missing values replaced by imputed values (Step 1); estimating treatment effects in each copy of the data (Step 2); averaging the estimated treatment effects to give overall estimated measure of association and calculating standard errors using Rubin's rules (Step 3) (Rubin, 1996; Rubin, 2004a). Applications of propensity score methods in data with missing values involve a similar approach: 1) creation of multiple copies of imputed data; 2) estimation of propensity scores and treatment effects in each of the imputed copies of the dataset (Qu and Lipkovich, 2009; Leyrat et al., 2019); and 3) pooling of treatment effects by averaging across the multiple datasets and estimation of standard errors using Ruben's rule (Crowe et al., 2010; Leyrat et al., 2019) (**Figure 3A**). An alternative approach is pooling the propensity scores from the multiple copies of data, in step 2, and conducting the analysis in the pooled data (**Figure 3B**); however, this method has been proved sub-optimal in terms of bias reduction (Leyrat et al., 2019).

ADVANTAGES AND LIMITATIONS OF PROPENSITY SCORE METHODS

Previous literature reviews of observational studies have found that results from both traditional regression and propensity scores analyses are similar (Shah et al., 2005; Stürmer et al., 2006a). These findings may be in part due to sub-optimal implementations of propensity score methods (Shah et al., 2005; Austin, 2008a; Ali et al., 2015); however, similarity of findings has been used to question the need for propensity score methods if they do not provide better ways to improve confounding control. Despite these findings, propensity score methods will remain advantageous for several reasons compared to covariate-adjustment techniques, which correct for covariate imbalances between treatment groups by conditioning them in the regression model for the outcome.

Transparency

Propensity score methods primarily aim at balancing treatment groups with respect to covariate distributions; when sufficient covariate balance is achieved, it is relatively easy to check and communicate the balance (Ali et al., 2015, Ali et al., 2016) by using simple graphical tools or quantitative statistics. In addition, propensity score methods, unlike regression adjustment, can

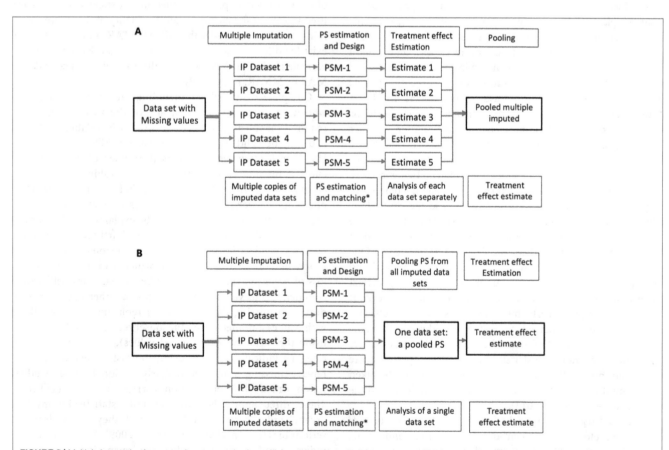

FIGURE 3 | Multiple imputation in propensity score methods; multiple copies of imputed data are created and propensity score is estimated using these datasets. Treatment effects are estimated in several datasets **(A)** and propensity scores from multiple datasets are pooled and treatment effect estimated in a single dataset **(B)**. *Other PS methods, stratification, IPTW, and covariate adjustment using PS could also be used instead of matching.

give investigators an insight into the quality of the data at hand. Inadequate overlap in propensity score distributions (also called poor "common support") between treatment groups should be considered as a warning that the data set at hand may not be sufficient to reliably address the causal question without "model-dependent" extrapolations based on untrustworthy assumptions (Dehejia and Wahba, 2002; Rubin, 2004b; Rubin, 2007; Ali et al., 2016). In some cases, the researcher might decide to focus on individuals only in the overlapping regions using propensity score matching or trimming; as a consequence, the conclusions of the findings should be restricted to individuals that are sufficiently represented in the overlapping regions of the propensity score distributions (Ali et al., 2016). Conventional regression methods do not provide the researcher with these possibilities. Furthermore, covariate balance in regression methods is a "black-box" and, irrespective of inadequate overlap (i.e., when the treated and untreated groups are disparate on pretreatment covariates), conventional models use extrapolations to estimate treatment effects that may not be generalizable to the entire population in the data set.

Design Tools

Similar to RCTs, propensity score methods can be considered as design tools for pre-processing of the data (matching, stratification, and weighting) without using any outcome information at this stage. As a result, formal causal inference models (also called the potential outcomes framework) (Rubin, 2005) can be applied to clearly specify the causal question without conflating with the modeling approach (Vandenbroucke et al., 2016); hence, it allows for a simple and transparent analysis. In addition, this approach minimizes bias from potential misspecification of the outcome model (Rubin, 2004b). Furthermore, matched, stratified, and weighted analyses do not make strong assumptions of linearity in the relationship of propensity score with the outcome. If a non-parametric pre-processing of the data using propensity score methods does not reduce model dependence, it is reasonable to accept that the data do not have enough information to reliably support the causal inference by any other statistical method. In fact, this knowledge in itself should still be useful and the conclusion may be correct (Rubin, 2004b; Ho et al., 2007; Rubin, 2007; Ali et al., 2016).

Dimension Reduction

Propensity score typically summarizes a large number of measured pretreatment covariates to a single score; hence, it is called a "summary score." This is particularly useful in high-dimensional data with a substantially large number of pretreatment covariates compared to the number of outcome events including rare events, typical of most medication safety studies in pharmacoepidemiology (Glynn et al., 2006). In this setting, maximum likelihood estimations used in conventional regression techniques such as logistic and Cox regression require several outcome events for each parameter included in the regression model; the rule of thumb is that ≥ 10 outcome events are required per confounder included in a model (Peduzzi et al., 1995; Peduzzi et al., 1996). On the other hand, Cepeda et al. (2003) suggested using propensity score when there are fewer than eight outcomes per included covariate to effectively improve estimation.

Doubly Robust Estimations

Generally, doubly roubst estimations (DR) estimation methods apply different procedures or models simultaneously and produce a consistent estimate of the parameter if either of the two models, not necessarily both, has been correctly specified (Imai and Ratkovic, 2014). Several applications of propensity scores have been described as DR in terms of estimating the effect of a certain treatment, including:

1) The combined use of propensity score methods (matching, regression, or weighting) with regression adjustments. These approaches use non-parametric pre-processing of the data to minimize imbalances in measured covariates and, if there are still residual differences, the covariates can be adjusted in the outcome model (Rubin and Thomas, 2000; Nguyen et al., 2017).

2) The combined use of propensity and prognostic score methods (Leacy and Stuart, 2014; Ali et al., 2018b); a prognostic score is any function of a set of covariates that when conditioned on creates independence between the potential outcome under the control (no treatment) condition and the unreduced covariates (Hansen, 2008). Hence, differences in outcomes between treated and untreated individuals can be attributed to the effect of the treatment under study. The two approaches could be combined in several ways such as full matching on a Mahalanobis distance combining the estimated propensity and prognostic scores; full matching on the estimated prognostic score within propensity score calipers; and subclassification on an estimated propensity and prognostic score grid with five subclasses, among others (Leacy and Stuart, 2014; Ali et al., 2018b). Methods combining propensity and prognostic scores were no less robust to model misspecification than single-score methods even when both prognostic and propensity score models were incorrectly specified in simulation and empirical studies (Leacy and Stuart, 2014).

3) The use of covariate balancing propensity score (CBPS) introduced by Imai and Ratkovic (2014) involves estimation of the propensity score such that the resulting covariate balance is optimized. This approach utilizes the dual characteristics of the propensity score as a covariate balancing score and the conditional probability of treatment assignment. Specifically, "the covariate balancing property (i.e., mean independence between the treatment status and measured covariates after inverse propensity score weighting) is used as condition to imply estimation of the propensity score while also incorporating the standard estimation procedure" (Imai and Ratkovic, 2014). Unlike other covariate balancing methods, a single model determines the treatment assignment mechanism and the covariate balancing weights. Once CBPS is estimated, various propensity score methods such as matching and weighting can be implemented without modification (Imai and Ratkovic, 2014). The basic idea of

CBPS is optimizing covariate balance so that even when the propensity score model is misspecified, there will still be a reasonable balance of the covariates between the treatment and comparator groups. Unlike standard DR estimators, however, the CBPS approach does not require estimation of the outcome model.

4) Calculation of DR estimators using different approaches, for example, using the propensity score, predicted, and observed outcome ($\hat{Y}$ and Y, respectively). This approach involves specifying regression models for the treatment (Z) and the outcome (Y) as a function of covariates (X) and combining these subject-specific values to calculate the DR estimate for each individual. First, treatment is modelled as a function of covariates to estimate propensity scores for each individual using the observed data. Second, the relationships between measured confounders and the outcome are modelled within treated and untreated groups separately. The resulting parameter estimates are then used to calculate predicted outcomes ($\hat{Y}_1$, $\hat{Y}_0$) for each individual in the population that is treated (setting Z = 1) and not treated (setting Z = 0) given covariate values. Third, the DR estimates of the outcome are calculated for each individual both in the presence and absence of treatment (DR_1 and DR_0, respectively) using the subject-specific predicted ($\hat{Y}$) and observed (Y) outcomes weighted by the propensity score. Finally, the means of DR_1 and DR_0 are calculated across the entire study population and these means will be used to calculate the effect of the treatment (Funk et al., 2011).

Unmeasured Confounding

Propensity score methods, like other conventional regression methods, can account for only measured confounding factors and not unmeasured factors (Rosenbaum and Rubin, 1983). Therefore, propensity score analyses are only as good as the completeness and quality of the potential confounding variables that are available to the researcher. The only way to convince a critical reader that the study is not subject to unmeasured confounding is to have a rich set of covariates for constructing the propensity score model. Therefore, it is important to provide a detailed account of the variables collected and included in the propensity score model (Ali et al., 2015).

Modifications of the standard propensity score applications have been suggested to further reduce the risk of unmeasured confounding including the use of high-dimensional propensity score and propensity score calibration. High-dimensional propensity score refers to the use of a large number (in the range of several hundreds) of covariates to improve control of confounding; the underlying assumption is that the variables may collectively be proxies for unobserved confounding factors (Schneeweiss et al., 2009; Rassen et al., 2011). Propensity score calibration refers to the use of a "gold standard" propensity score estimated in a separate validation study, with more detailed covariate information unmeasured in the main study, to correct the main-study effect of the drug on the outcome (Stürmer et al., 2005; Stürmer et al., 2007).

Furthermore, sensitivity analyses (Rosenbaum and Rubin, 1983; Rosenbaum, 2005) are useful to assess the plausibility of the assumptions underlying the propensity score methods and how violations of them might affect the conclusions drawn (Stuart, 2010). Methods to deal with unmeasured confounding are summarized in **Figure 1**.

Effect Modification

In estimating treatment effects, there is often an interest to explore if the effect of treatment varies among different subgroups (for example, men versus women) of the population under study, often called "treatment effect modification." There are many ways to utilize propensity score methods to adjust for confounding in a subgroup analysis; however, common implementation of propensity score matching in the medical literature is sub-optimal (Wang et al., 2017; Ali et al.,

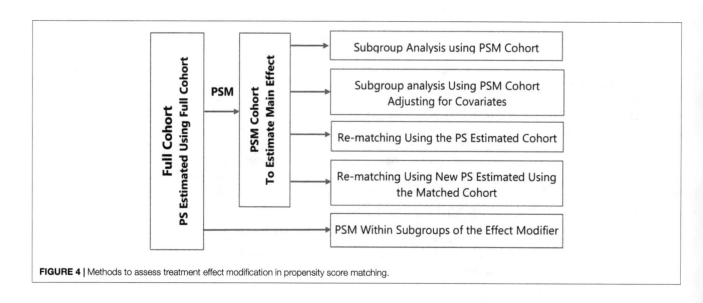

FIGURE 4 | Methods to assess treatment effect modification in propensity score matching.

TABLE 2 | Summary of considerations when planning, conducting, and reporting propensity score analysis.

Characteristics	What to consider	Methods available to deal with	What should or should not be done
Missing data	Missing data mechanism	Multiple imputation if missing at random (MAR)	Avoid complete case analysis and missing indicator category, the later may be biased even when MCAR assumption holds.
Variable selection	Potential confounders, intermediates, colliders	Clinical knowledge/expert opinion. Association between variables with outcome (and treatment). Balance diagnostics.	Avoid adjusting for intermediates, colliders, and strong instrumental variables the later (only when sure or suspect strong unmeasured confounding). Avoid the use of p-values, or step-wise variable selection methods.
Propensity score estimation	Variables included, interactions and higher order terms.	Logistic regression, Recursive partitioning, Neural network, Classification and regression trees, Random forest, and Boosting regression.	Report on the method used for estimation and variables included in the propensity score method.
Propensity score methods	The research question, the treatment effect estimand, and the extent of overlap.	Density plots of propensity scores.	Report the density plots or histograms in the propensity score distribution (preferably overlapping coefficients of the density plots).
Propensity score matching	Matching algorithm, matching with or with our replacement, and matching ratio	Exact (coarsened) matching, nearest neighbor matching (with or without caliper), stratified matching, and full matching. Matching ratio can be: 1-to-1 matching, 1-to- many matching, variable ratio matching, and full matching.	Report on the number of starting population, number matched, and number excluded (with their pre-treatment characteristics).
Propensity score stratification	Number of strata	Deciles and quintiles of propensity scores.	Report on the number of strata used and the covariate balance between treatment groups in each strata.
Regression adjustment using propensity score	Linear relationship between the outcome and the propensity core.		Report on whether linear relationship between the outcome and propensity core is checked and is fulfilled.
Inverse probability of treatment weighting	Whether there is sufficient overlap (positivity).	Weighted regression. Robust variance estimation or Bootstrapping for constructing confidence intervals.	Report on how weights are calculated, if weights are stabilized, the mean weights in both treatment groups, if trimming has been done.
Time-varying exposure	Whether there is time-varying confounding, and if any, whether it is affected by previous treatment.	Marginal Structural models using IPTW, G-formula and G-estimation of structural nested models.	If previous treatment affect time-varying confounding avoid matching, stratification and regression adjustment; apply MSM using IPTW.
Treatment effect modification	Identify potential effect modifier.	Matching on PS within strata of effect modifier, among others.	Avoid the use of stratified analysis using the PSM data without adjustment for covariates.
Multilevel treatment	Whether multilevel structure exists in the data, the number of clusters/levels	Multilevel propensity score methods.	Avoid use of single-level propensity score applications. Include multilevel structure at least in propensity score estimation or outcome analysis, preferably in both.
Multiple treatments	Number of treatment groups, whether there is order in the treatment categories (such as dosage).	Multiple matching and weighting: multinomial logistic regression, ordinal logistic regression, or generalized boosted model.	
Residual Confounding	Whether there is imbalance in covariates.	Doubly robust methods, propensity score calibration (PSC), high dimensional propensity score (HDPS) method.	Report on which method was used and why?
Unmeasured confounding	Whether there is potential unmeasured confounding, or whether the data contain proxies for unmeasured confounding.	Alternative methods such as instrumental variable methods, PSC, HDPS, or consider sensitivity analysis.	Report on the method used and the sensitivity analysis conducted.

2018a). The use of propensity score matched (PSM) cohort for subgroup analysis breaks the matched sets and might result in imbalance of covariates (Ali et al., 2018a). Depending on the frequency of treatment or outcome, small changes in the matched cohort might lead to large fluctuations for measures of association (Rassen et al., 2012).

To account for covariate imbalances, subgroup analyses of propensity score matched cohorts involve: i) adjusting for covariates in the outcome model or ii) re-matching within the subgroups either using the propensity score estimated in the full cohort or fitting new propensity score within subgroups (**Figure 4**) (Rassen et al., 2012; Wang et al., 2017). The choice of a specific method should take into account several factors: prevalence of the treatment and the outcome; strength of association between pretreatment covariates and the treatment; the true effect size within subgroups; and the amount of confounding within the subgroups (Wang et al., 2018).

REPORTING

The credibility of any research depends on a critical assessment by others of the strengths and weaknesses in study design, conduct, and analysis. Hence, transparent and adequate reporting of critical aspects of propensity score-based analysis (Ali et al., 2015), like other observational studies, helps readers follow "what was planned, what was done, what was found, and what conclusions were drawn" (Von Elm et al., 2007). It also makes it easier for other researchers to replicate the study findings using other data sources and to judge whether and how results can be included in systematic reviews (Von Elm et al., 2007). Despite substantial methodological developments and common applications of the propensity score methods, in general, reporting on important features of the propensity score analysis is poor, incomplete, and inconsistent in the medical literature (Austin, 2008a; Ali et al., 2015; Ali et al., 2016; Wang et al., 2017). This could in part be due to a lack of standards for the conduct and reporting of propensity score based studies in guidelines. Therefore, critical items relevant to propensity score analyses should be incorporated in guidelines on the conduct and reporting of observational studies, such as the STROBE statement (Von Elm et al., 2007; Ali et al., 2015) and the ENCePP guide on methodological standards in pharmacoepidemiology (Blake et al., 2012; Ali et al., 2015) to improve the quality of the conduct and reporting of propensity score based studies (Ali et al., 2015; Ali et al., 2016). **Table 2** summarizes important consideration when planning, conducting, and reporting propensity score analysis and list of items that should be reported are summarized by Ali et al. (2016).

CONCLUSION

Propensity score methods will remain important design and analytic tools to estimate effects of treatment from observational data. Preferably, they should be utilized in the design stage as tools for preprocessing of the data and they should be considered complementary tools, and not replacements, to conventional regression adjustments. In fact, when appropriate, propensity score methods should be used in combination with other model-based regression techniques. In addition, propensity score methods should not be regarded as magical remedies for the inadequacies of observational studies such as residual or unmeasured confounding (Rubin and Thomas, 2000; Ali et al., 2016). The ability of propensity score methods to overcome confounding is entirely dependent on the extent to which measured variables capture potential confounding. Taking full advantage of these methods requires explicit definition of the research question and appropriate choice of the propensity score method, transparent and detailed description of all subsequent statistical analyses to be conducted, and adequate reporting of the important aspects of the propensity score analyses (Ali et al., 2016).

AUTHOR CONTRIBUTIONS

MA, DP-A, RF, MB, and LS contributed to the conception and design of the study. MA wrote the first draft of the manuscript. DR and NB wrote sections of the manuscript. All authors contributed to manuscript revision and read and approved the submitted version.

FUNDING

This work is part of The 100 Million Brazilian Cohort project funded by the Wellcome Trust. Grant code: 202912/B/16/Z.

REFERENCES

Adelson, J. L., McCoach, D., Rogers, H., Adelson, J. A., and Sauer, T. M. (2017). Developing and applying the propensity score to make causal inferences: variable selection and stratification. *Front. Psychol.* 8, 1413. doi: 10.3389/fpsyg.2017.01413

Ali, M. S., Collins, G., and Prieto-Alhambra, D. (2017a). The "propensity score paradox": a threat to pharmaco-epidemiological studies? *Pharmacoepidemiol. Drug Saf.* 26:(Suppl.2):3–636. doi:10.1002/pds.4275

Ali, M. S., Douglas, I. J., Williamson, E., Prieto-Alhambra, D., and Smeeth, L., (2018a). "Evaluation of treatment effect modification in propensity score matching: An empirical example," in *Pharmacoepidemiology and drug safety* vol. 27. (NJ USA: Wiley 111 River St, Hoboken 07030-5774), 25–25.

Ali, M. S., Douglas, I. J., Williamson, E., Prieto-Alhambra, D., and Smeeth, L. (2018b). "A joint application of disease risk score and propensity score to control for confounding: A clinical example," in *Pharmacoepidemiology and drug safety* vol. 27. (NJ USA: Wiley 111 River St, Hoboken 07030-5774), 27–27.

Ali, M. S., Groenwold, R. H., Belitser, S. V., Pestman, W. R., Hoes, A. W., Roes, K. C., et al. (2015). Reporting of covariate selection and balance assessment in propensity score analysis is suboptimal: a systematic review. *J. Clin. Epidemiol.* 68, 122–131. doi: 10.1016/j.jclinepi.2014.08.011

Ali, M. S., Groenwold, R. H., and Klungel, O. H. (2016). Best (but oft-forgotten) practices: propensity score methods in clinical nutrition research-3. *Am. J. Clin. Nutr.* 104, 247–258. doi: 10.3945/ajcn.115.125914

Ali, M. S., Groenwold, R. H., Pestman, W. R., Belitser, S. V., Hoes, A. W., De Boer, A., et al. (2013). Time-dependent propensity score and collider-stratification bias: an example of beta 2-agonist use and the risk of coronary heart disease. *Eur. J Epidemiol.* 28, 291–299. doi: 10.1007/s10654-013-9766-2

Ali, M. S., Groenwold, R. H., Pestman, W. R., Belitser, S. V., Roes, K. C., Hoes, A. W., et al. (2014). Propensity score balance measures in pharmacoepidemiology: a simulation study. *Pharmacoepidemiol. Drug Saf.* 23, 802–811. doi: 10.1002/pds.3574

Ali, M. S., Khalid, S., Collins, G., and Prieto-Alhambra, D. (2017b). The comparative performance of logistic regression and random forest in propensity score methods: A simulation study. *Pharmacoepidemiol. Drug Saf.* 26:(Suppl.2):3–636. doi:10.1002/pds.4275

Ali, M. S., Khalid, S., Groenwold, R., Collins, G. S., Klungel, O., and Prieto-Alhambra, D. (2017c). Instrumental variables to test for unmeasured confounding: a precautionary note. *Pharmacoepidemiol. Drug Saf.* 26:(Suppl.2):3–636. doi:10.1002/pds.4275

Angrist, J. D., Imbens, G. W., and Rubin, D. B. (1996). Identification of causal effects using instrumental variables. *J. Am. Stat. Assoc.* 91, 444–455. doi: 10.1080/01621459.1996.10476902

Arpino, B., and Mealli, F. (2011). The specification of the propensity score in multilevel observational studies. *Comput. Stat. Data Anal.* 55, 1770–1780. doi: 10.1016/j.csda.2010.11.008

Austin, P. C. (2008a). A critical appraisal of propensity-score matching in the medical literature between 1996 and 2003. *Stat. Med.* 27, 2037–2049. doi: 10.1002/sim.3150

Austin, P. C. (2008b). The performance of different propensity-score methods for estimating relative risks. *J. Clin. Epidemiol.* 61, 537–545. doi: 10.1016/j.jclinepi.2007.07.011

Austin, P. C. (2009). Balance diagnostics for comparing the distribution of baseline covariates between treatment groups in propensity-score matched samples. *Stat. Med.* 28, 3083–3107. doi: 10.1002/sim.3697

Austin, P. C. (2011). An introduction to propensity score methods for reducing the effects of confounding in observational studies. *Multivariate Behav. Res.* 46, 399–424. doi: 10.1080/00273171.2011.568786

Austin, P. C. (2019). Assessing covariate balance when using the generalized propensity score with quantitative or continuous exposures. *Stat. Methods Med. Res* 28, 1365–1377. doi: 10.1177/0962280218756159

Austin, P. C., and Stuart, E. A. (2015). Moving towards best practice when using inverse probability of treatment weighting (iptw) using the propensity score to estimate causal treatment effects in observational studies. *Stat. Med.* 34, 3661–3679. doi: 10.1002/sim.6607

Bärnighausen, T., Tugwell, P., Røttingen, J.-A., Shemilt, I., Rockers, P., Geldsetzer, P., et al. (2017). Quasi-experimental study designs series—paper 4: uses and value. *J. Clin. Epidemiol.* 89, 21–29. doi: 10.1016/j.jclinepi.2017.03.012

Belitser, S. V., Martens, E. P., Pestman, W. R., Groenwold, R. H., De Boer, A., and Klungel, O. H. (2011). Measuring balance and model selection in propensity score methods. *Pharmacoepidemiol. Drug Saf.* 20, 1115–1129. doi: 10.1002/pds.2188

Blake, K. V., deVries, C. S., Arlett, P., Kurz, X., and Fitt, H. of Centres for Pharmacoepidemiology Pharmacovigilance, E. N. (2012). Increasing scientific standards, independence and transparency in post-authorisation studies: the role of the european network of centres for pharmacoepidemiology and pharmacovigilance. *Pharmacoepidemiol. Drug Saf.* 21, 690–696. doi: 10.1002/pds.3281

Brookhart, M. A., Schneeweiss, S., Rothman, K. J., Glynn, R. J., Avorn, J., and Stürmer, T. (2006). Variable selection for propensity score models. *Am. J. Epidemiol.* 163, 1149–1156. doi: 10.1093/aje/kwj149

Cepeda, M. S., Boston, R., Farrar, J. T., and Strom, B. L. (2003). Comparison of logistic regression versus propensity score when the number of events is low and there are multiple confounders. *Am. J. Epidemiol.* 158, 280–287. doi: 10.1093/aje/kwg115

Cole, S. R., and Hernán, M. A. (2008). Constructing inverse probability weights for marginal structural models. *Am. J. Epidemiol.* 168, 656–664. doi: 10.1093/aje/kwn164

Cole, S. R., Platt, R. W., Schisterman, E. F., Chu, H., Westreich, D., Richardson, D., et al. (2009). Illustrating bias due to conditioning on a collider. *Int. J. Epidemiol.* 39, 417–420. doi: 10.1093/ije/dyp334

Concato, J., Shah, N., and Horwitz, R. I. (2000). Randomized, controlled trials, observational studies, and the hierarchy of research designs. *N. Engl. J. Med.* 342, 1887–1892. doi: 10.1056/NEJM200006223422507

Crowe, B. J., Lipkovich, I. A., and Wang, O. (2010). Comparison of several imputation methods for missing baseline data in propensity scores analysis of binary outcome. *Pharm. Stat.* 9, 269–279. doi: 10.1002/pst.389

Cummings, P. (2013). Missing data and multiple imputation. *JAMA Pediatr.* 167, 656–661. doi: 10.1001/jamapediatrics.2013.1329

Dehejia, R. H., and Wahba, S. (2002). Propensity score-matching methods for nonexperimental causal studies. *Rev. Econ. Stat.* 84, 151–161. doi: 10.1162/003465302317331982

D'Agostino, Jr, R. B. (2007). Propensity scores in cardiovascular research. *Circulation* 115, 2340–2343. doi: 10.1161/CIRCULATIONAHA.105.594952

Eichler, H.-G., Abadie, E., Breckenridge, A., Flamion, B., Gustafsson, L. L., Leufkens, H., et al. (2011). Bridging the efficacy–effectiveness gap: a regulator's perspective on addressing variability of drug response. *Nat. Rev. Drug. Discov.* 10, 495. doi: 10.1038/nrd3501

Funk, M. J., Westreich, D., Wiesen, C., Stürmer, T., Brookhart, M. A., and Davidian, M. (2011). Doubly robust estimation of causal effects. *Am. J. Epidemiol.* 173, 761–767. doi: 10.1093/aje/kwq439

Glynn, R. J., Schneeweiss, S., and Stürmer, T. (2006). Indications for propensity scores and review of their use in pharmacoepidemiology. *Basic Clin. Pharmacol. Toxicol.* 98, 253–259. doi: 10.1111/j.1742-7843.2006.pto_293.x

Goldstein, H., Browne, W., and Rasbash, J. (2002). Multilevel modelling of medical data. *Stat. Med.* 21, 3291–3315. doi: 10.1002/sim.1264

Greenland, S. (2000). Principles of multilevel modelling. *Int. J. Epidemiol.* 29, 158–167. doi: 10.1093/ije/29.1.158

Greenland, S., and Morgenstern, H. (2001). Confounding in health research. *Annu. Rev. Public Health* 22, 189–212. doi: 10.1146/annurev.publhealth.22.1.189

Greenland, S., Robins, J. M., and Pearl, J. (1999). Confounding and collapsibility in causal inference. *Stat. Sci.* 14, 29–46. doi: 10.1214/ss/1009211805

Hansen, B. B. (2004). Full matching in an observational study of coaching for the sat. *J. Am. Stat. Assoc.* 99, 609–618. doi: 10.1198/016214504000000647

Hansen, B. B. (2008). The prognostic analogue of the propensity score. *Biometrika* 95, 481–488. doi: 10.1093/biomet/asn004

Hernán, M. Á., Brumback, B., and Robins, J. M. (2000). Marginal structural models to estimate the causal effect of zidovudine on the survival of hiv-positive men. *Epidemiology* 11(5), 561–570. doi: 10.1097/00001648-200009000-00012

Hirano, K., and Imbens, G. W. (2001). Estimation of causal effects using propensity score weighting: An application to data on right heart catheterization. *Health Serv. Outcomes Res. Methodol.* 2, 259–278. doi: 10.1023/A:1020371312283

Ho, D., Imai, K., King, G., and Stuart, E. (2007). Matching as nonparametric preprocessing for reducing model dependence in parametric causal inference. *Polit. Anal.* 15 (3), 199–236. doi:10.1093/pan/mpl013

Imai, K., and Ratkovic, M. (2014). Covariate balancing propensity score. *J. R. Stat. Soc. Series. B. Stat. Methodol.* 76, 243–263. doi: 10.1111/rssb.12027

Imai, K., and Van Dyk, D. A. (2004). Causal inference with general treatment regimes: Generalizing the propensity score. *J. Am. Stat. Assoc.* 99, 854–866. doi: 10.1198/016214504000001187

Imbens, G. W. (2000). The role of the propensity score in estimating dose-response functions. *Biometrika* 87, 706–710. doi: 10.1093/biomet/87.3.706

Imbens, G. W. (2004). Nonparametric estimation of average treatment effects under exogeneity: A review. *Rev. Econ. Stat.* 86, 4–29. doi: 10.1162/003465304323023651

Imbens, G. W., and Rubin, D. B. (2015). *Causal inference in statistics, social, and biomedical sciences an introduction.* Cambridge: Cambridge University Press. doi: 10.1017/CBO9781139025751

Joffe, M. M., and Rosenbaum, P. R. (1999). Invited commentary: propensity scores. *Am. J. Epidemiol.* 150, 327–333. doi: 10.1093/oxfordjournals.aje.a010011

Johnson, S. R., Tomlinson, G. A., Hawker, G. A., Granton, J. T., and Feldman, B. M. (2018). Propensity score methods for bias reduction in observational studies of treatment effect. *Rheum. Dis. Clin.* 44, 203–213. doi: 10.1016/j.rdc.2018.01.002

King, G., and Nielsen, R. (2016). Why propensity scores should not be used for matching. Copy at. *http://j.mp/1sexgVw Download Citation BibTex Tagged XML Download Paper 378.* doi: 10.1017/pan.2019.11

Leacy, F. P., and Stuart, E. A. (2014). On the joint use of propensity and prognostic scores in estimation of the average treatment effect on the treated: a simulation study. *Stat. Med.* 33, 3488–3508. doi: 10.1002/sim.6030

Lee, B. K., Lessler, J., and Stuart, E. A. (2010). Improving propensity score weighting using machine learning. *Stat. Med.* 29, 337–346. doi: 10.1002/sim.3782

Lee, B. K., Lessler, J., and Stuart, E. A. (2011). Weight trimming and propensity score weighting. *PloS One* 6, e18174. doi: 10.1371/journal.pone.0018174

Leyrat, C., Seaman, S. R., White, I. R., Douglas, I., Smeeth, L., Kim, J., et al. (2019). Propensity score analysis with partially observed covariates: How should multiple imputation be used? *Stat. Methods Med. Res* 28, 3–19. doi: 10.1177/0962280217713032

Li, F., Morgan, K. L., and Zaslavsky, A. M. (2018). Balancing covariates via propensity score weighting. *J. Am. Stat. Assoc.* 113, 390–400. doi: 10.1080/01621459.2016.1260466

Li, F., Zaslavsky, A. M., and Landrum, M. B. (2013). Propensity score weighting with multilevel data. *Stat. Med.* 32, 3373–3387. doi: 10.1002/sim.5786

Linden, A., and Samuels, S. J. (2013). Using balance statistics to determine the optimal number of controls in matching studies. *J. Eval. Clin. Pract.* 19, 968–975. doi: 10.1111/jep.12072

Lunt, M. (2013). Selecting an appropriate caliper can be essential for achieving good balance with propensity score matching. *Am. J. Epidemiol.* 179, 226–235. doi: 10.1093/aje/kwt212

Lunt, M., Solomon, D., Rothman, K., Glynn, R., Hyrich, K., Symmons, D. P., et al. (2009). Different methods of balancing covariates leading to different effect estimates in the presence of effect modification. *Am. J. Epidemiol.* 169, 909–917. doi: 10.1093/aje/kwn391

Makady, A., de Boer, A., Hillege, H., Klungel, O., Goettsch, W., and on behalf of GetReal Work Package 1. (2017). What is real-world data? a review of definitions based on literature and stakeholder interviews. *Value Health* 20, 858–865. doi: 10.1016/j.jval.2017.03.008

McCaffrey, D. F., Ridgeway, G., and Morral, A. R. (2004). Propensity score estimation with boosted regression for evaluating causal effects in observational studies. *Psychol. Methods* 9, 403. doi: 10.1037/1082-989X.9.4.403

Myers, J. A., Rassen, J. A., Gagne, J. J., Huybrechts, K. F., Schneeweiss, S., Rothman, K. J., et al. (2011a). Effects of adjusting for instrumental variables on bias and precision of effect estimates. *Am. J. Epidemiol.* 174, 1213–1222. doi: 10.1093/aje/kwr364

Myers, J. A., Rassen, J. A., Gagne, J. J., Huybrechts, K. F., Schneeweiss, S., Rothman, K. J., et al. (2011b). Myers et al. respond to "understanding bias amplification". *Am. J. Epidemiol.* 174, 1228–1229. doi: 10.1093/aje/kwr353

Nguyen, T.-L., Collins, G. S., Spence, J., Daurès, J.-P., Devereaux, P., Landais, P., et al. (2017). Double-adjustment in propensity score matching analysis: choosing a threshold for considering residual imbalance. *BMC Med. Res. Methodol.* 17, 78. doi: 10.1186/s12874-017-0338-0

Patrick, A. R., Schneeweiss, S., Brookhart, M. A., Glynn, R. J., Rothman, K. J., Avorn, J., et al. (2011). The implications of propensity score variable selection strategies in pharmacoepidemiology: an empirical illustration. *Pharmacoepidemiol. Drug Saf.* 20, 551–559. doi: 10.1002/pds.2098

Pearl, J. (2011). Invited commentary: understanding bias amplification. *Am. J. Epidemiol.* 174, 1223–1227. doi: 10.1093/aje/kwr352

Pearl, J. (2012). On a class of bias-amplifying variables that endanger effect estimates. arXiv e-prints e1203.3503. https://ui.adsabs.harvard.edu/abs/2012arXiv1203.3503P.

Peduzzi, P., Concato, J., Feinstein, A. R., and Holford, T. R. (1995). Importance of events per independent variable in proportional hazards regression analysis ii. accuracy and precision of regression estimates. *J. Clin. Epidemiol.* 48, 1503–1510. doi: 10.1016/0895-4356(95)00048-8

Peduzzi, P., Concato, J., Kemper, E., Holford, T. R., and Feinstein, A. R. (1996). A simulation study of the number of events per variable in logistic regression analysis. *J. Clin. Epidemiol.* 49, 1373–1379. doi: 10.1016/S0895-4356(96)00236-3

Platt, R. W., Schisterman, E. F., and Cole, S. R. (2009). Time-modified confounding. *Am. J. Epidemiol.* 170, 687–694. doi: 10.1093/aje/kwp175

Qu, Y., and Lipkovich, I. (2009). Propensity score estimation with missing values using a multiple imputation missingness pattern (mimp) approach. *Stat. Med.* 28, 1402–1414. doi: 10.1002/sim.3549

Rassen, J. A., Glynn, R. J., Brookhart, M. A., and Schneeweiss, S. (2011). Covariate selection in high-dimensional propensity score analyses of treatment effects in small samples. *Am. J. Epidemiol.* 173, 1404–1413. doi: 10.1093/aje/kwr001

Rassen, J. A., Glynn, R. J., Rothman, K. J., Setoguchi, S., and Schneeweiss, S. (2012). Applying propensity scores estimated in a full cohort to adjust for confounding in subgroup analyses. *Pharmacoepidemiol. Drug Saf.* 21, 697–709. doi: 10.1002/pds.2256

Robins, J. M., Hernan, M. A., and Brumback, B. (2000). Marginal structural models and causal inference in epidemiology. *Epidemiology* 11 (5), 550–560 doi: 10.1097/00001648-200009000-00011

Rosenbaum, P. R. (2005). Sensitivity analysis in observational studies. In: *Encyclopedia of statistics in behavioral science.* Eds. B. S. Everitt and D. C. Howell (John Wiley & Sons, Ltd.) 4, 1809–1814. doi: 10.1002/0470013192.bsa606

Rosenbaum, P. R., and Rubin, D. B. (1983). The central role of the propensity score in observational studies for causal effects. *Biometrika* 70, 41–55. doi: 10.1093/biomet/70.1.41

Rosenbaum, P. R., and Rubin, D. B. (1984). Reducing bias in observational studies using subclassification on the propensity score. *J. Am. Stat. Assoc.* 79, 516–524. doi: 10.1080/01621459.1984.10478078

Rosenbaum, P. R., and Rubin, D. B. (1985). Constructing a control group using multivariate matched sampling methods that incorporate the propensity score. *Am. Stat.* 39, 33–38. doi: 10.1080/00031305.1985.10479383

Rubin, D. B. (1996). Multiple imputation after 18+ years. *J. Am. Stat. Assoc.* 91, 473–489. doi: 10.1080/01621459.1996.10476908

Rubin, D. B. (1997). Estimating causal effects from large data sets using propensity scores. *Ann. Intern. Med.* 127, 757–763. doi: 10.7326/0003-4819-127-8_Part_2-199710151-00064

Rubin, D. B. (2001). Using propensity scores to help design observational studies: application to the tobacco litigation. *Health Serv. Outcomes Res. Methodol.* 2, 169–188. rubin2001using. doi: 10.1023/A:1020363010465

Rubin, D. B. (2004a). *Multiple imputation for nonresponse in surveys* Vol. 81. New York: John Wiley & Sons.

Rubin, D. B. (2004b). On principles for modeling propensity scores in medical research. *Pharmacoepidemiol. Drug Saf.* 13, 855–857. doi: 10.1002/pds.968

Rubin, D. B. (2005). Causal inference using potential outcomes: Design, modeling, decisions. *J. Am. Stat. Assoc.* 100, 322–331. doi: 10.1198/016214504000001880

Rubin, D. B. (2007). The design versus the analysis of observational studies for causal effects: parallels with the design of randomized trials. *Stat. Med.* 26, 20–36. doi: 10.1002/sim.2739

Rubin, D. B., and Thomas, N. (1996). Matching using estimated propensity scores: relating theory to practice. *Biometrics* 52, 249–264. doi: 10.2307/2533160

Rubin, D. B., and Thomas, N. (2000). Combining propensity score matching with additional adjustments for prognostic covariates. *J. Am. Stat. Assoc.* 95, 573–585. doi: 10.1080/01621459.2000.10474233

Schafer, J. L., and Kang, J. (2008). Average causal effects from nonrandomized studies: a practical guide and simulated example. *Psychol. Methods* 13, 279. doi: 10.1037/a0014268

Schneeweiss, S. (2006). Sensitivity analysis and external adjustment for unmeasured confounders in epidemiologic database studies of therapeutics. *Pharmacoepidemiol. Drug Saf.* 15, 291–303. doi: 10.1002/pds.1200

Schneeweiss, S., Gagne, J., Glynn, R., Ruhl, M., and Rassen, J. (2011). Assessing the comparative effectiveness of newly marketed medications: methodological challenges and implications for drug development. *Clin. Pharmacol. Ther.* 90, 777–790. doi: 10.1038/clpt.2011.235

Schneeweiss, S., Rassen, J. A., Glynn, R. J., Avorn, J., Mogun, H., and Brookhart, M. A. (2009). High-dimensional propensity score adjustment in studies of treatment effects using health care claims data. *Epidemiology* 20, 512. doi: 10.1097/EDE.0b013e3181a663cc

Setoguchi, S., Schneeweiss, S., Brookhart, M. A., Glynn, R. J., and Cook, E. F. (2008). Evaluating uses of data mining techniques in propensity score estimation: a simulation study. *Pharmacoepidemiol. Drug Saf.* 17, 546–555. doi: 10.1002/pds.1555

Shah, B. R., Laupacis, A., Hux, J. E., and Austin, P. C. (2005). Propensity score methods gave similar results to traditional regression modeling in observational studies: a systematic review. *J. Clin. Epidemiol.* 58, 550–559. doi: 10.1016/j.jclinepi.2004.10.016

Sibbald, B., and Roland, M. (1998). Understanding controlled trials. why are randomised controlled trials important? *BMJ* 316, 201. doi: 10.1136/bmj.316.7126.201

Sterne, J. A., White, I. R., Carlin, J. B., Spratt, M., Royston, P., Kenward, M. G., et al. (2009). Multiple imputation for missing data in epidemiological and clinical research: potential and pitfalls. *BMJ* 338, b2393. doi: 10.1136/bmj.b2393

Stuart, E. A. (2008). Developing practical recommendations for the use of propensity scores: Discussion of 'a critical appraisal of propensity score matching in the medical literature between 1996 and 2003'by peter austin, statistics in medicine. *Stat. Med.* 27, 2062–2065. doi: 10.1002/sim.3207

Stuart, E. A. (2010). Matching methods for causal inference: A review and a look forward. *Stat. Sci.* 25, 1. stuart2010matching. doi: 10.1214/09-STS313

Stürmer, T., Joshi, M., Glynn, R. J., Avorn, J., Rothman, K. J., and Schneeweiss, S. (2006a). A review of the application of propensity score methods yielded increasing use, advantages in specific settings, but not substantially different estimates compared with conventional multivariable methods. *J. Clin. Epidemiol.* 59, 437–4e1. doi: 10.1016/j.jclinepi.2005.07.004

Stürmer, T., Rothman, K. J., and Glynn, R. J. (2006b). Insights into different results from different causal contrasts in the presence of effect-measure modification. *Pharmacoepidemiol. Drug Saf.* 15, 698–709. doi: 10.1002/pds.1231

Stürmer, T., Schneeweiss, S., Avorn, J., and Glynn, R. J. (2005). Adjusting effect estimates for unmeasured confounding with validation data using propensity score calibration. *Am. J. Epidemiol.* 162, 279–289. doi: 10.1093/aje/kwi192

Stürmer, T., Schneeweiss, S., Rothman, K. J., Avorn, J., and Glynn, R. J. (2007). Performance of propensity score calibration—a simulation study. *Am. J. Epidemiol.* 165, 1110–1118. doi: 10.1093/aje/kwm074

Tarricone, R., Boscolo, P. R., and Armeni, P. (2016). What type of clinical evidence is needed to assess medical devices? *Eur. Respir. Rev.* 25, 259–265. doi: 10.1183/16000617.0016-2016

Uddin, M. J., Groenwold, R. H., Ali, M. S., de Boer, A., Roes, K. C., Chowdhury, M. A., et al. (2016). Methods to control for unmeasured confounding in pharmacoepidemiology: an overview. *Int. J. Clin. Pharmacol. Res.* 38, 714–723. doi: 10.1007/s11096-016-0299-0

Vandenbroucke, J. P., Broadbent, A., and Pearce, N. (2016). Causality and causal inference in epidemiology: the need for a pluralistic approach. *Int. J. Epidemiol.* 45, 1776–1786. doi: 10.1093/ije/dyv341

Von Elm, E., Altman, D. G., Egger, M., Pocock, S. J., Gøtzsche, P. C., Vandenbroucke, J. P., et al. (2007). The strengthening the reporting of observational studies in epidemiology (strobe) statement: guidelines for reporting observational studies. *PLoS Med.* 4, e296. doi: 10.1371/journal.pmed.0040296

Wang, S. V., He, M., Jin, Y., Wyss, R., Shin, H., Ma, Y., et al. (2017). A review of the performance of different methods for propensity score matched subgroup analyses and a summary of their application in peer-reviewed research studies. *Pharmacoepidemiol. Drug Saf.* 26, 1507–1512. doi: 10.1002/pds.4328

Wang, S. V., Jin, Y., Fireman, B., Gruber, S., He, M., Wyss, R., et al. (2018). Relative performance of propensity score matching strategies for subgroup analyses.

Am. J. Epidemiol. 187 (8): 1799–1807. doi: 10.1093/aje/kwy049

Weitzen, S., Lapane, K. L., Toledano, A. Y., Hume, A. L., and Mor, V. (2005). Weaknesses of goodness-of-fit tests for evaluating propensity score models: the case of the omitted confounder. *Pharmacoepidemiol. Drug Saf.* 14, 227–238. doi: 10.1002/pds.986

Westreich, D., Cole, S. R., Funk, M. J., Brookhart, M. A., and Stürmer, T. (2011). The role of the c-statistic in variable selection for propensity score models. *Pharmacoepidemiol. Drug Saf.* 20, 317–320. doi: 10.1002/pds.2074

Westreich, D., Lessler, J., and Funk, M. J. (2010). Propensity score estimation: neural networks, support vector machines, decision trees (cart), and meta-classifiers as alternatives to logistic regression. *J. Clin. Epidemiol.* 63, 826–833. doi: 10.1016/j.jclinepi.2009.11.020

Yuan, H., Ali, M. S., Brouwer, E. S., Girman, C. J., Guo, J. J., Lund, J. L., et al. (2018). Real-world evidence: What it is and what it can tell us according to the international society for pharmacoepidemiology (ispe) comparative effectiveness research (cer) special interest group (sig). *Clin. Pharmacol. Ther.* 104, 239–241. doi: 10.1002/cpt.1086

Zhang, X., Faries, D. E., Li, H., Stamey, J. D., and Imbens, G. W. (2018). Addressing unmeasured confounding in comparative observational research. *Pharmacoepidemiol. Drug Saf.* 27, 373–382. doi: 10.1002/pds.4394

21

Big Data's Role in Precision Public Health

Shawn Dolley*

Cloudera, Inc., Palo Alto, CA, United States

*Correspondence:
Shawn Dolley
shawn.dolley@gmail.com

Precision public health is an emerging practice to more granularly predict and understand public health risks and customize treatments for more specific and homogeneous subpopulations, often using new data, technologies, and methods. Big data is one element that has consistently helped to achieve these goals, through its ability to deliver to practitioners a volume and variety of structured or unstructured data not previously possible. Big data has enabled more widespread and specific research and trials of stratifying and segmenting populations at risk for a variety of health problems. Examples of success using big data are surveyed in surveillance and signal detection, predicting future risk, targeted interventions, and understanding disease. Using novel big data or big data approaches has risks that remain to be resolved. The continued growth in volume and variety of available data, decreased costs of data capture, and emerging computational methods mean big data success will likely be a required pillar of precision public health into the future. This review article aims to identify the precision public health use cases where big data has added value, identify classes of value that big data may bring, and outline the risks inherent in using big data in precision public health efforts.

Keywords: precision public health, big data, computational epidemiology, infectious disease surveillance, precision population health

INTRODUCTION

This review article aims to identify the precision public health use cases where big data has added value, identify classes of value that big data may bring, and outline the risks inherent in using big data in precision public health efforts. This article focuses on surveying current practice, with a breadth of examples. The article does not include a critical review of the methods included in the big data and precision public health published research. It is hoped this article may pave the way for future researchers to measure the strengths and weaknesses, robustness, and validity of individual studies, interventions and outcomes. With the breadth of practice defined here, such follow-on in-depth critical review could identify precision public health best practices in design, methods, implementation, and analysis.

METHODS

The terms "big data" and "precision public health"—two relatively new disciplines—often do not appear in the nomenclature of contemporary public health interventions and studies. Searching for the terms "big data" or "precision public health" returns a small fraction of the actual activity. Based on the lack of existing reviews and the complexity in identifying the intersection of precision public health and big data, the rationale of this narrative review article is to find examples of the use of big data in implementations of precision public health published in peer-reviewed academic journals.

The author (a) reviewed a large number of public health studies to look for precision and big data, as well as related and follow-on studies, (b) identified and searched for specific types of big data being applied to public health, and (c) searched for uses of data in precision public health to identify big vs. small data—always using the definition of these terms rather than relying on the presence of the terms "big data" or "precision public health."

Searches were performed using Google Scholar and Google. Examples of public health implementations—with and without big data—and precision public health implementations—with and without big data—only qualified for this article if they were published in peer-reviewed journals. In the presence of multiple qualifying examples, best attempts were made to limit examples to a single citation. In the presence of multiple examples, to reduce risk of bias and attempt to identify the most robust examples, the examples selected were those with the (a) most clearly identifiable public health use case, (b) clearest use of big data, (c) most "precision," (d) in journals with the highest impact factor, that were (e) the most recent—and in that order of priority. Searches were concluded by July 20, 2017.

Search terms used were as follows:

1. For identifying implementations using big data volume, the term "public health" and each of the following: "big data," "gene-wide," "genome," "genomic," "germline," "GWAS," "imaging," "molecular," "multi-omic," "pan-omic," "phenome," "PWAS," "translational," "video," "whole exome," and "whole genome."
2. For identifying implementations using big data variety, the term "public health" and each of the following: "big data," "drone," "Facebook," "Instagram," "IoT," "internet of things," "linked," "linked data," "patient-centered," "patient generated," "mobile," "mobile phone," "registry," "registries," "secondary use," "semantic," "sensors," "social media," "surveys," "Twitter," "UAV," "unmanned aerial vehicle," "variety," and "wearable."
3. For identifying implementations using big data velocity, the term "public health" and each of the following: "big data," "continuous," "monitor," "real-time," "sensor," "streams," "streaming," "velocity," and "video."
4. For identifying public health implementations—including programs, trials, innovations and experiments—using big data, the term "big data" and each of the following: "adverse drug event," "ADE," "adverse event," "cohort," "epidemic," "epidemiology," "health intervention," "health risk," "heterogeneous," "homogeneous," "human movement," "outcomes," "pandemic," "pharmaco-epidemiology," "population health," "precision public health," "prevention," "public health," "signal detection," "surveillance," "targeted intervention," "tracking," "vaccine," "vector," and "virus."

Google Scholar also provides lists of more recent studies which have cited the current study. These lists were reviewed to identify if more recent studies existed that provided better examples of pertinent characteristics.

This method has a number of limitations. Google Scholar has limitations, including relying on the end user to discriminate which studies returned are from peer-reviewed journals. No review protocol exists independent of this review article. No study selection or summary measures were collected, and no meta-analysis was performed. No study characteristics were collected. No assessment of the validity of included studies was performed beyond their inclusion in peer-reviewed academic journals. No assessment of cumulative level bias risk was performed. No additional analysis methods were used. The selection of studies included was not independently reviewed. The scope of this narrative review precludes enumerating additional limitations. Limitations aside, the result of these methods is a collection of studies or programs where big data and precision public health—as these terms are defined in this article—are being used together. Through implementing these methods, this review article is the first to identify the scope and scale of big data's role in precision public health, highlight classes of innovation, and identify the risks of using big data in this field.

PRECISION PUBLIC HEALTH

"Precision public health is a new field driven by technological advances that enable more precise descriptions and analyzes of individuals and population groups, with a view to improving the overall health of populations" (1). The term was coined in Australia by Dr. Tarun Weeramanthri in 2013, and first found in print in 2014 (2). Dr. Muin Khoury and Dr. Sandro Galea describe precision public health as "improving the ability to prevent disease, promote health, and reduce health disparities in populations by applying emerging methods and technologies for measuring disease, pathogens, exposures, behaviors, and susceptibility in populations; and developing policies and targeted implementation programs to improve health" (3). Precision public health leverages big data and its enabling technologies to achieve a previously impossible level of targeting or speed (4). The Bill & Melinda Gates Foundation adds that precision public health "requires robust primary surveillance data, rapid application of sophisticated analytics to track the geographical distribution of disease, and the capacity to act on such information" (5). Precision public health works because "more-accurate methods for measuring disease, pathogens, exposures, behaviors, and susceptibility could allow better assessment of population health and development of policies and targeted programs for preventing disease" (4). Arnett & Claas add "Precision public health is characterized by discovering, validating, and optimizing care strategies for well-characterized population strata" (6). As for the size of the strata, Colijn et al. state "precision approaches must act at the right scale, which will often be intermediate—between "one size fits all" medicine and fully individualized therapies" (7).

The prominence of the term "precision" in the new practices of precision medicine and precision public health will invariably raise questions about their similarity. While precision medicine requires genetic, lifestyle, and environmental data to meet goals of more customized and potentially individualized clinical treatments, precision public health is about increased accuracy and granularity in defining public cohorts and delivering target interventions of many types (4–6). Precision medicine and precision public health are independent.

BIG DATA IN HEALTHCARE AND PUBLIC HEALTH

Big data has recently become a ubiquitous approach to driving insights, innovation and new interventions across economic sectors (8, 9). The United States National Institute of Standards and Technology defines big data as follows: "Big Data consists of extensive datasets—primarily in the characteristics of volume, variety, velocity, and/or variability—that require a scalable architecture for efficient storage, manipulation, and analysis," (10). Decreases in costs of technology enabled the big data phenomenon to emerge (11). Data of "such a high volume, velocity and variety to require specific technology and analytical methods for its transformation into value" has a symbiotic relationship with the technology innovation on which it relies; the term big data often conflates the actual physical data with the unique technologies required to use it (12, 13).

In patient-specific healthcare, big data technology has helped enable greater scales of volume, variety and velocity (14, 15). Usable data *volume* has significantly increased in areas such as genomics (16, 17), molecular research (18, 19), medical image mining (20), and population health (21, 22). Enabling a *variety* of data to be integrated, for a more complete view of patient or population, has occurred in areas including air quality (23, 24), wearables (25, 26), patient generated content *via* the web (27), patient or physician movement (28, 29), medical studies (30), and critical care (31). Big data enabling increased *velocity* in healthcare was one of the earliest uses, in areas such as clinical prediction (32, 33), and diagnostics (15, 33). Current examples and future vision for use of big data exists in multiple and varying pathologies, including cancer (34), cardiology (35), epilepsy (36), family medicine (37), gastroenterology (38), nursing (39), pediatric ophthalmology (40), psychiatry (41, 42), and women's health (43) as examples.

Barrett et al. state succinctly: "Big data can play a key role in both research and intervention activities and accelerate progress in disease prevention and population health" (44). Big data shows utility across the entire spectrum of public health disciplines. This capability ranges from "monitoring population health in real-time" to building "definitive extents and databases on the occurrence of many diseases" (45). Public health subject areas that include examples of the use of big data include community health (46), environmental health science (24, 47), epidemiology (48), infectious disease (45), maternal and child health (49), occupational health and safety (50), and nutrition (51). There is optimism and evidence for big data's value in public health, both in research and in intervention (52).

BIG DATA IN PRECISION PUBLIC HEALTH

Today, use of big data has been shown to improve precision in select disciplines of public health. These areas include performing disease surveillance and signal detection (53, 54), predicting risk (55, 56), targeting interventions (6), and understanding disease (57). Research and proofs-of-concept with this data for these applications have been performed around the world. With the pace of technology innovation, and the speed at which precision health practitioners have embraced big data, there will likely be more public health disciplines, practices, approaches, and interventions implemented in the future or that are beyond the scope of this article (58, 59).

PERFORMING DISEASE SURVEILLANCE AND SIGNAL DETECTION

Disease surveillance and signal detection are among the most commonly cited and revolutionary of the big data use cases in precision public health (45, 60–62). Precision signal detection or disease surveillance using big data has shown efficacy in air pollution (23, 24), antibiotic resistance (63), cholera (64), dengue (65, 66), drowning (67), drug safety (68, 69), electromagnetic field exposure (70), Influenza A H1N1 (71), Lyme disease (72), monitoring food intake (73), and whooping cough (74).

Disease surveillance often includes tracking affected individuals, i.e., human carriers, patients, or victims (75). Stoddard et al. stated in 2009: "Human movement is a critical, understudied behavioral component underlying the transmission dynamics of many vector-borne pathogens" (76). In the effort to track disease spread by human vectors, a premium is placed on information that is more recent and granular (77, 78). Thus, access to huge volumes of streaming real-time data generated by humans seems at once an ideal signal repository for identifying and tracking affected individuals, and definitionally big data (78).

Indeed, big data supports alternate and in some ways superior methods to track affected individuals (45, 62). Because affected individuals move so quickly and at such a wide range, the real-time capabilities of big data and big data technology are now critical in this discipline (79, 80). Studies have shown efficacy using mobile phone data in tracking movement in cholera (81), dengue (82), Ebola (83), human immunodeficiency virus (HIV) (84), malaria (85), rubella (85), and schistosomiasis (86). Other mechanisms that have shown efficacy or promise in tracking movement of affected individuals include air travel data (87), GPS data-loggers (88), magnetometers (89), Twitter (71), and web searches (65).

PREDICTING RISK

Effective signal detection often leads to attempts to predict future signals (90, 91). Predicting public health risk leads to a chance to implement preventive interventions (56, 92). Models predicting either disease spread or outcomes, using traditional or non-big data sources, have been developed across the spectrum of public health crises, including dengue (93), HIV (94), influenza (95), malaria (96), Rift Valley Fever (97), and tuberculosis (98).

One early example of using big data for public health prediction, Google Flu Trends, was a well-publicized failure (99). Since that episode, approaches to predicting risk using the internet and social media have shown special care to include merging big data with non-social media data sources, avoid overfitting models with relatively few cases, and being conscious of the risks of big data (56, 100).

Big data has been used for risk prediction of spread or outcomes in public health topics such as air pollution (101), antibiotic resistance (102), avian influenza A (103), blood lead levels (104), child abuse (49), diabetes (105), Ebola (106), HIV (107), malaria (108), gestational diabetes (109), smoking progression (110), West Nile (111), and Zika (86, 112, 113).

TARGETING TREATMENT INTERVENTIONS

Applying treatment interventions to homogeneous cohorts within a larger heterogeneous population has been advocated since Lalonde's seminal report "A New Perspective on the Health of Canadians" in 1974 (114). Historical examples of adding precision to public health treatment populations include gonorrhea in the 1980s (115), HIV in the 1990s (116), breast cancer in the 2000s (117), and malaria in the 2010s (118). In 2010, the US Department of Health and Human Services said of those citizens with multiple chronic conditions: "Indeed, developing means for determining homogeneous subgroups among this heterogeneous population is viewed as an important step in the effort to improve the health status of the total population" (119).

Big data was leveraged in public health research identifying finer-grain treatment interventions in childhood asthma (120), childhood obesity (121), diarrhea (122), Hepatitis C (123), HIV (124), injectable drug use (125), malaria (126), opioid medication misuse (127), use of smokeless tobacco (128), and the Zika virus (129).

One clinical example at the intersection of identifying subpopulations for effective interventions and big data is personalized vaccinology or "vaccinomics" (130). Most vaccines today are applied in a one-size fits all model: the typical implementation assumes a homogenous population, uses the same vaccine and dosages for all patients, ignores replicated, empirical realities of a heterogeneous population, and does not use sophisticated genomic capabilities at hand (131, 132). While today's vaccines are applied homogeneously, the results are individual: "The response to a vaccine is the cumulative result of non-random interactions with host genes, epigenetic phenomena, metagenomics and the microbiome, gene dominance, complementarity, epistasis, coinfections, and other factors" (133). Vaccinomics would focus on homogeneous subpopulations treated with vaccines, dosages and approaches that would "hold the promise of moving away from one standard vaccine against all human populations…to one where vaccines can be relatively easily tailor-fitted to individual, community and population specificity" (134).

UNDERSTANDING DISEASE

Data volume and variety in epidemiology have grown consistently over time well before the age of big data (135–137). Contemporary exponential increases in data sizes, and perhaps more importantly increases in variety of data sources, make big data a valuable addition to the epidemiologist's toolkit (64, 138). Glymour states "We recommend that social epidemiologists take advantage of recent revolutionary improvements in data availability and computing

power to examine new hypotheses and expand our repertoire of study designs" (139). Big data may have added relevance in study designs that are patient-centric and precision-oriented (140).

"Person-oriented approaches, in contrast, focus on differences between individuals as characterized by configurations and patterns of variables. This is well in line with a precision-medicine approach to understanding disease risk, resilience, and treatment response in subpopulations of individuals" (140).

Big data is a component in studies that have shown new precision characteristics of such public health concerns as cholera (141), chikungunya (142), diabetes (143, 144), diarrhea (145), heatwave (146), influenza (147), opioid epidemic (148, 149), preterm birth (150), stunting (151), and Zika (152).

Table 1 summarizes the public health crises cited previously for which exists peer-reviewed research in at least two of the four precision public health disciplines. While the precision health research in **Table 1** and in this article has peer-reviewed and exhaustive methods, there are some opportunity gaps that future research should consider and include. **Table 2** lists critical gaps that occasionally exist in the research, grouped by precision public health discipline.

CONTRIBUTIONS OF BIG DATA

Big data offers special contributions to precision public health in enabling a wider view of health variables through linking disparate or novel data (44, 153, 154) and enabling large study populations with volumes of multiomic data to identify "molecular cohorts" (155).

The technologies behind big data make it much easier to integrate a variety of data within a study (156). For example, because big data does not require investment in an *a priori* data

TABLE 1 | Precision public health research leveraging big data.

| Public health crisis | Precision public health discipline | | | |
	Performing disease surveillance and signal detection	Predicting risk	Targeting treatment interventions	Understanding disease
Air pollution	(23, 24)	(101)		
Antibiotic resistance	(63)	(102)		
Diabetes		(105, 109)		(143, 144)
Diarrhea			(122)	(145)
Ebola	(83)	(106)		
HIV	(84)	(107)	(124)	
Influenza (multiple)	(71)	(103)		(147)
Malaria	(85)	(108)	(126)	
Opioid epidemic			(127)	(148, 149)
Zika	(86, 112, 113)		(129)	(152)

Research studies (by citation) applying precision with the help of big data to a public health crisis. Public health crises are only included if big data in precision public health examples exist in more than one precision public health discipline.

TABLE 2 | Potential gaps in research methods in precision public health using big data.

Study attribute	Precision public health discipline			
	Performing disease surveillance and signal detection	Predicting risk	Targeting treatment interventions	Understanding disease
Data	• Lack of clinical data, lack of attempt to build data sharing agreements to attain clinical data, or lack of attempt to use other methods to add phenotypic data about subjects • No addition of traditional surveillance approach data to test incremental improvement in hybrid approaches	• Lack of clinical data, lack of attempt to build data sharing agreements to attain clinical data, or lack of attempt to use other methods to add phenotypic data about subjects • Novel determinants may be missed by starting with too narrow a scope • Data collected in the coverage area may not be available in other areas	• Molecular substrate is missing entirely, or missing within specific ethnicities or other variables • Lack of showing positive treatment outcomes *via* electronic health records or detailed clinical data	• Data identifying more variety or precision in disease or vector etiology is not present when such precision is available/possible • Molecular substrate is missing entirely, or missing within specific ethnicities or other variables • Lack of adding other variables *ex post facto* to validate homogeneity of precision subgroups
Subjects	• Privacy risks not addressed; as precision increases, subjects could be uniquely identified • Children not included, either by design or due to big data constraints	• Children not included, either by design or due to big data constraints • Lack of "*n*" in the high risk areas limits validity measure results at subject or molecular levels • Lack of data collection from healthy or "healthier" subjects	• Privacy risks not addressed; as precision increases, subjects could be uniquely identified • Some study or disease types have low "*n*," cannot attain high confidence levels, with no guidance for future alternatives to increase confidence levels	• Lack of subject precision when such precision or finer-grain subject characterization is available/possible • Some study or disease types have low "*n*," cannot attain high confidence levels, with no guidance for future alternatives to increase confidence levels
Geography	• Study was conducted in a city and no design included for applying research approaches to rural areas • Limited coverage area • No mention of outcomes' ability to scale outside the study coverage area	• Lack of geographical precision when such precision is available/possible • Study was conducted in a city and no design included for applying research approaches to rural areas • Limited coverage area • No mention of outcomes' ability to scale outside the study coverage area	• Lack of plan on how to implement an intervention selectively to a high-risk geographic area or areas • Lack of discussion of variability of geographic attributes that affect intervention dynamics • Pilots may have been done so precisely that additional pilots in other continents or biomes need to be completed to increase validity	• Lack of geographic classification included in the research or lack of geographic precision • No concept of geography-as-phenotype; no epigenomic or exposomic component addressed
Scaling	• Sensor, UAV or other hardware is expensive, or additional hardware is needed • Study performed at a country or province level and not scalable to more precise geographies due to limitations of data availability or other factors	• Machine learning approach may have been selected *a priori* rather than as a result of testing multiple methods, limiting potential to scale the approach forward • No postulates for taking predictions and translating them to actions, such as prevention, intervention, programming or cures	• No postulates for taking research findings and translating them to actions, such as prevention, intervention, programming or cures • Study may be theoretical or not include an end-to-end pilot implementation • Pilot may be missing precision disease understanding that affects long-term outcomes • Lack of plan for iterative or long-term follow up	• No postulates for taking research findings and translating them to actions, such as prevention, intervention, programming or cures • Lack of plan to replicate disease understanding in cohorts that are more random, larger, or more homogeneous/specific

Critical features sometimes missing from precision public health studies leveraging big data, shown by public health discipline type.

schema, users can bring together a variety of different data and link it when the analytics are created (157). This enables researchers to link a mélange of unstructured disease and outcome data (158, 159). In their 2017 study, Harry Hemingway, in their completion of 33 studies using linked data with a total population of two million patients, said "Our findings clearly show that research using one of the NHS greatest assets—its data—is vital to innovate improvements in disease prevention, to make earlier diagnoses and to give the best treatments" (160). The inclusion of data variety increases the number of independent variables; one novel variable—or a combination of as yet uncompared

variables—could end up being significant in defining relevant precision subpopulations (161, 162).

Examples of data that has been linked to help identify more precise cohorts of populations include: longitudinal health claims data (163, 164); secondary use anonymized electronic health records (159, 165); cohort studies, health surveys, and registries (166–168); environmental variables (104); molecular data such as from the genome, exposome, microbiome, or transcriptome (169–172); "mhealth" wearable and sensor data (173); mobile phone sensing data and self-reports (174); online patient generated content (175); and the semantic web (176).

The explosion of new volumes of genomic "big data" helped make possible the precision medicine movement (177). One of precision medicine's promises was to lead to development of new treatments for subpopulations defined by their similarities at the molecular level (178, 179). Currently, translational efforts in precision medicine often work by identifying cohorts of patients who have or lack specific genomic or molecular biomarkers (132, 180). Since today's precision medicine works at the granularity of disease subtypes and population strata and not at the "n of one" level, contemporary precision medicine really is—when applied to community crises—an example of precision public health (2).

Researchers agree that only by using very large sample sizes will genomic studies have the proper statistical power (181, 182). "These large case–control studies are essential for boosting the statistical power needed to detect the genetic variants responsible for rare diseases and can provide the necessary knowledge for use in the clinical setting," (183). Big data has been a necessary component in the scale-up of genomic sample sizes, enabled by the decrease in cost of gene sequencing (183). Future versions of sovereign genomics programs in over ten countries have the potential to create data sets with millions of samples (184–186). These databases should be ideal platforms for research such as genome wide association studies, which have been used with over ten thousand cases per study in public health diseases such as Alzheimer's disease (25,000+ cases), autism (16,000 cases), high blood pressure (200,000+ cases), posttraumatic stress disorder (10,000+ cases), and smoking (50,000+ cases) (187–191).

The most sophisticated precision approaches to public health today at once include data from multiple omic disciplines, can make use of linked phenotype data, and leverage novel or recent types of computation (7, 132, 192, 193). In targeting interventions, *de novo* or improved computational methods like geospatial risk modeling, latent class modeling, social molecular pathological epidemiology, and agent-based modeling simulation all benefit from big data to better identify these "intermediate" subpopulations (49, 122, 126, 193–196).

RISKS

More work needs to be done both enumerating and evaluating the risks and challenges of using big data in precision public health.

1. Individuals could be stigmatized, even when not singularly identified, when they are stratified into small, observable cohorts, where they cannot maintain a "concealable stigmatized identity" (197).
2. Big data could enable non-consented individuals to identify patients' or citizens' identities either due to small cohorts or by "drilling through" the deeper and wider set of population data (198–200).
3. There are known drawbacks in increased reliance on a "high-risk" strategy, as originated by Rose, including ignoring population level determinants of health; taking focus away from a radical campaign that could have more sustainable positive effect for a larger population; risking missed interventions to borderline cases; or encouraging behaviors that continue to exist outside of social norms (201).

4. Big data risks targeting only relatively wealthier communities where data can be collected, or where big data expertise or distribution technologies are endemic (72, 202, 203).
5. For data collected through social media, crowdsourcing or similar channels, there may be more data about, in or from urban centers or areas of dense population, which will require additional computational governance (64).
6. Prevalence of large volumes of new types of individual health information available digitally risks that it could fall into the hands of unregulated commercial enterprises, or of insurance companies (204).
7. Experiencing governance gaps due to default use of existing governing legislation, rules or principles designed for data and technologies "that have now been superseded" by big data calls for more regulation (16, 205).
8. Applying novel big data without the appropriate controls, clinical interpretation, or statistical governance could lead to model overfitting, lack of accuracy, or results like Google Flu Trends, and could damage public faith in big data's ability to add precision to public health or trust in contributing their own data (99, 206–208).
9. Big data brings unique challenges in data quality. Cai and Zhu created a big data quality framework with no less than 14 attributes by which any big data's robustness should be assessed. Ignoring qualities like timeliness, accuracy, completeness or reliability leads to research weakness (209).
10. Performing healthcare research that includes big data is marked by, and needs, larger teams of diverse practitioners, often including informaticians, data scientists, computer scientists, physicians, researchers, and more—potentially leading to fewer studies and the challenges inherent in collaborating in large teams (59, 173).
11. Research that includes big data with high "variety" or linked data is likely to include a higher median number of data sources, which could require increased investment in cleaning and curating the data—resulting in slower scientific progress—or could compel the challenges of analyzing high dimensional data (210). For example, the high dimensionality of data found in both molecular and linked data incurs specific risk. Alyass et al. believe this data is "prone to high rates of false-positives due to chance alone…this requires researchers to adjust for multiple testing to control for type 1 error rates…or reduce dimensionality *via* sparse methods" (211).

CONCLUSION

Precision public health is exciting. Today's public health programs can achieve new levels of speed and accuracy not plausible a decade ago. Adding precision to many parts of public health engagement has led and will lead to tangible benefits. Precision can enable public health programs to maintain the same efficacy while decreasing costs, or hold costs constant while delivering better, smarter, faster, and different education, cures and interventions, saving lives.

Precision public health does not require big data. That said, the future of big data in precision public health is assured, based on its successes and acceleration of use to date. Big data and the methods created to make it useful allow precision public health practitioners to operate at the top of their license and can bring more insight to cohort membership, disease pathways and treatments. Big data enables lower costs and more precision to find, educate, track, and help each high-risk citizen. In the future, precision public health needs, imperatives, mandates and techniques will drive new capabilities into big data.

Using big data in precision public health has risks. A number of risks were identified here and future study will expand these or identify more. Protecting the dignity, privacy, security of citizens and patients, while finding truly meaningful significant outcomes in a reasonable timeframe will take effort on the part of each and every researcher in this space.

What are the calls to action? Investment has increased, but additional investment and research are needed in many areas. First, more experimentation is needed to understand how to best create and mobilize open data, open science, open source communities, and open collaboration platforms. For context, the Observational Health Data Sciences and Informatics collaborative is a thriving global open science community focused on large scale population health outcomes and prediction. If such a collaborative existed for precision public health, one imagines practitioners could leverage shared best practices, data, open software, and opportunities. Second, there are opportunity gaps in training precision public health workers in countries with a dearth of data scientists, on-premise data storage and computational assets, or access to big data. For example, communities suffering public health crises increasingly desire to "learn how to use the information and improve their ability to respond to future outbreaks in the region," rather than having their data removed for analysis by better funded nations (212). Third, follow-on research is needed in the area of big data in precision public health. Specifically, (a) best practices in performing data quality assessment along a broad range of attributes should be enumerated, (b) existing research should be scored along these attributes as well as those studies' compliance with statistical best practices specific to big data and high dimensionality, (c) each area of value delivery—disease surveillance, predicting risk, targeting intervention and understanding disease—needs their own full treatment with regard to methods, data sources, data management, and more, (d) some critical framework ought to be created and proposed to systematically measure precision

public health studies and programs, specific to and beyond big data, and (e) as precision public health becomes more mature, emerging trends should be noticed and evaluated. Fourth, more work is needed in areas of ethics, risk, and governance. The community should be watching for overreliance on big data-driven approaches that lead to decreases in radical whole-population solutions that increase baseline health norms. Fifth, the global economic opportunity of using big data prescriptively in public health has not been systematically measured, beyond specific country or disease successes. For context, organizations such as the United Nations, the World Bank, and the United States Agency for International Development have estimated economic impacts of individual epidemics. These or other institutions could convene a task force to estimate the economic benefit of applying precision to public health responses, as well as the relative contribution of big data. Sixth, precision public health centers of excellence in universities can help. Today, leaders in schools of public health are speaking and writing about precision public health; presumably academic courses, concentrations and centers will follow in stepwise progression. Seventh, new technical innovation must continue and needs investment. For example, this could include applying deep learning to precision public health use cases, or creating a novel free and open source data science software "pipeline" for geospatial event prediction.

Future precision public health will be transformative. It will include new applications, modifications, and uses of today's assets, including social media and communication platforms, unmanned aerial vehicles, mobile applications, mobile sequencing, self-screening, sensors, vaccine or drug internet-of-things inventions, and more. Tomorrow, we could be looking up, wondering if a high-resolution satellite is mapping our neighborhood to predict the path of an infectious disease, or if a drone is approaching with a targeted intervention. With future applications of precision public health and the speed of big data adoption, tomorrow's new public health students and young practitioners soon won't think of the discipline as precision public health. They will only think of it as public health.

AUTHOR CONTRIBUTIONS

The author confirms being the sole contributor of this work and approved it for publication.

REFERENCES

1. Baynam G, Bauskis A, Pachter N, Schofield L, Verhoef H, Palmer RL, et al. 3-Dimensional facial analysis—facing precision public health. *Front Public Health* (2017) 5:31. doi:10.3389/fpubh.2017.00031
2. Severi G, Southey MC, English DR, Jung CH, Lonie A, McLean C, et al. Epigenome-wide methylation in DNA from peripheral blood as a marker of risk for breast cancer. *Breast Cancer Res Treat* (2014) 148(3):665–73. doi:10.1007/s10549-014-3209-y
3. Khoury MJ, Galea S. Will precision medicine improve population health? *JAMA* (2016) 316(13):1357–8. doi:10.1001/jama.2016.12260
4. Khoury MJ, Iademarco MF, Riley WT. Precision public health for the era of precision medicine. *Am J Prev Med* (2016) 50(3):398. doi:10.1016/j.amepre.2015.08.031

5. Dowell SF, Blazes D, Desmond-Hellmann S. Four steps to precision public health. *Nat News* (2016) 540(7632):189. doi:10.1038/540189a
6. Arnett DK, Claas SA. Precision medicine, genomics, and public health. *Diabetes Care* (2016) 39(11):1870–3. doi:10.2337/dc16-1763
7. Colijn C, Jones N, Johnston IG, Yaliraki S, Barahona M. Toward precision healthcare: context and mathematical challenges. *Front Physiol* (2017) 8:136. doi:10.3389/fphys.2017.00136
8. LaValle S, Lesser E, Shockley R, Hopkins MS, Kruschwitz N. Big data, analytics and the path from insights to value. *MIT Sloan Manage Rev* (2011) 52(2):21.
9. Lohr S. The age of big data. *N Y Times* (2012) 11(2012):SR1. Available from: http://www.nytimes.com/2012/02/12/sunday-review/big-datas-impact-in-the-world.html (Accessed on February 26, 2017).
10. National Institute of Standards and Technology. *NIST Big Data Interoperability Framework: Volume 1, Definitions (NIST Special Publication 1500-1).* (2015).

Available from: http://nvlpubs.nist.gov/nistpubs/SpecialPublications/NIST. SP.1500-1.pdf

11. Cukier K, Mayer-Schoenberger V. The rise of big data: how it's changing the way we think about the world. *Foreign Aff* (2013) 92:28. doi:10.2469/dig.v43.n4.65

12. De Mauro A, Greco M, Grimaldi M. What is big data? A consensual definition and a review of key research topics. In: Giannakopoulos G, Sakas DP, Kyriaki-Manessi D, editors. *AIP Conference Proceedings*, Vol. 1644. Madrid: AIP (2015). p. 97–104. doi:10.1063/1.4907823

13. Hu H, Wen Y, Chua TS, Li X. Toward scalable systems for big data analytics: a technology tutorial. *IEEE Access* (2014) 2:652–87. doi:10.1109/ACCESS.2014.2332453

14. Andreu-Perez J, Poon CC, Merrifield RD, Wong ST, Yang GZ. Big data for health. *IEEE J Biomed Health Inform* (2015) 19(4):1193–208. doi:10.1109/JBHI.2015.2450362

15. Belle A, Thiagarajan R, Soroushmehr SM, Navidi F, Beard DA, Najarian K. Big data analytics in healthcare. *Biomed Res Int* (2015) 2015:370194. doi:10.1155/2015/370194

16. Locke AE, Kahali B, Berndt SI, Justice AE, Pers TH, Day FR, et al. Genetic studies of body mass index yield new insights for obesity biology. *Nature* (2015) 518(7538):197–206. doi:10.1038/nature14177

17. Visscher PM, Brown MA, McCarthy MI, Yang J. Five years of GWAS discovery. *Am J Hum Genet* (2012) 90(1):7–24. doi:10.1016/j.ajhg.2011.11.029

18. Altaf-Ul-Amin M, Afendi FM, Kiboi SK, Kanaya S. Systems biology in the context of big data and networks. *Biomed Res Int* (2014) 2014:11. doi:10.1155/2014/428570

19. Wilhelm M, Schlegl J, Hahne H, Gholami AM, Lieberenz M, Savitski MM, et al. Mass-spectrometry-based draft of the human proteome. *Nature* (2014) 509(7502):582–7. doi:10.1038/nature13319

20. Gillies RJ, Kinahan PE, Hricak H. Radiomics: images are more than pictures, they are data. *Radiology* (2015) 278(2):563–77. doi:10.1148/radiol.2015151169

21. Hripcsak G, Ryan PB, Duke JD, Shah NH, Park RW, Huser V, et al. Characterizing treatment pathways at scale using the OHDSI network. *Proc Natl Acad Sci U S A* (2016) 113(27):7329–36. doi:10.1073/pnas.1510502113

22. Slobogean GP, Giannoudis PV, Frihagen F, Forte ML, Morshed S, Bhandari M. Bigger data, bigger problems. *J Orthop Trauma* (2015) 29:S43–6. doi:10.1097/BOT.0000000000000463

23. Predić B, Yan Z, Eberle J, Stojanovic D, Aberer K. Exposuresense: integrating daily activities with air quality using mobile participatory sensing. *Pervasive Computing and Communications Workshops (PERCOM Workshops), 2013 IEEE International Conference*. IEEE (2013). p. 303–5.

24. Zheng Y, Liu F, Hsieh HP. U-air: When urban air quality inference meets big data. *Proceedings of the 19th ACM SIGKDD International Conference on Knowledge Discovery and Data Mining*. ACM (2013). p. 1436–44.

25. Chen M, Zhang Y, Li Y, Hassan MM, Alamri A. AIWAC: Affective interaction through wearable computing and cloud technology. *IEEE Wireless Commun* (2015) 22(1):20–7. doi:10.1109/MWC.2015.7054715

26. Jiang P, Winkley J, Zhao C, Munnoch R, Min G, Yang LT. An intelligent information forwarder for healthcare big data systems with distributed wearable sensors. *IEEE Syst J* (2016) 10(3):1147–59. doi:10.1109/JSYST.2014.2308324

27. Martínez P, Martínez JL, Segura-Bedmar I, Moreno-Schneider J, Luna A, Revert R. Turning user generated health-related content into actionable knowledge through text analytics services. *Comput Industry* (2016) 78:43–56. doi:10.1016/j.compind.2015.10.006

28. Frisby J, Smith V, Traub S, Patel VL. Contextual computing: a Bluetooth based approach for tracking healthcare providers in the emergency room. *J Biomed Inform* (2016) 65:97–104. doi:10.1016/j.jbi.2016.11.008

29. Qi B, Miao H, Yuan X, Xiao X. A patient tracking and positioning system based on improved DV-Hop algorithm. *Information and Communication Technology Convergence (ICTC), 2015 International Conference on*. IEEE (2015). p. 1297–9.

30. Gorenshteyn D, Zaslavsky E, Fribourg M, Park CY, Wong AK, Tadych A, et al. Interactive big data resource to elucidate human immune pathways and diseases. *Immunity* (2015) 43(3):605–14. doi:10.1016/j.immuni.2015.08.014

31. Celi LA, Mark RG, Stone DJ, Montgomery RA. "Big data" in the intensive care unit. Closing the data loop. *Am J Respir Crit Care Med* (2013) 187(11):1157–66. doi:10.1164/rccm.201212-2311ED

32. Bar-Or A, Healey J, Kontothanassis L, Van Thong JM. BioStream: a system architecture for real-time processing of physiological signals. *Engineering in Medicine and Biology Society, 2004. IEMBS'04. 26th Annual International Conference of the IEEE*. (Vol. 2), IEEE (2004). p. 3101–4.

33. Ahmad S, Ramsay T, Huebsch L, Flanagan S, McDiarmid S, Batkin I, et al. Continuous multi-parameter heart rate variability analysis heralds onset of sepsis in adults. *PLoS One* (2009) 4(8):e6642. doi:10.1371/journal.pone.0006642

34. Shaikh AR, Butte AJ, Schully SD, Dalton WS, Khoury MJ, Hesse BW. Collaborative biomedicine in the age of big data: the case of cancer. *J Med Internet Res* (2014) 16(4):e101. doi:10.2196/jmir.2496

35. Dilsizian SE, Siegel EL. Artificial intelligence in medicine and cardiac imaging: harnessing big data and advanced computing to provide personalized medical diagnosis and treatment. *Curr Cardiol Rep* (2014) 16(1):1–8. doi:10.1007/s11886-013-0441-8

36. Ben-Menachem E. Epilepsy in 2015: the year of collaborations for big data. *Lancet Neurol* (2016) 15(1):6. doi:10.1016/S1474-4422(15)00356-7

37. Phillips RL Jr, Bazemore AW, DeVoe JE, Weida TJ, Krist AH, Dulin MF, et al. A family medicine health technology strategy for achieving the triple aim for US health care. *Fam Med* (2015) 47(8):628.

38. Wooden B, Goossens N, Hoshida Y, Friedman SL. Using big data to discover diagnostics and therapeutics for gastrointestinal and liver diseases. *Gastroenterology* (2017) 152(1):53–67. doi:10.1053/j.gastro.2016.09.065

39. Westra BL, Clancy TR, Sensmeier J, Warren JJ, Weaver C, Delaney CW. Nursing knowledge: big data science—implications for nurse leaders. *Nurs Adm Q* (2015) 39(4):304–10. doi:10.1097/NAQ.0000000000000130

40. Clark A, Ng JQ, Morlet N, Semmens JB. Big data and ophthalmic research. *Surv Ophthalmol* (2016) 61(4):443–65. doi:10.1016/j.survophthal.2016.01.003

41. McIntyre RS, Cha DS, Jerrell JM, Swardfager W, Kim RD, Costa LG, et al. Advancing biomarker research: utilizing 'Big Data' approaches for the characterization and prevention of bipolar disorder. *Bipolar Disord* (2014) 16(5):531–47. doi:10.1111/bdi.12162

42. Passos IC, Mwangi B, Kapczinski F. Big data analytics and machine learning: 2015 and beyond. *Lancet Psychiatry* (2016) 3(1):13–5. doi:10.1016/S2215-0366(15)00549-0

43. Stein P, Falco L, Kuebler F, Annaheim S, Lemkaddem A, Delgado-Gonzalo R, et al. Digital womens health based on wearables and big data. *Fertil Steril* (2016) 106(3):e113. doi:10.1016/j.fertnstert.2016.07.339

44. Barrett MA, Humblet O, Hiatt RA, Adler NE. Big data and disease prevention: from quantified self to quantified communities. *Big data* (2013) 1(3):168–75. doi:10.1089/big.2013.0027

45. Hay SI, George DB, Moyes CL, Brownstein JS. Big data opportunities for global infectious disease surveillance. *PLoS Med* (2013) 10(4):e1001413. doi:10.1371/journal.pmed.1001413

46. Consolvo S, McDonald DW, Toscos T, Chen MY, Froehlich J, Harrison B, et al. Activity sensing in the wild: a field trial of UbiFit garden In: *Proceedings of the SIGCHI Conference on Human Factors in Computing Systems*. ACM (2008). p. 1797–806. doi:10.1145/1357054.1357335

47. Braem B, Latre S, Leroux P, Demeester P, Coenen T, Ballon P. Designing a smart city playground: real-time air quality measurements and visualization in the city of things testbed. *Smart Cities Conference (ISC2), 2016 IEEE International*. IEEE (2016). p. 1–2.

48. Lardon J, Abdellaoui R, Bellet F, Asfari H, Souvignet J, Texier N, et al. Adverse drug reaction identification and extraction in social media: a scoping review. *J Med Internet Res* (2015) 17(7):e171. doi:10.2196/jmir.4304

49. Daley D, Bachmann M, Bachmann BA, Pedigo C, Bui MT, Coffman J. Risk terrain modeling predicts child maltreatment. *Child Abuse Negl* (2016) 62:29–38. doi:10.1016/j.chiabu.2016.09.014

50. Bragazzi NL, Dini G, Toletone A, Brigo F, Durando P. Leveraging big data for exploring occupational diseases-related interest at the level of scientific community, media coverage and novel data streams: the example of silicosis as a pilot study. *PLoS One* (2016) 11(11):e0166051. doi:10.1371/journal.pone.0166051

51. Hood L, Lovejoy JC, Price ND. Integrating big data and actionable health coaching to optimize wellness. *BMC Med* (2015) 13(1):4. doi:10.1186/s12916-014-0238-7

52. Burke-Garcia A, Scally G. Trending now: future directions in digital media for the public health sector. *J Public Health* (2014) 36(4):527–34. doi:10.1093/pubmed/fdt125

53. Bansal S, Chowell G, Simonsen L, Vespignani A, Viboud C. Big data for infectious disease surveillance and modeling. *J Infect Dis* (2016) 214(Suppl 4):S375–9. doi:10.1093/infdis/jiw400

54. O'Shea J. Digital disease detection: a systematic review of event-based internet biosurveillance systems. *Int J Med Inform* (2017) 101:15–22. doi:10.1016/j.ijmedinf.2017.01.019

55. Chatterjee N, Shi J, García-Closas M. Developing and evaluating polygenic risk prediction models for stratified disease prevention. *Nat Rev Genet* (2016) 17(7):392–406. doi:10.1038/nrg.2016.27

56. Gandon S, Day T, Metcalf CJE, Grenfell BT. Forecasting epidemiological and evolutionary dynamics of infectious diseases. *Trends Ecol Evol* (2016) 31(10):776–88. doi:10.1016/j.tree.2016.07.010

57. Schneeweiss S. Improving therapeutic effectiveness and safety through big healthcare data. *Clin Pharmacol Ther* (2016) 99(3):262–5. doi:10.1002/cpt.316

58. Obermeyer Z, Emanuel EJ. Predicting the future—big data, machine learning, and clinical medicine. *N Engl J Med* (2016) 375(13):1216. doi:10.1056/NEJMp1606181

59. Gu D, Li J, Li X, Liang C. Visualizing the knowledge structure and evolution of big data research in healthcare informatics. *Int J Med Inform* (2017) 98:22–32. doi:10.1016/j.ijmedinf.2016.11.006

60. Eysenbach G. Infodemiology and infoveillance: framework for an emerging set of public health informatics methods to analyze search, communication and publication behavior on the Internet. *J Med Internet Res* (2009) 11(1):e11. doi:10.2196/jmir.1157

61. Nsoesie EO, Brownstein JS. Computational approaches to influenza surveillance: beyond timeliness. *Cell Host Microbe* (2015) 17(3):275–8. doi:10.1016/j.chom.2015.02.004

62. Salathé M. Digital pharmacovigilance and disease surveillance: combining traditional and big-data systems for better public health. *J Infect Dis* (2016) 214(Suppl_4):S399–403. doi:10.1093/infdis/jiw281

63. MacFadden DR, Fisman D, Andre J, Ara Y, Majumder MS, Bogoch II, et al. A platform for monitoring regional antimicrobial resistance, using online data sources: resistanceopen. *J Infect Dis* (2016) 214(Suppl 4):S393–8. doi:10.1093/infdis/jiw343

64. Chunara R, Andrews JR, Brownstein JS. Social and news media enable estimation of epidemiological patterns early in the 2010 Haitian cholera outbreak. *Am J Trop Med Hyg* (2012) 86(1):39–45. doi:10.4269/ajtmh.2012.11-0597

65. Chan EH, Sahai V, Conrad C, Brownstein JS. Using web search query data to monitor dengue epidemics: a new model for neglected tropical disease surveillance. *PLoS Negl Trop Dis* (2011) 5(5):e1206. doi:10.1371/journal.pntd.0001206

66. Gomide J, Veloso A, Meira W Jr, Almeida V, Benevenuto F, Ferraz F, et al. Dengue surveillance based on a computational model of spatio-temporal locality of Twitter. *Proceedings of the 3rd International Web Science Conference.* ACM (2011). 3 p.

67. Claesson A, Svensson L, Nordberg P, Ringh M, Rosenqvist M, Djarv T, et al. Drones may be used to save lives in out of hospital cardiac arrest due to drowning. *Resuscitation* (2017) 114:152–6. doi:10.1016/j.resuscitation.2017.01.003

68. Correia RB, Li L, Rocha LM. Monitoring potential drug interactions and reactions via network analysis of instagram user timelines. *Pacific Symposium on Biocomputing. Pacific Symposium on Biocomputing.* (Vol. 21), NIH Public Access (2016). 492 p.

69. Freifeld CC, Brownstein JS, Menone CM, Bao W, Filice R, Kass-Hout T, et al. Digital drug safety surveillance: monitoring pharmaceutical products in twitter. *Drug Safety* (2014) 37(5):343–50. doi:10.1007/s40264-014-0155-x

70. Joseph W, Aerts S, Vandenbossche M, Thielens A, Martens L. Drone based measurement system for radiofrequency exposure assessment. *Bioelectromagnetics* (2016) 37:195–9. doi:10.1002/bem.21964

71. Signorini A, Segre AM, Polgreen PM. The use of Twitter to track levels of disease activity and public concern in the US during the influenza A H1N1 pandemic. *PLoS One* (2011) 6(5):e19467. doi:10.1371/journal.pone.0019467

72. Pesälä S, Virtanen MJ, Sane J, Jousimaa J, Lyytikäinen O, Murtopuro S, et al. Health care professionals' evidence-based medicine internet searches closely mimic the known seasonal variation of lyme borreliosis: a register-based study. *JMIR Public Health Surveill* (2017) 3(2):e19. doi:10.2196/publichealth.6764

73. Alajajian SE, Williams JR, Reagan AJ, Alajajian SC, Frank MR, Mitchell L, et al. The lexicocalorimeter: gauging public health through caloric input and output on social media. *PLoS One* (2017) 12(2):e0168893. doi:10.1371/journal.pone.0168893

74. Ghosh S, Chakraborty P, Nsoesie EO, Cohn E, Mekaru SR, Brownstein JS, et al. Temporal topic modeling to assess associations between news trends and infectious disease outbreaks. *Sci Rep* (2017) 7:40841. doi:10.1038/srep40841

75. Wilson ME. Travel and the emergence of infectious diseases. *Emerg Infect Dis* (1995) 1(2):39. doi:10.3201/eid0102.950201

76. Stoddard ST, Morrison AC, Vazquez-Prokopec GM, Soldan VP, Kochel TJ, Kitron U, et al. The role of human movement in the transmission of vector-borne pathogens. *PLoS Negl Trop Dis* (2009) 3(7):e481. doi:10.1371/journal.pntd.0000481

77. Aarestrup FM, Koopmans MG. Sharing data for global infectious disease surveillance and outbreak detection. *Trends Microbiol* (2016) 24(4):241–5. doi:10.1016/j.tim.2016.01.009

78. Simonsen L, Gog JR, Olson D, Viboud C. Infectious disease surveillance in the big data era: towards faster and locally relevant systems. *J Infect Dis* (2016) 214(Suppl 4):S380–5. doi:10.1093/infdis/jiw376

79. Kraemer MU, Hay SI, Pigott DM, Smith DL, Wint GW, Golding N. Progress and challenges in infectious disease cartography. *Trends Parasitol* (2016) 32(1):19–29. doi:10.1016/j.pt.2015.09.006

80. Tatem AJ. Mapping population and pathogen movements. *Int Health* (2014) 6(1):5–11. doi:10.1093/inthealth/ihu006

81. Finger F, Genolet T, Mari L, de Magny GC, Manga NM, Rinaldo A, et al. Mobile phone data highlights the role of mass gatherings in the spreading of cholera outbreaks. *Proc Natl Acad Sci U S A* (2016) 113(23):6421–6. doi:10.1073/pnas.1522305113

82. Wesolowski A, Qureshi T, Boni MF, Sundsøy PR, Johansson MA, Rasheed SB, et al. Impact of human mobility on the emergence of dengue epidemics in Pakistan. *Proc Natl Acad Sci U S A* (2015) 112:11887–92. doi:10.1073/pnas.1504964112

83. Wesolowski A, Buckee CO, Bengtsson L, Wetter E, Lu X, Tatem AJ. Commentary: containing the ebola outbreak - the potential and challenge of mobile network data. *PLoS Curr* (2014) 6. doi:10.1371/currents.outbreaks.0177e7fcf52217b8b634376e2f3efc5e

84. Isdory A, Mureithi EW, Sumpter DJ. The impact of human mobility on HIV transmission in Kenya. *PLoS One* (2015) 10:e0142805. doi:10.1371/journal.pone.0142805

85. Wesolowski A, Buckee CO, Engø-Monsen K, Metcalf CJE. Connecting mobility to infectious diseases: the promise and limits of mobile phone data. *J Infect Dis* (2016) 214(Suppl 4):S414–20. doi:10.1093/infdis/jiw273

86. Mari L, Gatto M, Ciddio M, Dia ED, Sokolow SH, De Leo GA, et al. Big-data-driven modeling unveils country-wide drivers of endemic schistosomiasis. *Sci Rep* (2017) 7:489. doi:10.1038/s41598-017-00493-1

87. Huff A, Allen T, Whiting K, Breit N, Arnold B. FLIRT-ing with Zika: a web application to predict the movement of infected travelers validated against the current Zika virus epidemic. *PLoS Curr* (2016) 8. doi:10.1371/currents.outbreaks.711379ace737b7c04c89765342a9a8c9

88. Vazquez-Prokopec GM, Bisanzio D, Stoddard ST, Paz-Soldan V, Morrison AC, Elder JP, et al. Using GPS technology to quantify human mobility, dynamic contacts and infectious disease dynamics in a resource-poor urban environment. *PLoS One* (2013) 8(4):e58802. doi:10.1371/journal.pone.0058802

89. Nguyen KA, Watkins C, Luo Z. Co-location epidemic tracking on London public transports using low power mobile magnetometer. *arXiv preprint arXiv* (2017):1704.00148. doi:10.1109/IPIN.2017.8115963

90. Gubler DJ. Surveillance for dengue and dengue hemorrhagic fever. *Bull Pan Am Health Organ* (1989) 23(4):397–404.

91. Langmuir AD. William Farr: founder of modern concepts of surveillance. *Int J Epidemiol* (1976) 5(1):13–8. doi:10.1093/ije/5.1.13

92. Godman B, Finlayson AE, Cheema PK, Zebedin-Brandl E, Gutiérrez-Ibarluzea I, Jones J, et al. Personalizing health care: feasibility and future implications. *BMC Med* (2013) 11(1):179. doi:10.1186/1741-7015-11-179

93. Naish S, Dale P, Mackenzie JS, McBride J, Mengersen K, Tong S. Climate change and dengue: a critical and systematic review of quantitative modelling approaches. *BMC Infect Dis* (2014) 14(1):167. doi:10.1186/1471-2334-14-167

94. Isham V. Mathematical modelling of the transmission dynamics of HIV infection and AIDS: a review. *J Royal Stat Soc Ser A (Stat Soc)* (1988) 151(1):5–30. doi:10.2307/2982179

95. Nsoesie EO, Brownstein JS, Ramakrishnan N, Marathe MV. A systematic review of studies on forecasting the dynamics of influenza outbreaks. *Influenza Other Respi Viruses* (2014) 8(3):309–16. doi:10.1111/irv.12226

96. Zinszer K, Verma AD, Charland K, Brewer TF, Brownstein JS, Sun Z, et al. A scoping review of malaria forecasting: past work and future directions. *BMJ Open* (2012) 2(6):e001992. doi:10.1136/bmjopen-2012-001992

97. Linthicum KJ, Anyamba A, Tucker CJ, Kelley PW, Myers MF, Peters CJ. Climate and satellite indicators to forecast rift valley fever epidemics in Kenya. *Science* (1999) 285(5426):397–400. doi:10.1126/science.285.5426.397

98. Ozcaglar C, Shabbeer A, Vandenberg SL, Yener B, Bennett KP. Epidemiological models of *Mycobacterium tuberculosis* complex infections. *Math Biosci* (2012) 236(2):77–96. doi:10.1016/j.mbs.2012.02.003

99. Lazer D, Kennedy R, King G, Vespignani A. The parable of Google flu: traps in big data analysis. *Science* (2014) 343(6176):1203–5. doi:10.1126/science.1248506

100. Yang S, Santillana M, Brownstein JS, Gray J, Richardson S, Kou SC. Using electronic health records and Internet search information for accurate influenza forecasting. *BMC Infect Dis* (2017) 17(1):332. doi:10.1186/s12879-017-2424-7

101. Chen J, Chen H, Wu Z, Hu D, Pan JZ. Forecasting smog-related health hazard based on social media and physical sensor. *Inf Syst* (2017) 64:281–91. doi:10.1016/j.is.2016.03.011

102. Davis JJ, Boisvert S, Brettin T, Kenyon RW, Mao C, Olson R, et al. Antimicrobial resistance prediction in PATRIC and RAST. *Sci Rep* (2016) 6:27930. doi:10.1038/srep27930

103. Gilbert M, Golding N, Zhou H, Wint GW, Robinson TP, Tatem AJ, et al. Predicting the risk of avian influenza A H7N9 infection in live-poultry markets across Asia. *Nat Commun* (2014) 5:4116. doi:10.1038/ncomms5116

104. Sadler RC, LaChance J, Hanna-Attisha M. Social and built environmental correlates of predicted blood lead levels in the flint water crisis. *Am J Public Health* (2017) 107(5):763–9. doi:10.2105/AJPH.2017.303692

105. Phan TP, Alkema L, Tai ES, Tan KH, Yang Q, Lim WY, et al. Forecasting the burden of type 2 diabetes in Singapore using a demographic epidemiological model of Singapore. *BMJ Open Diabetes Res Care* (2014) 2(1):e000012. doi:10.1136/bmjdrc-2013-000012

106. Liu X, Speranza E, Muñoz-Fontela C, Haldenby S, Rickett NY, Garcia-Dorival I, et al. Transcriptomic signatures differentiate survival from fatal outcomes in humans infected with Ebola virus. *Genome Biol* (2017) 18(1):4. doi:10.1186/s13059-016-1137-3

107. Ireland ME, Schwartz HA, Chen Q, Ungar LH, Albarracín D. Future-oriented tweets predict lower county-level HIV prevalence in the United States. *Health Psychol* (2015) 34S:1252–60. doi:10.1037/hea0000279

108. Franke J, Gebreslasie M, Bauwens I, Deleu J, Siegert F. Earth observation in support of malaria control and epidemiology: MALAREO monitoring approaches. *Geospat Health* (2015) 10(1):335. doi:10.4081/gh.2015.335

109. White SL, Lawlor DA, Briley AL, Godfrey KM, Nelson SM, Oteng-Ntim E, et al. Early antenatal prediction of gestational diabetes in obese women: development of prediction tools for targeted intervention. *PLoS One* (2016) 11(12):e0167846. doi:10.1371/journal.pone.0167846

110. Pugach O, Cannon DS, Weiss RB, Hedeker D, Mermelstein RJ. Classification tree analysis as a method for uncovering relations between CHRNA5A3B4 and CHRNB3A6 in predicting smoking progression in adolescent smokers. *Nicotine Tob Res* (2017) 19(4):410–6. doi:10.1093/ntr/ntw197

111. Chuang TW, Wimberly MC. Remote sensing of climatic anomalies and West Nile virus incidence in the northern Great Plains of the United States. *PLoS One* (2012) 7(10):e46882. doi:10.1371/journal.pone.0046882

112. Bogoch II, Brady OJ, Kraemer MU, German M, Creatore MI, Brent S, et al. Potential for Zika virus introduction and transmission in resource-limited countries in Africa and the Asia-Pacific region: a modelling study. *Lancet Infect Dis* (2016) 16(11):1237–45. doi:10.1016/S1473-3099(16)30270-5

113. McGough SF, Brownstein JS, Hawkins JB, Santillana M. Forecasting Zika incidence in the 2016 Latin America outbreak combining traditional disease surveillance with search, social media, and news report data. *PLoS Negl Trop Dis* (2017) 11(1):e0005295. doi:10.1371/journal.pntd.0005295

114. Lalonde M. *A New Perspective on the Health of Canadians (The Lalonde Report)*. Ottawa: Minister of Supply and Services Canada (1974).

115. Hethcote HW, Yorke JA, Nold A. Gonorrhea modeling: a comparison of control methods. *Math Biosci* (1982) 58(1):93–109. doi:10.1016/0025-5564(82)90053-0

116. Richert CA, Peterman TA, Zaidi AA, Ransom RL, Wroten JE, Witte JJ. A method for identifying persons at high risk for sexually transmitted infections: opportunity for targeting intervention. *Am J Public Health* (1993) 83(4):520–4. doi:10.2105/AJPH.83.4.520

117. Gomez SL, Tan S, Keegan TH, Clarke CA. Disparities in mammographic screening for Asian women in California: a cross-sectional analysis to identify meaningful groups for targeted intervention. *BMC Cancer* (2007) 7(1):201. doi:10.1186/1471-2407-7-201

118. Bousema T, Griffin JT, Sauerwein RW, Smith DL, Churcher TS, Takken W, et al. Hitting hotspots: spatial targeting of malaria for control and elimination. *PLoS Med* (2012) 9(1):e1001165. doi:10.1371/journal.pmed.1001165

119. U.S. Department of Health and Human Services. *Multiple Chronic Conditions—A Strategic Framework: Optimum Health and Quality of Life for Individuals with Multiple Chronic Conditions*. Washington, DC: U.S. Department of Health and Human Services (2010).

120. Hose AJ, Depner M, Illi S, Lau S, Keil T, Wahn U, et al. Latent class analysis reveals clinically relevant atopy phenotypes in 2 birth cohorts. *J Allergy Clin Immunol* (2017) 139(6):1935–45. doi:10.1016/j.jaci.2016.08.046

121. Koning M, Hoekstra T, de Jong E, Visscher TL, Seidell JC, Renders CM. Identifying developmental trajectories of body mass index in childhood using latent class growth (mixture) modelling: associations with dietary, sedentary and physical activity behaviors: a longitudinal study. *BMC Public Health* (2016) 16(1):1128. doi:10.1186/s12889-016-3757-7

122. Lal A. Spatial modelling tools to integrate public health and environmental science, illustrated with infectious cryptosporidiosis. *Int J Environ Res Public Health* (2016) 13(2):186. doi:10.3390/ijerph13020186

123. Fraenkel L, Lim J, Garcia-Tsao G, Reyna V, Monto A, Bridges JF. Variation in treatment priorities for chronic hepatitis C: a latent class analysis. *Patient* (2016) 9(3):241. doi:10.1007/s40271-015-0147-7

124. Barral MF, Sousa AK, Santos AF, Abreu CM, Tanuri A, Soares MA. Identification of novel resistance-related polymorphisms in HIV-1 subtype C RT connection and RNAse H domains from patients under virological failure in Brazil. *AIDS Res Hum Retroviruses* (2017) 33(5):465–71. doi:10.1089/AID.2015.0376

125. Roth AM, Armenta RA, Wagner KD, Roesch SC, Bluthenthal RN, Cuevas-Mota J, et al. Patterns of drug use, risky behavior, and health status among persons who inject drugs living in San Diego, California: a latent class analysis. *Subst Use Misuse* (2015) 50(2):205–14. doi:10.3109/10826084.2014.962661

126. Bousema T, Okell L, Felger I, Drakeley C. Asymptomatic malaria infections: detectability, transmissibility and public health relevance. *Nat Rev Microbiol* (2014) 12(12):833–40. doi:10.1038/nrmicro3364

127. Cochran G, Hruschak V, Bacci JL, Hohmeier KC, Tarter R. Behavioral, mental, and physical health characteristics and opioid medication misuse among community pharmacy patients: a latent class analysis. *Res Soc Admin Pharm* (2016) 13(6):1055–61. doi:10.1016/j.sapharm.2016.11.005

128. Fu Q, Vaughn MG. A latent class analysis of smokeless tobacco use in the United States. *J Community Health* (2016) 41(4):850–7. doi:10.1007/s10900-016-0163-0

129. Castro LA, Fox SJ, Chen X, Liu K, Bellan SE, Dimitrov NB, et al. Assessing real-time Zika risk in the United States. *BMC Infect Dis* (2017) 17(1):284. doi:10.1186/s12879-017-2394-9

130. Poland GA, Ovsyannikova IG, Jacobson RM. Application of pharmacogenomics to vaccines. *Pharmacogenomics* (2009) 10(5):837–52. doi:10.2217/PGS.09.25

131. Pellegrino P, Falvella FS, Cheli S, Perrotta C, Clementi E, Radice S. The role of toll-like receptor 4 polymorphisms in vaccine immune response. *Pharmacogenomics J* (2016) 16(1):96–101. doi:10.1038/tpj.2015.21

132. Poland GA. The case for personalized vaccinology in the 21st century. *Presented at the National Vaccine Advisory Committee Meeting on February 7th, 2017*. (2017) Available from: https://www.hhs.gov/sites/default/files/poland_presentation.pdf

133. Poland GA, Ovsyannikova IG, Jacobson RM, Smith DI. Heterogeneity in vaccine immune response: the role of immunogenetics and the emerging field of vaccinomics. *Clin Pharmacol Ther* (2007) 82(6):653–64. doi:10.1038/sj.clpt.6100415

134. Nandy A, Basak SC. Viral epidemics and vaccine preparedness. *J Mol Pathol Epidemiol* (2017) 2:S1.

135. Arzberger P, Schroeder P, Beaulieu A, Bowker G, Casey K, Laaksonen L, et al. Promoting access to public research data for scientific, economic, and social development. *Data Sci J* (2004) 3:135–52. doi:10.2481/dsj.3.135

136. Hammond EC, Irwin J, Garfinkel L. Data-processing and analysis in epidemiological research. *Am J Public Health Nations Health* (1967) 57(11):1979–84. doi:10.2105/AJPH.57.11.1979

137. Lopez AD. The evolution of the global burden of disease framework for disease, injury and risk factor quantification: developing the evidence base for national, regional and global public health action. *Global Health* (2005) 1(1):5. doi:10.1186/1744-8603-1-5

138. Kao RR, Haydon DT, Lycett SJ, Murcia PR. Supersize me: how whole-genome sequencing and big data are transforming epidemiology. *Trends Microbiol* (2014) 22(5):282–91. doi:10.1016/j.tim.2014.02.011

139. Glymour MM, Osypuk TL, Rehkopf DH. Invited commentary: off-roading with social epidemiology—exploration, causation, translation. *Am J Epidemiol* (2013) 178(6):858–63. doi:10.1093/aje/kwt145

140. Johnson SB, Little TD, Masyn K, Mehta PD, Ghazarian SR. Multidisciplinary design and analytic approaches to advance prospective research on the multilevel determinants of child health. *Ann Epidemiol* (2017) 27(6):361–70. doi:10.1016/j.annepidem.2017.05.008

141. Geethanjali C, Bhanumathi S. Generating drug-gene association for Vibrio cholerae using ontological profile similarity. *Indian J Sci Technol* (2016) 9(33). doi:10.17485/ijst/2016/v9i33/99620

142. Rujirojindakul P, Chongsuvivatwong V, Limprasert P. Association of ABO blood group phenotype and allele frequency with chikungunya fever. *Adv Hematol* (2015) 2015:543027. doi:10.1155/2015/543027

143. Ross MC, Muzny DM, McCormick JB, Gibbs RA, Fisher-Hoch SP, Petrosino JF. 16S gut community of the Cameron County Hispanic cohort. *Microbiome* (2015) 3(1):7. doi:10.1186/s40168-015-0072-y

144. Scott RA, Scott LJ, Mägi R, Marullo L, Gaulton KJ, Kaakinen M, et al. An expanded genome-wide association study of type 2 diabetes in Europeans. *Diabetes* (2017) 66(11):2888–902. doi:10.2337/db16-1253

145. Bustamante M, Standl M, Bassat Q, Vilor-Tejedor N, Medina-Gomez C, Bonilla C, et al. A genome-wide association meta-analysis of diarrhoeal disease in young children identifies FUT2 locus and provides plausible biological pathways. *Hum Mol Genet* (2016) 25(18):4127–42. doi:10.1093/hmg/ddw264

146. Xiao J, Spicer T, Jian L, Yun GY, Shao C, Nairn J, et al. Variation in population vulnerability to heat wave in Western Australia. *Front Public Health* (2017) 5:64. doi:10.3389/fpubh.2017.00064

147. Barber MF, Elde NC. Escape from bacterial iron piracy through rapid evolution of transferrin. *Science* (2014) 346(6215):1362–6. doi:10.1126/science.1259329

148. Kringel D, Ultsch A, Zimmermann M, Jansen JP, Ilias W, Freynhagen R, et al. Emergent biomarker derived from next-generation sequencing to identify pain patients requiring uncommonly high opioid doses. *Pharmacogenomics J* (2016) 17(5):419–26. doi:10.1038/tpj.2016.28

149. Smith AH, Jensen KP, Li J, Nunez Y, Farrer LA, Hakonarson H, et al. Genome-wide association study of therapeutic opioid dosing identifies a novel locus upstream of OPRM1. *Mol Psychiatry* (2017) 22(3):346–52. doi:10.1038/mp.2016.257

150. Newnham JP, Kemp MW, White SW, Arrese CA, Hart RJ, Keelan JA. Applying precision public health to prevent preterm birth. *Front Public Health* (2017) 5:66. doi:10.3389/fpubh.2017.00066

151. Danaei G, Andrews KG, Sudfeld CR, Fink G, McCoy DC, Peet E, et al. Risk factors for childhood stunting in 137 developing countries: a comparative risk assessment analysis at global, regional, and country levels. *PLoS Med* (2016) 13(11):e1002164. doi:10.1371/journal.pmed.1002164

152. Faria NR, da Silva Azevedo RDS, Kraemer MU, Souza R, Cunha MS, Hill SC, et al. Zika virus in the Americas: early epidemiological and genetic findings. *Science* (2016) 352(6283):345–9. doi:10.1126/science.aaf5036

153. Hansen M, de Klerk N, Stewart L, Bower C, Milne E. Linked data research: a valuable tool in the ART field. *Hum Reprod* (2015) 30(12):2956–7. doi:10.1093/humrep/dev247

154. Millett ER, Quint JK, De Stavola BL, Smeeth L, Thomas SL. Improved incidence estimates from linked vs. stand-alone electronic health records. *J Clin Epidemiol* (2016) 75:66–9. doi:10.1016/j.jclinepi.2016.01.005

155. Saleheen D, Zhao W, Young R, Nelson CP, Ho WK, Ferguson JF, et al. Loss of cardio-protective effects at the ADAMTS7 locus due to gene-smoking interactions. *Circulation* (2017) 135(24):2336–53. doi:10.1161/CIRCULATIONAHA.116.022069

156. Strohbach M, Daubert J, Ravkin H, Lischka M. Big data storage. In: *New Horizons for a Data-Driven Economy*. Cham: Springer International Publishing (2016). p. 119–41. doi:10.1007/978-3-319-21569-3_7

157. Brennan PF, Bakken S. Nursing needs big data and big data needs nursing. *J Nurs Scholarsh* (2015) 47(5):477–84. doi:10.1111/jnu.12159

158. Miani C, Robin E, Horvath V, Manville C, Cave J, Chataway J. Health and healthcare: assessing the real world data policy landscape in Europe. *Rand Health Q* (2014) 4(2):15.

159. Bonner S, McGough AS, Kureshi I, Brennan J, Theodoropoulos G, Moss L, et al. Data quality assessment and anomaly detection via map/reduce and linked data: a case study in the medical domain. *Big Data (Big Data), 2015 IEEE International Conference*. IEEE (2015). p. 737–46.

160. Hemingway H, Feder GS, Fitzpatrick NK, Denaxas S, Shah AD, Timmis AD. Using nationwide 'big data' from linked electronic health records to help improve outcomes in cardiovascular diseases: 33 studies using methods from epidemiology, informatics, economics and social science in the ClinicAl disease research using LInked Bespoke studies and Electronic health Records (CALIBER) programme. *Programme Grants Appl Res* (2017) 5(4):doi:10.3310/pgfar05040

161. Collyer ML, Sekora DJ, Adams DC. A method for analysis of phenotypic change for phenotypes described by high-dimensional data. *Heredity* (2015) 115(4):357–65. doi:10.1038/hdy.2014.75

162. Mooney SJ, Westreich DJ, El-Sayed AM. Epidemiology in the era of big data. *Epidemiology* (2015) 26(3):390. doi:10.1097/EDE.0000000000000274

163. Lin KJ, Schneeweiss S. Considerations for the analysis of longitudinal electronic health records from claims data to study the effectiveness and safety of drugs. *Clin Pharmacol Ther* (2016) 100(2):147–59. doi:10.1002/cpt.359

164. Setiawan VW, Virnig BA, Porcel J, Henderson BE, Le Marchand L, Wilkens LR, et al. Linking data from the multiethnic cohort study to medicare data: linkage results and application to chronic disease research. *Am J Epidemiol* (2015) 181(11):917–9. doi:10.1093/aje/kwv055

165. Finlayson SG, LePendu P, Shah NH. Building the graph of medicine from millions of clinical narratives. *Sci Data* (2014) 1:140032. doi:10.1038/sdata.2014.32

166. Hall ES, Goyal NK, Ammerman RT, Miller MM, Jones DE, Short JA, et al. Development of a linked perinatal data resource from state administrative and community-based program data. *Matern Child Health J* (2014) 18(1):316–25. doi:10.1007/s10995-013-1236-7

167. Kent EE, Malinoff R, Rozjabek HM, Ambs A, Clauser SB, Topor MA, et al. Revisiting the surveillance epidemiology and end results cancer registry and Medicare health outcomes survey (SEER-MHOS) linked data resource for patient-reported outcomes research in older adults with cancer. *J Am Geriatr Soc* (2016) 64(1):186–92. doi:10.1111/jgs.13888

168. Sanmartin C, Decady Y, Trudeau R, Dasylva A, Tjepkema M, Finès P, et al. Linking the Canadian community health survey and the Canadian mortality database: an enhanced data source for the study of mortality. *Health Rep* (2016) 27(12):10.

169. Croes K, De Coster S, De Galan S, Morrens B, Loots I, Van de Mieroop E, et al. Health effects in the Flemish population in relation to low levels of mercury exposure: from organ to transcriptome level. *Int J Hyg Environ Health* (2014) 217(2):239–47. doi:10.1016/j.ijheh.2013.06.004

170. Findley K, Williams DR, Grice EA, Bonham VL. Health disparities and the microbiome. *Trends Microbiol* (2016) 24(11):847–50. doi:10.1016/j.tim.2016.08.001

171. Ou J, Carbonero F, Zoetendal EG, DeLany JP, Wang M, Newton K, et al. Diet, microbiota, and microbial metabolites in colon cancer risk in rural Africans and African Americans. *Am J Clin Nutr* (2013) 98(1):111–20. doi:10.3945/ajcn.112.056689

172. Rozek LS, Dolinoy DC, Sartor MA, Omenn GS. Epigenetics: relevance and implications for public health. *Annu Rev Public Health* (2014) 35:105–22. doi:10.1146/annurev-publhealth-032013-182513

173. Carreiro S, Chai PR, Carey J, Chapman B, Boyer EW. Integrating personalized technology in toxicology: sensors, smart glass, and social media applications in toxicology research. *J Med Toxicol* (2017) 13(2):166–72. doi:10.1007/s13181-017-0611-y

174. Triantafyllidis AK, Velardo C, Salvi D, Shah SA, Koutkias VG, Tarassenko L. A survey of mobile phone sensing, self-reporting, and social sharing for

pervasive healthcare. *IEEE J Biomed Health Inform* (2017) 21(1):218–27. doi:10.1109/JBHI.2015.2483902

175. Ji X, Chun SA, Cappellari P, Geller J. Linking and using social media data for enhancing public health analytics. *J Inform Sci* (2017) 43(2):221–45. doi:10.1177/0165551515625029

176. Xie L, Draizen EJ, Bourne PE. Harnessing big data for systems pharmacology. *Annu Rev Pharmacol Toxicol* (2017) 57:245–62. doi:10.1146/annurev-pharmtox-010716-104659

177. Mirnezami R, Nicholson J, Darzi A. Preparing for precision medicine. *N Eng J Med* (2012) 366(6):489–91. doi:10.1056/NEJMp1114866

178. Fradkin JE, Hanlon MC, Rodgers GP. NIH Precision Medicine Initiative: implications for diabetes research. *Diabetes Care* (2016) 39(7):1080–4. doi:10.2337/dc16-0541

179. Gligorijević V, Malod-Dognin N, Pržulj N. Integrative methods for analyzing big data in precision medicine. *Proteomics* (2016) 16(5):741–58. doi:10.1002/pmic.201500396

180. Vargas AJ, Harris CC. Biomarker development in the precision medicine era: lung cancer as a case study. *Nat Rev Cancer* (2016) 16(8):525–37. doi:10.1038/nrc.2016.56

181. Burton PR, Hansell AL, Fortier I, Manolio TA, Khoury MJ, Little J, et al. Size matters: just how big is BIG? Quantifying realistic sample size requirements for human genome epidemiology. *Int J Epidemiol* (2009) 38(1):263–73. doi:10.1093/ije/dyn147

182. Ma'n HZ, Junker A, Knoppers BM, Rahimzadeh V. Streamlining review of research involving humans: Canadian models. *J Med Genet* (2015) 52(8):566–9. doi:10.1136/jmedgenet-2014-102640

183. Peterson TA, Doughty E, Kann MG. Towards precision medicine: advances in computational approaches for the analysis of human variants. *J Mol Biol* (2013) 425(21):4047–63. doi:10.1016/j.jmb.2013.08.008

184. Althani A. Qatar biobank and Qatar genome programs road map. *J Tissue Sci Eng* (2015) 6:157. doi:10.4172/2157-7552.1000157

185. Nimmesgern E, Benediktsson I, Norstedt I. Personalized medicine in Europe. *Clin Transl Sci* (2017) 10(2):61–3. doi:10.1111/cts.12446

186. Stephens ZD, Lee SY, Faghri F, Campbell RH, Zhai C, Efron MJ, et al. Big data: astronomical or genomical? *PLoS Biol* (2015) 13(7):e1002195. doi:10.1371/journal.pbio.1002195

187. Escott-Price V, Bellenguez C, Wang L-S, Choi S-H, Harold D, Jones L, et al. Gene-wide analysis detects two new susceptibility genes for Alzheimer's disease. *PLoS One* (2014) 9(6):e94661. doi:10.1371/journal.pone.0094661

188. Ehret GB, Ferreira T, Chasman DI, Jackson AU, Schmidt EM, Johnson T, et al. The genetics of blood pressure regulation and its target organs from association studies in 342,415 individuals. *Nat Genet* (2016) 48(10):1171–84. doi:10.1038/ng.3667

189. Justice AE, Winkler TW, Feitosa MF, Graff M, Fisher VA, Young K, et al. Genome-wide meta-analysis of 241,258 adults accounting for smoking behaviour identifies novel loci for obesity traits. *Nat Commun* (2017) 8:14977. doi:10.1038/ncomms14977

190. The Autism Spectrum Working Group of the Psychiatric Genomics Consortium. Meta-analysis of GWAS of over 16,000 individuals with autism spectrum disorder highlights a novel locus at 10q24. 32 and a significant overlap with schizophrenia. *Mol Autism* (2017) 8:21. doi:10.1186/s13229-017-0137-9

191. Chen CY, Stein M, Ursano R, Cai T, Gelernter J, Heeringa S, et al. Genome-wide association study of posttraumatic stress disorder symptom domains in two cohorts of United States army soldiers. *Biol Psychiatry* (2017) 81(10):S91–2. doi:10.1016/j.biopsych.2017.02.236

192. Hamada T, Keum N, Nishihara R, Ogino S. Molecular pathological epidemiology: new developing frontiers of big data science to study etiologies and pathogenesis. *J Gastroenterol* (2016) 52(3):265–75. doi:10.1007/s00535-016-1272-3

193. Nishi A, Milner DA Jr, Giovannucci EL, Nishihara R, Tan AS, Kawachi I, et al. Integration of molecular pathology, epidemiology and social science for global precision medicine. *Expert Rev Mol Diagn* (2016) 16(1):11–23. doi:10.1586/14737159.2016.1115346

194. Jung T, Wickrama KAS. An introduction to latent class growth analysis and growth mixture modeling. *Soc Personality Psychol Compass* (2008) 2(1):302–17. doi:10.1111/j.1751-9004.2007.00054.x

195. Speybroeck N, Van Malderen C, Harper S, Müller B, Devleesschauwer B. Simulation models for socioeconomic inequalities in health: a systematic review. *Int J Environ Res Public Health* (2013) 10(11):5750–80. doi:10.3390/ijerph10115750

196. Zhang X, Pérez-Stable EJ, Bourne PE, Peprah E, Duru OK, Breen N, et al. Big data science: opportunities and challenges to address minority health and health disparities in the 21st Century. *Ethn Dis* (2017) 27(2):95–106. doi:10.18865/ed.27.2.95

197. Quinn DM, Chaudoir SR. Living with a concealable stigmatized identity: the impact of anticipated stigma, centrality, salience, and cultural stigma on psychological distress and health. *J Pers Soc Psychol* (2009) 97(4):634. doi:10.1037/a0015815

198. Narayanan A, Shmatikov V. Myths and fallacies of personally identifiable information. *Commun ACM* (2010) 53(6):24–6. doi:10.1145/1743546.1743558

199. Ohm P. Broken promises of privacy: responding to the surprising failure of anonymization. *Ucla L Rev* (2009) 57:1701.

200. Sweeney L. Weaving technology and policy together to maintain confidentiality. *The J Law Med Ethics* (1997) 25(2-3):98–110. doi:10.1111/j.1748-720X.1997.tb01885.x

201. Rose G. Sick individuals and sick populations. *Int J Epidemiol* (2001) 30(3):427–32. doi:10.1093/ije/30.3.427

202. Andrejevic M. Big Data, big questions| the big data divide. *Int J Commun* (2014) 8:1673–89.

203. Lupton D. Health promotion in the digital era: a critical commentary. *Health Promot Int* (2015) 30(1):174–83. doi:10.1093/heapro/dau091

204. Kostkova P, Brewer H, de Lusignan S, Fottrell E, Goldacre B, Hart G, et al. Who owns the data? Open data for healthcare. *Front Public Health* (2016) 4:7. doi:10.3389/fpubh.2016.00007

205. Vayena E, Salathé M, Madoff LC, Brownstein JS. Ethical challenges of big data in public health. *PLoS Comput Biol* (2015) 11(2):e1003904. doi:10.1371/journal.pcbi.1003904

206. Belgrave D, Henderson J, Simpson A, Buchan I, Bishop C, Custovic A. Disaggregating asthma: big investigation versus big data. *J Allergy ClinImmunol* (2017) 139(2):400–7. doi:10.1016/j.jaci.2016.11.003

207. Mascalzoni D, Dove ES, Rubinstein Y, Dawkins HJ, Kole A, McCormack P, et al. International charter of principles for sharing bio-specimens and data. *Eur J Hum Genet* (2015) 23(6):721. doi:10.1038/ejhg.2014.197

208. Santillana M, Nguyen AT, Louie T, Zink A, Gray J, Sung I, et al. Cloud-based electronic health records for real-time, region-specific influenza surveillance. *Sci Rep* (2016) 6:25732. doi:10.1038/srep25732

209. Cai L, Zhu Y. The challenges of data quality and data quality assessment in the big data era. *Data Sci J* (2015) 14:2. doi:10.5334/dsj-2015-002

210. Johnstone IM, Titterington DM. Statistical challenges of high-dimensional data. *Philos Trans A Math Phys Eng Sci* (2009) 367:4237–53. doi:10.1098/rsta.2009.0159

211. Alyass A, Turcotte M, Meyre D. From big data analysis to personalized medicine for all: challenges and opportunities. *BMC Med Genomics* (2015) 8(1):33. doi:10.1186/s12920-015-0108-y

212. Maxmen A. Massive Ebola data site planned to combat outbreaks. *Nat News* (2017) 549(7670):15. doi:10.1038/nature.2017.22545

22

Cost-Effectiveness Analysis of Influenza A (H1N1) Chemoprophylaxis in Brazil

Luisa von Zuben Vecoso[1]*, Marcus Tolentino Silva[2], Mariangela Ribeiro Resende[1], Everton Nunes da Silva[3] and Tais Freire Galvao[1]*

[1] University of Campinas, Campinas, Brazil, [2] Universidade de Sorocaba, Sorocaba, Brazil, [3] University of Brasilia, Brasilia, Brazil

*Correspondence:
Tais Freire Galvao
taisgalvao@gmail.com
Luisa von Zuben Vecoso
luisavecoso@gmail.com

Background: Oseltamivir and zanamivir are recommended for treating and preventing influenza A (H1N1) worldwide. In Brazil, this official recommendation lacks an economic evaluation. Our objective was to assess the efficiency of influenza A chemoprophylaxis in the Brazilian context.

Methods: We assessed the cost-effectiveness of oseltamivir and zanamivir for prophylaxis of influenza for high risk population, compared to no prophylaxis, in the perspective of Brazilian public health system. Quality-adjusted life years (QALY) and effectiveness data were based on literature review and costs in Brazilian real (BRL) were estimated from official sources and micro-costing of 2016's H1N1 admissions at a university hospital. We used a decision-tree model considering prophylaxis and no prophylaxis and the probabilities of H1N1, ambulatory care, admission to hospital, intensive care, patient discharge, and death. Adherence and adverse events from prophylaxis were included. Incremental cost-effectiveness ratio was converted to 2016 United States dollar (USD). Uncertainty was assessed with univariated and probabilistic sensitivity analysis.

Results: Adherence to prophylaxis was 0.70 [95% confidence interval (CI) 0.54; 0.83]; adverse events, 0.09 (95% CI 0.02; 0.18); relative risk of H1N1 infection in chemoprophylaxis, 0.43 (95% CI 0.33; 0.57); incidence of H1N1, 0.14 (95% CI 0.11; 0.16); ambulatory care, 0.67 (95% CI 0.58; 0.75); hospital admission, 0.43 (CI 95% 0.39; 0.42); hospital mortality, 0.14 (CI 95% 0.12; 0.15); intensive care unit admission, 0.23 (95% CI 0.20; 0.27); and intensive care mortality, 0.40 (95% CI 0.29; 0.52). QALY in H1N1 state was 0.50 (95% CI 0.46; 0.53); in H1N1 inpatients, 0.23 (95% CI 0.18; 0.28); healthy, 0.885 (95% CI 0.879; 0.891); death, 0. Adverse events estimated to affect QALY in −0.185 (95% CI −0.290; −0.050). Cost for chemoprophylaxis was BRL 39.42 [standard deviation (SD) 17.94]; ambulatory care, BRL 12.47 (SD 5.21); hospital admission, BRL 5,727.59 (SD 7,758.28); intensive care admission, BRL 19,217.25 (SD 7,917.33); and adverse events, BRL 292.05 (SD 724.95). Incremental cost-effectiveness ratio was BRL −4,080.63 (USD −1,263.74)/QALY and −982.39 (USD −304.24)/H1N1 prevented. Results were robust to sensitivity analysis.

Conclusion: Chemoprophylaxis of influenza A (H1N1) is cost-saving in Brazilian health system context.

Keywords: cost-effectiveness, cost-utility, neuraminidase inhibitor, prophylaxis, influenza, Brazil, Unified Health System

INTRODUCTION

Influenza A (H1N1) prophylaxis with neuraminidase inhibitors is recommended by the World Health Organization (WHO), and health agencies of most developed and underdeveloped countries (World Health Organization, 2010; World Health Organization, 2019). Population at risk for influenza A complications includes pregnant and postpartum women, the elderly, children, indigenous people, immunosuppressed persons, health professionals, and long-term residents among others (Uyeki et al., 2018; Martinez et al., 2019). Influenza A accounted for 97% of the specimen circulating in the firsts months of 2019, of which 60% were influenza A (H1N1) 2009 pandemic (World Health Organization, 2019). Deaths associated with respiratory diseases from seasonal influenza accounts 300,000 to 650,000 annually (Iuliano et al., 2018). Higher burden of death is observed in less developed regions and in the elderly (Iuliano et al., 2018).

Complete efficacy data of neuraminidase inhibitors were published in 2014 and updated in 2016 (Jefferson et al., 2014a; Jefferson et al., 2014c; Heneghan et al., 2016). Before this effort, 60% of the patient data from phase III clinical trials have never been published; previous evidence could have been biased in favor of chemoprophylaxis (Jefferson et al., 2014b). Biases and conflicts of interests involved in research on influenza treatment and prevention translate into a need for studies on the drugs' clinical performance vis-à-vis health systems' financial investments (Jefferson et al., 2014b). Economic evaluations that take into consideration complete efficacy evidence are not available.

The efficiency of Influenza A (H1N1) chemoprophylaxis is also absent in in the Brazilian context, in which it is recommended and funded by the Ministry of Health (Brasil. Ministério da Saúde, 2017). Our objective was to assess the cost-effectiveness of influenza A (H1N1) chemoprophylaxis in the Brazilian public health system.

METHODS

Target Population and Subgroups

Our target population were non-vaccinated or vaccinated for less than 15 days, people groups with high risk for influenza complications (the elderly, children, indigenous people, obese individuals, people with chronic diseases or immunodeficiency, pregnant or puerperal women), health care and laboratory workers exposed to samples or cases of influenza, and residents of nursing homes or inpatients during an outbreak (Brasil. Ministério da Saúde. Secretaria de Vigilância em Saúde, 2017).

Setting and Location

The Unified Health System (*Sistema Único de Saúde*, SUS) is a public and universal health system (Paim et al., 2011). SUS is the public health sector responsible for primary care, access to medicines, immunization programs, complex services (cancer treatment and HIV/AIDS care), sanitary regulation, and sentinel surveillance, which monitors influenza by means of mandatory reports on flu syndrome and severe acute respiratory syndrome (World Health Organization, 2010). Access to these services has been largely improving since the system's birth in 1988 (Paim et al., 2011). Despite this gradual improvement over the decades, SUS is systematically underfunded (Paim et al., 2011).

Study Perspective

We adopted the SUS perspective and considered costs in the SUS context and excluded societal costs such as absence from work and patient personal costs. This involved costs for drug acquisition, health care services expenditure in cases of symptomatic diseases (ambulatory treatment, medical consultation, hospital admission, and procedures), and treatment of prophylaxis-related adverse events.

Comparators

We assessed influenza A (H1N1) chemoprophylaxis in the aforementioned high-risk population, comparing oseltamivir and zanamivir prophylaxis with no prophylaxis.

Oseltamivir is an oral antiviral drug that inhibits the neuraminidase surface enzyme [Anatomical Therapeutic Chemical (ATC) code: J05AH02]. Its market availability was scientifically supported by experimentally infecting healthy subjects with influenza A and B (EPAR summary for the public, 2015). The drug effectively prevented influenza A infection after individuals were exposed to it (Jefferson et al., 2006), and was also able to reduce cases of symptomatic influenza within households (Dobson et al., 2015), as well as the time for alleviation of symptoms in infected adults. Oseltamivir significantly increased the incidence of nausea, vomit, and psychiatric events (Jefferson et al., 2006). Adults and children with more than 40 kg should take a 75 mg dose orally every 12 h, for 10 days. For children below this weight, the dosage is adjusted to 3–3.5 mg/kg for infants; 30 mg for children up to 15 kg; 45 mg, for over 15 to 23 kg; and 60 mg, until 40 kg (Brasil. Ministério da Saúde. Secretaria de Vigilância em Saúde, 2017).

Zanamivir is an antiviral selective neuraminidase inhibitor (ATC code: J05AH01) administered intranasally (Relenza, 2015). *In vitro* assays showed that low concentrations of the drug were able to inhibit influenza A and B neuraminidase.

Symptom duration was reduced in healthy adults (median reduction 1.5 days; 1.0–2.5 days), but the mean time for symptom alleviation in elderly (>65 years) and in 5 or 6 year-old children was not significantly reduced. It has no documented benefits against non-febrile disease (body temperature < 37.8°C) (Relenza, 2015). Zanamivir is employed only in cases where oral oseltamivir is not feasible. Adults and children older than 5 years should receive two 5 mg inhalations per day for 10 days (Brasil. Ministério da Saúde. Secretaria de Vigilância em Saúde, 2017).

Time Horizon and Discount Rate
We evaluated the outcomes of influenza A (H1N1) prophylaxis based on the duration of influenza infection, which is less than 21 days. No discount rate was applied.

Choice of Health Outcomes
Quality-adjusted life years (QALY) was the primary outcome. Willingness-to-pay (WTP) threshold was considered to be 30,000 Brazilian real (BRL) per QALY (Soarez and Novaes, 2017). Prevented influenza A (H1N1) was also assessed, as a secondary outcome.

Measurement of Effectiveness
Search Strategy
Data on oseltamivir's and zanamivir's effectiveness in preventing symptomatic flu and its complications was gathered from search on the literature held on March, 2017. The following search strategy was employed in the MEDLINE (via PubMed) database: (oseltamivir OR tamiflu OR zanamivir OR relenza OR "neuraminidase inhibitors") AND (H1N1 OR influenza) AND ("clinical trial"[Filter] OR "systematic"[Filter] OR cost OR economic). The same strategy was adjusted to Embase, Scopus, and Cochrane Library databases. Additional searches were performed to ascertain effectiveness and cost data in the Brazilian scenario. Results were imported to Covidence (www.covidence.org) for identifying duplications; pair selection was performed by two independent researchers. Systematic reviews, randomized clinical trials, and observational studies were included.

Complementary non-systematic searches were performed in order to gather specific data on prevalence, hospitalization, death in hospital, and other variables included in the model. Information was also collected from SUS electronic systems whenever needed. When estimates from different studies were available, random-effect meta-analysis was performed using *Stata* (version 14.2).

Quality Assessment of Included Studies
We assessed the quality of all the included studies using standard instruments: A MeaSurement Tool to Assess systematic Reviews (AMSTAR 2) for systematic reviews (Shea et al., 2017), Newcastle–Ottawa scale for cohort and case–control studies (Wells et al., 2000), and the Joanna Briggs Institute checklist for prevalence studies (Munn et al., 2015).

Estimating Resources and Costs
Costs of oseltamivir and zanamivir acquisition were obtained from 2016 purchase data, provided by the Brazilian Ministry of Health, using information made available by the Pharmaceutical Assistance Department. Health care assistance costs were obtained from the SUS reimbursement system (http://sigtap.datasus.gov.br/tabela-unificada/app/sec/inicio.jsp). We considered the dosage and administration according to Brazilian guidelines (Brasil. Ministério da Saúde. Secretaria de Vigilância em Saúde, 2017).

Health expenditures were obtained from micro-costing of all inpatients admitted in 2016 for H1N1 treatment at the Clinics' Hospital of the University of Campinas, Campinas, São Paulo — a 400-beds high complexity hospital.

Currency, Price Date, and Conversion
Costs were calculated in BRL acquisitive value in 2016. Costs gathered from the literature from previous years were corrected to 2016 using the Brazilian consumer's price index (*Índice de Preços ao Consumidor*, IPCA) (https://ww2.ibge.gov.br/home/estatistica/indicadores/precos/inpc_ipca/defaultinpc.shtm). The obtained incremental cost-effectiveness ratio (ICER) was converted to United States dollars (USD) using the exchange rate for July 1st, 2016 provided by Brazil's Central Bank (1 USD = 3.229 BRL) (https://www4.bcb.gov.br/pec/taxas/ingl/ptaxnpesq.asp?id = quotations).

Choice of Model
TreeAge Pro 2018 (R.2.0) software was used to build a decision-tree model. Two scenarios were considered: chemoprophylaxis and no chemoprophylaxis. In both scenarios, the following probabilities were assessed: H1N1 infection, ambulatory care, hospital admission, intensive care admission, patient discharge, and death. In the prophylaxis scenario, we included adherence to prophylaxis and incidence of adverse events (**Figure 1**).

Costs for outcomes were calculated considering that all flu cases were influenza A (H1N1) type; half-cycle correction was used to calculate costs for cases with death as the final outcome. Clinical plausibility was evaluated by an infectious disease specialist doctor, who was part of the research team (MRR) and had experience in influenza management.

Assumptions
We considered that all symptomatic patients would seek outpatient care. Hospital admission was assumed as a probability for those seeking ambulatory care, and admission to the intensive care unit as a probability for people admitted to the hospital. Death was assumed as possible only for people admitted to the hospital or to the intensive care. Subjects who did not develop flu were considered healthy. No sequelae or late effects of influenza were considered.

Analytical Methods
Uncertainties of the model were estimated according to variations in the adopted parameters. A tornado diagram of minimum and maximum values was used for univariate sensitivity analysis.

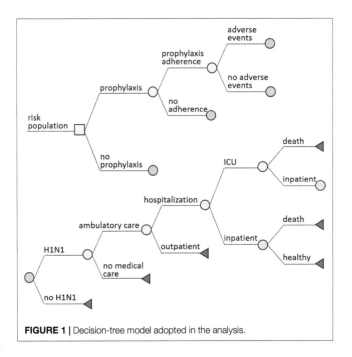

FIGURE 1 | Decision-tree model adopted in the analysis.

Sensitivity-enhancing model parameters were chosen for best- and worst-case scenario analyses.

Probabilistic sensitivity analysis was performed using Monte Carlo, employing a 10,000 simulation count and threshold analysis to identify the maximum cost of the technology, all other parameters unchanged (*ceteris paribus*). We used variables as distribution; beta distribution was adopted for probabilities and outcomes, gamma for costs, and log-normal for relative risk (Bilcke et al., 2011).

Ethics Approval Statement

The study was approved by the University of Campinas Ethics Committee, report number 2,357,158 issued on October, 30th 2017. The study was exempt from consent procedure, once patient data would be from medical records.

RESULTS

Study Parameters
Effectiveness Data
Probabilities of efficacy adopted are described in **Table 1**.

TABLE 1 | Probabilities of outcomes, distribution parameters adopted in the analytical model, and sources.

Variable	Effect (95%CI)	Distribution parameters[a]	Source	Quality of evidence
Prophylaxis adherence	0.70 (0.54; 0.83)	$\alpha = 26$ $\beta = 11$	Proportion of health professionals that completed post-exposure prophylaxis during 2009 pandemic in a hospital in Melbourne, Australia (Upjohn et al., 2012)	5/9 [b]
Adverse events incidence	0.09 (0.02; 0.18)	Mean = 0.09 SD = 0.06	Sum of risk differences for significant adverse events (headache, nausea, and psychiatric events) (Jefferson et al., 2014a)	High-quality review [c]
Prevention of H1N1 with chemoprophylaxis	0.43 (0.33; 0.57)[d]	$\mu = -0.84$ $\sigma = 0.14$[e]	Meta-analysis of 7 clinical trials for the prophylaxis with oseltamivir or zanamivir in the general population (Jefferson et al., 2014a)	High-quality review [c]
H1N1 in risk population	0.14 (0.11; 0.16)	Mean = 0.14 SD = 0.02	Meta-analysis of 20 incidence studies on febrile acute respiratory syndrome in households (Lau et al., 2012)	Critically-low quality review [c]
Ambulatory care	0.67 (0.58; 0.75)	Mean = 0.67 SD = 0.04	Meta-analysis comprising 38 studies on the incidence of symptoms after experimental infection with influenza (Carrat et al., 2008)	Critically-low quality review [c]
Hospital admission	0.43 (0.39; 0.42)	$\alpha = 1,911$ $\beta = 2,809$	Proportion of hospital admission among confirmed H1N1 cases in 2010, Parana, Brazil (Lenzi et al., 2012)	8/10 [f]
Death in hospital	0.14 (0.12; 0.15)	$\alpha = 258$ $\beta = 1,653$	Mortality in hospital among confirmed H1N1 cases in 2010, Parana, Brazil (Lenzi et al., 2012)	8/10 [f]
Intensive care unit admission	0.23 (0.20; 0.27)	$\alpha = 148$ $\beta = 484$	Proportion of intensive care admission among inpatients of the Clinics' Hospital of the University of Sao Paulo during 2009 pandemic (Calmona, 2013)	8/9 [b]
Death in intensive care unit	0.40 (0.29; 0.52)	$\alpha = 25$ $\beta = 38$	Mortality among H1N1 patients in 11 intensive care units during 2009 pandemic, Parana, Brazil (Duarte et al., 2009)	8/10 [f]

[a]beta distribution. [b]Joanna Briggs Institute checklist. [c]AMSTAR 2. [d]relative risk. [e]log-normal distribuiton. [f]Newcastle-Ottawa scale. CI, confidence interval; SD, standard deviation.

Prophylaxis adherence was considered to be 70%, according to adherence data from health professionals exposed to H1N1 virus during the 2009 pandemic (Upjohn et al., 2012). The incidence of adverse events among those who adhered to the prophylaxis was estimated as 9%, based on the incidence of headaches, nausea and psychiatric events—the most frequent and significant adverse events (**Appendix A**).

Risk of H1N1 infection in the high-risk population was considered to be 14%, based on the incidence of symptomatic infection among households which had contact with infected patients (Lau et al., 2012). The relative risk of H1N1 infection with prophylaxis was considered to be 0.43 [95% confidence interval (CI) 0.33; 0.57], according to meta-analysis for the prophylaxis with the antivirals (Jefferson et al., 2014a) (**Data Sheet S1**). Since scientific evidence showed no efficacy for preventing complications (a proxy for seeking for medical care), hospital or intensive care admission and death from influenza (Jefferson et al., 2014a; Jefferson et al., 2014c; Heneghan et al., 2016), these variables had the same probability in both prophylaxis and no prophylaxis branches: the probability of seeking medical care (ambulatory care) was 0.67, the incidence of symptomatic illness after experimental influenza infection (Carrat et al., 2008), assuming that all people who developed symptoms would seek medical care.

Incidence of hospital (43%), and intensive care (23%) admission, hospital (23%), and intensive care mortality (40%) were based on Brazilian studies held during the 2009–2010 pandemics (Duarte et al., 2009; Lenzi et al., 2012; Calmona, 2013). Complete quality assessment of studies that provided data to the model are available at **Data Sheet S2**.

Utility

QALY for H1N1 infections managed in outpatient services was 0.50 and those admitted to hospital or intensive care was 0.23 based on a study with patients infected with H1N1 during the 2009 pandemic (Hollmann et al., 2013). Adverse events reduced QALY in 0.195 (**Appendix A**). The QALY for the healthy state was 0.885, the mean QALY measured in two population-based Brazilian studies (Zimmermann et al., 2016; Silva et al., 2017). QALY for death was 0 (**Table 2**).

Costs

Cost with prophylaxis was BRL 39.42, based on average expenditure of Brazilian Ministry of Health with the antivirals (**Appendix B**). Treatment of prophylaxis' adverse cost BRL 292.05, calculated from the cost of each main adverse event (headache, nausea, and psychiatric event) weighted to each adverse event incidence (**Appendix A**).

Outpatient care cost BRL 12.47 according to SUS reimbursement for an urgent care consultation. Cost of hospital admission was estimated in BRL 5,727.59 and for intensive care, BRL 19,217.25 (**Table 3**).

Incremental Costs and Outcomes

The prophylaxis scenario was undominated, while no prophylaxis was absolutely dominated (**Table 4**). The incremental cost of prophylaxis was BRL −54.45, and QALY increased 0.013, resulting in an ICER of BRL −4,080.63 per QALY (USD −1,263.74/QALY). For the secondary outcome prevention of H1N1 infection, incremental QALY was 0.055, and ICER was BRL −982.39 per prevented case (USD −304,24/prevented H1N1).

Characterizing Uncertainty
Univariate Sensitivity Analysis

The tornado-diagram sensitivity analysis demonstrated the robustness of our model when using expected intervals for each variable (**Figure 2**). None of the variables changed the cost-effectiveness profile of the technology given the adopted WTP threshold (BRL 30,000.00/QALY). The ICER remained robust after best- and worst-case scenario analysis with highest impact variables in the tornado (**Table 5**). Threshold analysis led to BRL 134.00 limit for chemoprophylaxis cost-effectiveness.

PROBABILISTIC SENSITIVITY ANALYSIS

In the probabilistic sensitivity analysis, 68% of ICER would be in fourth quadrant (higher effectiveness and lower cost) and 18% of ICER, in first quadrant (higher cost and effectiveness). The probability of the technology being under the WTP threshold (BRL 30.000/QALY) was 97.9% (**Table 6**, **Figure 3**).

TABLE 2 | Utilities considered in the model.

Health state	QALY (95%CI)	Mean (SD)[a]	Source	Quality of evidence
H1N1 outpatient	0.50 (0.46; 0.53)	0.50 (0.02)	QALY for outpatients infected with H1N1 during the 2009 pandemic, Spain (Hollmann et al., 2013)	7/10 [b]
H1N1 inpatient	0.23 (0.18; 0.28)	0.23 (0.03)	QALY for inpatients infected with H1N1 during the 2009 pandemic, Spain (Hollmann et al., 2013)	7/10 [b]
Adverse events	−0.195 (−0.290; −0.050)[c]	−0.195 (0.121)	Reducion in QALY (Lindner et al., 2009; Araujo et al., 2014) weighted to the incidence of each adverse event (Jefferson et al., 2014a) (Appendix A)	Low quality[d]
Healthy	0.885 (0.879; 0.891)	0.885 (0.003)	Weighted mean QALYy assessed by Brazilian population-based studies (Zimmermann et al., 2016; Silva et al., 2017)	8/9 [e]
Death	0	0	-	

[a]beta distribution. [b]Newcastle-Ottawa scale. [c]reduction on QALY due to adverse events. [d]data from previous economic evaluation which used multiple sources. [e]Joanna Briggs Institute checklist (both studies had this score). QALY, quality-adjusted life years; SD, standard deviation.

TABLE 3 | Costs included in the model, in Brazilian real.

Cost item	Mean (SD)[a]	Source
Chemoprophylaxis	39.42 (17.94)	Brazilian Ministry of Health's costs with oseltamivir and zanamivir acquisition, 2016 (Appendix B)
Ambulatory care	12.47 (5.21)	Procedure code 03.01.06.002-9 — urgent care with 24-hour observation, with specialized care (SIGTAP database)[b]
Hospitalization	5,727.59 (7,758.28)	Micro-costing of inpatients with H1N1 in 2016 at Clinics' Hospital of the University of Campinas
Intensive care unit	19,217.25 (7,917.33)	Micro-costing of intensive care unit in patients with H1N1 in 2016 at the Clinics' Hospital of the University of Campinas
Adverse events	292.05 (724.95)	Cost of each event in proportion to incidence (Appendix A)

[a]gamma distribution. [b]available from: http://sigtap.datasus.gov.br/tabela-unificada/app/sec/inicio.jsp; SD, standard deviation.

TABLE 4 | Costs, effectiveness and incremental cost-effectiveness ratio (ICER) of prophylaxis compared to no prophylaxis.

Scenario	Cost (BRL)	QALY	Prevented H1N1
Prophylaxis	230.83	0.832	0.915
No prophylaxis	285.29	0.819	0.860
Incremental	−54.45	0.013	0.055
ICER (BRL)		−4,080.63	−982,39
ICER (USD)		−1,263.74	−304.24

QALY, quality-adjusted life years; BRL, Brazilian real (1 USD = 3.229 BRL); USD, United States dollar.

DISCUSSION

H1N1 prophylaxis compared to no prophylaxis was cost-saving in the context of the Brazilian health system for both QALY and prevention of H1N1 outcomes. The mean cost calculated from micro-costing are aligned to previous Brazilian studies that

TABLE 5 | Incremental cost-effectiveness ratio for best- and worst-case scenarios (variables with the highest impact in the univariate sensitivity analysis).

Variable	Best-case scenario	Worst-case scenario
Incidence of adverse event	−24,783.28	−2,956.06
Cost of adverse events	−5,435.36	1,307.65
Utility reduction in case of adverse events	−7,650.05	−2,383.32
Cost of prophylaxis	−5,399.30	−2,249.13

estimated the cost of hospital admission to influenza A (H1N1) (Silva et al., 2012).

The chemoprophylaxis reduces the cost and the increases the effectiveness of influenza A (H1N1) prevention. Its effect on QALY (0.013), however, may be clinically irrelevant. In any case, preventing a single influenza A (H1N1) case by means of prophylaxis could save nearly BRL 1,000. At the same time, Brazil has no official WTP threshold (Soarez and Novaes, 2017). Whether present represents a cost-effective alternative is subject for debate. Effects of neuraminidase inhibitors on prophylaxis came from clinical trials in which exposure to H1N1 and treatment onsets were highly controlled. The effectiveness for chemoprophylaxis is limited to strict conditions according to a mathematical modelling and computer simulations, and stockpiling for this situation is questioned (Parra-Rojas et al., 2018). Despite a protocol to start the drug in the first 24 hours post-exposure, pragmatic clinical trial revealed late initiation of oseltamivir at the hospital setting without reduction of clinical failures among the assessed groups (Ramirez et al., 2018). This potentially unrealistic efficacy data may have inflated the effects of prophylaxis.

We obtained influenza prevention efficacy data from systematic reviews carried out as the offspring of a Cochrane Collaboration and The BMJ campaign to obtain complete clinical trials data from Roche, the drug manufacturer. The campaign's efforts led to the publication of the systematic review in 2014; it was then updated in 2016, with no changes in the results (Jefferson et al., 2014a; Jefferson et al., 2014c; Heneghan et al., 2016). Sixty percent of patient data in phase III clinical trials had never been published, suggesting that

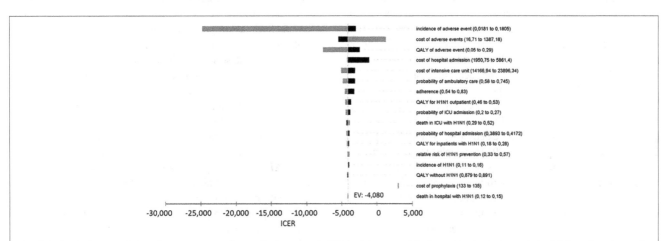

FIGURE 2 | Univariate sensitivity analysis of incremental cost-effectiveness ratio (ICER) of chemoprophylaxis compared to no prophylaxis. QALY, quality-adjusted life years; ICU, intensive care unit.

TABLE 6 | Probabilities (p) of incremental cost-effectiveness ratio (ICER) in each quadrant according to 10,000 Monte Carlo simulations, chemoprophylaxis versus no prophylaxis.

Quadrant	Incremental effect	Incremental cost	ICER	n	p
IV	>0	<0	Superior	6,849	0.6849
I	>0	>0	<30.000	1,793	0.1793
III	<0	<0	>30.000	153	0.0153
I	>0	>0	>30.000	57	0.0057
III	<0	<0	<30.000	749	0.0749
II	<0	>0	Inferior	399	0.0399

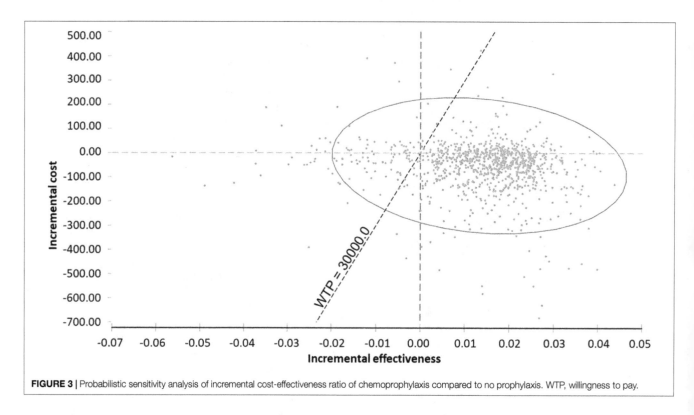

FIGURE 3 | Probabilistic sensitivity analysis of incremental cost-effectiveness ratio of chemoprophylaxis compared to no prophylaxis. WTP, willingness to pay.

previously-published research was biased in favor of the technology (Jefferson et al., 2014a). Publication bias was reduced once all clinical trials with the drugs were taken into consideration in such efforts (Jefferson et al., 2014a; Jefferson et al., 2014c; Heneghan et al., 2016).

Some of our probabilities were based on data from studies held during the 2009 influenza A (H1N1) pandemic, a period marked by greater virulence of influenza in Brazil and worldwide (Ministério da Saúde, 2012). In 2009, cases of severe acute respiratory syndrome in Brazil reached more than 44 per 100,000 inhabitants; later in 2010, its occurrence decreased to 4.6 cases per 100.000 inhabitants, finally reaching 2.5 in 2011. Influenza vaccine has been part of programmed vaccination for the elderly (>65 years of age) since 1999, and its use was expanded in 2010 to people >60 years of age. In 2011, pregnant women, children between six months and two years of age, indigenous people and health workers were included; since then, vaccine coverage has hovered above 80% (Ministério da Saúde, 2012). The probabilities adopted in our model led to more severe consequences for influenza, favoring the prophylaxis performance. We assumed that all patients with symptoms would seek for medical care, therefore we did not consider "out-of-pocket" expenses in cases

that patients would treat themselves without seeking for medical consult, as did an economic study of dengue in Brazil (Godoi et al., 2018). Adherence to prophylaxis was based on health professionals during the 2009 pandemic, period with greater concern about infection. Such assumptions and use data from the pandemia brought to a more conservative scenario that probably does not reflect the current scenario, where more people vaccinated and greater herd immunity is granted. Deterministic and probabilistic sensitivity analysis attested robustness of cost-effectiveness when probabilities of infection, hospital admission, and death by H1N1 ranged, partially circumventing these limitations.

The primary outcome of our study was based on QALY from the Spanish context, due to lack of utility data for influenza in Brazil. QALY for healthy state was based in Brazilian population data (Zimmermann et al., 2016; Silva et al., 2017). We evaluated the prevention of influenza as a secondary outcome, which does not involve population perception and favored prophylaxis. The Brazilian protocol for influenza states that chemoprophylaxis should be administered to non-vaccinated or vaccinated for less than 15 days people (Brasil. Ministério da Saúde. Secretaria de Vigilância em Saúde, 2017). Data on the effectiveness of the antiviral drugs segregated by vaccination status were not available for a specific analysis of the target-population not under the vaccine's effect. Influenza vaccination showed to reduce healthcare utilization in the elderly (Doyon-Plourde et al., 2019), as well as antibiotic usage in health adults (Buckley et al., 2019). While maintaining consistency with the national guideline, ignoring the effect of vaccination in our model may have favored the need and effectiveness of the chemoprophylaxis.

Our study is similar to previous health economic evaluations on influenza chemoprophylaxis, which also adopted a decision-tree model with a time horizon shorter than one year and favored the prophylaxis. In the Canadian health system, post-exposure prophylaxis in institutionalized and vaccinated elderly was dominant for preventing influenza-like illnesses when compared to no prophylaxis (Risebrough et al., 2005). This evaluation was based on three alternatives – prophylaxis with amantadine, prophylaxis with oseltamivir and no prophylaxis – and predicted viral resistance and adverse effects on the amantadine branch, influenza-like illnesses, complications, death, survival, and treatment in hospital or institution (Risebrough et al., 2005). The research was sponsored by oseltamivir manufacturer, F. Hoffmann-La Roche.

In the United Kingdom, post-exposure prophylaxis for inter-family contacts was probably cost-effective in the context of the National Health System, considering 2002's cost data (Sander et al., 2006). The model compared prophylaxis to no prophylaxis with or without oseltamivir treatment in the case of symptomatic influenza, and predicted complications, outpatient care, hospital admission, recovery and death, and assessed QALY and avoided cases of influenza-like illness. Probabilistic and sensitivity analysis attested the robustness of the model (Sander et al., 2006). The study was also sponsored by F. Hoffmann-La Roche, and the last author was an employee of the company.

United States analysis of post-exposure prophylaxis with oseltamivir in children up to 12 years was cost-effective in the perspectives of society and the payer, with 2008's costs (Talbird et al., 2009). The model compared prophylaxis to no prophylaxis and predicted development of influenza, hospital admission, outpatient care, death, and survival (Talbird et al., 2009). The research was commissioned by Roche, and the last author was its employee.

The National Health System in the United Kingdom funded a systematic review about efficacy and effectiveness of seasonal

and post-exposure prophylaxis, with subsequent analysis of cost-effectiveness using amantadine, oseltamivir, and zanamivir in vaccinated and non-vaccinated individuals (Tappenden et al., 2009). Six subgroups were considered: children, adults and elderly, in high-risk or healthy states, using cost data for 2006. Influenza-like illnesses, search for outpatient care, antiviral treatment, complications, death, and survival were considered in the analysis (Tappenden et al., 2009). The model predicted adverse effects to amantadine, vaccination, and prophylaxis abandonment ranging from 1.3% to 14.7%. Post-exposure prophylaxis was under 30,000.00 British pounds/QALY for non-vaccinated children and the elderly. None of these economic assessments considered herd immunity, adverse events of the studied drugs, and the complete efficacy data with lower risk of publication bias (Jefferson et al., 2014a; Jefferson et al., 2014c; Heneghan et al., 2016).

CONCLUSION

Post-exposure prophylaxis for influenza A (H1N1) is cost-saving in the context of the Brazilian public health system. Current Brazilian guidance for influenza A (H1N1) prevention is supported by the findings, but a lack of national efficacy and effectiveness data is noticed. Both oseltamivir and zanamivir are already incorporated for this purpose, changes to current guidelines are unnecessary.

AUTHOR CONTRIBUTIONS

LV, TG and MS designed the work, LV collected the data, LV and TG did the analyses and drafted the work, MS, ES and MR interpreted the data and revised the work critically. All authors approved the version to be published and agree to be accountable for all aspects of the work.

FUNDING

The study was funded by HAOC – PROADI SUS. Nonfinancial support was provided by Clinics' Hospital and Faculty of Pharmaceutical Sciences of the University of Campinas.

REFERENCES

(2019). Antiviral drugs for treatment and prophylaxis of seasonal influenza. *Med. Lett. Drugs Ther.* 61 (1563), 1–4.

Araujo, R., de Nardi Chagas, K., Nabeshima, C., Pepe, C., Bernardino, G., and Donato, B. (2014). Cost-effectiveness of dasatinib versus nilotinib for the secondline treatment of patients with chronic myeloid leukemia (CML) under the brazilian private healthcare system. *JBES Braz. J. Health Econ. J. Bras. Econ. Saúde* 6 (3).

Bilcke, J., Beutels, P., Brisson, M., and Jit, M. (2011). Accounting for methodological, structural, and parameter uncertainty in decision-analytic models: a practical guide. *Med. Decis. Making* 31 (4), 675–692. doi: 10.1177/0272989X11409240

Brasil. Ministério da Saúde. Secretaria de Vigilância em Saúde (2017). "Departamento de Vigilância das Doenças Transmissíveis," in *Protocolo de tratamento de Influenza 2017* (Brasília: Ministério da Saúde). bvsms.saude.gov.br/bvs/publicacoes/protocolo_tratamento_influenza_2017.pdf.

Brasil. Ministério da Saúde (2017). "Portaria N° 2.436, de 21 de setembro de 2017," in *Aprova a Política Nacional de Atenção Básica, estabelecendo a revisão de diretrizes para a organização da Atenção Básica, no âmbito do Sistema Único de Saúde (SUS)*, vol. 183. (Brasília: Diário Oficial da União). http://pesquisa.in.gov.br/imprensa/jsp/visualiza/index.jsp?jornal=1&pagina=68&data=22/09/2017.

Buckley, B. S., Henschke, N., Bergman, H., Skidmore, B., Klemm, E. J., Villanueva, G., et al. (2019). Impact of vaccination on antibiotic usage: a systematic review and meta-analysis. *Clin. Microbiol. Infect.* doi: 10.1016/j.cmi.2019.06.030

Calmona, C. O. (2013). *Influenza A H1N1 no Hospital das Clínicas da Faculdade de Medicina da Universidade de São Paulo (HC/FMUSP); perfil clínico dos casos atendidos e utilização de serviços hospitalares.* São Paulo: Universidade de São Paulo.

Carrat, F., Vergu, E., Ferguson, N. M., Lemaitre, M., Cauchemez, S., Leach, S., et al. (2008). Time lines of infection and disease in human influenza: a review of volunteer challenge studies. *Am. J. Epidemiol.* 167 (7), 775–785. doi: 10.1093/aje/kwm375

Dobson, J., Whitley, R. J., Pocock, S., and Monto, A. S. (2015). Oseltamivir treatment for influenza in adults: a meta-analysis of randomised controlled trials. *Lancet* 385 (9979), 1729–1737. doi: 10.1016/S0140-6736(14)62449-1

Doyon-Plourde, P., Fakih, I., Tadount, F., Fortin, E., and Quach, C. (2019). Impact of influenza vaccination on healthcare utilization - a systematic review. *Vaccine* 37 (24), 3179–3189. doi: 10.1016/j.vaccine.2019.04.051

Duarte, P. A. D., Venazzi, A., Youssef, N. C. M., Oliveira, M. C d, Tannous, L. A, Duarte, C. B., et al. (2009). Outcome of influenza A (H1N1) patients admitted to intensive care units in the Paraná state, Brazil. *Rev. Bras. Ter. Intensiva* 21, 231–236. doi: 10.1590/S0103-507X2009000300001

EPAR summary for the public (2015). *Tamiflu - oseltamivir.* Londvon: European Medicines Agency. http://www.ema.europa.eu/ema/index.jsp?curl=pages/medicines/human/medicines/000402/human_med_001075.jsp.

Godoi, I. P., Da Silva, L. V. D., Sarker, A. R., Megiddo, I., Morton, A., Godman, B., et al. (2018). Economic and epidemiological impact of dengue illness over 16 years from a public health system perspective in Brazil to inform future health policies including the adoption of a dengue vaccine. *Expert Rev. Vaccines* 17 (12), 1123–1133. doi: 10.1080/14760584.2018.1546581

Heneghan, C. J., Onakpoya, I., Jones, M. A., Doshi, P., Del Mar, C. B., Hama, R., et al. (2016). Neuraminidase inhibitors for influenza: a systematic review and meta-analysis of regulatory and mortality data. *Health Technol. Assess.* 20 (42), 1–242. doi: 10.3310/hta20420

Hollmann, M., Garin, O., Galante, M., Ferrer, M., Dominguez, A., and Alonso, J. (2013). Impact of influenza on health-related quality of life among confirmed (H1N1)2009 patients. *PLoS One* 8 (3), e60477. doi: 10.1371/journal.pone.0060477

Iuliano, A. D., Roguski, K. M., Chang, H. H., Muscatello, D. J., Palekar, R., Tempia, S., et al. (2018). Estimates of global seasonal influenza-associated respiratory mortality: a modelling study. *Lancet* 391 (10127), 1285–1300. doi: 10.1016/S0140-6736(17)33293-2

Jefferson, T., Demicheli, V., Rivetti, D., Jones, M., Di Pietrantonj, C., and Rivetti, A. (2006). Antivirals for influenza in healthy adults: systematic review. *Lancet* 367 (9507), 303–313. doi: 10.1016/S0140-6736(06)67970-1

Jefferson, T., Jones, M. A., Doshi, P., Del Mar, C. B., Hama, R., Thompson, M. J., et al. (2014a) Neuraminidase inhibitors for preventing and treating influenza in healthy adults and children. *Cochrane Database Syst. Rev.* 2014 (4), Cd008965. doi: 10.1002/14651858.CD008965.pub4

Jefferson, T., Jones, M. A., Doshi, P., Del Mar, C. B., Hama, R., Thompson, M. J., et al. (2014b). Risk of bias in industry-funded oseltamivir trials: comparison of core reports versus full clinical study reports. *BMJ Open* 4 (9), e005253. doi: 10.1136/bmjopen-2014-005253

Jefferson, T., Jones, M., Doshi, P., Spencer, E. A., Onakpoya, I., and Heneghan, C. J. (2014c). Oseltamivir for influenza in adults and children: systematic review of clinical study reports and summary of regulatory comments. *BMJ* 348, g2545. doi: 10.1136/bmj.g2545

Lau, L. L., Nishiura, H., Kelly, H., Ip, D. K., Leung, G. M., and Cowling, B. J. (2012). Household transmission of 2009 pandemic influenza A (H1N1): a systematic review and meta-analysis. *Epidemiology* 23 (4), 531–542. doi: 10.1097/EDE.0b013e31825588b8

Lenzi, L., Mello, A. M., Silva, L. R., Grochocki, M. H. C., Pontarolo, R., and Pandemic influenza, A. (2012). (H1N1) 2009: risk factors for hospitalization. *J. Bras. Pneumol.* 38, 57–65. doi: 10.1590/S1806-37132012000100009

Lindner, L. M., Marasciulo, A. C., Farias, M. R., and Grohs, G. E. M. (2009). [Economic evaluation of antipsychotic drugs for schizophrenia treatment within the brazilian healthcare system]. *Rev. Saude Publica* 43, 62–69. doi: 10.1590/S0034-89102009000800010

Martinez, A., Soldevila, N., Romero-Tamarit, A., Torner, N., Godoy, P., Rius, C., et al. (2019). Risk factors associated with severe outcomes in adult hospitalized patients according to influenza type and subtype. *PLoS One* 14 (1), e0210353. doi: 10.1371/journal.pone.0210353

Ministério da Saúde (2012). "Secretaria de Vigilância em Saúde. Informe Técnico de Influenza," in *Vigilância de Síndrome Respiratória Aguda Grave (SRAG), de Síndrome Gripal (SG) e de internações por CID J09 a J18.* Brasília: Ministério da Saúde. http://portalsaude.saude.gov.br/images/pdf/2014/maio/22/informe-influenza-2009-2010-2011-220514.pdf.

Munn, Z., Moola, S., Lisy, K., Riitano, D., and Tufanaru, C. (2015). Methodological guidance for systematic reviews of observational epidemiological studies reporting prevalence and cumulative incidence data. *Int. J. Evid. Based Healthc.* 13 (3), 147–153. doi: 10.1097/XEB.0000000000000054

Paim, J., Travassos, C., Almeida, C., Bahia, L., and Macinko, J. (2011). The Brazilian health system: history, advances, and challenges. *Lancet* 377 (9779), 1778–1797. doi: 10.1016/S0140-6736(11)60054-8

Parra-Rojas, C., Nguyen, V. K., Hernandez-Mejia, G., and Hernandez-Vargas, E. A. (2018). Neuraminidase inhibitors in influenza treatment and prevention(-)is it time to call it a day? *Viruses* 10 (9), E454. doi: 10.3390/v10090454

Ramirez, J., Peyrani, P., Wiemken, T., Chaves, S. S., and Fry, A. M. (2018). A randomized study evaluating the effectiveness of oseltamivir initiated at the time of hospital admission in adults hospitalized with influenza-associated lower respiratory tract infections. *Clin. Infect. Dis.* 67 (5), 736–742. doi: 10.1093/cid/ciy163

Relenza (2015). *Summary of Product Characteristics.* SmPC: medical products agency in Sweden. https://lakemedelsverket.se/LMF/Lakemedelsinformation/?nplid=19990209000018&type=product.

Riseborough, N. A., Bowles, S. K., Simor, A. E., McGeer, A., and Oh, P. I. (2005). Economic evaluation of oseltamivir phosphate for postexposure prophylaxis of influenza in long-term care facilities. *J. Am. Geriatr. Soc.* 53 (3), 444–451. doi: 10.1111/j.1532-5415.2005.53162.x

Sander, B., Hayden, F. G., Gyldmark, M., and Garrison, L. P., Jr. (2006). Postexposure influenza prophylaxis with oseltamivir: cost effectiveness and cost utility in families in the UK. *Pharmacoeconomics* 24 (4), 373–386. doi: 10.2165/00019053-200624040-00007

Shea B. J., R. B., Wells, G., Thuku, M., Hamel, C., Moran, J., Moher, D., et al. (2017). AMSTAR 2: a critical appraisal tool for systematic reviews that include randomised or non-randomised studies of healthcare interventions, or both. *BMJ* 358, j4008. doi: 10.1136/bmj.j4008

Silva, C. S., Haddad, MdCL., and de Carvalho Silva, L. G. (2012). [Cost of hospitalization of patients with influenza A (H1N1) in a public university hospital]. *Ciênc. Cuidado Saúde* 11 (3), 481–488. doi: 10.4025/cienccuidsaude.v11i3.13729

Silva, M. T., Caicedo Roa, M., and Galvao, T. F. (2017). Health-related quality of life in the Brazilian Amazon: a population-based cross-sectional study. *Health Qual Life Outcomes* 15 (1), 159. doi: 10.1186/s12955-017-0734-5

Soarez, P. C. D., and Novaes, H. M. D. (2017). Limiares de custo-efetividade e o Sistema Único de Saúde. *Cad. Saude Publica* 33 (4), e00040717. doi: 10.1590/0102-311x00040717

Talbird, S. E., Brogan, A. J., and Winiarski, A. P. (2009). Oseltamivir for influenza postexposure prophylaxis: economic evaluation for children aged 1-12 years in the U.S. *Am. J. Prev. Med.* 37 (5), 381–388. doi: 10.1016/j.amepre.2009.08.012

Tappenden, P., Jackson, R., Cooper, K., Rees, A., Simpson, E., Read, R., et al. (2009). Amantadine, oseltamivir and zanamivir for the prophylaxis of influenza (including a review of existing guidance no. 67): a systematic review and economic evaluation. *Health Technol. Assess.* 13 (11), iii, ix–xii, 1–246. doi: 10.3310/hta13110

Upjohn, L. M., Stewardson, A. J., and Marshall, C. (2012). Oseltamivir adherence and tolerability in health care workers treated prophylactically after occupational influenza exposure. *Am. J. Infect. Control* 40 (10), 1020–1022. doi: 10.1016/j.ajic.2011.11.014

Uyeki, T. M., Bernstein, H. H., Bradley, J. S., Englund, J. A., File, T. M., Fry, A. M., et al. (2018). Clinical practice guidelines by the infectious diseases society of America: 2018 update on diagnosis, treatment, chemoprophylaxis, and institutional outbreak management of seasonal influenzaa. *Clin. Infect. Dis.* 68 (6), e1–e47. doi: 10.1093/cid/ciy866

Wells, G., Shea, B., O'connell, D., Peterson, J., Welch, V., Losos, M. et al., (2000) *The Newcastle-Ottawa Scale (NOS) for assessing the quality of nonrandomised studies in meta-analyses.* Available from: http://www.ohri.ca/programs/clinical_epidemiology/oxford.asp.

World Health Organization (2010). Pharmacological Management of Pandemic

Influenza A (H1N1) 2009. Available from: http://www.who.int/csr/resources/publications/swineflu/h1n1_use_antivirals_20090820/en/.

World Health Organization (2019). Influenza update – 337. 18 March 2019 – Update number 337, based on data up to 03 March 2019 2019. Available from: https://www.who.int/influenza/surveillance_monitoring/updates/latest_update_GIP_surveillance/en/.

Zimmermann, I. R., Silva, M. T., Galvao, T. F., and Pereira, M. G. (2016). Health-related quality of life and self-reported long-term conditions: a population-based survey. *Rev. Bras. Psiquiatr.* doi: 10.1590/1516-4446-2015-1853

APPENDIX

Appendix A. Cost and Utility of Adverse Events

We used the risk difference of each significant adverse event reported in the systematic review (Jefferson et al., 2014a) to calculate the probabilities of adverse events.

Event	Risk difference, % (95%CI)	Weight (%)	Costs		QALY	
			Raw	Weighted	Raw	Weighted
Headache	3.15 (0.88; 5.78)	33.7	16.71[a] (Araujo et al., 2014)	5.625	−0.050 (Araujo et al., 2014)	−0.017
Nausea	5.15 (0.86; 9.51)	55.0	235.06[a] (Araujo et al., 2014)	129.33	−0.290 (Araujo et al., 2014)	−0.160
Psychiatric[b]	1.06 (0.07; 2.76)	11.3	1,387.18[c] (Lindner et al., 2009)	157.10	−0.167 (Lindner et al., 2009)	−0.019
Total	9.36 (1.81; 18.05)	100.0	–	292.05[d]	–	−0.1953

[a]2014's costs corrected to 2016. [b]"suspected serious psychotic/suicidal adverse events (including hallucination, psychosis, schizophrenia, paranoia, aggression/hostility and attempted suicide)" (Jefferson et al., 2014a). [c]2009's costs corrected to 2016. [d]Standard deviation = 736.34. QALY, quality-adjusted life years.

Appendix B. Expenditure With Acquisition of Oseltamivir and Zanamivir by the Pharmaceutical Services Department, Brazilian Ministry of Health in 2016

It is worth noting that we did not consider stockpiling costs and loss due to product expiration, since such data was unavailable. This would be important information for calculating the total cost of chemoprophylaxis.

Medicine	Unity	Unity price	Prophylaxis price[a]	Expenditure[b]	Weighted price of prophylaxis (BRL)
Oseltamivir 30 mg	Capsule	2.18	21.78[c]	3,036,670	2.58
Oseltamivir 45 mg	Capsule	3.27	32.70	2,578,500	3.28
Oseltamivir 75 mg	Capsule	4.29	42.92	20,057,500	33.53
Zanamivir 5 mg	Kit	63.92	63.92[d]	1,000	0.02
Total				25,673,670	**39.42**

BRL, Brazilian real; [a]standard deviation = 17.94. [b]expenditure in BRL from 01/01/2016 to 08/23/2017. [c]minimum value adopted on the univariate sensitivity analysis. [d]maximum value adopted on the univariate sensitivity analysis.

23

Comprehending the Health Informatics Spectrum: Grappling with System Entropy and Advancing Quality Clinical Research

Matthew I. Bellgard[1]*, Nigel Chartres[2], Gerald F. Watts[3,4], Steve Wilton[1,5,6], Sue Fletcher[1,5,6], Adam Hunter[1] and Tom Snelling[7,8,9]

[1] Centre for Comparative Genomics, Murdoch University, Murdoch, WA, Australia, [2] Health Informatics Society of Australia, North Melbourne, VIC, Australia, [3] School of Medicine, University of Western Australia, Perth, WA, Australia, [4] Lipid Disorders Clinic, Cardiometabolic Service, Royal Perth Hospital, Perth, WA, Australia, [5] Centre for Neuromuscular and Neurological Disorders, University of Western Australia, Nedlands, WA, Australia, [6] Perron Institute for Neurological and Translational Science, Nedlands, WA, Australia, [7] Princess Margaret Hospital for Children, Perth, WA, Australia, [8] Wesfarmers Centre of Vaccines and Infectious Diseases, Telethon Kids Institute, University of Western Australia, Perth, WA, Australia, [9] Menzies School of Health Research and Charles Darwin University, Darwin, NT, Australia

Keywords: health, informatics, clinical research, information communication technology, clinical practice

*Correspondence:
Matthew I. Bellgard
mbellgard@ccg.murdoch.edu.au

Clinical research is complex. The knowledge base is information and data rich where value and success depend upon focused, well designed connectivity of systems achieved through stakeholder collaboration. Quality data, information, and knowledge must be utilized in an effective, efficient, and timely manner to affect important clinical decisions and communicate health prevention strategies. In recent decades, it has become apparent that information communication technology (ICT) solutions potentially offer multidimensional opportunities for transforming health care and clinical research. However, it is also recognized that successful utilization of ICT in improving patient care and health outcomes depends on a number of factors such as the effective integration of diverse sources of health data; how and by whom quality data are captured; reproducible methods on how data are interrogated and reanalyzed; robust policies and procedures for data privacy, security and access; usable consumer and clinical user interfaces; effective diverse stakeholder engagement; and navigating the numerous eclectic and non-interoperable legacy proprietary health ICT solutions in hospital and clinic environments (1, 2). This is broadly termed health informatics (HI).

We outline three scenarios from across the health spectrum where these issues are exemplified: (i) for a given clinical trial methodology and study design, the nature of how quality data is captured, by whom, how it is aggregated, reused and repurposed is just as critical as the data content itself. This becomes critical with the desire to simultaneously evaluate and optimize the effective and cost-effective use of new medications (3); (ii) in a systems biology context, clever strategies to combine disparate datasets at the gene, gene expression, protein as well as at a protein–protein interaction levels are essential to unlock underlying molecular mechanisms that affect routine clinical decisions (4); and (iii) in evidence-based medicine, encoding expert clinical knowledge into decision support systems and data standards for collecting diverse patient's physiological measurements are critical to ensure effective cross jurisdictional data sharing for diseases (5).

These three examples highlight the potential broad spectrum of the role of ICT in health. Simply stated, at one end of the spectrum, health ICT systems are critical for the routine day-to-day running of hospitals and clinics. These systems are used by various health stakeholders for a diverse range of clinical services and administrative procedures. More recently, there is an increasing demand to reuse and repurpose health data contained within these ICT systems for clinical research and reporting such as compliance, efficiency metrics, funding of health programs, epidemiological studies, and health promotion. On the other end of the spectrum, clinical research embeds ICT and its application involving bioinformaticians, biostatisticians, and analytic workflow environments within research projects. There is a growing demand to embed outputs of this research as evidence to inform health-care policy and improve clinical practice.

The significant challenge is how we bridge these two ends of the spectrum. While the overall driver of improved patient outcomes is shared, the demands placed on available ICT systems for data capture, access, and analysis are usually beyond what they were originally designed for. We contend that the field of HI is the important bridge that delivers the promise spanning ICT spectrum in both health care and clinical research. We now explore the challenges in HI that need to be overcome.

KEY HI CHALLENGES WITHIN THE CURRENT ENVIRONMENT

Key Challenge 1: Defining HI

There are numerous broad definitions of HI. One such definition is that HI is "an evolving scientific discipline that deals with the collection, storage, retrieval, communication and optimal use of health and related data, information and knowledge" (6). The discipline draws on computational and information science methodologies and technologies to support clinical decision-making to improve health care. Such a broad definition has both advantages and disadvantages. On the one hand, this definition is a "catch all" for the spectrum of ICT in health care and clinical research. On the other, such a broad definition impacts a diverse range of health-related stakeholders from researchers, clinicians, nurses, public, allied health, health professionals, government departments, administrators, and software engineers. This presents a significant challenge of ensuring effective communication and uptake of robust HI.

Key Challenge 2: Current Health ICT Ecosystems

In reality, health ICT ecosystems are largely fragmented (7, 8). For example, typically within a hospital ICT system environment, there are stand-alone systems, meaning that important health data are also siloed. Depending on the nature of these systems (some of which are as simple as spreadsheets), it is highly likely to contain significant data entry errors, duplications, inconsistencies, and incompleteness. The key challenge here is that fragmented ICT systems impedes the ability to monitor chronic diseases, effectively follow-up patients after hospital discharge, prevent avoidable complications (for example, hospital readmissions), or enable longitudinal epidemiological studies. This has a flow on cost burden effect and can inhibit efficiency

gains within the health system. In Australia, numerous health-care business units (such as radiology, pharmacy, pathology, and radio oncology) typically have their own ICT systems that do not interface with each other, and most hospital systems do not interact with external systems, such as general practice clinics or private clinic rooms. Therefore, ownership and management of data become an important barrier between health-care business units and affect the quality of patient care. Furthermore, when proprietary systems are deployed and hosted by third parties, the ability of the client to exercise their ownership rights over their data requires clarification at the outset of the hosting arrangements.

Key Challenge 3: Underlying Causes of Issues with Current ICT Ecosystems

Many papers and conferences addressing significant issues inherent in the challenges of introducing successful ICT ecosystems into the health sector continue to identify some key underlying causes for system failures and continuing difficulties in achieving meaningful connectivity within the health-care system, for example, see Ref. (9). These issues generally fall under the following 10 headings.

Leadership and Governance

Currently, the required degree of alignment of shared leadership and appropriate governance arrangements, across the many areas of responsibility, needed for systems synergies, are limited. Program management is equally important to project management to ensure shared learning of technical and interpersonal expertise.

Policy and Funding Models

Although health reform agendas mean to streamline policy-making and funding models, many stakeholders consider that very little has really been achieved that delivers any significant improvements into the way health systems operate. In this context, there are significant funding and resourcing pressures on any given state/national health system. The nature of these pressures unfortunately means that the focus reverts back to a business-as-usual paradigm within health systems. Furthermore, the current budgetary and operational pressures on the health sector restrict the ability of leadership within the sector to respond to contemporary challenges.

Regulatory Impediments

Existing and complex regulatory environments are viewed as a major issue where very little practical and beneficial change has been able to be introduced.

Productivity and Performance

It is recognized that significant progress has been made in reporting/compliance arrangements and systems that are focusing on transparency and accountability of health-care service providers. Given the current widespread lack of active use of data standards utilized within the fragmented health ICT ecosystem, it is difficult to harness the big data opportunities inherently available in health-care performance metrics (10).

As such it is neither feasible nor practical to be able to use performance metrics to assess productivity in meaningful depth that could introduce transformative efficiencies into service delivery models.

Standards

Globally, there is much valuable work on developing open standards in health, for example, Ref. (11, 12). However, there remain many challenges in their widespread adoption related to limited funding, limited leadership capacity, widespread agreement, and limited workforce skills and resources. A particular issue concerns the focus on data collection and data entry rather than what we refer to as a more holistic approach to data management including the *purposeful application of collected data* to improve health outcomes.

Business Models and Processes—The Illusion of Risk Free Procurement

A significant barrier to the successful deployment of new systems is managing the transition from legacy ICT systems and data management processes in delivery of health services. This has further exacerbated the disparity between implemented ICT solutions and the business models and processes, which they purport to support. For instance, the procurement processes of health ICT solutions should be continually reviewed and iteratively refined along the dimensions of digital disruption, accountability, risk assessment, risk mitigation, risk averse strategies.

Evidence of potential suboptimal processes is highlighted by the patient journey through the health system, which invariably spans organizational and operational boundaries whose systems are typically not seamlessly connected to support the overall delivery of health care (9). In the case of rare disease diagnosis, a patient's navigation through the health system is referred to more as an odyssey than a journey (3).

In addition, business model and process reform which is required systemically throughout the health system and much of which depends upon regulatory reform, is considered one of the most significant barriers to any beneficial transformation of the health system.

Sociotechnical Complexities

Sociotechnical complexities (complexities that span societal and technical boundaries) are inextricably linked to many aspects of business models and their associated business processes. Many of these complexities are inherently cultural in nature, in so far as many health workforce participants operate within long standing conventionally designed systems ecosystems. So while some progress continues to be achieved in specific situations, the big breakthroughs can only be achieved through large-scale business model and process reform as driven by regulatory change. If these are not addressed, then, for example, emerging trends such as patient empowerment *via* the measured self (13), the Internet of things (5), and personalized medicine will only see these complexities exacerbated (14).

Another key aspect of this concerns a real focus on business models, business processes, and systems, which collectively enable much more community engagement at all levels in consultation on matters such as prevention, patient care, diagnosis, treatment, management, privacy, and consent.

Infrastructure Component Connectivity

Technical and communication infrastructure is no longer viewed as the major issue as it was in recent times. It is clear that more effort needs to be made to connect existing infrastructure components to enable better communication between health-care service providers and so achieve more coordination of services.

Workforce

A barrier to success exists in the form of limited staff capacity across a range of administrative, clinical, research and technology disciplines to overcome the significant business-as-usual pressures of national health systems. This must be addressed to implement transformative change. ICT systems inherently can track performance, which can give rise to fear of inappropriate exposure for suboptimal clinical decision-making.

Clinical Research

There are limited virtual spaces where the health sector can interface with the research sector. Health departments do not have infrastructure to provide analytic environments for their big data, academic environments are typically not structured to handle health data, despite possessing the analytic capabilities.

CASE STUDY: DEMENTIA

The Organisation for Economic Co-operation and Development (OECD) has recognized that there is clear potential to improve science and innovation systems through big data and open science for the prevention and care of dementia. In 2010, 35 million people worldwide were diagnosed with dementia with annual health costs estimated at USD 604 billion with the number of people diagnosed to exceed 115 million by 2050. The multifactorial nature of the condition requires the collection, storage, and processing of increasingly large and very heterogeneous datasets (behavioral, genetic, -omics, environmental, epigenetic, clinical data, brain imaging, and so forth) (10).

To successfully apply informatics systems to big data, current barriers, issues, and challenges need to be recognized and addressed along with implementing key critical success factors. For example, the OECD identified data sharing as the most significant barrier in managing dementia (15). The root cause of this significant barrier arises from current cultural, technical, administrative, regulatory, infrastructure, and financial obstacles that need to be overcome. In addition, data standards, data sharing, new analytic approaches, security and protecting privacy, along with approaches for engaging stakeholders and the public are critical factors for effectively and successfully harnessing big data. Hence, the future opportunity for big data in improving health-care systems requires carefully crafted strategies at both

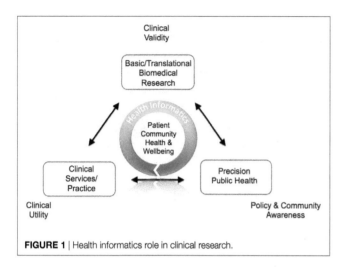

FIGURE 1 | Health informatics role in clinical research.

policy and ICT implementation levels across a broad range of HI challenges. In particular, regard needs to be paid to the established discipline of data governance, which is particularly important for providing a solid structural basis for managing human resources, processes, and technologies (1, 2).

THE FUTURE CONTRIBUTION OF HI TO IMPROVING HEALTH OUTCOMES

A learning health-care system requires a number of critical ingredients that can improve care of patients. These entail definition of clinical context, accurate collection of patient characteristics and outcome data, availability of decision support systems, utilization and application of real world data, and effective engagement of all stakeholders.

Introducing a Guiding Model for the Role of HI to Span the Spectrum of ICT in Clinical Research

Owing to the current complexities and issues inherent in making substantial progress in improving health outcomes through the deployment of ICT enabling systems it is clear that there needs to be a better understanding of the role which HI plays.

Figure 1 provides an overview of a proposed guiding model highlighting the ideal role that HI plays in health care. Within this model, for example, clinical research will generate and analyze data such as a personalized genome sequence, to obtain clinical validity of candidate pathogenic mutations (16). The identified pathogenic mutation data are captured as one of myriad of patient phenotypes and patient reported outcomes to ascertain clinical utility, such as in a disease registry, e.g., Ref. (17, 18), as part of clinical services and practice, in a personalized medicine context (14). In the third axes, pathogenic mutations data can be aggregated in a de-identified manner across geographical

locations to inform policy and community awareness (19) and undertaking important population health research.

CONCLUSION AND FUTURE PERSPECTIVE: STRATEGIES FOR SHAPING EFFECTIVE AND SUSTAINABLE SYSTEMS

From our experience, there are three key linked and iterative strategies for shaping and delivering successful systems. These are to:

- Facilitate a vision for shaping successful sustainable synergistic systems through shared leadership enabling collaborative stakeholder engagement;
- Recognize and address complexity through engaging stakeholders and the health workforce in identifying issues, problems, barriers, and potential solutions; and
- Create clever connected communities for the purposes of identifying and introducing innovative and informed investments in synergistic systems.

These, necessarily, need to be very skilfully planned, managed, and executed, which requires professional systems thinking HI practitioners who also have a very pragmatic working knowledge of the health system. This topic will be the subject of further commentary.

Information communication technology solutions must be discussed in an open and willing environment where risk is understood and carefully managed to facilitate strategic planning. These solutions must be designed to be able to apply open data standards and open system principles that promote interoperability, service oriented architectures, application programming interfaces, and appropriate assessment of legacy ICT systems (12, 20).

AUTHOR CONTRIBUTIONS

All the authors have contributed to this work.

FUNDING

The authors gratefully acknowledge the combined support-in-part funding for this work. This includes the RD-Connect-European Union Seventh Framework Programme (FP7/2007–2013 program HEALTH. 2012.2. 1.1-1-C) under grant agreement number 305444: RD Connect: an integrated platform connecting databases, registries, biobanks, and clinical bioinformatics for rare disease research, the financial support of Australian National Health and Medical Research Council (APP1055319) under the NHMRC–European Union Collaborative Research Grants scheme, the Wellcome Trust [REF 104746], and the Australian Bioinformatics Facility funded through Bioplatforms Australia Pty. Ltd., an Australian National Collaborative Research Infrastructure Strategy initiative.

REFERENCES

1. Chartres N. *Data Governance, HISA Thought Leadership Series.* Vol. 1. Melbourne: HISA (2012).

2. Chartres N. *Data Governance: Data Governance Journeys – Enabling Improved Healthcare Outcomes, HISA Thought Leadership Series.* Vol. 1. Melbourne: HISA (2013).

3. Hilbert JE, Ashizawa T, Day JW, Luebbe EA, Martens WB, McDermott MP, et al. Diagnostic odyssey of patients with myotonic dystrophy. *J Neurol* (2013) 260(10):2497–504. doi:10.1007/s00415-013-6993-0

4. Wolkenhauer O, Auffray C, Jaster R, Steinhoff G, Dammann O. The road from systems biology to systems medicine. *Pediatr Res* (2013) 73(4 Pt 2):502–7. doi:10.1038/pr.2013.4

5. Bellgard MI, Napier KR, Bittles AH, Szer J, Fletcher S, Zeps N, et al. Design of a framework for the deployment of collaborative independent rare disease-centric registries: Gaucher disease registry model. *Blood Cells Mol Dis* (2017). doi:10.1016/j.bcmd.2017.01.013

6. HISA. *Australias Digital Health Future: Vision for Cohesive Collaborative & Constructive Digital Disruption in Healthcare.* Melbourne: HISA (2015).

7. Srinivasan U, Rao S, Ramachandran D, Jonas D. *Flying Blind: Australian Consumers and Digital Health: Australian Health Data Series, Health Market Quality Research Program.* Vol. 1. Sydney: CMCRC (2016).

8. Gibson CJ, Dixon BE, Abrams K. Convergent evolution of health information management and health informatics: a perspective on the future of information professionals in health care. *Appl Clin Inform* (2015) 6(1):163–84. doi:10.4338/ACI-2014-09-RA-0077

9. Chartres N. *Patient Journeys: A Synopsis of HIC2013.* Vol. 4. New South Wales: PulseIT Magazine (2013).

10. OECD. Unleashing the power of big data for Alzheimer's disease and dementia research: main points of the OECD expert consultation on unlocking global collaboration to accelerate innovation for Alzheimer's disease and dementia. *OECD Digital Economy Papers.* No. 233. Paris: OECD Publishing (2014). doi:10.1787/5jz73kvmvbwb-en

11. Robinson PN, Kohler S, Bauer S, Seelow D, Horn D, Mundlos S. The human phenotype ontology: a tool for annotating and analyzing human hereditary disease. *Am J Hum Genet* (2008) 83(5):610–5. doi:10.1016/j.ajhg.2008.09.017

12. Wilkinson MD, Dumontier M, Aalbersberg IJ, Appleton G, Axton M, Baak A, et al. The FAIR guiding principles for scientific data management and stewardship. *Sci Data* (2016) 3:160018. doi:10.1038/sdata.2016.18

13. Mishali M, Omer H, Heymann AD. The importance of measuring self-efficacy in patients with diabetes. *Fam Pract* (2011) 28(1):82–7. doi:10.1093/fampra/cmq086

14. Bellgard MI, Sleeman MW, Guerero FD, Fletcher S, Baynam G, Goldblatt J, et al. Rare disease research roadmap: navigating the bioinformatics and translational challenges for improved patient health outcomes. *Health Policy Technol* (2014) 3(4) 325–335. doi:10.1016/j.hlpt.2014.08.007

15. Anderson G, Oderkirk J, editors. Dementia research and care: can big data help? Paris: OECD Publishing (2015). doi:10.1787/9789264228429-en

16. Salgado D, Bellgard MI, Desvignes JP, Beroud C. How to identify pathogenic mutations among all those variations: variant annotation and filtration in the genome sequencing era. *Hum Mutat* (2016) 37(12):1272–82. doi:10.1002/humu.23110

17. Bellgard MI, Macgregor A, Janon F, Harvey A, O'Leary P, Hunter A, et al. A modular approach to disease registry design: successful adoption of an internet-based rare disease registry. *Hum Mutat* (2012) 33(10):E2356–66. doi:10.1002/humu.22154

18. Bellgard M, Walker CM, Napier K, Lamont L, Hunter A, Render L, et al. Design of the familial hypercholesterolaemia Australasia network registry: creating opportunities for greater international collaboration. *J Atheroscler Thromb* (2017). doi:10.5551/jat.37507

19. Bladen CL, Salgado D, Monges S, Foncuberta ME, Kekou K, Kosma K, et al. The TREAT-NMD DMD global database: analysis of more than 7,000 Duchenne muscular dystrophy mutations. *Hum Mutat* (2015) 36(4):395–402. doi:10.1002/humu.22758

20. Bellgard M, Beroud C, Parkinson K, Harris T, Ayme S, Baynam G, et al. Dispelling myths about rare disease registry system development. *Source Code Biol Med* (2013) 8(1):21. doi:10.1186/1751-0473-8-21

24

Fusogenic Liposomes Increase the Antimicrobial Activity of Vancomycin Against *Staphylococcus aureus* Biofilm

Andreia Borges Scriboni[1], Verônica Muniz Couto[2], Lígia Nunes de Morais Ribeiro[2], Irlan Almeida Freires[3], Francisco Carlos Groppo[1], Eneida de Paula[2], Michelle Franz-Montan[1]* and Karina Cogo-Müller[1,4]*

[1] *Department of Physiological Sciences, Piracicaba Dental School, University of Campinas, Piracicaba, Brazil,* [2] *Department of Biochemistry and Tissue Biology, Biology Institute, University of Campinas, Campinas, Brazil,* [3] *Department of Oral Biology, University of Florida College of Dentistry, Gainesville, FL, United States,* [4] *Faculty of Pharmaceutical Sciences, University of Campinas, Campinas, Brazil*

*Correspondence:
Michelle Franz-Montan
michelle@fop.unicamp.br
Karina Cogo-Müller
karina.muller@fcf.unicamp.br

Objective: The aim of the present study was to encapsulate vancomycin in different liposomal formulations and compare the *in vitro* antimicrobial activity against *Staphylococcus aureus* biofilms.

Methods: Large unilamellar vesicles of conventional (LUV VAN), fusogenic (LUV$_{fuso}$ VAN), and cationic (LUV$_{cat}$ VAN) liposomes encapsulating VAN were characterized in terms of size, polydispersity index, zeta potential, morphology, encapsulation efficiency (%EE) and *in vitro* release kinetics. The formulations were tested for their Minimum Inhibitory Concentration (MIC) and inhibitory activity on biofilm formation and viability, using methicillin-susceptible *S. aureus* ATCC 29213 and methicillin-resistant *S. aureus* ATCC 43300 strains.

Key Findings: LUV VAN showed better %EE (32.5%) and sustained release than LUV$_{fuso}$ VAN, LUV$_{cat}$ VAN, and free VAN. The formulations were stable over 180 days at 4°C, except for LUV VAN, which was stable up to 120 days. The MIC values for liposomal formulations and free VAN ranged from 0.78 to 1.56 µg/ml against both tested strains, with no difference in the inhibition of biofilm formation as compared to free VAN. However, when treating mature biofilm, encapsulated LUV$_{fuso}$ VAN increased the antimicrobial efficacy as compared to the other liposomal formulations and to free VAN, demonstrating a better ability to penetrate the biofilm.

Conclusion: Vancomycin encapsulated in fusogenic liposomes demonstrated enhanced antimicrobial activity against mature *S. aureus* biofilms.

Keywords: fusogenic liposomes, cationic liposomes, *Staphylococcus aureus*, vancomycin, biofilm

INTRODUCTION

Staphylococcus aureus (*S. aureus*) is a Gram-positive microorganism responsible for the majority of nosocomial and community-acquired infections. Notably, *S. aureus* infections remain a global public health issue highly costly for the healthcare system, with increasing morbidity and mortality rates worldwide (Chakraborty et al., 2012; Honary et al., 2013; Elkhodairy et al., 2014; Holland et al., 2014). Today, over 90% of *S. aureus* strains are found to be resistant to methicillin (methicillin resistant *S. aureus*—MRSA), penicillin, aminoglycosides, macrolides, lincosamides, and other beta-lactams (Chakraborty et al., 2012; Muppidi et al., 2012; Sande et al., 2012; Elkhodairy et al., 2014; Shi et al., 2014).

In this scenario of microbial resistance, vancomycin (VAN) is considered a first-choice antibiotic for the treatment of methicillin-resistant *S. aureus* (MRSA) infections (Pumerantz et al., 2011; Honary et al., 2013; Holland et al., 2014; Men et al., 2016; Gudiol et al., 2017). While VAN remains a first-choice antibiotic for the treatment of MRSA infections, its therapeutic efficacy is limited due to its high molecular weight (1,449.2 g mol^{-1}) and hydrophilicity restricting the drug interaction with bacterial cells and hindering its penetration into biofilms (Howden et al., 2010; Nicolosi et al., 2010; Butler et al., 2014; Moghadas-Sharif et al., 2015). In addition to that, VAN systemic side effects are another limiting factor, which include severe watery diarrhea, kidney failure (Pumerantz et al., 2011; Rose et al., 2012; Honary et al., 2013), ototoxicity, neutropenia, fever, anaphylaxis, thrombocytopenia, and phlebitis (McAuley, 2012).

Bacterial biofilms are characterized by the aggregation of specific bacterial species adhered to a substrate, forming highly organized microbial communities (Khameneh et al., 2014; McCarthy et al., 2015). Biofilm-forming bacteria display a differentiated phenotype compared to planktonic cells and have the ability to produce an extracellular polymeric matrix composed mainly of polysaccharides (Khameneh et al., 2014; Dong et al., 2015; McCarthy et al., 2015). This scaffold provides an extremely robust defense mechanism, which hinders antibiotic penetration into the biofilm structure, substantially reducing the susceptibility of bacterial cells to exogenous agents (Dong et al., 2015; McCarthy et al., 2015; Moghadas-Sharif et al., 2015).

The shortcomings of VAN traditional treatment along with the increased microbial resistance rates, and difficulty to treat biofilms have encouraged the development of drug-carrier systems such as VAN-loaded liposomal formulations (Kadry et al., 2004; Drulis-Kawa et al., 2009; Nicolosi et al., 2010; Lankalapalli et al., 2015). It has been shown that the liposomal sustained release of VAN (i) enhances antibacterial efficacy due to higher interaction of the antibiotic molecule with bacterial cells (Kim and Jones, 2004); (ii) improves pharmacokinetics (Ma et al., 2011); (iii) reduces toxicity (Sande et al., 2012); and (iv) increases the antimicrobial spectrum of action against Gram-negative bacteria (Nicolosi et al., 2010). Furthermore, liposomes can facilitate antibiotic penetration into bacterial cells and, therefore, increase drug concentration in the biofilm inner layers (Moghadas-Sharif et al., 2015). Despite these reports, only a few studies have evaluated the effects of liposomal formulations on the inhibition of biofilm development

and viability, particularly *Staphylococcus* biofilms (Ma et al., 2011; Moghadas-Sharif et al., 2015).

The liposome composition can be specifically modulated in terms of morphology to favor the adsorption onto, or fusion with, the microbial cell membrane. Likewise, vesicle surfaces can be changed based on the characteristics of the infectious agent (Nicolosi et al., 2010). Among some types of liposomes with the ability of interacting with bacterial biofilm cells are fusogenic and cationic liposomes (Kim et al., 1999; Nicolosi et al., 2010). Fusogenic liposomes are vesicles that may fuse with biological membranes, thereby increasing drug contact and delivery into cells. They consist of lipids, such as dioleoyl-phosphatidylethanolamine (DOPE) and cholesterol hemisuccinate (CHEMS), which provide increased fluidity to the lipid bilayer and may destabilize biological membranes (Nicolosi et al., 2010; Aoki et al., 2015; Nicolosi et al., 2015). Because of their composition, fusogenic liposomes are normally in the liquid crystalline phase and, under specific chemical conditions, e.g., acidic milieu or in the presence of cations (Forier et al., 2014) they can lose the bilayer arrangement and fuse. Cationic liposomes are composed of lipids with a positive residual charge, such as stearylamine (SA), dimethyldioctadecylammonium bromide (DDBA), dimethylaminoethane carbamoyl cholesterol (DC-chol), and dioleoyltrimethylammoniumpropane (DOTAP), which provides specific electrostatic interaction with bacterial cell wall and biofilms, both negatively charged (Kim et al., 1999; Torchilin, 2012; Zhang et al., 2014; Moghadas-Sharif et al., 2015).

While fusogenic and cationic liposomes have proven advantages in interacting with bacterial cells and formed biofilms, there is still no consensus on the ideal composition of liposome-encapsulated VAN formulations able to prolong drug release and increase its antimicrobial efficacy. Thus, in the present study we developed and characterized large unilamellar vesicles of conventional (LUV VAN), fusogenic (LUV$_{fuso}$ VAN), and cationic (LUV$_{cat}$ VAN) liposomes encapsulating vancomycin hydrochloride. The *in vitro* antimicrobial activity of these formulations on *S. aureus* biofilms was further determined and compared.

MATERIALS AND METHODS

Materials

VAN hydrochloride was kindly provided by Teuto/Pfizer Laboratory (Anápolis, GO, Brazil). HEPES buffer, cholesterol (Chol), alpha-tocopherol (α-T) and egg phosphatidylcholine (EPC) were purchased from Sigma-Aldrich (St. Louis, MO, USA) and chloroform was obtained from Merck (Darmstadt, Germany). Dioleoylphosphatidylethanolamine (DOPE), dipalmitoylphosphatidylcholine (DPPC), cholesterol hemisuccinate (CHEMS) and stearylamine (Sa) were purchased from Avanti Polar Lipids Inc. (Alabaster, AL USA).

Preparation of Liposomal Formulations

Conventional (LUV VAN), fusogenic (LUV$_{fuso}$ VAN) and cationic (LUV$_{cat}$ VAN) liposomal formulations were prepared containing 10 mg/ml VAN. Plain, VAN-free formulations were used as negative controls in the experiments (LUV, LUV$_{fuso}$, and LUV$_{cat}$). All liposomal formulations were prepared with 10 mM lipid concentration, with the following composition: LUV–EPC : Chol:α-T (4:3:0.07, mol%) (Cereda et al., 2006); LUV$_{fuso}$–DOPE : DPPC : CHEMS:α-T (4:2:4:0.07, mol%) (Nicolosi et al., 2010); LUV$_{cat}$–EPC : Sa:Chol:α-T (1:0.5:0.5:0.07, mol%) (Kadry et al., 2004), respectively. All formulations were prepared in HEPES buffer (80 mM) containing 150 mM NaCl (pH 7.4).

Preparation of liposomal formulations was carried out as previously described, with modifications (Cereda et al., 2006). Briefly, the lipids were dissolved in chloroform, evaporated under nitrogen flow to obtain the lipid film, and vacuumed for 2 h to ensure complete solvent removal. Subsequently, the film was hydrated in HEPES buffer with or without VAN hydrochloride solution. Then the suspension was vortexed for 5 min to form large multilamellar vesicles (MLVs). The suspensions were extruded under nitrogen flow at high pressure (Extruder Emulsiflex C5, Avestin, Inc., Ottawa, ON, Canada) 12 times using polycarbonate membrane initially with 400 nm pores, and then, with 100 nm pores, to obtain small unilamellar vesicles. The extrusion of LUV$_{fuso}$ formulation was performed in water bath at 50°C, which is higher than the DPPC phase transition temperature (Nicolosi et al., 2010).

Characterization of Liposomal Formulations
Morphological Analysis
The morphology of the different types of VAN-containing liposomes or plain liposomes was analyzed by Transmission Electron Microscopy (TEM) (906 LEO-ZEISS, Jena, Germany) at 80 kV. Briefly, one drop of each formulation was added to a copper-coated grid with 200 mesh for 10 s (Electron Microscopy Sciences, Fort Washington, PA). Subsequently, uranyl acetate aqueous solution (2%, w/v) was added and kept at room temperature for 4 h.

Determination of Size, Polydispersity Index, Zeta Potential and Stability of Liposomes
Liposomal vesicles were diluted in deionized water for evaluation of the average size (nm), polydispersity index (PDI), and zeta potential (mV) by the dynamic light scattering using Nano ZS equipment (Malvern Instruments Ltd., Worcestershire, UK, England) at 25°C in triplicate. To evaluate stability of liposomes, these parameters were monitored during 180 days at 4°C.

Vancomycin Encapsulation Efficiency
The encapsulation efficiency (%EE) of VAN into liposomal formulations was determined by the ultrafiltration–centrifugation method (Da Silva et al., 2016) (35). Unencapsulated VAN was separated from encapsulated VAN by ultracentrifugation (Optima L-90K Ultracentrifuge, Beckman Coulter Inc. Pasadena, California, USA) at 120,000g for 2 h at 10°C. Aliquots from the supernatant were diluted in deionized water and analyzed spectrophotometrically at 280 nm (Varian Cary⁺ 50 UV-vis,

Varian Inc., Palo Alto, CA, USA). The %EE was calculated based on the concentration of unencapsulated VAN over the concentration of VAN in solution, using the formula as follows:

$$\%EE = \frac{[VAN\,solution] - [unencapsulated\,VAN]}{[VAN\,solution]} \times 100$$

Evaluation of Vancomycin Release *In Vitro*
The drug release assay was performed using the Franz vertical diffusion cell (Franz, 1975), which consists of two compartments—one donor and one receptor—separated by a regenerated cellulose membrane (Spectra/Por® 2) with molecular exclusion limit of 12,000–14,000 Da (Spectrum Laboratories Inc., Rancho Dominguez, CA, USA) (de Araujo et al., 2008; Da Silva et al., 2016). An aliquot of 1 ml of the liposomal suspensions was added to the donor compartment, while the receptor compartment was filled with 4 ml of buffer (pH 7.4), maintained at 37°C and 400 rpm agitation. Aliquots of the receptor medium were removed throughout the 10-hour experiment and analyzed by spectrophotometry at 280 nm (Varian Cary® 50 UV-Vis, Varian Inc., Palo Alto, CA, USA). The collected volume was replaced with fresh medium due to the dilution effect.

Evaluation of Antimicrobial Activity
Microorganisms and Growth Conditions
Methicillin-susceptible *S. aureus* (MSSA) ATCC 29213 and methicillin-resistant *S. aureus* (MRSA) ATCC 43300 strains were used in this study. Microorganisms were maintained in Tryptone Soy Broth (TSB) (Difco®, New Jersey, USA) with 20% glycerol at −80°C, and cultivated onto Tryptone Soy Agar (Difco®, New Jersey, USA) plates at 37°C. Mueller Hinton Broth (MHB) (Difco®, New Jersey, USA) was used in the MIC assay, while Brain Heart Infusion (Difco®, New Jersey, USA) plus 1% D-glucose (Sigma-Aldrich, St. Louis, MO, USA) was used in the biofilm killing assays.

Experimental Groups
Test formulations consisted of VAN-containing and VAN-free LUV, LUV$_{fuso}$ and LUV$_{cat}$. The experimental groups were set as follows: A—culture medium, test formulation and inoculum; B—culture medium, control formulation and inoculum; C—culture medium, free VAN solution and inoculum; D—culture medium, HEPES buffer (vehicle) and inoculum; E—culture medium and test formulation; F—culture medium and inoculum; and G—culture medium alone.

Minimum Inhibitory Concentration (MIC)
The MIC was determined by the microdilution method, as previously described by the CLSI (2012), using Mueller-Hinton Broth. The formulations were added to 96-well microplates and serially diluted to obtain concentrations ranging from 0.025 to 50 µg/ml. From 18–24 h agar cultures, three to five colonies of *S. aureus* were dispersed into saline solution and bacterial inoculum was adjusted using a spectrophotometer (λ 625nm, OD 0.1, 1 to 2 × 10^8 CFU/ml). Then, the inoculum was diluted and

transferred to the wells at a final concentration of 5×10^4 CFU/ml. The plates were incubated at 37°C for 24 h and the absorbance was read at 620 nm (Biochrom ASYS UVM 340, Biochrom, Cambridge, England). The MIC was defined as the lowest concentration of the formulation which inhibited visible bacterial growth. The experiments were performed in six replicates.

Inhibitory Effects on Biofilm Formation

The liposomal formulations were tested for their ability to inhibit biofilm formation and adherence according to the protocol proposed by Graziano et al. (2015) and Wu et al. (2013). First, BHI medium supplemented with 1% glucose and S. aureus cell suspension (final concentration of 5×10^4 CFU/ml) were added to 96-well U-bottom microplates. Right after, the test formulations were added to the wells and plates were then incubated for 24 h, at 37°C. After this period, the supernatant was removed, and the wells were washed three times with distilled water to remove loosely bound or non-adhered cells. Biofilms were stained with 0.4% crystal violet, solubilized with 98% ethanol and read in a microplate reader at 575 nm (Asys UVM 340, Biochrom, Cambridge, England).

Inhibitory Effects on Biofilm Viability

The liposomal formulations were next tested for their inhibitory effects on biofilm viability, as previously described (Graziano et al., 2015) (39). Cellulose acetate membranes (25 mm diameter, 0.2 μM pores) (Sartorius Stedim GmbH, Guxhagen, Hessen, Germany) were used as substrates for S. aureus biofilm formation. The membranes were placed in 6-well plates containing BHI medium supplemented with 1% glucose and bacterial suspension (approximately 1×10^6 CFU/ml in each well). The plates were incubated at 37°C for 24 h. Then the membranes were transferred to new plates containing fresh BHI plus 1% glucose, and biofilms were treated with the formulations at $1 \times$ MIC, $10 \times$ MIC, and $50 \times$ MIC for 24 h. Treated biofilm-coated membranes were gently washed (three times) through immersion into 5 ml of 0.9% NaCl. Then, the membranes were transferred to other tubes containing freshly 5 ml of 0.9% NaCl and then sonicated with six pulses of 9.9 s, 5 s time-interval, 5% amplitude (VibraCell 400W, Sonics & Materials Inc., Newtown, CT, USA) and vortexed at 3,800 rpm for 30 s. Ten-microliter aliquots were collected from each tube, serially diluted, and plated for CFUs onto TSA. The plates were incubated at 37°C for 24 h.

Statistical Analysis

The data distribution was analyzed using the Shapiro–Wilks test. The variables size, PDI, zeta potential, and %EE, were compared using unpaired t-test. Stability parameters for liposomes and the biofilm data were compared using analysis of variance (ANOVA) followed by Tukey's post-hoc test. The drug release profile was analyzed by two-way ANOVA followed by Tukey's post-hoc test. Statistical analyses were performed on Origin 8.0 (Microcal TM Software Inc., EUA) and GraphPad Prism 6.0 (San Diego, California, USA). The data were presented as mean and standard deviation (SD), with a 5% significance level. All data are representative of three independent experiments.

RESULTS

Characterization of Liposomal Formulations

TEM images confirmed that the liposomal vesicles had spherical shape with clear edges. Vesicle size in all formulations ranged between 100 and 200 nm. Micrographs of all liposomal formulations are presented in **Figure 1**. As exemplified in **Figures 1C, D**, some fusogenic vesicles were found to merge with each other, which typically characterizes this type of liposome.

The means and standard deviations of size, PDI, zeta potential and %EE of the liposomal formulations are given in **Table 1**. Comparisons were made between plain and VAN-containing liposomes. No differences in size were found while PDI values increased for VAN-containing formulations in comparison to plain controls ($p < 0.05$). Moreover, as expected, the zeta potential values confirmed the presence of negative charges on LUV and LUV_{fuso} liposomes and positive charges on LUV_{cat}. The encapsulation decreased the negative zeta potentials of LUV_{fuso} VAN liposomes ($p < 0.05$), while it increased the positive zeta potential in LUV_{cat} VAN, as compared to their respective controls ($p < 0.05$). Higher %EE values were observed for LUV VAN, followed by LUV_{fuso} VAN and LUV_{cat} VAN.

The stability of the formulations was determined from measurements of size, PDI and zeta potential (**Figures 2A–C**) during storage at 4°C. In general, LUV_{cat} VAN, LUV_{fuso} VAN and LUV VAN kept their size during the 180-day experimental period ($p > 0.05$). LUV VAN showed an increase in size after 7 days of storage ($p < 0.05$) but kept their size in the other time points. LUV_{cat} VAN also changed in size after 60 and 90 days ($p < 0.05$). However, these alterations were no greater than 10% of the initial size. No significant changes in PDI and Zeta values were found during the experiment ($p > 0.05$). It is also worth noting that, although with an increasingly trend, PDI values were found to be under 0.2, as required for a monodisperse size distribution.

The release kinetics of VAN in solution and encapsulated in the liposomal formulations was determined in vitro. As seen in **Figure 3**, encapsulated VAN formulations showed prolonged releases overtime as compared to free VAN ($p < 0.05$).

The LUV VAN formulation showed slower release profile than the other liposomes ($p < 0.05$), whereas LUV_{fuso} VAN and LUV_{cat} VAN were found to have very similar release kinetics ($p > 0.05$). As expected, VAN-free formulations showed greater percent release at all timepoints, with a significant difference from the other liposomal formulations ($p < 0.05$).

Antimicrobial Activity

Free and encapsulated VAN LUV formulations affected bacterial growth in both MSSA (29213) and MRSA (43300) strains, with MIC values ranging between 0.78 and 1.56 μg/ml. These findings are in line with the information provided by the CLSI concerning S. aureus susceptibility to VAN (CLSI, 2012).

Next, the formulations were tested for their inhibitory effects on S. aureus ATCC 29213 biofilm adherence and formation. As shown in **Figure 4**, treatment with all formulations inhibited biofilm formation in a dose-dependent

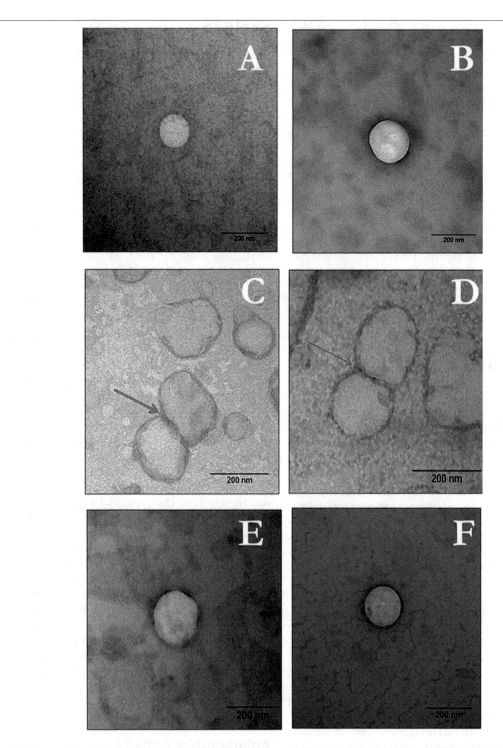

FIGURE 1 | TEM images of LUV VAN, LUV$_{fuso\ VAN}$, and LUV$_{ca}$ VAN. The left panel represents plain vesicles and the right panel indicated VAN-containing LUVs as follows: **(A, B)** LUV; **(C, D)** LUV$_{fuso}$; and **(E, F)** LUV$_{cat}$. Bars indicate 200 nm, with 100,000× magnification).

fashion. Free VAN was found to inhibit biofilm formation at MIC (1.56 µg/ml) and higher concentrations as compared to the untreated biofilm control, while the inhibitory effects of liposome-encapsulated VAN were only seen from 2 × MIC (3.13 µg/ml).

These results corroborate those of the *in vitro* release kinetics assay (**Figure 3**), in which encapsulated VAN showed a late release profile as compared to free VAN. These can be attributed to the % amount of VAN encapsulated into the liposomes, so that just a fraction amount of VAN is available to immediately

TABLE 1 | Mean (± SD) of the size (nm), polydispersity index (PDI), zeta potential (mV) and encapsulation efficiency (%EE) of the liposomal formulations developed in this study.

Formulation	Size (nm ± SD)	PDI (± SD)	Zeta Potential (mV ± SD)	%EE (± SD)
LUV	157.53 ± 2.58	0.09 ± 0.03	−19.2 ± 5.5	–
LUV VAN	152.60 ± 0.80	0.17 ± 0.01*	−16.9 ± 0.5	32.5 ± 0.1
LUV$_{fuso}$	161.87 ± 2.45	0.14 ± 0.02	−48.6 ± 4.9	–
LUV$_{fuso}$ VAN	153.37 ± 0.70	0.20 ± 0.01*	−41.3 ± 2.3*	11.4 ± 0.1
LUV$_{cat}$	130.97 ± 1.59	0.13 ± 0.01	50.6 ± 3.5	–
LUV$_{cat}$ VAN	139.73 ± 2.55	0.18 ± 0.02*	62.5 ± 5.6*	10.1 ± 0.1

The asterisk "*" indicates statistically significant difference between plain (LUV, LUV$_{FUSO}$, LUV$_{CAT}$) and their respective vancomycin-containing liposomes (LUV VAN, LUV$_{FUSO}$ VAN, LUV$_{CAT}$ VAN), p < 0.05 (unpaired t-test).

act. Thus, it is likely that a lower amount of VAN molecules was initially released from the liposomal formulations, thereby slowing up their overall antimicrobial effects.

The inhibitory effects of the formulations on biofilm viability were also investigated. **Figure 5** shows the mean (± SD) CFU/ml (Log$_{10}$) of biofilms treated for 24 h at 1 × MIC, 10 × MIC, and 50 × MIC. The data was compared among treatment groups and the untreated control. At 1 × MIC, only LUV$_{cat}$ VAN caused a significant decrease in the number of viable biofilm cells ($p <$ 0.01). Nevertheless, at 10 × MIC and 50 × MIC all formulations showed significant inhibitory effects as compared to the untreated control ($p <$ 0.05). Free VAN was not able to affect biofilm viability significantly at 10 × MIC (p > 0.05), but it did at 50 × MIC (p < 0.05). When liposomal formulations were compared among themselves, we observed that LUV$_{fuso}$ VAN had the most

noticeable inhibitory potential on mature biofilms, followed by LUV$_{cat}$ VAN and LUV VAN, with significant differences among them (p < 0.05).

The effects on mature biofilms treated with LUV$_{cat}$ VAN and free VAN were found to be similar at 50 × MIC (p > 0.05) and greater than those promoted by LUV VAN ($p <$ 0.05). LUV$_{fuso}$ VAN was the most active formulation against *S. aureus* biofilm viability when compared to the other groups ($p <$ 0.05). LUV$_{fuso}$ VAN reduced biofilm viability by 3.5 Log$_{10}$ CFU/ml (35×); LUV$_{cat}$ VAN and free VAN caused a reduction of 2.5 Log$_{10}$ CFU/ml (25×), while LUV VAN reduced biofilm viability by 1 log$_{10}$ CFU/ml (10×) in comparison to the control.

DISCUSSION

Nosocomial and community-acquired MRSA infections remain a major concern in global health and have driven the adoption of public policies and medical research in this field (Honary et al., 2013; Elkhodairy et al., 2014; Holland et al., 2014). Evidence has shown the promising results of liposomal vesicles as drug carriers for pharmaceutical application (Kim et al., 1999; Nicolosi et al., 2010; Ma et al., 2011) (25, 26, 30). Herein, we report the development, characterization, and antimicrobial properties of experimental formulations containing VAN encapsulated into conventional, fusogenic and cationic liposomes. We compared the different formulations and demonstrated that the drug-delivery liposomes were more active than VAN in solution in reducing mature biofilm, with better efficacy for LUV$_{fuso}$ VAN.

Our goal when selecting the liposomal formulations was to achieve greater interaction with bacterial cells and, thereby, facilitate penetration into mature biofilms. Conventional (LUV)

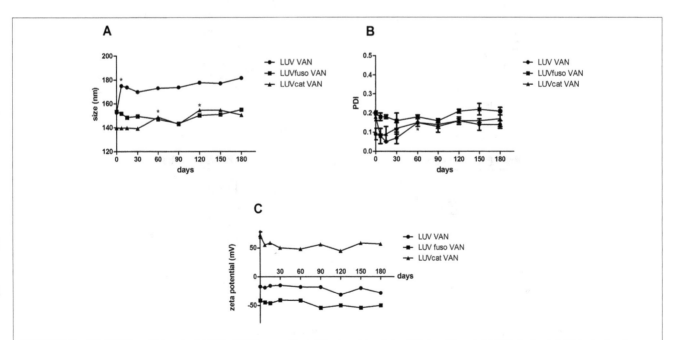

FIGURE 2 | Size **(A)**, PDI **(B)** and Zeta potential **(C)** for VAN liposomal formulations analyses during 180 days. The asterisk "*" indicates statistically significant difference between the drug treatment and its respective untreated control at $p < 0.05$ (One-way ANOVA, followed by Tukey's post-hoc test).

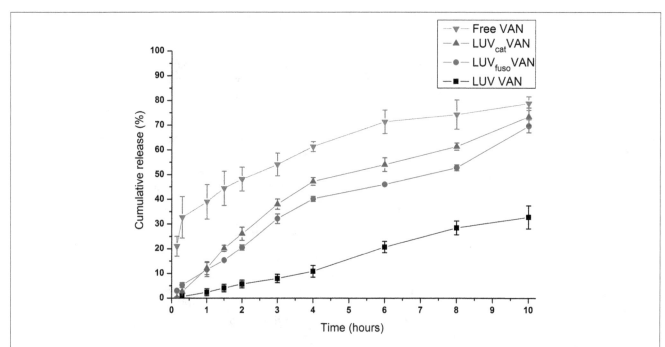

FIGURE 3 | *In vitro* release kinetics of VAN in solution and encapsulated in the liposomal formulations, at 37°C. Two-way ANOVA, Tukey, P < 0.05. There were statistical difference between groups, as follows: LUV VAN × LUV_fuso VAN—from 1 to 10 h; LUV VAN × LUV_cat VAN—from 1 to 10h; LUV VAN × free VAN—from 0.15 to 10 h; LUV_fuso VAN × free VAN—from 0.15 to 8 h; LUVcat VAN × free VAN—from 0.15 to 8 h.

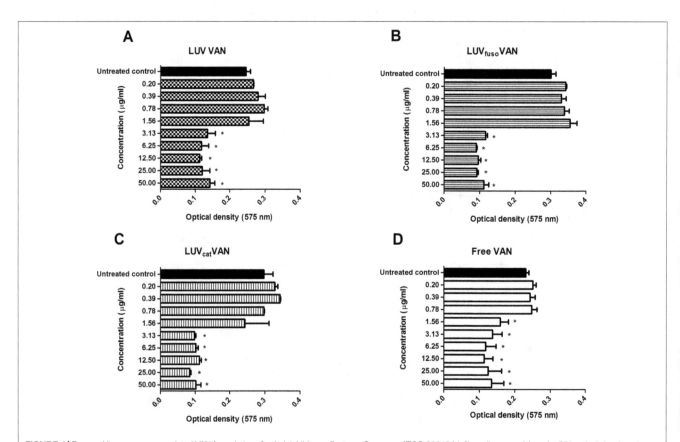

FIGURE 4 | Free and liposome-encapsulated VAN formulations for their inhibitory effects on S. *aureus* ATCC 29213 biofilm adherence. Mean (± SD) optical density values of S. *aureus* biofilms treated with different concentrations of VAN encapsulated into LUV VAN **(A)**, LUV_fuso VAN **(B)**, LUV_cat VAN **(C)**, or free VAN solution **(D)**. The asterisk "*" indicates statistically significant difference between the drug treatment and its respective untreated control at $p < 0.05$ (One-way ANOVA, followed by Tukey's post-hoc test).

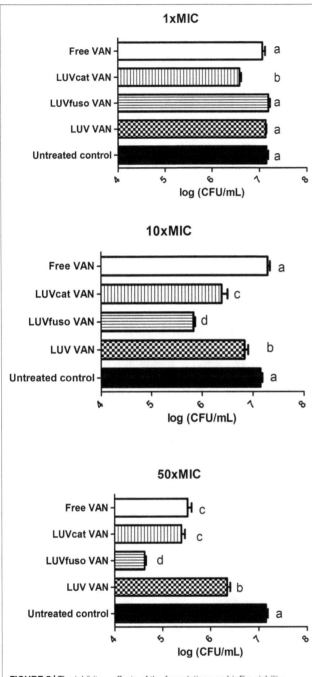

FIGURE 5 | The inhibitory effects of the formulations on biofilm viability. Inhibitory effects of liposomal and plain formulations on *S. aureus* ATCC 29213 mature biofilm viability at 1 × MIC, 10 × MIC, and 50 × MIC. The values are expressed as mean (± SD) of CFU/ml. Different letters indicate significant differences between groups ($p < 0.05$ One-way ANOVA, with Tukey's post-hoc test).

bilayers due to the presence of DOPE. Additionally, EPC and CHEMS contribute to greater stability of the formulation (Aoki et al., 2015; Nicolosi et al., 2015). LUV_{cat} liposomes contained stearylamine, EPC, and cholesterol in their composition. Sa is a positively charged lipid that facilitates, through electrostatic interactions, adsorption in the negatively charged bacterial biofilm (Balazs and Godbey, 2011). In order to prevent lipid oxidation, the antioxidant alpha-tocopherol was added to all liposomal formulations (de Paula et al., 2012).

The effect of VAN encapsulation was observed in changes in the Zeta values and size distribution in comparison to controls (**Table 1**). Such changes may have occurred because encapsulated VAN has a tendency to be located in the aqueous core or adjacent lipid-water interface near the polar head groups (Bozzuto and Molinari, 2015). This molecular location of VAN in liposomes could contribute to the reduction of size distribution homogeneity and enhance electrostatic attraction among liposomes, as VAN is positively charged. Similar results concerning vesicle size and PDI were also found with tetraether lipid liposomes (Uhl et al., 2017). Moreover, after 180 days of storage (4°C) the structural properties of the liposomes were maintained after VAN encapsulation, presenting desirable size and monodisperse distribution, as required for a drug delivery system.

LUV VAN and LUV_{cat} VAN showed higher %EE (32.5% and 10.1%, respectively) than those already reported (2.0% and 5.0%, respectively) using equivalent (conventional, cationic) liposomes, but prepared by sonication and containing 20 mg/ml VAN (Kadry et al., 2004). On the other hand, Nicolosi et al. (2010) observed greater %EE (65.8%) for fusogenic liposomes (prepared by the reverse-phase evaporation method) as compared to our findings (11.4%) (Nicolosi et al., 2010). According to the authors, the preparation method and drug concentration in the liposomal suspension may have influenced the high upload (Muppidi et al., 2012).

In this study, no significant difference was observed in the release kinetics of VAN-containing LUV_{fuso} and LUV_{cat}. Both formulations released 12% of VAN after 1 h, whereas LUV VAN released 2% and free VAN 33%. The differences in the drug controlled release profile among the liposomal formulations may be a result of their diverse %EE (Lankalapalli et al., 2015; Liu et al., 2015). Recently (Lankalapalli et al., 2015), evaluated the release kinetics of VAN from conventional liposomes EPC : Chol liposomes with VAN (10 mg/ml), prepared by the ethanol injection method. The authors observed similar results to those found in our study regarding VAN release from LUV VAN liposomes, and different results with regard to release of free VAN, which was about 42% after 22 h. This divergence may be related to the free VAN concentration used in the donor compartment, which was 100 mg/ml in the study by Lankalapalli et al. and 10 mg/ml in our study.

It is also known that VAN exerts antibacterial action by inhibiting the synthesis of cell wall peptidoglycans (Howden et al., 2010). This drug has a high affinity to the D-Ala-D-Ala residue from the peptidoglycan precursor, lipid II, thereby blocking the addition of final precursors by transglycosylation and transpeptidation, which ultimately interrupts cell wall formation.

liposomes contain a mixture of EPC and cholesterol, which increases the rigidity and stability of the vesicles (de Paula et al., 2012). LUV_{fuso} liposomes contain DOPE in their composition, which promotes destabilization of the lipid bilayer (towards inverse hexagonal structures) at acidic pH as it occurs in infected tissue. The use of DPPC was required for stabilization of the lipid

In *S. aureus*, peptidoglycan biosynthesis takes place in the cell division septum in a specific site of the cytoplasmic membrane (Howden et al., 2010). Thus, in order to promote its effects on the cell wall, VAN molecules should penetrate approximately 20 layers of peptidoglycan to reach the division septum and bind to the protein fraction (L-lysine-D-alanyl-D-alanine) of murein monomers used as a substrate for glycosyltransferases. Depending on the bacterial cell cycle phase, the division septum can be completely formed or under formation (Nicolosi et al., 2010). Hence, the distance between the cell wall and the plasma membrane is shorter at the early phases of bacterial growth, which might have contributed to the bactericidal effects of free VAN. However, when bacterial growth reaches a final stage, the division septum is completely formed. As a result, the distance between the cell wall and the plasma membrane is wider, which may hinder the action of free VAN. In this case scenario, it is believed that encapsulated VAN could more effectively penetrate the cell wall and reach the periplasmic space, therefore promoting its antibacterial effects (Sande et al., 2012; Nicolosi et al., 2015). Such increased penetration can explain the improved antibiofilm activity observed in our study for the liposomal formulations.

The MIC values of liposome-encapsulated VAN on *S. aureus* ATCC 29213 observed in our study are in agreement with those found by Kadry et al. (2004). These authors reported MIC values of 0.75 µg/ml and 1.50 µg/ml for cationic and conventional liposomes, respectively. Another study found that encapsulation of VAN into conventional liposomes reduced by 2 the MIC against MRSA strains as compared to free VAN (Sande et al., 2012). This liposomal formulation was composed of DSPC : DCP:Chol (7:2:1, mol%) containing VAN at 50 mg/ml, which was 5 times higher than the VAN concentration used in our study.

Our findings indicate that free VAN at MIC had better inhibitory effects on early stages of biofilm formation than had the liposomal formulations. The latter inhibited biofilm adherence only from 2 × MIC, probably due to the encapsulation of vancomycin into the liposomes, with less free drug available to interact with forming biofilm. On the other hand, the liposomal formulations showed improved antibacterial activity than free VAN against mature biofilms, particularly LUV$_{fuso}$ VAN which was the most effective. Therefore, encapsulated VAN showed greater bactericidal effects on mature biofilms probably due to its increased ability to penetrate the peptidoglycan layers, whereas free VAN remained trapped in the cell wall.

Fusogenic liposomes have an increased potential to interact with extracellular matrix and cell wall due to their ability to merge with lipid membranes (Forier et al., 2014; Nicolosi et al., 2015). These vesicles are composed of lipids that promote destabilization of the lipid bilayers (Forier et al., 2014) and their fusion with the bacterial cell wall was previously proved through flow cytometry, lipid-mixing assay, electronic transmission microscopy and immunochemistry (Beaulac et al., 1998; Sachetelli et al., 2000; Forier et al., 2014; Wang et al., 2016). These vesicles can pass through the cell wall and deliver VAN into the periplasmic space, thereby making it easier for the drug to reach the division septum

and block peptidoglycan biosynthesis (Howden et al., 2010; Sande et al., 2012; Nicolosi et al., 2015). Besides, cationic liposomes may have a higher affinity for negatively charged biofilms, which can decrease VAN delivery time into the infectious focus (Kim et al., 1999; Kadry et al., 2004). Accordingly, these liposomes probably release VAN in the vicinities of the bacterial cell wall due to the affinity with its negative charge, resulting in inhibition of cell wall biosynthesis.

There are other studies with VAN-loaded liposomal formulations (Ma et al., 2011; Barakat et al., 2014), but very few tested the ability in inhibit or eradicate *S. aureus* biofilm, which is a more resistant form of growth and much less sensitive to antibiotics. In the present study, we compared two formulations that are claimed to be effective against bacterial growth: fusogenic and cationic vesicles. Both formulations were effective in reducing mature biofilm, but with superiority to fusogenic vesicles.

To the best of the author´s knowledge, there are only two studies that encapsulate vancomycin into fusogenic liposomes (Nicolosi et al., 2010; Garcia et al., 2017), but none of them tested the activity against *S. aureus*. In addition, there are other non-fusogenic VAN-loaded liposomes that were tested against *S. aureus*, but very few aimed to test against biofilm (Ma et al., 2011; Barakat et al., 2014). Other drug delivery systems have also been proposed to improve drug delivery at sites of infection and to overcome antimicrobial resistance, such as injectable and biodegradable hydrogels (Zhao et al., 2017; Qu et al., 2018; Liang et al., 2019; Qu et al., 2019), polymeric nanoparticles (Lakshminarayanan et al., 2018), metal-based nanoparticles (Brown et al., 2012; Noronha et al., 2017), carbon-based nanoparticles (Zhao et al., 2017; Jiang et al., 2018), etc. Contributing to the development and comparison of antibiotics delivery systems, the present study showed that the liposomes here tested can reduce the formation and viability of mature biofilm, in a way superior to free vancomycin.

CONCLUSION

We demonstrated the successful development, characterization and stability of LUV, LUV$_{fuso}$ and LUV$_{cat}$ encapsulated VAN formulations. Liposomes improved the antimicrobial activity of vancomycin against *S. aureus* biofilm, with better efficacy for fusogenic vesicles. Future studies are needed to validate this formulation as a candidate for *S. aureus* infection control.

AUTHOR CONTRIBUTIONS

AS: Conception and design of the project. Acquisition of data. Analysis and interpretation of data. Writing and revision of the manuscript. Approval of the final version of the manuscript. VC: Acquisition of data. Analysis and interpretation of data. Final approval of the version to be published. LR: Acquisition of data. Analysis and interpretation of data. Writing and revision of the manuscript. Approval of the final version of the manuscript. IF: Writing and revision of the manuscript. Approval of the final version of the manuscript. FG: Conception and design of the project. Analysis and interpretation of data. Approval of the final version. EP: Conception and design of the project. Analysis and interpretation of data. Writing and revision of the manuscript. Approval of the final version. MF-M: Conception and design of the project. Analysis and interpretation of data. Writing and revision of the manuscript. Approval of the final version. KC-M: Conception and design of the project. Coordination and execution of the experiments. Analysis and interpretation

of data. Writing and revision of the manuscript. Approval of the final version of the manuscript.

ACKNOWLEDGMENTS

The authors thank the São Paulo Research Foundation (FAPESP, grant no. 2014/14457-5) for financial support and Teuto/Pfizer for kindly donating the vancomycin.

REFERENCES

Aoki, A., Akaboshi, H., Ogura, T., Aikawa, T., Kondo, T., and Tobori, N. (2015). Preparation of pH-sensitive anionic liposomes designed for drug delivery system (DDS) application. *J. Oleo. Sci.* 64, 233–242. doi: 10.5650/jos.ess14157

Balazs, D. A., and Godbey, W. (2011). Liposomes for use in gene delivery. *J. Drug Delivery* 2011, 326497. doi: 10.1155/2011/326497

Barakat, H. S., Kassem, M. A., El-Khordagui, L. K., and Khalafallah, N. M. (2014). Vancomycin-eluting niosomes: a new approach to the inhibition of staphylococcal biofilm on abiotic surfaces. *AAPS PharmSciTech.* 15 (5), 1263–1274. doi: 10.1208/s12249-014-0141-8

Beaulac, C., Sachetelli, S., and Lagace, J. (1998). In-vitro bactericidal efficacy of sub-MIC concentrations of liposome-encapsulated antibiotic against Gram-negative and Gram-positive bacteria. *J. Antimicrob. Chemother.* 41 (1), 35–41 doi: 10.1093/jac/41.1.35

Bozzuto, G., and Molinari, A. (2015). Liposomes as nanomedical devices. *Int. J. Nanomed.* 10, 975–999. doi: 10.2147/IJN.S68861

Brown, A. N., Smith, K., Samuels, T. A., Lu, J., Obare, S. O., and Scott, M. E. (2012). Nanoparticles functionalized with ampicillin destroy multiple-antibiotic-resistant isolates of Pseudomonas aeruginosa and Enterobacter aerogenes and methicillin-resistant Staphylococcus aureus. *Appl. Environ. Microbiol.* 78 (8), 2768–2774. doi: 10.1128/AEM.06513-11

Butler, M. S., Hansford, K. A., Blaskovich, M. A., Halai, R., and Cooper, M. A. (2014). Glycopeptide antibiotics: back to the future. *J. Antibiot.* 67, 631–644. doi: 10.1038/ja.2014.111

Cereda, C. M., Brunetto, G. B., de Araújo, D. R., and de Paula, E. (2006).Liposomal formulations of prilocaine, lidocaine and mepivacaine prolong analgesic duration. *Can. J. Anaesth.* 53, 1092–1097. Available at: https://www.ncbi.nlm.nih.gov/pubmed/17079635. doi: 10.1007/BF03022876

Chakraborty, S. P., Sahu, S. K., Pramanik, P., and Roy, S. (2012). In vitro antimicrobial activity of nanoconjugated vancomycin against drug resistant Staphylococcus aureus. *Int. J. Pharm.* 436, 659–676. doi: 10.1016/j.ijpharm.2012.07.033

CLSI (2012). "Performance Standards for Antimicrobial Susceptibility Testing - Twenty-Second Informational Supplement": In *M100-S25*, vol. 32, 3.

Da Silva, C. M. G., Fraceto, L. F., Franz-Montan, M., Couto, V. M., Casadei, B. R., Cereda, C. M. S., et al. (2016). Development of egg PC/cholesterol/α-tocopherol liposomes with ionic gradients to deliver ropivacaine. *J. Liposome Res.* 26 (1), 1–10. doi: 10.3109/08982104.2015.1022555

de Araujo, D. R., Cereda, C. M. S., Brunetto, G. B., Vomero, V. U., Pierucci, A., Neto, H. S., et al. (2008). Pharmacological and local toxicity studies of a liposomal formulation for the novel local anaesthetic ropivacaine. *J. Pharm. Pharmacol.* 60 (11), 1449–1457. doi: 10.1211/jpp/60.11.0005

de Paula, E., Cereda, C. M., Fraceto, L. F., de Araújo, D. R., Franz-Montan, M., Tofoli, G. R., et al. (2012). Micro and nanosystems for delivering local anesthetics. *Expert Opin. Drug Deliv.* 9, 1505–1524. doi: 10.1517/17425247.2012.738664

Dong, D., Thomas, N., Thierry, B., Vreugde, S., Prestidge, C. A., and Wormald, P. J. (2015). Distribution and Inhibition of Liposomes on Staphylococcus aureus and Pseudomonas aeruginosa Biofilm. *PloS One* 10, e0131806. doi: 10.1371/journal.pone.0131806

Drulis-Kawa, Z., Dorotkiewicz-Jach, A., Gubernator, J., Gula, G., Bocer, T., and Doroszkiewicz, W. (2009). The interaction between Pseudomonas aeruginosa cells and cationic PC : Chol:DOTAP liposomal vesicles versus outer-membrane structure and envelope properties of bacterial cell. *Int. J. Pharm.* 367, 211–219. doi: 10.1016/j.ijpharm.2008.09.043

Elkhodairy, K. A., Afifi, S. A., and Zakaria, A. S. (2014). A promising approach to provide appropriate colon target drug delivery systems of vancomycin HCL: pharmaceutical and microbiological studies. *Biomed. Res. Int.* 2014, 182197. doi: 10.1155/2014/182197

Forier, K., Raemdonck, K., De Smedt, S. C., Demeester, J., Coenye, T., and Braeckmans, K. (2014). Lipid and polymer nanoparticles for drug delivery to bacterial biofilms. *J. Control Release* 190, 607–623. doi: 10.1016/j.jconrel.2014.03.055

Franz, T. J. (1975). Percutaneous absorption on the relevance of in vitro data. *J. Invest. Dermatol.* 64, 190–195. Available at: https://www.ncbi.nlm.nih.gov/pubmed/123263. doi: 10.1111/1523-1747.ep12533356

Garcia, C. B., Shi, D., and Webster, T. J. (2017). Tat-functionalized liposomes for the treatment of meningitis: An in vitro study. *Int. J. Nanomed.* 12, 3009–3021. doi: 10.2147/IJN.S130125

Graziano, T. S., Cuzzullin, M. C., Franco, G. C., Schwartz-Filho, H. O., de Andrade, E. D., Groppo, F. C., et al. (2015). Statins and antimicrobial effects: simvastatin as a potential drug against Staphylococcus aureus biofilm. *PloS One* 10, e0128098. doi: 10.1371/journal.pone.0128098

Gudiol, C., Cuervo, G., Shaw, E., Pujol, M., and Carratalà, J. (2017). Pharmacotherapeutic options for treating Staphylococcus aureus bacteremia. *Expert Opin. Pharmacother.* 18, 1947–1963. doi: 10.1080/14656566.2017.1403585

Holland, T. L., Arnold, C., and Fowler, V. G. (2014). Clinical management of Staphylococcus aureus bacteremia: a review. *JAMA* 312, 1330–1341. doi: 10.1001/jama.2014.9743

Honary, S., Ebrahimi, P., and Hadianamrei, R. (2013).Optimization of size and encapsulation efficiency of 5-FU loaded chitosan nanoparticles by response surface methodology. *Curr. Drug Deliv.* 10, 742–752. Available at: https://www.ncbi.nlm.nih.gov/pubmed/24274636. doi: 10.1001/jama.2014.9743

Howden, B. P., Davies, J. K., Johnson, P. D., Stinear, T. P., and Grayson, M. L. (2010). Reduced vancomycin susceptibility in Staphylococcus aureus, including vancomycin-intermediate and heterogeneous vancomycin-intermediate strains: resistance mechanisms, laboratory detection, and clinical implications. *Clin. Microbiol. Rev.* 23, 99–139. doi: 10.1128/CMR.00042-09

Jiang, L., Su, C., Ye, S., Wu, J., Zhu, Z., Wen, Y., et al. (2018). Synergistic antibacterial 2nanostructures. *Nanotechnology* 29 (50), 505102. doi: 10.1088/1361-6528/aae424

Kadry, A. A., Al-Suwayeh, S. A., Abd-Allah, A. R., and Bayomi, M. A. (2004). Treatment of experimental osteomyelitis by liposomal antibiotics. *J. Antimicrob. Chemother.* 54, 1103–1108. doi: 10.1093/jac/dkh465

Khameneh, B., Zarei, H., and Bazzaz, B. S. F. (2014). The effect of silver nanoparticles on Staphylococcus epidermidis biofilm biomass and cell viability. *Nanomed. J.* 1, 302–307. doi: 10.7508/NMJ.2015.05.003

Kim, H. J., and Jones, M. N. (2004). The delivery of benzyl penicillin to Staphylococcus aureus biofilms by use of liposomes. *J. Liposome Res.* 14, 123–139. doi: 10.1081/LPR-200029887

Kim, H. J., Michael Gias, E. L., and Jones, M. N. (1999). "The adsorption of cationic liposomes to Staphylococcus aureus biofilms": In *Colloids and Surfaces A: Physicochemical and Engineering Aspects*. doi: 10.1016/S0927-7757(98)00765-1

Lakshminarayanan, R., Ye, E., Young, D. J., Li, Z., and Loh, X. J. (2018). Recent advances in the development of antimicrobial nanoparticles for combating resistant pathogens. *Adv. Healthc. Mater.* 7 (13), e1701400 doi: 10.1002/adhm.201701400

Lankalapalli, S., Vinai Kumar Tenneti, V. S., and Nimmali, S. K. (2015). Design and development of vancomycin liposomes. *Ind. J. Pharm. Educ. Res.* 49, 208–215. doi: 10.5530/ijper.49.3.6

Liang, Y., Zhao, X., Ma, P. X., Guo, B., Du, Y., and Han, X. (2019). pH-responsive injectable hydrogels with mucosal adhesiveness based on chitosan-grafted-dihydrocaffeic acid and oxidized pullulan for localized drug delivery. *J. Colloid Interface Sci.* 536 (15), 224–234. doi: 10.1016/j.jcis.2018.10.056

Liu, J., Wang, Z., Li, F., Gao, J., Wang, L., and Huang, G. (2015). Liposomes for systematic delivery of vancomycin hydrochloride to decrease nephrotoxicity: characterization and evaluation. *Asian J. Pharm. Sci.* 10 (3), 212–222. doi: 10.1016/j.ajps.2014.12.004

Ma, T., Shang, B. C., Tang, H., Zhou, T. H., Xu, G. L., Li, H. L., et al. (2011). Nano-hydroxyapatite/chitosan/konjac glucomannan scaffolds loaded with cationic liposomal vancomycin: preparation, in vitro release and activity against Staphylococcus aureus biofilms. *J. Biomater Sci. Polym. Ed.* 22, 1669–1681. doi: 10.1163/092050611X570644

McAuley, M. A. (2012). Allergic reaction or adverse drug effect: correctly classifying vancomycin-induced hypersensitivity reactions. *J. Emerg. Nurs.* 38, 60–62. doi: 10.1016/j.jen.2011.09.010

McCarthy, H., Rudkin, J. K., Black, N. S., Gallagher, L., O'Neill, E., and O'Gara, J. P. (2015). Methicillin resistance and the biofilm phenotype in Staphylococcus aureus. *Front. Cell Infect. Microbiol.* 5, 1. doi: 10.3389/fcimb.2015.00001

Men, P., Li, H. B., Zhai, S. D., and Zhao, R. S. (2016). Association between the AUC0-24/MIC ratio of vancomycin and its clinical effectiveness: a systematic review and meta-analysis. *PloS One* 11, e0146224. doi: 10.1371/journal.pone.0146224

Moghadas-Sharif, N., Fazly Bazzaz, B. S., Khameneh, B., and Malaeekeh-Nikouei, B. (2015). The effect of nanoliposomal formulations on Staphylococcus epidermidis biofilm. *Drug Dev. Ind. Pharm.* 41, 445–450. doi: 10.3109/03639045.2013.877483

Muppidi, K., Pumerantz, A. S., Wang, J., and Betageri, G. (2012). Development and stability studies of novel liposomal vancomycin formulations. *ISRN Pharm.* 2012, 636743. doi: 10.5402/2012/636743

Nicolosi, D., Scalia, M., Nicolosi, V. M., and Pignatello, R. (2010). Encapsulation in fusogenic liposomes broadens the spectrum of action of vancomycin against Gram-negative bacteria. *Int. J. Antimicrob. Agents* 35, 553–558. doi: 10.1016/j.ijantimicag.2010.01.015

Nicolosi, D., Cupri, S., Genovese, C., Tempera, G., Mattina, R., and Pignatello, R. (2015). Nanotechnology approaches for antibacterial drug delivery: preparation and microbiological evaluation of fusogenic liposomes carrying fusidic acid. *Int. J. Antimicrob. Agents* 45, 622–626. doi: 10.1016/j.ijantimicag.2015.01.016

Noronha, V. T., Paula, A. J., Durán, G., Galembeck, A., Cogo-Müller, K., Franz-Montan, M., et al. (2017). Silver nanoparticles in dentistry. *Dent. Mater.* 33, 1110–1126. doi: 10.1016/j.dental.2017.07.002

Pumerantz, A., Muppidi, K., Agnihotri, S., Guerra, C., Venketaraman, V., Wang, J., et al. (2011). Preparation of liposomal vancomycin and intracellular killing of meticillin-resistant Staphylococcus aureus (MRSA). *Int. J. Antimicrob. Agents* 37, 140–144. doi: 10.1016/j.ijantimicag.2010.10.011

Qu, J., Zhao, X., Liang, Y., Zhang, T., Ma, P. X., and Guo, B. (2018). Antibacterial adhesive injectable hydrogels with rapid self-healing, extensibility and compressibility as wound dressing for joints skin wound healing. *Biomaterials.* 183, 185–199. doi: 10.1016/j.biomaterials.2018.08.044

Qu, J., Zhao, X., Liang, Y., Xu, Y., Ma, P. X., and Guo, B. (2019). Degradable conductive injectable hydrogels as novel antibacterial, anti-oxidant wound dressings for wound healing. *Chem. Eng. J.* 362, 548–560. doi: 10.1016/j.cej.2019.01.028

Rose, W. E., Fallon, M., Moran, J. J., and Vanderloo, J. P. (2012). Vancomycin tolerance in methicillin-resistant Staphylococcus aureus: influence of vancomycin, daptomycin, and telavancin on differential resistance gene expression. *Antimicrob. Agents Chemother.* 56, 4422–4427. doi: 10.1128/AAC.00676-12

Sachetelli, S., Khalil, H., Chen, T., Beaulac, C., Sénéchal, S., and Lagacé, J. (2000). Demonstration of a fusion mechanism between a fluid bactericidal liposomal formulation and bacterial cells. *Biochim. Biophys. Acta - Biomembr.* 1463 (2), 254–266. doi: 10.1016/S0005-2736(99)00217-5

Sande, L., Sanchez, M., Montes, J., Wolf, A. J., Morgan, M. A., Omri, A., et al. (2012). Liposomal encapsulation of vancomycin improves killing of methicillin-resistant Staphylococcus aureus in a murine infection model. *J. Antimicrob. Chemother.* 67, 2191–2194. doi: 10.1093/jac/dks212

Shi, J., Mao, N. F., Wang, L., Zhang, H. B., Chen, Q., Liu, H., et al. (2014). Efficacy of combined vancomycin and fosfomycin against methicillin-resistant Staphylococcus aureus in biofilms in vivo. *PloS One* 9, e113133. doi: 10.1371/journal.pone.0113133

Uhl, P., Pantze, S., Storck, P., Parmentier, J., Witzigmann, D., Hofhaus, G., et al. (2017). Oral delivery of vancomycin by tetraether lipid liposomes. *Eur. J. Pharm. Sci.* 108, 111–118. doi: 10.1016/j.ejps.2017.07.013

Torchilin, V. (2012). "Liposomes in Drug Delivery," in *Fundamentals and Applications of Controlled Release Drug Delivery.* Eds. J. Siepmann, R. A. Siegel, M. J. Rathbone (Springer), 289–328.

Wang, Z., Ma, Y., Khalil, H., Wang, R., Lu, T., Zhao, W., et al. (2016). Fusion between fluid liposomes and intact bacteria: Study of driving parameters and in vitro bactericidal efficacy. *Int. J. Nanomed.* 11, 4025–4036. doi: 10.2147/IJN.S55807

Wu, W. S., Chen, C. C., Chuang, Y. C., Su, B. A., Chiu, Y. H., and Hsu, H. J. (2013). Efficacy of combination oral antimicrobial agents against biofilm-embedded methicillin-resistant Staphylococcus aureus. *J. Microbiol. Immunol. Infect.* 46, 89–95. doi: 10.1016/j.jmii.2012.03.009

Zhang, L., Yan, J., Yin, Z., Tang, C., Guo, Y., Li, D., et al. (2014). Electrospun vancomycin-loaded coating on titanium implants for the prevention of implant-associated infections. *Int. J. Nanomed.* 9, 3027–3036. doi: 10.2147/IJN.S63991

Zhao, X., Wu, H., Guo, B., Dong, R., Qiu, Y., and Ma, P. X. (2017). Antibacterial anti-oxidant electroactive injectable hydrogel as self-healing wound dressing with hemostasis and adhesiveness for cutaneous wound healing. *Biomaterials.* 122, 34–47. doi: 10.1016/j.biomaterials.2017.01.011

Permissions

List of Contributors

May Oo Lwin, Karthikayen Jayasundar, Anita Sheldenkar, Kosala Subasinghe and Schubert Foo
Wee Kim Wee School of Communication and Information, Nanyang Technological University (NTU), Singapore

Chee Fu Yung and Jie Chen
KK Women's and Children's Hospital (KKH), Singapore

Peiling Yap, Huarong Xu, Siaw Ching Chai and Brenda Sze Peng Ang
Tan Tock Seng Hospital (TTSH), Singapore

Udeepa Gayantha Jayasinghe and Ashwin Kurlye
Institute of Media Innovation (IMI), Singapore

Natália Karol de Andrade, Rogério Heládio Lopes Motta, Caio Chaves Guimarães and Jimmy de Oliveira Araújo
Division of Pharmacology, Anesthesiology and Therapeutics, Faculdade São Leopoldo Mandic, Instituto de Pesquisas São Leopoldo Mandic, Campinas, Brazil

Cristiane de Cássia Bergamaschi and Luciane Cruz Lopes
Pharmaceutical Science Graduate Course, University of Sorocaba, Sorocaba, Brazil

Luciana Butini Oliveira
Division of Paediatric Dentistry, Faculdade São Leopoldo Mandic, Instituto de Pesquisas São Leopoldo Mandic, Campinas, Brazil

Estêvão Luiz Carvalho Braga
Department of General and Specialized Surgery, Anesthesiology, Fluminense Federal University, Niterói, Brazil

Ismar Lima Cavalcanti
Department of General and Specialized Surgery, Anesthesiology, Fluminense Federal University, Niterói, Brazil
Coordination for Education, Brazilian National Cancer Institute (INCA), Rio de Janeiro, Brazil

Fernando Lopes Tavares de Lima and Mario Jorge Sobreira da Silva
Coordination for Education, Brazilian National Cancer Institute (INCA), Rio de Janeiro, Brazil

Rubens Antunes da Cruz Filho
Department of Clinical Medicine, Fluminense Federal University, Niterói, Brazil

Nubia Verçosa
Department of Surgery, Anesthesiology, Federal University of Rio de Janeiro, Rio de Janeiro, Brazil

Caron M. Molster and Karla Lister
Office of Population Health Genomics, Public Health Division, Department of Health Western Australia, Perth, WA, Australia

Selina Metternick-Jones
Sir Charles Gairdner Hospital, Perth, WA, Australia

Gareth Baynam
Office of Population Health Genomics, Public Health Division, Department of Health Western Australia, Perth, WA, Australia
Genetic Services WA, Perth, WA, Australia
School of Paediatrics and Child Health, University of Western Australia, Perth, WA, Australia
Institute for Immunology and Infectious Diseases, Murdoch University, Perth, WA, Australia
Telethon Kids Institute, University of Western Australia, Perth, WA, Australia
Western Australian Register of Developmental Anomalies, Perth, WA, Australia
Spatial Sciences, Department of Science and Engineering, Curtin University, Perth, WA, Australia

Angus John Clarke
Division of Cancer and Genetics, School of Medicine, Cardiff University, Cardiff, UK

Volker Straub
Institute of Human Genetics, University of Newcastle upon Tyne, Newcastle upon Tyne, UK

Hugh J. S. Dawkins
Office of Population Health Genomics, Public Health Division, Department of Health Western Australia, Perth, WA, Australia
Centre for Comparative Genomics, Murdoch University, Perth, WA, Australia
Centre for Population Health Research, Curtin University, Perth, WA, Australia
School of Pathology and Laboratory Medicine, University of Western Australia, Perth, WA, Australia

Nigel Laing
Centre for Medical Research, Harry Perkins Institute of Medical Research, University of Western Australia, Perth, WA, Australia
Neurogenetics Unit, Department of Diagnostic Genomics, PathWest Laboratory Medicine, Department of Health Western Australia, Perth, WA, Australia

Andressa Wanneska Martins da Silva, Elza Ferreira Noronha and Maria Inês de Toledo
Tropical Medicine, Faculty of Medicine, University of Brasília, Brasília, Brazil

Micheline Marie Milward de Azevedo Meiners
College of Pharmacy, Faculty of Ceilândia, University of Brasília, Brasília, Brazil

Adrian P. Brown, Anna M. Ferrante, Sean M. Randall, James H. Boyd and James B. Semmens
Centre for Population Health Research, Curtin University, Bentley, WA, Australia

Aryane Alves Vigato, Naially Cardoso de Faria, Mirela Inês de Sairre and Daniele Ribeiro de Araujo
Human and Natural Sciences Center, ABC Federal University, Santo André, Brazil

Samyr Machado Querobino
Department of Biomedical Sciences, State University of Minas Gerais, Passos, Brazil

Ana Carolina Bolela Bovo Candido and Lizandra Guidi Magalhães
Research Group on Natural Products, Center for Research in Sciences and Technology, University of Franca, Franca, Brazil

Cíntia Maria Saia Cereda and Giovana Radomille Tófoli
São Leopoldo Mandic Research Unit, São Leopoldo Mandic Faculty, Campinas, Brazil

Leonardo Fernandes Fraceto
Department of Environmental Engineering, State University "Júlio de Mesquita Filho", Sorocaba, Brazil

Estefânia Vangelie Ramos Campos
Human and Natural Sciences Center, ABC Federal University, Santo André, Brazil
Department of Environmental Engineering, State University "Júlio de Mesquita Filho", Sorocaba, Brazil

Ian Pompermayer Machado
Department of Fundamental Chemistry, Institute of Chemistry, University of São Paulo, São Paulo, Brazil

Katrina Spilsbury, Janine Alan and James B. Semmens
Centre for Population Health Research, Curtin University, Perth, WA, Australia

Diana Rosman
Centre for Population Health Research, Curtin University, Perth, WA, Australia
Data Linkage, Department of Health WA, Perth, WA, Australia

Anna M. Ferrante and James H. Boyd
PHRN Centre for Data Linkage, Centre for Population Health Research, Curtin University, Perth, WA, Australia

Gabrielle Kéfrem Alves Gomes, Mariana Linhares Pereira, Cristina Sanches and André Oliveira Baldoni
Grupo de Pesquisa em Epidemiologia e Avaliação de Novas Tecnologias em Saúde, Universidade Federal de São João del-Rei, Divinópolis, Brazil

Tarun Stephen Weeramanthri
Department of Health, Government of Western Australia, Perth, WA, Australia
Cooperative Research Centre for Spatial Information, Carlton, VIC, Australia

Peter Woodgate
Cooperative Research Centre for Spatial Information, Carlton, VIC, Australia
Global Spatial Network Board, Cooperative Research Centre for Spatial Information, Carlton, VIC, Australia

Clare Yuen Zen Lee
School of Pharmacy, Monash University Malaysia, Bandar Sunway, Malaysia

Pairote Chakranon
Faculty of Pharmacy, Silapakorn University, Pathom, Thailand

Shaun Wen Huey Lee
School of Pharmacy, Monash University Malaysia, Bandar Sunway, Malaysia
Asian Centre for Evidence Synthesis in Population, Implementation and Clinical Outcomes (PICO), Health and Well-being Cluster, Global Asia in the 21st Century (GA21) Platform, Monash University Malaysia, Selangor, Malaysia
School of Pharmacy, Taylor's University, Subang Jaya, Malaysia

Malcolm Campbell
GeoHealth Laboratory, Department of Geography, University of Canterbury, Christchurch, New Zealand

Bruna Carolina de Araújo, Roberta Crevelário de Melo, Maritsa Carla de Bortoli, José Ruben de Alcântara Bonfim and Tereza Setsuko Toma
Department of Health, Institute of Health, Government of the State of São Paulo, São Paulo, Brazil

Dimitris Ballas
Department of Geography, University of Sheffield, Sheffield, UK
Department of Geography, University of the Aegean, Mytilene, Greece

Renata Lima
LABiToN – Laboratory of Bioactivity Assessment and Toxicology of Nanomaterials, University of Sorocaba, Sorocaba, Brazil

Fernando Sá Del Fiol
CRIA – Antibiotic Reference and Information Center, University of Sorocaba, Sorocaba, Brazil

Victor M. Balcão
PhageLab – Laboratory of Biofilms and Bacteriophages, i(bs)2 – intelligent biosensing and biomolecule stabilization research group, University of Sorocaba, Sorocaba, Brazil
Department of Biology and CESAM, University of Aveiro, Campus Universitário de Santiago, Aveiro, Portugal

Lakkhina Troeung, Angelita Martini and David B. Preen
Centre for Health Services Research, School of Population Health, The University of Western Australia, Perth, WA, Australia

Nita Sodhi-Berry
Centre for Health Services Research, School of Population Health, The University of Western Australia, Perth, WA, Australia
Occupational Respiratory Epidemiology, School of Population Health, The University of Western Australia, Perth, WA, Australia

Eva Malacova
Centre for Health Services Research, School of Population Health, The University of Western Australia, Perth, WA, Australia
Department of Health, Safety and Environment, School of Public Health, Curtin University, Perth, WA, Australia

Hooi Ee
Department of Gastroenterology, Sir Charles Gairdner Hospital, Queen Elizabeth II Medical Centre, Nedlands, WA, Australia

Peter O'Leary
Health Policy and Management, Faculty of Health Sciences, School of Public Health, Curtin University, Perth, WA, Australia
School of Women's and Infants' Health, The University of Western Australia, Perth, WA, Australia

Iris Lansdorp-Vogelaar
Department of Public Health, Erasmus MC University Medical Centre, Rotterdam, Netherlands

Natália Gibim Mellone, Marcus Tolentino Silva, Mariana Del Grossi Paglia, Luciane Cruz Lopes, Sílvio Barberato-Filho, Fernando de Sá Del Fiol and Cristiane de Cássia Bergamaschi
Pharmaceutical Science Graduate Course, University of Sorocaba, Sorocaba, Brazil

Yuanzhi Liu, Xiaoyan Zhong, Qiming Wei and Yilan Huang
Department of Pharmacy, The Affiliated Hospital of Southwest Medical University, Luzhou, China

Junyi Zhao
Department of Pharmacy, The Affiliated Hospital of Southwest Medical University, Luzhou, China
College of Pharmacy, Southwest Medical University, Luzhou, China

Izabela Fulone, Silvio Barberato-Filho and Luciane Cruz Lopes
Pharmaceutical Sciences Graduate Course, University of Sorocaba, UNISO, Sorocaba, Brazil

Jorge Otavio Maia Barreto
Fiocruz School of Government, Fiocruz Brasília, Oswaldo Cruz Foundation, Brasília, Brazil

Marcel Henrique de Carvalho
Veredas Institute, Brasília, Brazil

Edward Mezones-Holguin
Universidad San Ignacio de Loyola (USIL), Centro de Excelencia en Estudios Económicos y Sociales en Salud, Lima, Peru

Rocio Violeta Gamboa-Cardenas
Seguro Social en Salud (EsSalud), Hospital Nacional Guillermo Almenara Irigoyen, Servicio de Reumatologia, Lima, Peru

Gadwyn Sanchez-Felix
Seguro Social en Salud (EsSalud), Hospital Nacional Edgardo Rebagliati Martins, Servicio de Dermatología, Lima, Peru

José Chávez-Corrales
Seguro Social en Salud (EsSalud), Hospital Nacional
Edgardo Rebagliati Martins, Servicio de Reumatologia,
Lima, Peru

**Luis Miguel Helguero-Santin and Luis Max Laban
Seminario**
Universidad Nacional de Piura (UNP), Facultad de
Ciencias de la Salud, Sociedad Científica de Estudiantes
de Medicina (SOCIEMUNP), Piura, Peru

**Paula Alejandra Burela-Prado, Maribel Marilu
Castro-Reyes and Fabian Fiestas**
Seguro Social en Salud (EsSalud), Instituto de
Evaluación de Tecnologías Sanitarias e Investigación
(IETSI), Lima, Peru

Elizabeth Williamson
Faculty of Epidemiology and Population Health,
London School of Hygiene and Tropical Medicine,
London, United Kingdom

M Sanni Ali
Faculty of Epidemiology and Population Health,
London School of Hygiene and Tropical Medicine,
London, United Kingdom
Nuffield Department of Orthopaedics, Rheumatology
and Musculoskeletal Sciences (NDORMS), Center for
Statistics in Medicine (CSM), University of Oxford,
Oxford, United Kingdom
Centre for Data and Knowledge Integration for
Health (CIDACS), Instituto Gonçalo Muniz, Fundação
Osvaldo Cruz, Salvador, Brazil

Liam Smeeth
Faculty of Epidemiology and Population Health,
London School of Hygiene and Tropical Medicine,
London, United Kingdom
Centre for Data and Knowledge Integration for
Health (CIDACS), Instituto Gonçalo Muniz, Fundação
Osvaldo Cruz, Salvador, Brazil

Dandara Ramos, Nivea Bispo and Julia M. Pescarini
Centre for Data and Knowledge Integration for
Health (CIDACS), Instituto Gonçalo Muniz, Fundação
Osvaldo Cruz, Salvador, Brazil

Daniel Prieto-Alhambra
GREMPAL Research Group (Idiap Jordi Gol) and
Musculoskeletal Research Unit (Fundació IMIM-Parc
Salut Mar), Universitat Autònoma de Barcelona,
Barcelona, Spain

Luciane Cruz Lopes
University of Sorocaba–UNISO, Sorocaba, São Paulo,
Brazil

Maria Y. Ichihara and Mauricio L. Barreto
Centre for Data and Knowledge Integration for
Health (CIDACS), Instituto Gonçalo Muniz, Fundação
Osvaldo Cruz, Salvador, Brazil
Institute of Public Health, Federal University of Bahia
(UFBA), Salvador, Brazil

Rosemeire L. Fiaccone
Centre for Data and Knowledge Integration for
Health (CIDACS), Instituto Gonçalo Muniz, Fundação
Osvaldo Cruz, Salvador, Brazil
Institute of Public Health, Federal University of Bahia
(UFBA), Salvador, Brazil
Department of Statistics, Federal University of Bahia
(UFBA), Salvador, Brazil

Shawn Dolley
Cloudera, Inc., Palo Alto, CA, United States

**Luisa von Zuben Vecoso, Mariangela Ribeiro
Resende and Tais Freire Galvao**
University of Campinas, Campinas, Brazil

Marcus Tolentino Silva
Universidade de Sorocaba, Sorocaba, Brazil

Everton Nunes da Silva
University of Brasilia, Brasilia, Brazil

Matthew I. Bellgard and Adam Hunter
Centre for Comparative Genomics, Murdoch
University, Murdoch, WA, Australia

Nigel Chartres
Health Informatics Society of Australia, North
Melbourne, VIC, Australia

Gerald F. Watts
School of Medicine, University of Western Australia,
Perth, WA, Australia
Lipid Disorders Clinic, Cardiometabolic Service, Royal
Perth Hospital, Perth, WA, Australia

Steve Wilton and Sue Fletcher
Centre for Comparative Genomics, Murdoch
University, Murdoch, WA, Australia
Centre for Neuromuscular and Neurological Disorders,
University of Western Australia, Nedlands, WA,
Australia
Perron Institute for Neurological and Translational
Science, Nedlands, WA, Australia

**Andreia Borges Scriboni, Francisco Carlos Groppo
and Michelle Franz-Montan**
Department of Physiological Sciences, Piracicaba
Dental School, University of Campinas, Piracicaba,
Brazil

Tom Snelling
Princess Margaret Hospital for Children, Perth, WA, Australia
Wesfarmers Centre of Vaccines and Infectious Diseases, Telethon Kids Institute, University of Western Australia, Perth, WA, Australia
Menzies School of Health Research and Charles Darwin University, Darwin, NT, Australia

Verônica Muniz Couto, Lígia Nunes de Morais Ribeiro and Eneida de Paula
Department of Biochemistry and Tissue Biology, Biology Institute, University of Campinas, Campinas, Brazil

Irlan Almeida Freires
Department of Oral Biology, University of Florida College of Dentistry, Gainesville, FL, United States

Karina Cogo-Müller
Department of Physiological Sciences, Piracicaba Dental School, University of Campinas, Piracicaba, Brazil
Faculty of Pharmaceutical Sciences, University of Campinas, Campinas, Brazil

Index

Printed in the USA
CPSIA information can be obtained
at www.ICGtesting.com
JSHW051409091023
49903JS00006B/343